Theory and practice of
Histotechnology

Theory and practice of
Histotechnology

DEZNA C. SHEEHAN, H.T.(ASCP)

Program Director, School of Histotechnology;
Assistant to the Director for Administration,
Laboratory of Surgical Pathology, Hospital of
the University of Pennsylvania,
Philadelphia, Pennsylvania

BARBARA B. HRAPCHAK, M.Sc., M.T.(ASCP)

Education Coordinator, Histologic Technique,
Ohio State University Hospitals;
Department of Pathology, Ohio State University,
Columbus, Ohio

SECOND EDITION

with 170 *illustrations, including* 2 *color plates*

The C. V. Mosby Company

ST. LOUIS • TORONTO • LONDON   1980

COVER ILLUSTRATION: a rapid mucin stain

Courtesy of Miss Gerre G. Wells, H.T.(ASCP), Education
Coordinator, School of Histotechnology, University of Tennessee,
Memphis, Tennessee

SECOND EDITION

The C. V. Mosby Company
11830 Westline Industrial Drive, St. Louis, Missouri 63141

Library of Congress Cataloging in Publication Data

Sheehan, Dezna C   1911-
   Theory and practice of histotechnology.

   Includes bibliographies and index.
   1.   Histology, Pathological—Technique.
I.   Hrapchak, Barbara B., 1945-   joint author.
II.   Title.   [DNLM: 1.   Histological technics.
2.   Stains and staining—Laboratory manuals.   QS525
S541t]
RB43.S44   1980   616'.018   80-11807
ISBN 0-8016-4573-5

GW/CB/B   9   8   7   6   5   4   3   2   01/C/264

Contributors

FREIDA L. CARSON, Ph.D.

Histopathology Department, Baylor University
Medical Center, Dallas, Texas

SIDNEY A. COLEMAN, M.D.

Cytology Laboratory, University of Tennessee,
Memphis, Tennessee

HELEN N. FUTCH, M.Ed.

Pathology Department, The University of Texas,
M. D. Anderson Hospital and Tumor Institute,
Houston, Texas

ROBERT HRAPCHAK, Ph.D.

Chemical Abstracts Service, Inc., Columbus,
Ohio

MARGARET S. JUDGE, H.T.(ASCP)

The University of Texas Health Science Center,
San Antonio, Texas

NESTOR G. MENOCAL, B.S., H.T.(ASCP)

Research Specialist on Ophthalmology,
University of Pennsylvania, Philadelphia,
Pennsylvania

NAN PILLSBURY, Ph.D.

Supervisor, Electron Microscopy Section,
Surgical Pathology Department, Hospital of the
University of Pennsylvania, Philadelphia,
Pennsylvania

LYN RICHARDSON, H.T.(ASCP)

Department of Anatomy, The University of
Texas Health Science Center, San Antonio,
Texas

JOHN SPAIR, Jr., H.T.(ASCP)

Surgical Pathology Laboratory, Hospital of the
University of Pennsylvania, Philadelphia,
Pennsylvania

MARIA SUGULAS, H.T.(ASCP)

The University of Texas Medical Branch,
Department of Anatomy, Galveston, Texas

DOLORES B. VENTURA, H.T.(ASCP)

Department of Ophthalmology and Pathology,
University of Pennsylvania, Philadelphia,
Pennsylvania

ANTHONY R. VILLANUEVA, H.T.(ASCP), B.Sc., M.A.

Director, Histology Division, Bone and Mineral
Research Laboratory, Henry Ford Hospital,
Detroit, Michigan

MYRON YANOFF, M.D.

Laboratory of Ophthalmic Pathology, Scheie
Eye Institute, Philadelphia, Pennsylvania

To
H. T. Enterline, M.D.
A pathologist who has constantly recognized
the need for professional growth in his histotechnologists,
has given them this opportunity, and has
worked diligently to support the growth of professionalism
in histotechnology throughout the United States

Foreword

The pathologist responsible for tissue diagnoses is heavily dependent on the competence of his histotechnologist. The ability to consistently turn out slides of high quality, well sectioned and well stained, on a wide variety of tissue is indeed an art. To develop skill in this art requires not only training in basic principles, but also experience, attention to detail, knowledge of the chemical rationale of the staining procedures carried out, and the ability to recognize quickly the probable cause of technical difficulties encountered in the daily work of the laboratory and to expediently remedy these difficulties.

I believe that information required by the histotechnologist is well supplied in this book. Mrs. Sheehan has had an enormous practical experience in this field and has also dedicated herself, for many years, not only to the training of histotechnologists in her own school of histotechnology, but also nationally, having been involved in several committees formed to upgrade the education of histotechnologists and to promote the recognition of histotechnology as a paramedical professional discipline. Ably assisted by Mrs. Hrapchak, she has developed this text for use with her own students as a ready

way of presenting information in understandable form and in sufficient detail so that common errors can be avoided. The original *Notebook for Students of Histologic Technique* by Mrs. Sheehan was augmented and amended over the years and was followed by the first edition of *Theory and Practice of Histotechnology* by Sheehan and Hrapchak. The result, in my mind, has been a very practical and extremely helpful book that tells what should be done and emphasizes common sources of error. The second edition adds completed information on many subjects briefly covered in the first edition and adds many chapters on the theory and practice of new technics in the laboratory. It should be extremely useful, not only to the histotechnologist in training, but also as a ready reference for the practicing or teaching histotechnologist.

H. T. Enterline, M.D.

Professor of Pathology,
University of Pennsylvania;
Director of Surgical Pathology and Cytology,
Director, School of Histotechnology,
Hospital of the University of Pennsylvania,
Philadelphia, Pennsylvania

Preface

The unpublished *Notebook for Students of Histologic Technique* by Dezna Sheehan was used in many laboratories over numerous years as a ready reference for both students and staff histotechnologists. The first edition of *Theory and Practice of Histotechnology* by Sheehan and Hrapchak was a sequel to the original notebook and answered a long-felt need of both small and large histopathology laboratories for an explanation of the theory of special staining technics.

This second edition expands on this subject, adds new subject matter, and completes information on many subjects briefly covered in the first edition. Chapters on enzyme histochemistry, immunohistochemistry, electron microscopy, eye pathology technics, inorganic chemistry, organic chemistry, and quality control are new to this edition. Chapters on mineralized bone and nerve tissue have been revised and expanded. Knife sharpening has been added to the chapter on instrumentation. Cytology technics, excerpts on safety, and a glossary of terms commonly used in the histopathology laboratory have been added to the chapter containing miscellaneous information.

In preparing this second edition of *Theory and Practice of Histotechnology*, we have considered the need of the student preparing for both levels of certification in Histologic Technique, H.T.(ASCP), and Histotechnology, H.T.L.(ASCP), by the Board of Registry. We have also carefully studied the needs of the education coordinator in educational programs accredited by CAHEA and residents in histopathology laboratories, as well as the important line technologist who, with the pathologist, is part of the team providing good patient care. The photomicrographs demonstrate the technics required for Board of Registry certification and many other technics so necessary to the pathologist for good patient diagnosis.

Acknowledgment is gratefully given to the artist, William M. Baldwin, III, Ph.D., for his keen understanding of the work he was required to illustrate and to Frances A. Pukas for her illustrations of incorrect and correct embedding and the proper cutting of a Technicon clock. We are also deeply grateful to Dr. Robert Hrapchak, Polly Stanton, M.T.(ASCP), and Doremus Brownback for the many hours spent in proofreading the manuscript.

We sincerely hope this book will be valuable to each of you in your daily professional pursuits.

Dezna C. Sheehan
Barbara B. Hrapchak

Contents

Introduction

The great development of pathologic anatomy in the second half of the nineteenth century was a natural consequence of the stimulus given it by the masters of the first half of the century.

Virchow's doctrine of cellular pathology, published in 1858, led to the recognition of microscopic pathology as a fundamental discipline in medicine. It was the recognition of this new field of microscopic examination of tissue that led to the birth of histotechnology.

It is difficult to realize that the all-important pioneer work of a century ago was accomplished without the many technical devices we know today and was performed largely on teased-out, unstained specimens floated onto thick, uneven slides.

Schliden, in 1842, complaining of a lack of histologic methods, suggested freehand cutting of tissues with a razor. Although the sliding microtome, with vertical feed screw, called a "cutting engine" had been developed in 1798 by Adams, the use of this instrument made little headway. The advance came with the use of embedding material to permeate and hold soft tissues firmly. In 1873, Fleming wrote first of embedding in soap and then, in 1876, of embedding in turpentine paraffin. Duval introduced celloidin in 1879, and this was followed by the use of chloroform paraffin by Klebs, in 1881. It was the introduction of Klebs' chloroform paraffin that made possible the cutting of serial sections. The freezing method was used in 1871 by Rutherford (though Bardeen attributed the method to Stilling during 1846), and Boyle cut sections of frozen eyes in 1863.

The first rotary microtomes were invented independently by Pfeifer at the Johns Hopkins University in 1883, and by Minot at Harvard University in 1886.

To alcohol, oldest of the fixatives, Hanover added chromic acid in 1844, followed by Flemming's chrome osmic acetic acid. In 1894, Zenker used potassium dichromate and mercuric dichloride for tissue fixation. Formalin was added in 1893 by J. Blum. In the last half of the century many other fixatives commonly used today, such as Carnoy's, Bouin's, and so forth came into use.

Various methods of processing tissue were devised. Prior to 1930 and the advent of the Autotechnicon, tissues were processed by moving them manually through fixative, graded alcohols, clearing agent, and several changes of paraffin for tissue impregnation. After these steps were completed, tissues were embedded in paper boats and the blocks were trimmed to cutting size and mounted on either metal or fiber block pivots for sectioning. This process took a minimum of several days, depending on the workday of the technologist.

From the methods of a century ago, histotechnology has advanced to a paramedical science of automation and sophisticated technics to aid the pathologist in patient diagnosis. Therefore, the histotechnologist, who is on the "team," should not only know what to do, but should also understand the theory of what he or she is doing. The chapters that follow cover the theory as well as the practice of histotechnology.

CHAPTER 1

Instrumentation

AUTOMATIC TISSUE CHANGERS
Autotechnicon (Mono and Duo)

The Autotechnicon,* the oldest of the commercial tissue changers, is a valuable instrument in the histopathology laboratory. It is particularly so in large hospitals where an abundant volume of tissue is processed daily.

The Autotechnicon consists of a timing clock that is cut to determine immersion periods of the tissues; reagent beakers of glass or plastic, which contain the reagents required by the particular technique being used; a beaker platform for precise alignment of beakers; a master shift carriage to automatically transfer tissues from one fluid to the next, in order, at time intervals predetermined by the timing clock; individual beaker covers, or a central cover to prevent evaporation of fluids; a displacer rotor, which provides constant rotation of the tissue basket during immersion in the fluids; a receptacle basket of stainless steel; stainless steel receptacles, or cassettes, for carrying the tissue during the processing and paraffin baths.

The pathologist cuts the pieces of tissue and places them in the tissue receptacle with an identifying number. The receptacle basket is attached to the displacer rotor on an arm of the master shift carriage. The tissue basket rotates slowly during immersion and travels clockwise in an orbit, moving progressively from one reagent beaker to another through the various processing stages. The sequence and duration of

---

*Technicon Instruments Corp., Tarrytown, N.Y.

immersion periods are determined by the pathologist and are precisely maintained by the clock mechanism. The timing mechanism is an alternate-current electric clock controlled by a timing disc, which permits a definite sequence of varying time intervals to be preset. The disc is calibrated over 24 hours and further subdivided into 5-minute intervals. When operating, it revolves on the clock face until a timing notch is encountered. At this point, a timing lever falls into the notch, starting the mechanism that raises the tissue basket from one fluid, shifts it, and immerses it into the next in line. The basket is of stainless steel, with die-cut perforations. The firm closure of the cassette guards against the possibility of specimen loss or mix up. The snap-action opening facilitates removal of tissue when the receptacle is coated with paraffin from the paraffin bath. The cassettes are fully perforated at the top, bottom, and sides, permitting free passage and draining of fluids.

The care of the Autotechnicon is extremely important. Paraffin should be kept in the paraffin baths and removed from all other areas of the instrument with soft cloths soaked in xylene. The receptacles and basket should be soaked in xylene and washed in very hot soapy water to remove all residual paraffin. Individual lids or the large lid to cover beakers must be kept free of paraffin at all times.

Lillie states "to remove paraffin from metal embedding molds, Technicon tissue carriers (including the nylon-plastic carriers furnished by the Technicon Company), boil them for 5 to 10 minutes completely immersed in a tall metal vessel containing about 10 to 12 gm (a level tablespoonful, or 16 ml) of powdered Oakite, Calgonite, or other technical sodium phosphate detergent in about a liter of water. Then cool until the paraffin can be removed as a solid cake; rinse and dry. The greasy film left by xylene cleaning is absent with this method, and the danger of working with an inflammable solvent is eliminated." (Peers, J. H.: Am. J. Clin. Pathol. **21:**794, 1951.)

Use of automatic tissue changers (see Chapter 3 for additional precautions)

I. Instruments must be quality controlled:
   A. Monthly or bimonthly maintenance check by electricians depending on use of instrument.
   B. Wires and plugs must be clean and free from paraffin.
   C. Total instrument must be dust free and free from paraffin.

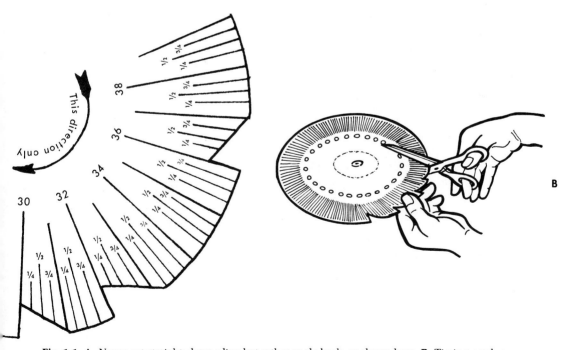

Fig. 1-1. A, Never cut straight along a line but rather angle back, as shown here. **B,** Timing notches are easily cut with ordinary scissors.

D. Clocks (if used) must be evenly cut.
  1. Cutting the 24-hour disc for Technicon (Fig. 1-1, *black*)—The timing disc is divided by 24 radial lines representing 1-hour intervals. With a red pencil, mark off the desired time intervals starting from zero, which should represent the time at which the tissues are placed on the Autotechnicon. Make cuts 9 mm deep at each of the red pencil marks. The cut should not follow the radial line, but angle back. Now make the longer angle cut, remembering that the shallower the angle, the less wear on the timing gears. A correctly cut disc will have one less notch than the number of steps used in the process—12 steps and 11 cuts.
  2. Cutting the clocks for Autotechnicon Mono or Duo—A clock cutter is found at the rear of these instruments. Mark the clock and cut it with the clock cutter. A correctly cut disc will have one less notch than the number of steps used in the process—12 steps and 11 cuts.
E. Baskets and cassettes must be clean and free of paraffin to allow for free exchange of fluids.
F. Baskets must be firmly attached to rotors to prevent spilling.
G. Small pieces of paper may be used to identify the specimen. Large pieces of paper hinder the penetration of the fluid.
H. Tissues must not overlap in the receptacle, since this produces poor penetration of fluid and paraffin.
I. The fluid level must always be higher than the level of the receptacles.
J. The tissues must never be more than 3 mm in thickness.
K. Always use clean tissue cassettes. Paraffin-coated cassettes inhibit fluid penetration.
L. *Change all fluids* on the instrument in accordance with the work volume in the laboratory. It is poor economy to skimp on clean reagents for processing tissue.
M. When changing solutions, the beakers should be thoroughly washed and dried and the instrument completely cleaned.
II. Handling automatic tissue changer problems
A. If a basket of tissue is caught up in the air and the tissue dries out, place the tissue in the following solution overnight:

Sodium carbonate	0.6 gm
Distilled water	42 ml
Absolute alcohol	18 ml

Process the following day on the standard 16-hour procedure, starting in 80% alcohol.
B. If the tissue goes back into the fixative after the paraffin:
  1. Rinse in 95% alcohol.
  2. Rinse in absolute alcohol.
  3. Rinse in xylene.
  4. 30 minutes of paraffin under vacuum.
  5. 30 minutes of fresh paraffin under vacuum.
  6. 30 minutes of fresh paraffin under vacuum.
C. If the tissue goes back into the 80% alcohol (first beaker on instrument) after paraffin:
  1. Rinse in absolute alcohol.
  2. Rinse in absolute alcohol.
  3. Rinse in xylene.
  4. 30 minutes of paraffin under vacuum.
  5. 30 minutes of fresh paraffin under vacuum.
  6. 30 minutes of fresh paraffin under vacuum.
D. If the tissue is in 80% alcohol, or 95% alcohol, instead of paraffin, in the morning:
  1. Check to see if the clock is properly set.
  2. Check to see if the clock is tight.
  3. Check the master switch.
  4. Proceed through remaining alcohols, clearing agent, and paraffin.

Autotechnicon Ultra

The newest Autotechnicon is the Autotechnicon Ultra for automatic vacuum processing of histologic tissue specimens for pathologic interpretation (Fig. 1-2).

The required reagents for the 12-station processing cycle are contained in stainless-steel beakers that sit in a well of mineral oil around a circular deck. As with previously described Technicon tissue processors, the tissues are loaded into small perforated cassettes or receptacles, which are transported in a perforated basket. The loaded basket hangs from a vacu-

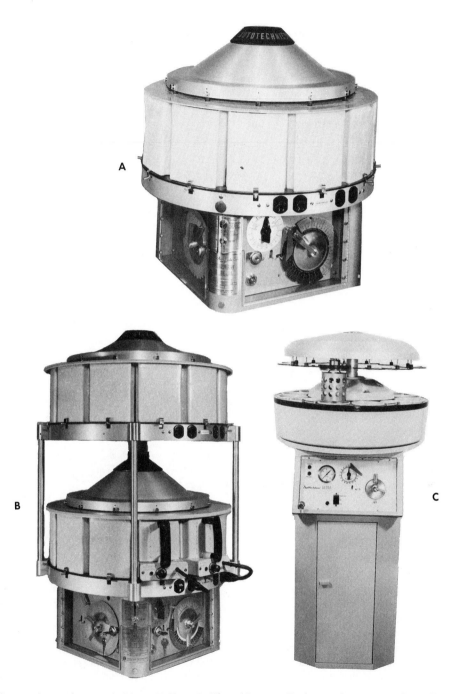

Fig. 1-2. Autotechnicon. **A,** Mono; **B,** Duo; **C,** Ultra. (Courtesy Technicon Instruments Corp., Tarrytown, N.Y.)

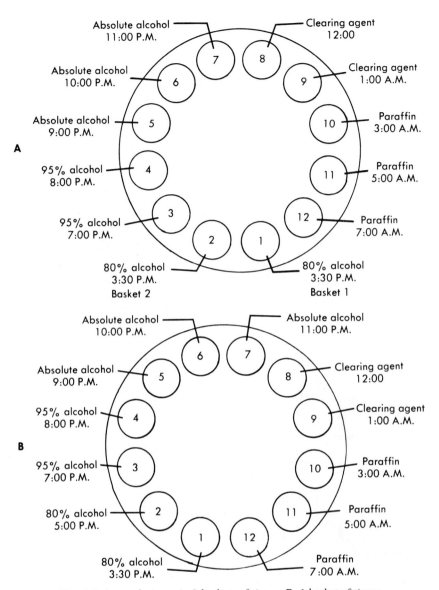

Fig. 1-3. Autotechnicon. **A,** 2 baskets of tissue; **B,** 1 basket of tissue.

um-sealing head attached to a superstructure that descends, rises, and rotates according to a program controlled by a timing clock. In moving from one station to another, the basket rises vertically, hovers briefly over the vacated beaker to drain off fluids and then moves through an arc of 30 degrees and descends to immersion depth in the next beaker in line.

During immersion, gentle heat, vacuum, and vertical oscillation operate to speed the exchange of fluids between tissues and reagents for 10 changes of the programmed sequence. The tissue basket then arrives at the first of two paraffin beakers. The final change shifts it to the second paraffin beaker, completing the processing cycle. The tissues remain in the thermostatically controlled beaker, under vacuum, until the technologist is ready to take them to the embedding bench. (See Figs. 1-3 to 1-7.)

The Autotechnicon Ultra is a tissue processor built along the classical line of the original processor. It contains, however, three completely new devices:

1. The fixative, dehydrating, clearing, and impregnating agents are all submerged in a constant-temperature mineral-oil bath.

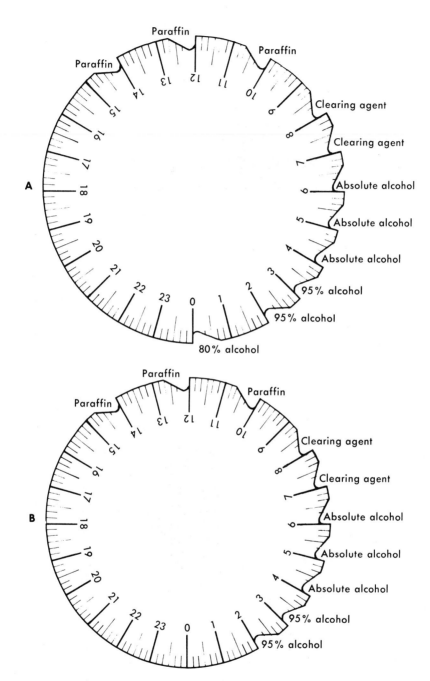

Fig. 1-4. Autotechnicon (old black instrument). **A,** 1 basket of tissue; **B,** 2 baskets of tissue.

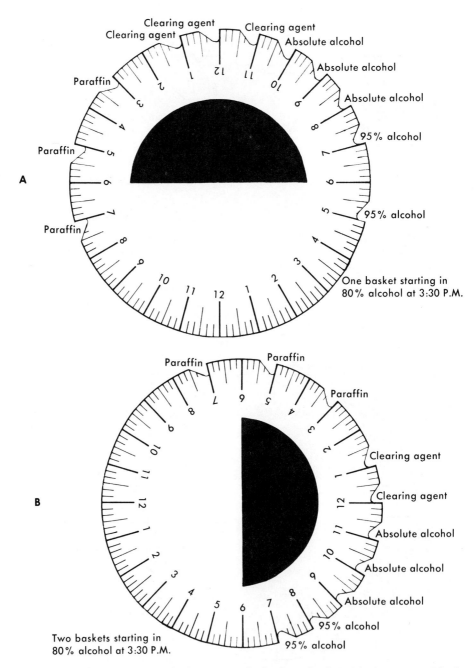

Fig. 1-5. Autotechnicon Duo. **A,** 1 basket upper, 1 basket lower level; **B,** 2 baskets upper, 2 baskets lower level.

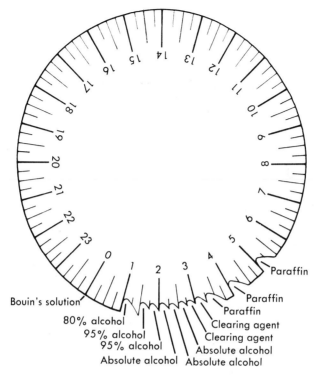

Fig. 1-6. RUSH SPECIMENS Autotechnicon Mono or Duo (6-hour technic).

With this bath, the reagents remain at a constant temperature of 38° to 40° C and the paraffin bath remains at 58° to 60° C.

2. The device for holding the basket containing the tissue cassettes is suspended under a vacuum head that provides 15 inches (380 mm) of mercury pressure throughout the processing cycle.

3. The instrument can be operated manually or automatically and the constant temperature of the mineral oil can be changed to suit the operator, or it can be shut off completely. In addition to this, the vacuum head can be adjusted for varying pressure, or if one deems advisable, the instrument may be operated without vacuum.

Lipshaw automatic tissue processors

There are five models of automatic tissue processors, the two most popular being the Trimatic and the 1000 model. The Trimatic may be used for conventional overnight processing, fast tissue processing under vacuum and heat, or automatic staining. The basket continually agitates and there is a 45-second pause over each beaker to allow for good drainage and prevent fluid carry-over. There are four thermal baths supplied as standard equipment for heating paraffin or solutions with each instrument. The Trimatic will accommodate up to three baskets, each holding approximately 36 capsules. The instrument may be used for automatic staining with slide carriers holding 42 slides. The instrument may be mounted on a portable floor cabinet or used on a laboratory bench.

The standard Lipshaw automatic tissue processor is 4 feet, 9 inches long and may be mounted on a laboratory shelf or placed on a worktable or mounted on a special processing stand (Fig. 1-8).

Fisher Tissuematon

The Model 60 Fisher Tissuematon (Fig. 1-9) carries 44 tissue specimens through a preprogrammed sequence of preparatory steps. The tissues are automatically fixed, dehydrated, infiltrated with embedding medium, and ready for sectioning and examination.

Histomatic TM tissue processor

This model automatically fixes, dehydrates, clears, and infiltrates tissue specimens in an enclosed system. Model 166 Histomatic (Fig. 1-10) automatically processes specimens in up to 120

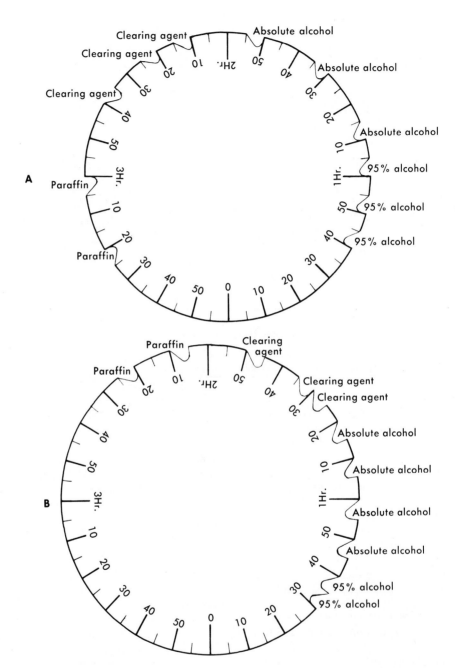

Fig. 1-7. RUSH SPECIMENS Autotechnicon Ultra. **A,** 4-hour technic; **B,** 3-hour technic; **C,** 2-hour technic; **D,** 1-hour technic.

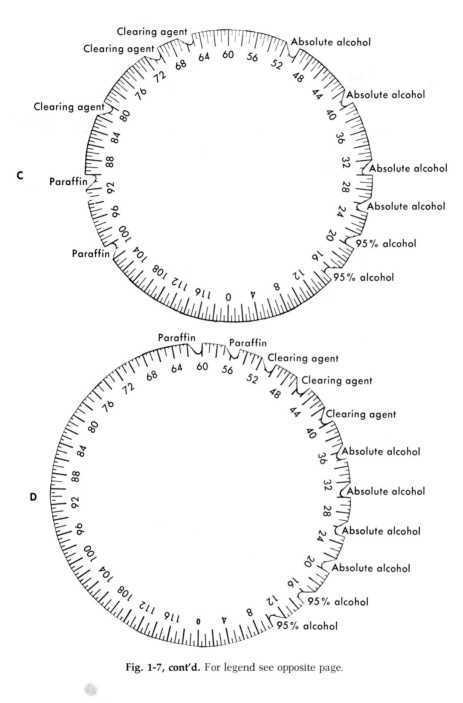

Fig. 1-7, cont'd. For legend see opposite page.

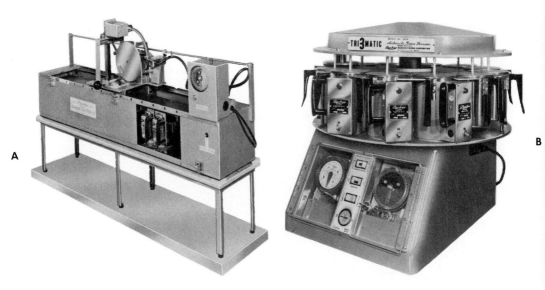

Fig. 1-8. A, Lipshaw Model 1000. **B,** Lipshaw Trimatic model. (Courtesy Lipshaw Manufacturing Corp., Detroit, Mich.)

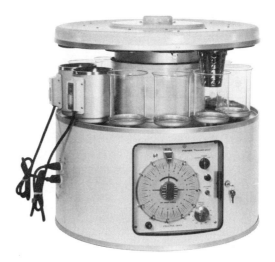

Fig. 1-9. Fisher Tissuematon. (Courtesy Fisher Scientific Co., Pittsburgh, Pa.)

tissue cassettes at one time, immerses them in a series of solvents for fixing, dehydrating, and clearing, and finally immerses them in paraffin for infiltration. The 120-cassette capacity of the Histomatic is double that of most traditional processors.

The Histomatic concept is a totally enclosed system with minimum air exposure. Histomatic introduces a truly major innovation in tissue processors: All processing takes place in an enclosed system. Tissue, solvents, and infiltrating media are inside the Histomatic system—not in open containers exposed to the air.

The laboratory. No noxious fumes escape, and there is no chance of fume buildup or explosions. All solvent fumes are channeled to one exhaust port, which can be easily vented to the outside.

Solvents for fixing, dehydrating, and clearing plus media for infiltration automatically flow into and out of a stationary tissue compartment. The Histomatic features a 2-minute drain period

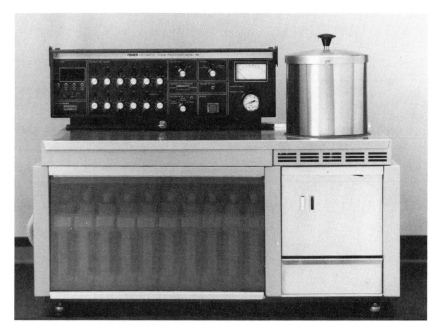

Fig. 1-10. Fisher Model 166 Histomatic Tissue Processor.

after each solvent cycle to assure minimum contamination of subsequent solvents.

Once you put tissues into the Histomatic tissue compartment, they are not fully exposed to air until the completely processed specimens are removed from the final infiltration bath. If the power fails, tissues remain safe inside the tissue compartment. As added protection, all valves will automatically close. When power is restored, the system will automatically resume the program sequence where it was interrupted.

Programming for operating conditions. The operator programs sequence and time period for each solvent/infiltrating-medium stage by presetting controls on the control panel. Conventional timing discs are not needed. A clear plastic window may then be locked over the control panel to prevent accidental or unauthorized program changes.

The following operating conditions may be selected:

Processing time. Can be set for anywhere from 10 minutes to 4 hours per cycle by 12 individual control timers, one for each of 10 solvent and 2 paraffin cycles. Tissues can be processed with or without vacuum—vacuum with all 12 stations or vacuum only on paraffin.

Number of solvent cycles. Use up to 10 solvents for fixing, dehydrating and clearing cy-

cles. To skip any solvent cycle, just set its individual control time to OFF.

Solvents are contained in ten 2-liter polyethylene reservoir containers. They are frontloaded and attached to the system by a series of permanently mounted screw caps. Bottles can be easily removed, refilled, or replaced. They are enclosed behind a transparent plastic sliding door. Solutions may be changed while machine is processing. Machine may be partially cleaned without disturbing processing. Additional tissue may be processed during the day on a short cycle.

Number of infiltration cycles. Use one or two infiltrating cycles with media from two paraffin wells preheated to 63° C.

Paraffin wells, contained in a slide-out drawer, can be easily drained and filled in place.

Temperature. Use the solvent heat control to apply gentle heat directly to the tissue compartment during all solvent cycles. Or you may opt to apply no heat at all. Thermostatically controlled system is factory-set to 40° ± 1° C, but is screwdriver adjustable over a 30° to 45° C range.

Infiltrating media (already preheated in paraffin wells) are automatically heated during infiltration in tissue compartment to factory-set temperature of 59° ± 1° C; screwdriver adjustable over 50° to 60° C range.

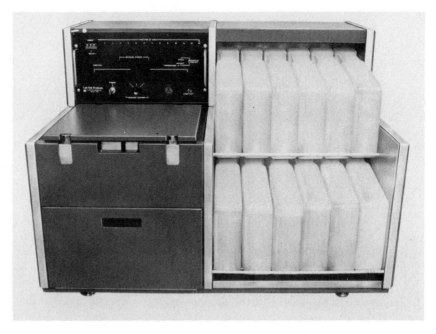

Fig. 1-11. Tissue-Tek III V.I.P. (Vacuum Infiltration Processor).

Tissue-Tek III V.I.P. (Vacuum Infiltration Processor)

The new Tissue-Tek III V.I.P. (Fig. 1-11) operates on the fluid-exchange principle. The tissue specimens are retained in one location while the processing fluids, paraffin, and cleaning agent are exchanged by alternation of vacuum and pressure in the proper sequence. This procedure ensures quality-processed tissue specimens and permits faster, safer, and more efficient tissue processing.

Light-emitting diode displays on the control panel indicate exact instrument status such as time remaining in delay cycle, processing cycle, and temperatures.

The V.I.P. is designed to accommodate most processing fluids and paraffins used in processing tissues. There are ten 1-gallon (3.8-liter) containers for processing fluids and an additional 1-gallon (3.8-liter) container for cleaning fluids. The oven holds two 1-gallon (3.8-liter) paraffin reservoirs. A consistent oven temperature is maintained to assure proper paraffin conditions. Fluid and paraffin are sequentially drawn from the containers into a central processing retort by vacuum and are returned to their respective containers by pressure. The vacuum/pressure cycle ensures thorough fluid and paraffin penetration during processing.

Air is blown through the transfer lines after each fluid transfer to assure clean, dry tubing. A charcoal filter is available to provide closed system and to eliminate fumes and noxious odors. An audible and visible alarm system is provided to alert operators to power loss, instrument malfunction, processing problems, and system interruptions.

A printed circuit board can be programmed for the desired time sequence; the processing cycle can be delayed up to 99.9 hours. A special programmable cleaning cycle prepares the unit for the next processing cycle.

The retort chamber can process over 300 specimens simultaneously on a regular long cycle or single immediate biopsy on a rapid cycle. It has two locking latches and an interlock for sealed security during processing.

USE OF CLINICAL FREEZING MICROTOME

Fresh or fixed tissues may be placed directly on the freezing chamber of a clinical freezing microtome, frozen with carbon dioxide, and sectioned with little damage to the tissue. The method is rapid and its usage can avoid the use of fixatives, especially when the fixatives would affect using the tissue later for fluorescence microscopy or microincineration. There are several disadvantages to this method:

1. Distortion from both the cutting and freezing
2. Difficulty in cutting sections much larger than 2 × 2 cm
3. Considerable skill required to prepare sections thinner than 15 μm

Method of preparing sections

Fresh material may be cut, but better sections are obtained after tissue has been fixed in formalin and washed before freezing. If tissues are in alcohol, they should be hydrated to water and washed before freezing. Trim the tissue to 2 × 2 cm and 3 to 5 mm in thickness. Cut a circle of filter paper, wet it, and place it on the freezing chamber. Lay tissue on paper and add enough water to surround it. Proceed in the following manner:

1. Freeze with a rapid on-and-off gas flow of CO_2 by holding a small beaker over the tissue and object holder to aid in even hardening and freezing.
2. The knife should enter a point of the tissue on a square block, rather than the full width of the tissue. If a capsule, skin, or mucous membrane is present, it should face the knife, either on the shorter width, or on the left of the longer width, so that the cut is made from the capsule into the tissue to prevent the capsule from tearing away from the tissue.
3. The knife must be cool to prevent the sections from sticking to it and the tissue must be held firmly against the chamber until freezing begins.
4. Freeze the tissue hard and cut the sections when it has thawed down to the right consistency. As the block warms up and reaches the proper temperature, make the required number of sections by drawing the knife slowly and evenly through the tissue. Cut the required number of sections with an even and slow stroke. Remove from the knife with a finger moistened with distilled water and place the sections in distilled water at room temperature (25° C). If the block is frozen too hard, the sections crumble; if it is not frozen hard enough, the tissues are injured and jammed together.
5. The average thickness of sections is 15 μm. Very hard or dense tissue may not allow cutting at less than 18 to 20 μm. Considerable skill is required to cut thinner sections. The rate of cutting is very important. Sections, when cut too fast, tend to curl or break into shreds. Slow, even cutting permits warming of the cut surface of the block, a controlling factor in procuring a pliable section, free from undulations. This pliability prevents disintegration of the section when it is placed in water. Uneven sections are usually the result of freezing the block too hard and applying too much speed and unnecessary pressure, particularly when firm tissue is being cut. Sections that float rigidly are too thick, and when selecting sections for staining, choose complete sections that fold and unfold freely in the water.
6. All set screws holding the freezing equipment and the knife must be tight to avoid vibration when frozen sections are being cut.

Attaching frozen sections to slides

Celloidin method

1. Float the section on slide from water. Spread it out smoothly with camel's hair brush. Blot with bibulous paper.
2. Cover section with 95% alcohol for 30 seconds and blot with bibulous paper.
3. Flow 0.5% celloidin solution over tissue and slide and drain off the excess fluid at once.
4. Blow briskly on the section and immediately immerse the slide in distilled water.
5. The section is now attached to the slide by the thin layer of celloidin and may be stained by most of the usual staining methods, since celloidin does not prevent the penetration of stains and does not interfere with the visibility of the section. Avoid drying at any stage by proceeding quickly. If the tissue was not properly fixed before sectioning, or if it contains mucoid material, the 30 seconds in 95% alcohol in the first step prevents the tissue from sticking to the bibulous paper.
6. For clearing after staining and dehydrating, use oil of origanum or oil of thyme followed by xylene and mounting.

THE MICROTOME CRYOSTAT

The preparation of frozen sections by the method previously described (if one uses a clinical or standard freezing microtome, freezes the tissue with carbon dioxide, and cuts the sections at room temperature) has many disadvantages.

1. If the tissue has not been fixed, it is ex-

tremely difficult to cut, even when a freezing attachment to keep the knife cool is used.

2. Thin sections of unfixed tissue are limited in thinness, since most standard or clinical freezing microtomes can only be set at multiples of 5 μm and the tissue is too friable to produce good sections at this thickness.

3. The limit of thinness of fixed tissue is 10 to 15 μm, and most tissues are cut between 15 and 25 μm.

4. Under these conditions, therefore, fixation is necessary but provides multiple barriers to procedures involving enzyme histochemistry, fluorescence microscopy, autoradiography, and protein and inorganic histochemistry.

The cryostat is a refrigerated cabinet containing a microtome cooled by a mechanical refrigeration unit. It has been described as a rapid and easy means of preparing large, thin, unwrinkled sections of single or multiple pieces of fresh frozen tissue. We believe, however, that it is an instrument requiring an acquired skill before it can be operated efficiently. Since no skill requiring manual dexterity can develop fully without practice over a reasonable period of time, previous experience of section cutting with conventional microtomes is invaluable to the technologist using the cryostat, since the quality of the final section will depend on his or her experience and skill.

The instrument

There are many good cryostats sold in the laboratory market today. In preparing each of these for use, however, one should lubricate all moving surfaces with a silicone lubricant provided for this purpose. If there is insufficient lubricant, the microtome is stiff and difficult to operate. This problem may be alleviated by a few drops of absolute alcohol being placed on the moving surfaces to remove ice-crystal formation, followed by drying and oiling of the surfaces with the silicone lubricant.

The microtome is enclosed in a deep-freeze box and in most instances is mounted in the freezing compartment at a 45-degree angle. When originally plugged into the electrical socket, the microtome will take approximately 4 hours to reach the required temperature of $-10°$ C. Place the microtome knife in the knife holder and keep an extra knife in the freezing compartment for immediate use. It is essential to use a cold knife. If the knife temperature is higher than $-5°$ C, the temperature of the tissue block must be lower than $-10°$ C. In our laboratory, our cryostats are used at $-20°$ C. The efficiency of the cryostat depends on the tissue temperature, chamber temperature, and knife temperature and is least dependent on cutting-room temperature.

Knife angles are not critical and an angle of approximately 30 degrees provides a base line for cutting the majority of tissue. This angle is from knife tilt only and not the angle of the cutting facet. If the knife angle is too shallow, the tissue will pass over the knife without producing a section and give off a rubbing sound. Too steep an angle gives rise to compression, and although there is obviously an optimal knife angle for each type of tissue, deviation from the 30-degree angle is undesirable unless difficulties arise in cutting the tissue.

Cutting technic

1. Set the knife angle and the thickness scale. Each division on the scale is equal to 2 μm; therefore if the scale is set at 2, the tissue will be cut at 4 μm.

2. Place sufficient Lab-Tek OCT, an embedding medium for freezing tissue, on the object holder. Freeze it slightly in liquid nitrogen, which is kept in a widemouthed thermos container. Place the tissue in the slightly frozen OCT, add more OCT around and over the tissue and freeze solid in liquid nitrogen.

3. A device may be made in the following manner for freezing tissue in liquid nitro-

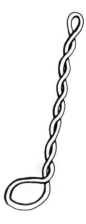

Fig. 1-12. Chuck holder for freezing tissue for the cryostat technic.

gen: We take two strands of heavy wire about 50 cm in length and continually curve the strands together until they reach 23 to 25 cm in length. Bend and curve the remaining wire into a circle to hold the object holder. This holder is indispensable for suspending the tissue down into the liquid nitrogen for rapid freezing of tissue from surgical cases (Fig. 1-12).

4. Transfer the frozen tissue on the object holder to the microtome head. Be sure the head is in the upper position and the drive wheel locked.

5. Tighten the clamp to hold the object holder firmly in place. Pull the knife holding clamp back so that there is 6 mm clearance between the subsequent down-travel of the block and the knife.

6. Release the lock of the drive wheel and bring the knife to within 1 or 2 mm of the tissue and adjust the block to the knife so that it is precisely parallel.

7. Bring the tissue almost into contact with the knife edge, release the ratchet from the micrometer wheel at the rear of the microtome, and advance the wheel clockwise by hand until the tissue begins to section. Trim off the face of the tissue until the desired cutting plane is reached.

8. Return the ratchet to the teeth of the micrometer wheel, clear the knife entirely free of tissue debris, and turn the drive wheel slowly until the leading edge of the section begins to cut.

9. With a fine camel's hair brush, gently stroke the section onto the microtome knife as the tissue moves down over the knife. Alternately, an antiroll plate device may be used.

10. A clean slide, at room temperature, is placed a tiny distance over the frozen section and the section will be attracted directly to the warm slide. Do not use pressure, since this will cause distortion or stretching artifacts. The slide may be held in the hand or attached to a suction-pickup device. Once mounted, the tissue slides may be stained or stored in a Deepfreeze for future use.

Microtome cryostat knives

Either a wedge-shaped knife or a slightly hollow–ground knife should be used. The wedge-shaped knife holds an edge longer under constant use, whereas the hollow-ground knife can be made sharper. A knife 185 mm in length is most suitable, but the ends should be covered with a slotted piece of plastic tubing to prevent accidents.

When paraffin-embedded sections are being cut, the soft tissues such as liver, kidney, spleen, and so forth usually are cut more easily than are hard tissues such as the uterus, skin, breast, and so on, which are normally more difficult to cut. With the cryostat, the reverse is true. The hard tissues cut easily and the soft tissues are more difficult to cut. It may be necessary to cut the soft tissue at a temperature of $-5°$ C. The exception is brain, which will cut well at $-20°$ C.

All frozen sections from surgery are cut on the cryostat and stained in the following manner to provide a rapid section for a permanent frozen-section record.

Sheehan rapid hematoxylin and eosin stain for frozen sections

1. Acetone for 30 seconds.
2. Xylene. Agitate until slide clears.
3. Absolute alcohol. Agitate until slide clears.
4. 95% alcohol. Agitate until slide clears.
5. 70% alcohol. Agitate until slide clears.
6. Tap water. Agitate until slide clears.
7. Delafield's hematoxylin for 1 minute.
8. Tap water. Rinse well.
9. Tap water. Rinse well.
10. Ammonia water until blue.
11. Tap water. Rinse well.
12. 95% alcohol. Agitate until slide clears.
13. Alcoholic eosin for 10 seconds.
14. 95% alcohol, 4 dips.
15. 95% alcohol, 4 dips.
16. Absolute alcohol, 4 dips.
17. Absolute alcohol, 4 dips.
18. Absolute alcohol and xylene (equal parts). Agitate until slide clears.
19. Absolute alcohol and xylene (equal parts). Agitate until slide clears.
20. Xylene.
21. Xylene.
22. Mount in synthetic resin in xylene.

Solutions
Ammonia water: 25 drops of concentrated ammonium hydroxide in 500 ml of tap water
Alcoholic eosin (this formula is well used in the routine H & E stain as well as this rapid stain)
Stock solutions
1% aqueous eosin Y
1% aqueous phloxine

Working solution

Stock eosin	100 ml
Stock phloxine	10 ml
95% ethanol	780 ml
Glacial acetic acid	4 ml

Delafield's hematoxylin (p. 142)

THE COMPOUND MICROSCOPE (Fig. 1-13)

The compound microscope is one of the very important instruments used in the histopathology laboratory. Knowledge of the instrument and its use and care is fundamental. The component parts of the microscope are as follows:

A light source
Condenser
Stage
Objectives
Nosepiece
Body tube
Eyepiece (or ocular)

The light source

In modern instruments the light source is supplied by low-voltage electric bulbs operated by a transformer that can be adjusted to the intensity of light required.

"Of great importance to microscopy is the behavior of refraction. In fact, the refractive behavior of light brings about the formation of images; therefore, refraction might be considered the single most important underlying concept in the functioning of the microscope. Refraction is the bending of a ray of light when it strikes a new optical medium at any angle other than the 'normal.' When one discusses microscopy, the new optical medium will consist of an interface of glass and air, air and glass, glass and glass, and other interfaces such as optical cements, mounting media, and immersion oils. The 'normal,' when one refers to a lens, is a line perpendicular to the tangent of the curved surface" (Wilson, M. B.).

Optical media	Refractive index
Air	1.000
Immersion substances	
Ethanol	1.330
Water	1.336
Xylene	1.49 to 1.50
Cedar oil	1.50 to 1.51
Immersion oil	1.515 to 1.52
Glass (slide and cover glass)	1.51

Condenser

The substage condenser is the first part of the lens system. The functions of the substage condenser are threefold:

1. To concentrate light upon the tissue specimen
2. To produce an adequate area of illumination upon the tissue specimen
3. To furnish strongly convergent light to the tissue so that full resolving power of objectives may be used.

To give even illumination, the condenser must be accurately centered with respect to the axis of the objective. The common mechanism provided on the complete substage for the centering of the condenser is a pair of centering screws.

The regulation of light illuminating an object is the function of the diaphragm. The intensity of illumination is, in part, regulated by the field diaphragm of the condenser. The aperture diaphragm regulates the convergence of the cone of light rays from the condenser. The purpose is to match the numerical aperture of the condenser to the numerical aperture of the objective that will give optimal image quality.

The stage

The stage of the microscope sits above the condenser with an opening through which the light passes. One of the most useful accessories on a microscope is a mechanical stage. It is a mechanism for moving the slide by rack and pinion or screw movement slowly in either of two mutually perpendicular directions. Mechanical stages are built into microscopes or

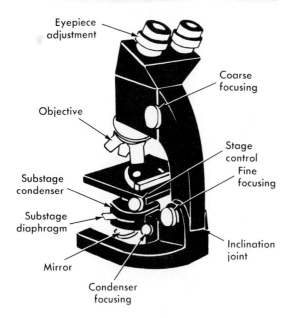

Fig. 1-13. The compound microscope.

added on. The mechanical stage is particularly helpful when one needs to search a specimen to make certain no part has been missed. On some mechanical stages a Vernier is located to make it possible to note the position of the slide in each direction. If the position of the field on each scale is noted, the slide can be immediately replaced in the same location to relocate the same field.

Objectives

The objectives are the second lens system of the compound microscope. The objective is the lens at the lower end of the body tube and has a major responsibility for the magnification and resolution of the image. It is the most important component of the microscope.

Either achromatic or apochromatic objections may be chosen. For routine microscopy in a histopathology laboratory, the less expensive achromatic objectives are most commonly used. These are corrected for two colors, red and blue. The most highly corrected are the apochromatic objectives, which are corrected for three colors. Plan apochromats provide a perfectly flat field of view and are ideally suited for photomicrography.

The numerical aperture (N.A.) of the objective is fundamentally important, since the microscope's ability to resolve is entirely dependent on the N.A., which is engraved on the side of the objective. Numerical aperture is the sine (sine u) of the half-aperture angle multiplied by the refractive index (n) of the medium filling the space between the cover glass and the front lens.

$$N.A. = n \times \sin u$$

Nosepiece

The nosepiece on the microscope revolves and can handle multiple objectives. The objectives, when possible, should remain screwed into the nosepiece to avoid damage.

Body tube

The body tube is monocular or binocular. Better vision results when it is possible to use both eyes simultaneously. A binocular body on the microscope permits the use of both eyes and gives some appearance of depth. The standard body tube is 16 cm in length.

Eyepieces (oculars)

The eyepieces are the third lens system on a compound microscope. The primary function of the eyepiece is to magnify the image of the specimen produced at the rear of the objective so that the eye can come closer to the image. The binocular bodies usually have inclined eyepiece tubes for greater comfort of the user. The binocular body has two adjustments, one changes the distance between the eyepieces until both eyes see a single field. This is an interpupillary adjustment that sets the centers of the lenses in the two eyepieces at exactly the same distance apart as the centers of the observer's eyes. The other adjustment compensates for any difference between the observer's eyes. To make this adjustment the microscope is focused sharp to the right eye. Then the right eye is closed and the adjustment on the left eyepiece turned until the image is sharp for the left eye. Both eyes should then see the image equally well.

FLUORESCENCE MICROSCOPY

An object fluoresces when it absorbs ultraviolet light reflected on it or transmitted through it and then emits the energy in visible lights of a specific violet, blue, green, yellow, orange, or red color. These substances, present in some tissues, are called *fluorophors*. Secondary fluorescence can be induced by the use of *fluorochromes*, which are strongly fluorescent dyes or chemicals that are applied to the tissue specimen.

See p. 311 for information on the equipment and reagents used in fluorescence procedures.

PHASE MICROSCOPY

Phase microscopy is the preferred microscope method for the study of unstained cells. Apparatus for phase microscopy is simple, relatively inexpensive, and easy to use and can be added to any conventional microscope. It may be used to study living material, cytoplasm, nucleus, cell inclusions, and the action of physical and chemical agents on tissue. However, the use of phase microscopy is not limited to the study of living cells or to unstained fixed tissue sections. The method is particularly useful to visualize tissue components that are essentially transparent and cannot be studied with bright-field microscopy.

A standard binocular microscope can be converted to a phase microscope by replacement of the standard condenser and objectives with special phase equipment. A phase-telescope eyepiece is also available.

It is possible to determine the approximate

refractive index of living and fixed tissue components with the aid of the phase-contrast microscope.

POLARIZING MICROSCOPY

The use of polarized light in the histopathology laboratory is distinctly valuable in the examination of doubly refractile particles such as crystals and some lipids, and it may also be used to study myelinated nervous tissue, collagen, and cross-striated muscle.

Lillie writes: "Polarized light may be produced by use of discs of Polaroid material, by interposition of a series of obliquely placed thin cover glasses, or by use of a Nicol prism. The polarizing device is set at any convenient place between the light source and the study slide. Also required is a second polarizing device, called an analyzer, that is usually placed over the microscope ocular."

When a ray of plane-polarized light, which vibrates in one plane, falls on the object, it is split into two rays, one ray obeying the law of refraction and the other passing through at a different velocity. After emerging from the object, the two rays are recombined.

Bright apple-green birefringence of amyloid is easily seen after Congo red and Sirius red staining.

CARE OF MICROSCOPE

1. The microscope is a precision instrument that must be handled skillfully and carefully.
2. It must be kept scrupulously clean in every detail.
3. Aside from cleaning the outer surface of the lenses, the objectives should remain in the nosepiece. A soft camel's hair brush should be used to remove dust from the objectives, and they can then be polished with lens paper or soft old linen.
4. The top lens of the eyepiece can be dusted with a camel's hair brush and then polished with lens paper or soft old linen.
5. "Prisms should never be touched, and cleaning should be confined to blowing off the dust with a rubber bulb fitted with a small-bore metal tube, since the slightest misalignment of the prisms will cause enormous eye fatigue." (Culling)
6. Never use facial tissues to clean optical glass. Use lens paper only!
7. If it is necessary to use a liquid to clean the dry objectives, Mallinckrodt's lens cleaner is excellent for this purpose.

8. When immersion oil is used, it may be cleaned off with a small amount of xylene followed by polishing with lens paper.

MICROTOMES

The first microtome, called a cutting engine, was made by Cummings in 1770, followed by Adam's cutting engine in 1798, which was essentially the first sliding microtome. Pritchard, in 1835, fastened Cumming's model to the edge of the table with a clamp and used a separate two-handled knife for cutting sections. In 1839, Chevalier introduced the word "microtome." Rotary microtomes were invented independently by Pfeifer at the Johns Hopkins University in 1883 and by Minot at Harvard University in 1886. Bausch and Lomb Optical Company manufactured the sliding microtome in 1882, and Spencer Lens Company produced the Clinical Microtome in 1901 followed by the large Spencer Rotary Microtome in 1910 (Richards) (American Optical Co., Buffalo, N.Y.).

The following microtomes are used in histopathology laboratories:

1. Standard rotary microtome for paraffin sectioning
2. Rustproof rotary microtome for cryostat sectioning
3. Clinical freezing microtome for cutting fresh and fixed tissues; primarily used for cutting tissue for fat stains
4. Sliding microtome for cutting celloidin-embedded material
5. Ultrathin sectioning microtome used with either a diamond or glass knife in electron microscopy
6. The JB-4 "Porter-Blum" microtome for plastic and paraffin sectioning (Ivan Sorvall, Inc., Newtown, Conn.)

With good care, a microtome will have a long useful life. The following maintenance should be carefully carried out and recorded:

1. Thorough daily cleaning of rotary microtomes used for paraffin sectioning. Soft cloths moistened with xylene, followed by thorough oiling of the knife-holder slides, will keep the instrument free of paraffin and rust. Do not use xylene on the painted surfaces, since it will remove the finish.
2. Use two drops of Bear Brand oil (Norton Company, Troy, N.Y., formerly Pike Oil), on inner oil pits (check manufacturer's diagram) requiring oil. This should be done every week or so on instruments that receive average use daily.

3. Grease inner surfaces with a good light neutral grease every 3 months if the instrument is used daily, or every 6 months if it is used less than daily.
4. Keep the instrument covered and free from dust when not in use.

MICROTOME KNIVES

Microtome knives must be kept in perfect condition if the technologist is to produce good histologic preparations for patient diagnosis. The sharpening of microtome knives is a skilled technology and may be done in the laboratory with the many adequate and good instruments sold today (see discussion on knife sharpening, below), or, if technical time is costly, it may be done commercially by many companies supplying laboratory needs. C. L. Sturkey (P.O. Box 59, Perkiomenville, Pa. 18074) manufactures microtome knives and does an excellent job of both reconditioning and sharpening microtome knives. They are picked up and delivered in the metropolitan Philadelphia area, but may be serviced by mail anywhere in the country. We highly recommend this service. It is economical and expedient in a laboratory where technical time is expensive and at a premium.

The wedge-shaped knife is used for cutting paraffin-embedded material on a rotary microtome, for cryostat sectioning, and for cutting fresh and fixed tissues on a clinical freezing microtome. The plano-concave knife is used for celloidin sectioning.

The standard microtome knife has a wedge angle of about 15 degrees. A bevel angle between the cutting facets for knives of American manufacture varies between 27 and 32 degrees. For the best possible sections of a given specimen, the knife should be adjusted to the proper tilt for the particular specimen. For an average specimen this tilt should be enough to give a clearance angle of 3 to 8 degrees (Richards).

KNIFE SHARPENERS

Lyn Richardson, Margaret S. Judge, and Maria Sugulas, with permission of The American Society for Medical Technology

Sharpening by hand

The single most important step in the laboratory is to produce a knife edge that will cut thin sections without knife marks or compression. An adequate tissue section may still be obtained with a sharp knife despite poor fixation and processing. The implications are obvious. If a section can be obtained, a diagnosis is possible.

The techniques for producing sharp knives were applied by hand for hundreds of years. Stone and leather were used to grind and polish steel to a keen edge. Until the development of automatic knife sharpeners, sharpening by hand was considered a vital skill of the histologist.

Hand-sharpening tools commonly used are hones with coarse to fine abrasive surfaces and strops. A hone is either a natural or synthetic abrasive stone or glass plate that is used to form a bevel or wedge tip on the microtome knife and to remove nicks. A hone should be at least 2.5 × 20 × 30 cm long to prevent uneven wear of the knife.

Excellent oil stones are produced in the United States and may be purchased as a unit* consisting of three stone grades that rotate through an oil bath to which they are attached. The three stone grades are (1) coarse (synthetic) for grinding a new bevel and removing large nicks, (2) medium (synthetic) for removing the serrated edge resulting from coarse honing and, (3) fine Arkansas oil stone (natural) for finishing the edge.

Some technologists prefer the water stones because a stream of water can be used while one is honing to wash away metal and abrasive particles that might damage the knife edge.

If a glass plate is to be used as a hone, it must be ground with a carborundum paste, oil or water mixture, and another sheet of glass to produce an abrasive surface. The ground plate is used with an abrasive or soap mixture to hone the knife. A carborundum paste is recommended for fast grinding and Diamantine for finishing. A neutral soap solution may also be used for finishing.

The hones must be kept flat to prevent uneven grinding along the knife edge. Diamond rubbing blocks† are available for resurfacing and finishing all worn hones. The hone, regardless of type, must be washed and dried with a lint-free cloth after resurfacing or honing.

Strops are used to finish the knife edge. This final polishing step forms a facet or secondary bevel at the tip of the bevel (Fig. 1-14). The stropping procedure is the actual sharpening step. The strop gives under the pressure of the knife, and the bevel angle at the very tip in-

---

* Lipshaw Manufacturing Co., Detroit, MI 48210
† Norton Co., Troy, NY 12181.

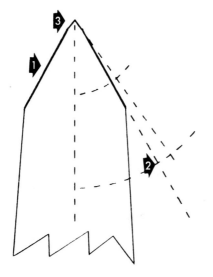

Fig. 1-14. 1, Primary bevel (hone). **2,** Bevel angle. **3,** Secondary bevel (strop). (From Judge, S., Richardson, L., and Sugulas, M.: Knife sharpening made easy, Bellaire, Texas, 1978, The American Society for Medical Technology.)

creases slightly to create a very small facet, which becomes the cutting surface. The facet appears as a fine white line when viewed through the microscope at 100× magnification. Excess stropping will round the edge and dull the knife. Six to 12 strokes on either side of the knife are usually sufficient.

Some strops are embedded with diamond particles. These strops are excellent but should be used cautiously. Five strokes on either side of the knife are recommended.

Strops are leather (horsehide, calfskin, and pigskin) or linen. There are three types of strops: (1) the hanging strop (razor strop), (2) the saddleback strop, a strop stretched across a heavy frame and made taut by turning an extending screw at one end, (3) the block strop, a strop mounted on a felt-padded wood block. The block strop is recommended for better support of the knife.

Linen cloth, when fastened to a stropping frame and stretched to its maximum, serves as a fine finishing strop. The linen strop produces a sharp edge and is sometimes used alone to strop a knife that is slightly dull.

Whether honing, stropping or doing both, a round metal back must be slipped onto a wedge or plano-concave knife. A handle is locked into one end of the knife beforehand. The honing back lifts the knife to the correct bevel angle

when the knife is laid across the hone or strop. The bevel must lay flat on the surface in order to grind the bevel to the edge without changing the angle. This is extremely important and should be checked before honing. The honing back is fitted to the knife at the factory and the two should be returned for refitting if the bevel is not flush with a flat surface. Any movement of the knife back on the knife should be corrected. If loose, the back may be closed slightly by pressing in a vise. When the knife back becomes worn, it should be replaced, since a worn back will cause a change in the bevel angle.

Although a variety of opinions exists among technologists on the choice of hones, strops, and abrasives and when or how to use them, the following basic rules should be observed:

1. Choose the finest quality hones, strops, and abrasives available.
2. Clean the knife thoroughly before sharpening.
3. Check the honing back for wear and fit.
4. Always slide the indicated end of the honing back onto the knife. The American Optical and Schmid honing backs are rounded at the insertion end. The Lipshaw back is not marked. One end should be marked with a file or diamond pen to ensure proper placement when the insertion end is not indicated.
5. Check the hone for uneven wear. Grind flat and resurface with a rubbing block, if necessary, and wash well with hot water.
6. Check that the bevel lays flat on the hone after the back is fitted to the knife.
7. Lubricate the hone with light machine oil or soap and water depending on the type of stone used.
8. Hone and strop the knife with the least amount of pressure. The weight of the knife is usually sufficient. The only time pressure should be applied is while honing a curved edge. In that case, apply pressure to the knife back along the high areas.
9. Use a microscope to check the progress of the knife edge at 100× magnification. A fine bright line should be visible. This is the secondary bevel.
10. Remove any abrasive along the knife edge after a change of hones and before stropping.
11. Examine the strop for nicks and replace if damaged. Keep the strop free of foreign matter. Lubricate the strop occasionally

with saddlesoap or neat's-foot oil and allow to dry overnight.

American Optical Automatic Knife Sharpener

Over the years there were several instruments developed for sharpening microtome knives, but they were manually operated. The American Optical knife sharpener was one of the first automatic sharpeners for use in the histopathology laboratory. American Optical has since manufactured the 925 and the 935 models. These instruments are simply constructed, easy to repair, and easy to operate.

The basic operation of the sharpener employs the use of a rectangular glass plate that remains stationary, while the knife and holder move back and forth across it, turning from side to side. American Optical supplies with each piece of equipment the following items:

1. Two glass plates

2. A coarse and fine abrasive for use on the plates
3. The glass honing compound, for the refinishing of the plates
4. The redressing pad that is also used in the refinishing procedure
5. The knife inspection block that is recommended for use when the knife is examined under the microscope

The knife should always be carefully inspected microscopically for assessment of the condition of the cutting edge. This is the only way to adequately judge the completeness of the sharpening process. It is imperative that students and technologists become familiar with the appearance of the knife edge either by "reflected light," that is using a lamp located above the knife or by "transmitted light" with the light coming from below. When examining the knife edge by either of these methods, use the 10× objective and the 10× eyepieces, to give a resul-

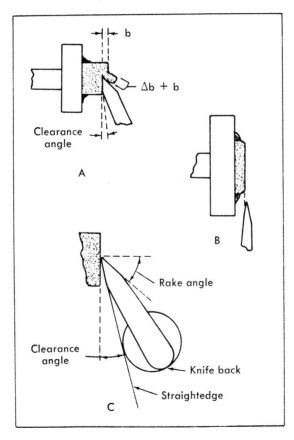

Fig. 1-15. A, Diagram showing clearance angle and increase in section thickness from compression. **B,** Wedging effect when there is no clearance angle. **C,** How to set clearance angle. (From Richards, O. W.: Effective use and proper care of the A.O. Microtome, Buffalo, N.Y., 1959 and 1975, American Optical Scientific Instrument Division.)

tant magnification of 100. The wooden knife inspection block holds the knife at the proper angle for viewing. (See Figs. 1-15 to 1-20.)

The following is the recommended procedure for sharpening on the Model 925.

Coarse honing operation

1. Inspect the knife for the presence and size of nicks.
2. Place the glass hone plate in the upper position. The proper positioning of the glass plate is essential for correct coarse honing, following the instructions of the manufacturer.

3. Attach the knife with the American Optical trademark to the right; this puts the handle slot to the left. Check to see that the knife holder is correctly and securely fastened to the shaft. Then with the two clamps facing up and the clamp screws loosened, install the knife so that the end with the AO trademark is to the right. This places the slotted end of the knife to the left, while facing the instrument. Tighten the two clamp screws until the knife is safely but temporarily fastened. *Note:* Always sharpen the longest knives first.
4. Center the knife in the holder using a ruler.

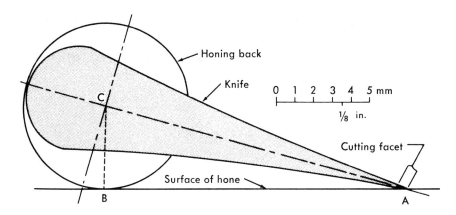

Fig. 1-16. Knife and honing back drawn to scale to show extent and formation of cutting bevel and facets. (From Richards, O. W.: Effective use and proper care of the A.O. Microtome, Buffalo, N.Y., American Optical Scientific Instrument Division.)

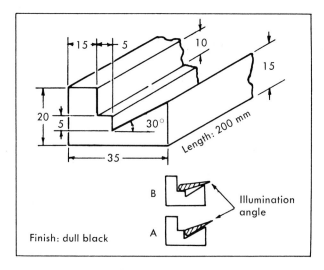

Fig. 1-17. Block for supporting microtome knife (dimensions in millimeters). **A,** Position for examining sharpness. **B,** Position for observation of polish. (From Richards, O. W.: Effective use and proper care of the A.O. Microtome, Buffalo, N.Y., American Optical Scientific Instrument Division.)

This is to ensure proper balance of the knife during the honing procedure. Using a ruler adjust the knife's position until the same distance is measured from the outside edge of each clamp to each end of the knife. Gradually tighten the clamp screws, alternating from one to the other until the knife is held firmly in place.

5. Thoroughly shake the coarse abrasive no. 937. Shake the abrasive thoroughly until all of the particles are in suspension.

6. Apply the coarse abrasive to the plate. This is accomplished by squeezing a narrow ribbon, about the width of a pencil, of the coarse abrasive across the plate. The ribbon should be approximately equal in length to the knife that is being sharpened. Remem-

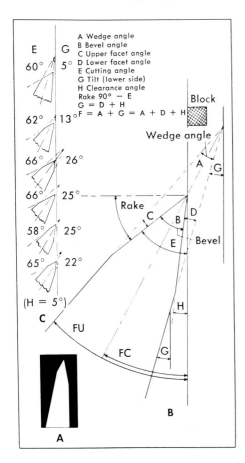

Fig. 1-18. A, Impression made by knife's cutting edge showing unequal sharpening. **B,** Geometry of knife-edge angles. **C,** Rake and tilt angles for a clearance angle of 5 degrees for proper placing of knives with unequal facets. (From Richards, O. W.: Effective use and proper care of the A.O. Microtome, Buffalo, N.Y., American Optical Scientific Instrument Division.)

ber to apply the coarse abrasive at least 2.5 cm inside the front edge of the plate. It is imperative that the plate not become dry while the sharpening procedure is in use.

7. First time setting is 60 minutes. Close the Plexiglas cover and turn on the switch. The knife is then automatically stroked against the high-frequency vibrating glass plate. After the equivalent of three full strokes on one side, a cam follower automatically turns the knife and hones the other cutting facet with three strokes. This cycle is repeated continuously for 60 minutes.

8. Remove the knife carefully. At the end of the cycle, the knife holder will stop in a raised horizontal position. *Note:* If the holder should stop upside down, with the knife clamps facing downward, turn the automatic timer knob beyond the 10-minute setting. Wait until the knife starts to move upward and then go through a half cycle and stop it in the correct raised position.

9. Clean the knife and inspect its condition. It will be necessary to wipe the knife with a clean cloth moistened with a solvent such as xylene. Then inspect the cutting facet under the microscope at 100×.

10. Clean the glass plate—continue coarse honing. To clean the glass plate, merely wash it under hot running tap water using a detergent to remove the abrasive and fine metal particles. Then wipe the plate so it is completely dry. Now apply fresh coarse abrasive and continue honing as required. Periodically inspect to check the progress of the knife. Remember to add abrasive as needed and to wash the plate when the abrasive becomes nearly black in color.

After the coarse honing procedure has been completed, it is then necessary to put a fine finished edge on the knife. This is accomplished by the use of the fine honing procedure.

Fine honing procedure

1. Check the knife for cleanliness. It is essential that all traces of the coarse abrasive are removed from the knife, the knife holder, and the glass honing plate before beginning the fine honing. Be sure to check and clean them thoroughly. If the same glass honing plate is to be used, remove it and wash the plate under hot running tap water using an

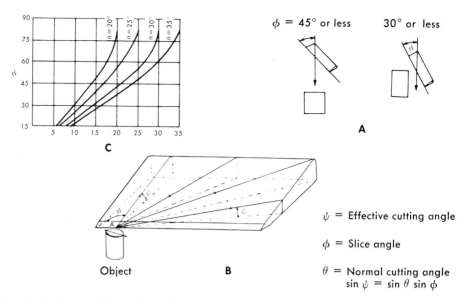

Fig. 1-19. A, Showing slice angle, ϕ, for square and rectangular blocks. **B,** Decreased wedging with small slice angles. **C,** Relations between them plotted from data of Preston (1933). (From Richards, O. W.: Effective use and proper care of the A.O. Microtome, Buffalo, N.Y., American Optical Scientific Instrument Division.)

ordinary detergent and carefully dry the plate.

2. Place the glass honing plate in the lower position. After inspecting the glass plate for evidence of wear, place it in the lower position.

3. Attach and center the knife. Install and center the knife the same way as the coarse honing procedure. Always double check to make sure that the clamp screws are tight. A loose knife might cause a serious accident.

4. Shake the fine abrasive no. 938.

5. Apply the fine abrasive to the glass plate.

6. Set the timer for 30 minutes when beginning the fine honing operation. Be sure to keep the Plexiglas cover closed while the instrument is running.

7. Clean the knife and inspect the condition of the edge. It is imperative that all abrasive be removed from the edge of the knife before it is inspected under the microscope at 100×. Look carefully for any small nicks that are still evident in the knife edge. The removal of such nicks, and not the width of the fine facets, determines the progress of the sharpening procedure.

8. Continue the fine honing procedure. Experience with models 925 and 935 will soon enable the technologist or student to estimate how much more time is needed to achieve the desired results. Remember that microscopic examination is still the final determining factor. Add the abrasive as required and periodically check that the plate is not a grayish color from the buildup of metal particles. Should this occur, the plate should be washed and fresh abrasive applied.

9. After fine honing is complete, the knife should be cleaned and carefully wiped dry. Where the atmosphere is corrosive and the knife is to be stored for any length of time, lubricate the knife with a good grade of light, neutral oil. The knife should never be stropped.

The honing action of the knife against the frosted glass plate will eventually cause a "shiny" path to be worn on the face of the plate as wide as the length of the knife.

Redressing the plates

Follow manufacturer's instructions.

Cleaning and lubrication

1. *Cleaning.* The Plexiglas cover and the outside enameled surfaces should be kept clean. Use warm water and detergent to keep these areas clean. Then sponge out and wipe dry the catch-basin on the hone table after each sharpening session. The knife holder, knife-

Fig. 1-20. A, Microtome knife-edge from the Shandon-Elliott Microsharp technic. **B,** Microtome knife-edge using 6 μm diamond compound. **C,** Microtome knife-edge finished with 1 μm diamond compound. **D,** Microtome knife-edge before sharpening. **E,** Microtome knife-edge during sharpening. **F,** Microtome knife-edge at completion of sharpening procedure. (From Judge, S., Richardson, L., and Sugulas, M.: Knife sharpening made easy, Bellaire, Texas, 1978, The American Society for Medical Technology.)

holder shaft, and the exposed fittings are of a noncorrosive material and require no attention other than normal cleaning.

2. *Lubrication.* Lubricate the instrument approximately once each month, more if used extensively. Lifetime Oilite bearings are used throughout the instrument; therefore only a few points require lubrication. Place just a drop or two of Bear Brand oil on the following:
   a. Round felt pad beneath the worm gear of the motor.
   b. The two brass bearings of the pivot points between the carrier arm assembly and the slide castings.
   c. The brass bearing at the end of the motor crank arm.
   d. The two slide rods. For this area, use Molykote spray graphite lubricant, which is usually available locally.

A modified procedure using diamond compound has also been developed for use on the American Optical sharpeners, as follows.

Richardson's modified coarse honing

1. Place the frosted glass plate in the coarse honing position.
2. Apply a small amount of 6 μm diamond compound to the plate.
3. Lubricate the diamond compound with lubricating fluid.
4. Rub the lubricated compound over the plate.
5. Allow the knife to recondition for 20 minutes.
6. Remove the knife from the sharpener and clean it with xylene.

7. Check the edge under the microscope to ensure that reconditioning is complete.

Since the surface for fine honing is critical, smooth plate glass is used for this modified procedure. Plate glass is obtainable from glass and window dealers, cut to the correct size. The cost per plate is approximately $2.00.

Richardson's modified fine honing procedure

1. Place the plate glass in the coarse honing position.
2. Apply an ample amount of 1 μm diamond compound to the plate glass, using a small amount of lubricating fluid.
3. Allow the knife to finish for 30 minutes to remove barbs and rough edges.
4. Wipe the plate clean with a lint-free towel and lower the plate to the fine-honing position.
5. Apply a small amount of 1 μm diamond compound to the plate, spreading the compound evenly. Do not apply any lubricating fluid in this final step.
6. Allow the knife to finish for 60 minutes.
7. Remove the knife and clean it with xylene. Check it again under the microscope.

The results of this modified procedure are excellent, even though the time involved will be a factor to consider in some laboratories. However, this procedure will be of value where improved sectioning, fewer recuts and better results are more important factors than the time involved.

Helpful hints

The following are helpful hints for the American Optical knife sharpeners:

1. Carefully measure the knife length and find the center of the knife. Score the center of the knife with a diamond-point pencil. Align this score with the center mark on the knife holder of models 925 and 935. Earlier models do not have a center mark on the knife holder; so it must be marked in the same manner as the knife.
2. A vortex mixer can be used to stir abrasives.
3. Place a small marble in the bottom of the abrasive bottle to aid in mixing.
4. When cleaning knives, never wipe across the knife. Always wipe up, away from the knife edge.
5. Coarse honing procedures produce a uniformly rough edge microscopically, and the technologist should become familiar with the appearance of the knife edge.
6. Do not remove the knife holder from the knife during sharpening procedures.

This can cause minor changes in the knife position from one time to another.

7. The knife-viewing block should be altered to hold the knives with the knife holder attached. This is easily accomplished if one cuts away the front edge so that the knife back rests on the slot.
8. Use one side of the plate for coarse honing and one side for fine honing. This eliminates the possibility of contaminating the fine-honing side with coarse abrasive. Mark the edges of the plate with dark nail polish; then seal the marks with a coat of clear nail polish.
9. To eliminate as many variables as possible, assign knives to the plates. A usual ratio would be one plate for each three to four knives. Post a chart showing which knives are to be sharpened on which plate. Plates and knives should be numbered.
10. If adequate redressing is not obtainable with the automatic redressing attachment on the Model 935, as has been the case in some laboratories, the hand-honing procedure should be followed.
11. Be sure to watch for worn areas where the knife holder might drag on the plate when using knives other than American Optical.

Hacker Perma-Sharp Microtome Knife Sharpener

The Perma-Sharp knife sharpener was designed on principles used in the razor-blade industry.

The knife bevel is maintained at a 24-degree angle each time the knife is passed through the circular rotating hones. The strops are set to polish an additional 3-degree facet at the tip of the bevel to produce a finely polished cutting edge. The double bevel produced is like that of a razor blade. A result of this design is the elimination of costly reconditioning of knives to reestablish the correct bevel angle. The 24-degree bevel facet on a knife sharpener on the Perma-Sharp becomes wider as the knife loses its width because of the loss of metal during the honing step. However, the final 3-degree facet remains the same so that the cut tissue always passes over a very small surface.

Sharpening time on the Perma-Sharp can be reduced to a few minutes, once the theory of operation is understood and the technic is mastered. The reduction in time and money spent to sharpen microtome knives has made the Perma-Sharp knife sharpener a widely accepted tool for obtaining good tissue sections.

The maintenance of this instrument is minimal. The Perma-Sharp does not involve lapping bars to flatten worn plates, or messy abrasive mixtures to grind and polish knives sharpened on rotating plates. On the Perma-Sharp, the knife is passed through low-speed circular hones and strops to achieve a fine edge. The circular hones withstand months, or even years, of use before the honing surfaces need redressing. A simple redressing device can be purchased from the manufacturer to redress the hones on all Perma-Sharp models. The life of the stropping wheels is determined by frequency of use. Even with frequent use, the strops will last for years.

An inexpensive abrasive wax stick is used on the circular strops for the final polishing step. All that is necessary to maintain them is an occasional removal of the wax buildup.

The Perma-Sharp knife sharpener is a relatively simple and effective means for producing excellent cutting surfaces on knives of standard shapes that are less than 25 cm (250 mm) in length and a minimum of 2 cm in width.

The operation of the Perma-Sharp sharpener does require some dexterity, since the knife is moved along the carrier bar by the operator who has also set the knife's position for the correct bevel.

For Perma-Sharp, there are several important points that must be covered:

1. Examine the knife to be sharpened before proceeding.
2. If the knife is badly damaged, it will need additional honing to wear away the damage.
3. If the knife is new, or being sharpened on the Perma-Sharp for the first time, it will need additional honing to establish a new bevel.
4. A felt marking pen may be used to mark the knife bevel to the edge of the knife approximately 2.5 cm from either end of the knife. When the marks are ground off by the hones, the new bevel is complete It is ready to pass through the strops.
5. Always slide the knife into the holder with the same end to the left. The knife may be marked with a diamond marking pen, or use the drill hole found on most knives.
6. Always clean the knife with a wipe soaked in a solvent, such as xylene, to remove paraffin and debris.

Instruction for the Perma-Sharp MK-4

The Model MK-4 Hacker Perma-Sharp has a number of improvements that make this knife sharpener easier to operate than previous models MK-1 to MK-3. On the MK-1 to MK-3 models, rapid on-off switching is required to run the strops at slow speed while the final polishing step of stropping is done. The end result depends on the dexterity of the operator.

On the MK-4, the addition of the variable slow-speed control allows an inexperienced operator to produce a highly-polished edge. When properly adjusted and operated, the MK-4 will sharpen knives that cut sections as thin as 2 μm.

The MK-4 is a well-constructed, quality microtome knife sharpener that can produce excellent knives when properly used.

The sharpening instructions for the Hacker Perma-Sharp MK-4 are as follows:

1. Turn switch to N, or full-speed position. Apply abrasive compound stick lightly across each rotating strop once only. (*Note:* Apply abrasive once for every six to eight knives sharpened. This will depend on the number of stropping strokes used on each knife. The wax in the abrasive tends to build up on the strops if applied too frequently. The abrasive becomes embedded in the wax, thereby reducing abrasive polishing action.) Switch the instrument off.
2. Clamp the knife in the holder.
3. Turn the vertical control knob at the top front of the panel from the left to the right until the knife edge clears the intersection of the hones. Do this before the knife is moved between the hones to prevent jamming.
4. Slide the knife between the hones until the left end of the knife holder is approximately 6 mm from the sharpener's side. The gauge reading will then be made along the actual cutting surface of the knife. If the center of the knife is higher than the outer edges, additional honing will produce a straight edge.
5. Attach the centrality gauge to the knife. Keep your hands away from the instrument or table during the next steps, since a false gauge reading could result.
6. Face the sharpener in line with the gauge. View the gauge from a position above the center line for accuracy.
7. Center the knife between the hones by

turning the horizontal control knob (front side panel) with the right hand. After every left or right turn of the knob, tilt the knife lightly back and forward against the hones. When the bubble positions on the gauge are an equal distance from the center line proceed to the next step.

8. Position the knife between the hones for the correct bevel by turning the vertical control knob, top front panel. Tilt the knife lightly backward and forward against the hones after every right or left turn. When the knife is positioned for the correct bevel, the bubble of the gauge will touch the outside edge of the black lines on either side of the center line when the knife is tilted. Repeat steps 7 and 8 until a correct setting is obtained.

9. Remove the centrality gauge and move the knife away from the hones.

10. Switch the instrument to N position. Allow hones to reach maximum speed. Slide knife edge just inside rotating hones. Tilt knife forward and quickly move knife across back hone with light pressure. Do not pause or apply uneven pressure. Tilt knife back with knife edge just inside hones. Move the knife quickly across front hone.

11. Inspect the knife. If nicks are still visible, repeat the honing step. If knife is being sharpened on this instrument for the first time, repeat the honing step to complete new bevel. Do not hone more than necessary—one pass on either side of the knife is usually sufficient. The knife will have a rough burr or serrated edge when the bevel is complete.

12. Move the knife along the carrier bar to the strops. Do not strike the knife edge against the hones.

13. Move the knife evenly along the back strop, using moderate pressure. Before the knife leaves the strop, tilt the knife back and move it across the front strop. Repeat this process 10 times. The knife edge will have a fine burr at this point. *Note:* If the knife does leave the strops, there is a danger of strop damage. The knife edge may strike the side of a strop on subsequent passes.

14. Switch the instrument off. Continue stropping until strops slow to a stop. Strop the knife twice on the stationary strops. This step further removes the burr.

15. Switch the instrument to *P*. Turn the speed-control knob, at the left of the top panel, to slow the strops down to approximately one revolution per minute. Strop 10 times on either side of the knife. When the strops rotate at very slow speeds, they remove the fine burr and polish the final facet of the knife. Use light pressure. Too much pressure may cause the strops to stall. Increase the speed of the strops slightly if stalling occurs with light pressure.

16. Switch the instrument off. Move the knife to the right end of the carrier bar. Carefully move the knife holder to an upright position. Grip the knife holder. Turn the Allen screw counterclockwise to loosen the clamp. Use great care in removing the knife.

17. Remove abrasive from the knife edge with Scott's Micro Assembly Wipes No. 5310 (p. 444) dipped in xylene or other solvent. Wipe toward the edge with short strokes to prevent damage to the edge. It is important to remember that once the knife is removed from the holder, it must be recentered and repositioned if further sharpening is necessary.

An alternate stropping method:

1. Strop 10 times on each side at maximum speed.

2. Reduce speed to medium. Strop 10 times on each side.

3. Reduce speed to slow (approximately 60 RPM). Strop 10 times on each side.

The edge will be sharp; so handle the knife with care.

Maintenance

Maintenance is essential for the proper operation of the equipment. The following maintenance instructions are for models MK-1 to MK-4.

1. Remove the cabinet and vacuum-clean it at least once a year to avoid creating a fire hazard from accumulated dust. Remove and empty the dust tray at least once a month. The handle for the tray is at the left base of the cabinet.

2. Remove abrasive buildup on strops. Clamp an old knife in the holder and adjust according to standard procedures. Bypass the hones and strop hard against strops when they are rotating at full speed. Or, remove the rod from an American Optical knife handle and run the round grip end

along the strops. Hold the rod firmly and apply moderate pressure along each strop.

3. Apply a few drops of light machine oil to the carrier bar once a week. Do not drip on hones or strops. Spread along bar with Scott's Micro Assembly Wipes No. 5310. Remove excess. Slide holder along the bar several times.

4. Check the diameter of the hones with the special gauge supplied with the sharpener.
   a. Move the carrier bar fully forward by turning the horizontal control.
   b. Insert gauge between the hones and the motors so that the base of the gauge rests on both shafts with the gauge pen across both wheels.
   c. Rock the gauge back and forth. If there is no movement of the handle, the hones are less than 14.83 cm in diameter and must be replaced.

5. To remove small irregularities, hones may need redressing if they are new or rough. A simple redressing device is now available from Hacker Instruments. Instructions are included or you may have the Hacker representative redress the hones for a fee.

6. Replace the synchronization belt at the left of strops if it becomes worn. Unplug the instrument, remove the cover, and cut the old belt. Stretch the new belt over one strop. Twist the belt into a figure 8 and stretch the end over the other strop. Make certain the center rod is between the belt.

7. Remove the horizontal and vertical controls and oil the threads. Do not apply grease. Remove any grease found on the rod ends because grease will cause slippage of the control rods during sharpening.

8. Make sure that your Perma-Sharp distributor* stocks hones, strops, and belts so that you have quick access to parts when they are needed.

Helpful hints

1. Impossible to center the knife. Make certain the knife is positioned in the V groove on the lower clamp of the centrality gauge.
2. Wavy knife edge. Uneven pressure applied to hones. Hone again using light, even pressure until the knife has a straight edge. Strop as usual.

---

*International Micro Optical, Inc., 5 Daniel Rd., Fairfield, N.J. 07006.

3. Too much pressure has been applied at the ends of the knife during honing step. This will not interfere with the actual cutting surface of the knife. The knife may be honed until the edge is straight from end to end. Strop at least 20 times to remove rough burr. Polish on slow-moving strops.

4. Knife edge is dull or leaves knife marks after sharpening.
   a. Make certain knife is firmly clamped in holder. Any movement of the knife could affect the sharpening process as well as the sharpness.
   b. The new bevel may not extend to the knife edge. Mark bevel with a felt-tipped pen from top of bevel to knife edge 2.5 cm from either end. When honing step grinds away the mark completely, the bevel is complete. Proceed to stropping steps.
   c. Excess stropping may dull the knife. Resharpen, or use the solutions given above.
   d. Buildup of wax on strops will reduce the polishing action. See maintenance instructions for method of removal. Apply abrasive lightly to the strops before resharpening.

5. Knife holder does not slide smoothly along carrier bar.
   a. See maintenance instructions.
   b. Inspect the carrier bar. If it is bent or damaged, it must be replaced.

6. The controls turn during sharpening procedure. Unscrew control knobs and pull them out completely. Remove grease and clean rod threads in xylene. Dry and apply oil to threads as described in maintenance procedures.

Shandon-Elliott Sharpeners
MK I and MK II

The Shandon-Elliott MK I was one of the first automatic knife sharpeners of this type to be sold in the United States. The MK II model, however, was the first sharpener to catch on. The MK II was to revolutionize knife sharpening within a short period of time after it was on the market. This instrument has a simple construction, is easy to repair, and easy to operate.

The instrument consists of a round glass plate 36.83 cm in diameter. It also has a knife pressure adjustment, which adjusts the amount of pressure with which the knife rests on the sharpening surface. With this particular instrument, the plate rotates in a circular manner while the knife changes from side to side to assure that each edge is sharpened evenly. A speed control is built into the instrument so that the knife will change back and forth at a fast or slow setting, depending on the desired sharpening procedure.

It is the technologist's responsibility to choose which abrasive is best suited to current needs. There are, however, two main considerations that govern the choice of abrasives:

1. Straightness of cutting edge
2. Condition of edge

The four recommended grades of abrasive that come with the knife sharpener are as follows:

1. Aluminum Oxide 2F, or coarse abrasive—to be used only when the edge is badly nicked or for the reconditioning of the glass plate.
2. Aluminum Oxide Optical 50, or medium abrasive—this is used until a straight edge and new facets are obtained.
3. Aluminum Oxide 1200, or fine abrasive—this is for polishing the knife edge.
4. Polishing Alumina 350—this grade is for daily maintenance of the knife edge.

The actual procedures to be followed can be varied at the discretion of the user.

Autosharp III

Shandon-Elliott brought out a new model the Autosharp III. It has all the same features, except that now instead of two glass plates, a glass and copper plate* are used. Also, instead of powdered abrasives, a 3 μm diamond compound is used, and this is called the "Microsharp Technique." This was a revolutionary step in knife sharpening. Expectations were that an excellent edge could be achieved in 5 minutes. Again, technologists found disappointment in the time frame. However, this procedure produced far superior knife edges than have ever been produced before.

Autosharp IV

Since the development of the MK II and Autosharp III knife sharpeners, Shandon-Elliott has brought out a new model called the Autosharp IV.

This new instrument is basically the same as the other two models except for the following:

1. The change-over control is designed for 5-, 10-, or 25-second intervals.
2. The knife-damping device has been eliminated.

3. The bevel setting is now in degrees instead of in numbers.
4. The knife-alignment device has been eliminated.
5. The use of the glass plate has been eliminated. Instead of glass plates, two copper* microsharp plates are used.
6. Powdered abrasives have been replaced by an 8 μm diamond compound for reconditioning and a 3 μm diamond compound for finishing.

A modified Autosharp IV knife sharpening technic
John Spair, Jr.

1. Clean knife thoroughly with xylene, check under microscope (10×) to determine condition of knife edge. If knife has a smooth edge with no visible knicks, go directly to the finishing procedure. If knife has knicks or burrs, first take burrs off with a wooden tongue depressor, and then go to the reconditioning procedure doing the following finishing procedure.
2. If a knife needs reconditioning, you shall determine the time it takes to get out knicks on a time scale of 5 to 30 minutes. If a knife needs longer than 30 minutes, you might want to use a glass plate and a powdered abrasive (coarse) to grind your edge down and then go through the reconditioning procedure and finishing. You might also want to send your knife out to a professional knife sharpening company if you are pressed for time or do not have the materials available. Under normal conditions you should never have any knife that is so badly knicked that it needs this special treatment, unless, of course, carelessness is involved by the technologist.

Reconditioning

1. Apply a small amount (no more than 2.5 cm) of 8 μm Shandon-Elliott diamond compound to a *red*-backed copper* plate, or whatever you have designated for this purpose.
2. Lubricate the diamond compound with 25 drops of Microsharp Lubricating Fluid, and spread evenly over the plate.
3. Set facet angle for whatever is indicated on the knife box. (We have found a 35 degree to be satisfactory for all our knives.)
4. Set the pressure control to maximum.

*Recently copper plates have been replaced by iron plates.

* Recently copper plates have been replaced by iron plates.

5. Set the change over to 25 seconds.
6. Allow the knife to sharpen from 5 to 30 minutes. Remember that experience is the best judge for this step. In the beginning it may be better to keep checking the knife microscopically before finishing the edge. It is also a wise idea to mark your knife box according to the procedure or time you used so that you can always refer to it should the need arise. I find that most knicked knives usually need no longer than 15 minutes unless it is a bone knife.
7. When the time goes off, stop the machine in the forward position to remove your knife, and clean the knife off with xylene.

Polishing procedure

1. Apply a small amount (no more than 2.5 cm) of Shandon-Elliott 3 μm diamond compound to a *green*-backed iron plate, or whatever you have designated for this purpose.
2. Lubricate the diamond compound with Microsharp Lubricating fluid, about 25 drops, and spread evenly over the plate.
3. Set facet angle the same as you set it for the reconditioning procedure.
4. Set pressure control for *medium* pressure.
5. Set the change over control to 10 seconds.
6. Set the time for 10 minutes and run.
7. When machine has stopped, reset the pressure to minimum, the change-over to 5 seconds, and the timer for 15 minutes and let run.
8. Take knife off the machine when it is in the forward position. Clean it with xylene and take knife clamp off knife.
9. Check the knife under the microscope. The edge should look completely straight if you have done everything right. If there are any small knicks because you did not give it enough time on the reconditioning procedure, mark these areas with a pencil so that the cutter may avoid these areas. Spread a thin film of oil on the knife edge to preserve the knife and return to the box. Mark the knife accordingly.

Troubleshooting methods. The troubleshooting methods are divided into three sections.

The first section to be discussed will be the *knife holders*. There are at present three types of holders—the standard holder that most laboratories use, the holder for drilled knives, and the universal holder that is provided with the Autosharp IV.

The main problem encountered with the knife holder is a technical error. The standard holder is placed on a knife without a set pattern. In other words, the same holder is not used with the same knife. This created numerous problems, such as double bevels, and even gouged plates. Since the holder is not centered correctly each time, the same problems arose.

This is solved easily when one numbers both the knife holder and the knife, so that the same holder will always be used with the same knife. The holder is scored and the knife is scored; doing so ensures that the knife is placed in the holder the same way each time.

To ensure a correct bevel and not an uneven one, the holder with the knife in position and locked down is measured on both sides to eliminate the chance of having the knife unevenly balanced in the holder.

The standard holder cannot be used on the Autosharp IV without some difficulty. It tends to become loose and let the knife slip out and gouge the plate. The holder can be modified by one of two ways. First, the notch in the holder can be scored deeper, or second, a small hole can be drilled into the notch to lock the holder to the locking screw.

The second holder is the one for drilled knives. This was believed to be the answer. However, not all companies manufacture drilled knives. The problem that arose using the drilled knives was unusual. The knife tended to gouge the plate. If the knife is placed in the same holder the same way each time, most gouging would be eliminated. Therefore, the holder and knives should be marked to ensure uniformity.

The universal holder, the third type, was introduced with the advent of the Autosharp IV. It has been observed that this holder will not hold a knife the same way twice. Because of the construction of the holder, knives can lean forward or backward, depending on the angle at which they are locked in. It is difficult to consistently tighten the screws evenly on either side of the holder. To help eliminate this problem, the knife should be marked so it faces the same way every time it is placed in the holder. This does not eliminate the problem of the knife tilting differently each time.

Now that all the holders have been briefly discussed, here is a simple check list to follow before one starts to sharpen a knife:

1. Place the numbered holder with the properly numbered knife.
2. Make sure that the score on the holder matches the score on the knife.

3. Measure both sides of the knife to ensure equal distance. Also measure the distance from the edge of the holder to the edge of the knife. This will ensure the equal distance of the holder and knife edge. This will help eliminate placing the knife in the holder at an incorrect angle.
4. Clamp the knife in the knife sharpener. Do not tighten excessively. Overtightening of the clamp might cause it to break.

Now that the holder and knife are properly aligned, there should be no more problems that would cause the Microsharp plate to gouge. This does not always hold true.

It is also essential to watch for wear inside the device. One laboratory was repeatedly gouging the plate. This did not occur when the knife first started, but after it had been sharpening for a while. The problem was simple but not obvious. The alignment device was too small. This made the screw in the knife holder loosen after the knife had been rotating. This, in turn, allowed the knife to slip forward and gouge the plate. There are two ways to correct this. First, simply file the device so that the screw will not loosen and, second, have the company replace the alignment device.

The second section to be discussed, the *Microsharp copper plates,* is of utmost importance to the technologist.

With proper care and maintenance of these plates, excellent knives can be obtained.

Many problems have been encountered with the use of these plates. There are two main problems that should be considered. First is the flatness of the plates; second is the ease with which the plate can be gouged.

Flatness is one of the selling points for the use of the copper plate. The manufacturer stresses the fact that the copper plate will not wear like previously used glass plates. For the most part, this is a true claim. However, the copper plate does and will wear. It has been observed that some copper plates are shipped warped or not flat from the factory. The plates are either convex (high) so that the middle of the knife is ground down or concave (bellied) so that only the ends sharpen. The interesting aspect of this problem is that the knife only shows these defects on pretreatment with either the glass plate and abrasive or the new procedures using large-mesh diamond compounds for reconditioning on the copper plate.

Now the question is raised that perhaps the first plate was not flat or the knife was warped. It is a proved fact that just one diamond compound will not reveal bevel defects. The knife is merely ground to fit the plate.

1. Alignment device out of adjustment
2. Screws in the knife holder loose
3. Bevel setting not locked
4. Incorrect bevel setting—the knife should always be sharpened on the same setting
5. Knife without an established bevel

What to do with a gouged plate

If the gouge in the plate is not of major damage, we recommend that you, the technologist, repair it. There are several ways to accomplish this. First, if the gouge is relatively small, a piece of Scotch Brite may be used to flatten the area. A second method is the use of an emery board or a fine piece of sandpaper. Should the damage be more serious, other steps must be taken to recondition the plate. One method is the use of a diamond bar. It has been found, however, that in a busy laboratory it is too time consuming and also causes the delicate Microsharp machines to break down more, requiring the need for repair more often than usual. Another method is the use of coarse and fine sandpaper. The plate can be ground down with an aluminum oxide type of coarse sandpaper wrapped around a level, flat piece of wood you can get from your maintenance department. After you have ground down the plate enough to get out your deep gouges, you can then finish the plate with a smooth finish with a fine aluminum oxide sandpaper wrapped around your wood. This should take you no longer than a half hour. It is advisable to wear a face mask so that you won't inhale the copper dust, or you may finish it underneath a hood.

To ensure that a proper bevel is maintained, the knife should always be sharpened on the same plate. This can be accomplished by numbering the plate and recording both this number and the bevel setting on the knife box.

The third section deals with the use or misuse of diamond compounds. Numerous laboratories have reported inadequate results with recommended sharpening times and many laboratories are sharpening as long as 2 hours. This is not so much a procedural error as it is a technical error. Some of the causes of this error are as follows:

1. Contamination of plate or compound with dust, grit, and the like
2. Improper lubrication
3. Inadequate cleaning of plate
4. Too much or too little diamond compound

Employing the proper maintenance and cleaning procedures will help eliminate these errors, with these recommended technics:

1. Make sure sharpener cover is kept closed, no sand from the gouge repair remains on the plate, and the compound is kept in a clean place. When using two grades of diamond compound, care must be taken not to carry over the large grade of compound to the finer grade plate. If the larger compound is carried over to the next plate, the knives will not finish properly.

2. Lubrication must be adequate for proper flow on the plate to allow movement of metal particles away from the knife path. The plate should never be allowed to become dry or have a heavy buildup of black material.

3. The plate should be cleaned immediately if there is a buildup of black metal particles. Always use Scott's Micro Assembly Wipes No. 5310 (p. 444) or lint-free cloth. Never use gauze. The plate need not be scrubbed, but it should be cleaned enough to remove metal particles. This can be accomplished with the use of xylene.

4. Too much diamond compound can cause the formation of a vacuum between the knife and the plate, resulting in the gouging of the plate or unnecessary popping when lifting off the plate.

Too little diamond compound results in prolonged sharpening with a buildup of metal particles which could result in damaging the knife edge instead of sharpening it.

There is a fourth section that must be considered when you sharpen a knife. This is the use of a microscope. It is essential that the microtome knife edge be checked prior to sharpening, during the sharpening procedure, and after the completion of the procedure.

It is a hard and fast rule in many laboratories that all knives will be checked under the microscope with a 10× objective and a 10× ocular.

The following simple troubleshooting methods can be used as a guideline before, during, and after sharpening of a microtome knife.

1. Knives—check knife edge under scope at 100× and be sure knife is thoroughly cleaned.

2. Holders—check alignment and tightness of screws.

3. Dust—make sure no dust, lint, or debris is on the plate or other parts of mechanism (particularly arm).

4. Alignment device—be sure it is tight and in proper alignment.

5. Plate setting—double-check the knife setting on the box with the plate-position setting. Be sure to use the gauge when changing plates or instruments. The gauge enhances the accuracy of the bevel settings when changing plates or instruments. This problem arose because of the differences in the thickness of the plates. For this reason it is extremely important to use the gauge when the plates or instruments are changed. Unfortunately the gauge will not fit on the Mark IV model. Extreme care must be taken to maintain the correct bevel when this instrument is used.

6. Place the knife on the instrument and tighten the screw-locking device.

7. Follow any procedure, be it the recommended procedure, a modified procedure, or your own procedure. But be sure your laboratory's procedure is followed by all personnel, to ensure reproduction of results.

8. Lower the knife slowly onto the plate by intermittently pushing the on and off switch (MK II), the power switch for the MK III, or the start switch for the Autosharp IV, to be sure the knife is riding straight and is not going to gouge the plate.

9. Double-check the pressure control and the change-over control with the procedure to be followed.

10. Clean and check the knife under the scope at 100× after completing the sharpening procedure.

Shandon-Elliott Autosharp IV automatic knife sharpener

The Autosharp IV requires less attention than the previously discussed other models. There are, however, a few simple maintenance requirements:

1. Wipe the excess off the copper plates, especially underneath where petroleum jelly has been applied.

2. Clean the drip tray.

3. Apply one drop of machine oil to the central drive pin about every 6 months.

It is recommended that technologists adhere strictly to the following rules:

1. Always close the lid of the instrument during operation and when it is not in use.

2. Keep both the inside and outside of the

instrument free from dust and abrasives by regular cleaning.

3. Keep the instrument in the most dust-free area available.

4. Remove all traces of oil, abrasives, cleaning fluid, and so forth from the instrument regularly, using a series of lint-free cloths or cleaning tissues.

5. Clean all knives thoroughly with xylene before attempting to fit them to the machine.

6. Ensure that both the back of the plate and the drip tray are entirely free from abrasive and dirt, in order to avoid rapid wear of the nylon buttons.

Reconditioning of copper plates
John Spair, Jr.

The Microsharp copper plates is of the utmost importance to the technologist. With proper care and maintenance of these plates, you will get excellent knives.

Make up a maintenance schedule, according to your usage, since the plate will and does wear and flatness of the plate is very important.

Occasionally, you will want to recondition the whole plate to ensure that you have flatness. This can be checked by means of a carpenter's level. Make sure first that the surface you are putting the plate on is level before you begin.

For those in between small repairs, such as small scratches or a small gouge, you can use an emery board, a piece of Scotch Brite, or a piece of very fine aluminum oxide type of sandpaper. Before reusing the plate, make sure you have absolute cleanliness either using soap and water or xylene. There are also other ways to clean the plates, it depends on the technologist's preference.

There are various methods of reconditioning the copper plates on the market today. One way is to send the plate to be repaired back to the manufacturer for a cost of about $60. Another is by using the diamond bar. Sending the plate out to be reconditioned can be expensive, especially if you have a large volume of knives. I have found also that using the diamond bar method takes too much time and causes extensive wear and tear on your machines, therefore requiring constant repairs. They are delicate machines that should be used for the delicate knife sharpening they were intended for.

My method of reconditioning the copper plates, involves using graded kinds of aluminum oxide sandpaper. There are two ways to do this.

The hand method takes about 20 minutes and involves wrapping the sandpaper around a flat piece of wood and reconditioning in a circular motion, periodically checking the flatness with your level. A better and ideal way is by means of a small electric finishing sander. I recommend an electric sander made by Rockwell International (Pittsburgh, Pa.). It is the Double Insulated Finishing Sander, Model 330, bloc sander. It is very simple to operate and small enough to hold in one hand by anyone. It measures about 22 cm high by 12.7 cm long. Read your instruction manual for operation, and recondition your plate, checking flatness again by using your level. Always use coarse sandpaper for difficult jobs, and always use very fine sandpaper to finish and polish, and clean plate thoroughly. For safety purposes, wear a mask of some kind when sanding to avoid inhaling copper dust.

The sanding procedure takes between 10 to 20 minutes to complete a plate and will cost practically nothing compared to some other methods.

Periodically check your flatness and recondition thoroughly when needed. Make your minor repairs by the afore-mentioned methods to keep plates always in good condition and to ensure good knives.

Copper plates will last a long time. Eventually they will need resurfacing with new copper when the layer wears down. This should be done by the manufacturer. The layer of copper could last you from 3 to 5 years.

Care of the microtome knife

Microtome knives should involve the following:

1. Oil them before placing them in storage boxes to prevent rust and corrosion. This is always necessary, but it is particularly so in areas where the humidity is high.

2. Remove the oil with facial tissue paper moistened with xylene and then remove the xylene with the paper moistened with absolute alcohol prior to using the knife for cutting sections.

BUEHLER ISOMET LOW SPEED SAW

It is now possible to rapidly cut gross undecalcified hard tissues, such as bone, using the Buehler Isomet Low Speed Saw (Fig. 1-21). The resulting cut specimens are thin and free of burning or deformation. The thin specimen of bone may then be rapidly decalcified and processed in the normal way, and several days will

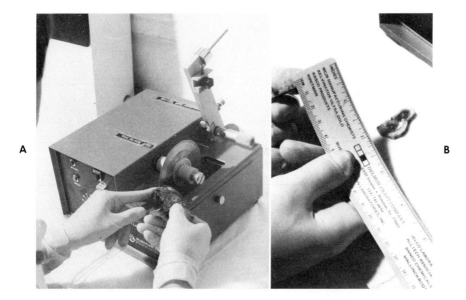

Fig. 1-21. A, Buehler Isomet Low Speed Saw. **B,** Specimen of gross undecalcified hard tissue cut by this saw.

be cut from the usual processing time. The technic is presently being used routinely in the Histopathology Laboratory at M. D. Anderson Tumor Institute in Houston, Texas, as well as in the Surgical Pathology Laboratory at the University of Pennsylvania Hospital in Philadelphia, Pennsylvania.

FUME-GARD

Fume-Gard is a compact, portable hood that takes up little bench space. No outside venting is required, since two activated charcoal filters capture objectionable fumes and filtered clean air exits from the machine. It is not designed to be used with microorganisms and is not explosion proof.

The horizontal Fume-Gard filters clean air through the rear of the machine, allowing observation of operation from a top and frontal viewpoint.

The vertical Fume-Gard draws odors upward through the filters, thus taking up less bench space, permitting viewing from all sides, and leaving a full frontal view.

The dual Fume-Gard is complete with two blower assemblies, filters, and hood. The length is 137.16 cm.

F fine-particle filter is an accessory for Fume-Gard. It removes fine powders and dust, controlling the spread of fine materials. It is especially useful for weighing or mixing dry chemi-

cals. It minimizes clean-up time by retaining particles on filter for easy disposal (Fig. 1-22).

HONEYWELL GLS 360 SLIDE STAINER (FORMERLY SKI STAINER)

This is a continuous feed automatic slide stainer that processes up to 360 histologic and cytologic slides an hour. All slides are processed identically; time of immersion of each slide in a given jar is equal, resulting in consistent quality staining.

Continuous feed eliminates batching. Technologists can process any number of slides any time of the day. Without batching, this stainer virtually eliminates nonproductive waiting periods. The completed slide is ready for coverslipping 20 minutes after it is placed on the stainer.

A continuous feed keeps each slide in its proper sequence throughout the entire staining process. Because slides are physically attached to a noiseless chain drive, they will not get accidentally switched.

The stainer saves time and reagents. It is dependable and easy to operate (Fig. 1-23).

The following is the hematoxylin and eosin procedure for Honeywell GLS 360 Slide Stainer (formerly SKI Stainer).

Turn on at least 15 minutes before use.
Check that all containers are seated well.
Check that water flow is on gently.
Check temperature 70° to 72° C.

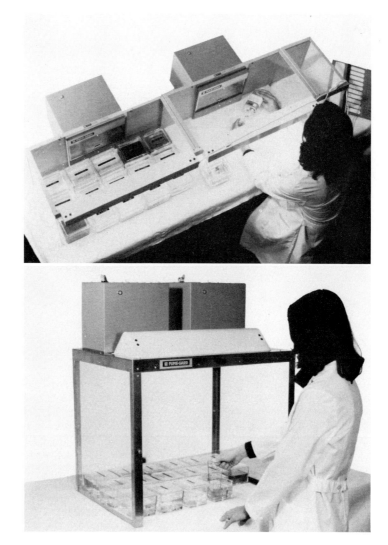

Fig. 1-22. Fume-Gard (Courtesy Lerner Laboratories, Stamford, Ct.)

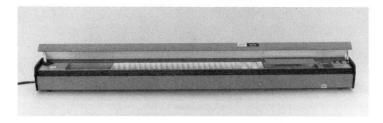

Fig. 1-23. Honeywell GLS 360 Slide Stainer.

Jar number	Staining agents
1	Jar inverted
2	No. 1 xylene—change daily by moving it to no. 3 position
3	No. 2 xylene
4	No. 3 xylene
5	Anhydrol*—change daily
6	95% Anhydrol—change daily
7	70% Anhydrol—change daily
8	Running water
9	No. 1 Hematoxylin, filter daily, throw out no. 1 daily
10	No. 2 Move up to no. 1 daily
11	No. 3 Move up to no. 2 daily
12	No. 4 Move up to no. 3 daily
13	No. 5 Move up to no. 4 daily
14	No. 6 Fresh each day—move up to no. 5 daily
15	Running water
16	Running water
17	0.25% hydrochloric acid in 70% Anhydrol—change when dirty or colored
18	Running water
19	0.5% alkaline alcohol—change daily
20	80% alcohol—change daily
21	70%—change daily
22	No. 1 Eosin-phloxine—change daily
23	No. 2 Same as above—move up to no. 1
24	No. 3 Same as above—move up to no. 2
25	No. 4 Eosin-phloxine—fresh daily; move up to no. 3
26	95% Anhydrol—change daily

Jars 10 and 11: pH 2.5 (Harris's or Delafield's)

Jars 22–25: pH 5.0

Jar number	Staining agents
27	Anhydrol—change daily
28	Anhydrol—fresh daily; move up to no. 1
29	Big container fresh Monday and Thursday of equal parts of tetrahydrofuran and xylene; fill daily to one quarter from top
30	Transfer slides to stainless steel xylene containers. Turn off when all slides have been stained. Check for staining results (1 in 20 slides)

CAUTION: Fill all containers to *TOP LINE.*
Leave daily changes empty overnight.
Refill first of all in morning.
Empty all containers on Friday and clean all well.
Leave all containers empty over the weekend unless you know of staining for Saturday morning.
Keep all stock bottles filled.

REFERENCES

Culling, C. F. A.: Handbook of histopathological and histochemical techniques, ed. 3, London, 1974, Butterworth & Co. (Pubs.) Ltd.

Judge, S., Richardson, L., and Sugulas, M.: Knife sharpening made easy, Bellaire, Texas, 1978, The American Society for Medical Technology.

Lillie, R. D., and Fullmer, H. M.: Histopathological technic and practical histochemistry, ed. 4, New York, 1976, McGraw-Hill Book Co.

Richards, O. W.: The effective use and proper care of the A.O. Microscope, Buffalo, N.Y., 1959, American Optical Corp., Scientific Instrument Division.

Richards, O. W.: The effective use and proper care of the A.O. Microtome, Buffalo, N.Y., 1959 and 1975, American Optical Corp., Scientific Instrument Division.

Thompson, S. W.: Selected histochemical and histopathological methods, Springfield, Ill., 1966, Charles C Thomas, Publisher.

*Anhydrol is a cheaper substitute for absolute ethanol.

CHAPTER 2

Fixation

AIM OF FIXATION AND CHOICE OF FIXING AGENT

Protoplasm, the only known form of matter in which life is manifested, is mainly composed of proteins, lipids, carbohydrates, and inorganic salts. The chief aim of fixation is the coagulation or precipitation of these protoplasmic substances, which renders the cells and tissue elements resistant to further changes from the reagents to which they are subjected before microscopic sections can be prepared. The various substances used for fixing fresh tissues possess the properties of killing, penetrating, and hardening in different degrees. A good fixative, therefore, will penetrate tissue and kill it quickly, will preserve the tissue elements, particularly the nuclei in the condition in which they are at the moment the fixing agent acts on them, and will harden or affect them so that they will not be altered by the various processes

of dehydrating, clearing, impregnation, embedding, staining, and mounting.

The finished microscopic tissue slide, on which a diagnosis may be made, can only be of value to the pathologist if the tissue is properly fixed. Fixation, the stabilization of protein, is the singularly most important step in producing good histologic slides. The choice of a fixative will depend on the nature of the pathologic lesion present in the tissue. An excellent example of this is clearly seen in the demonstration of chromaffin cells for the diagnosis of pheochromocytoma, where, without immediate fixation in a primary chromate fixative such as Orth's fluid, the technics for proving this diagnosis cannot be done (Sheehan). The student of histologic technic must be aware of this fact, since all fixatives are not compatible with all staining methods. In many instances, the fixative acts as a mordant for the staining; in others, it inhibits staining. For example, Bouin's fluid (picric acid) acts as a mordant for basic aniline dyes such as those used for trichrome stains; Zenker's fluid (mercuric chloride) is a mordant for metachromatic staining as well as for Giemsa staining of bone marrow. Adversely, if tissues have been fixed in any aqueous fixative, uric acid crystals cannot be demonstrated, since this technic requires fixation in absolute alcohol. When cytoplasmic inclusions are to be demonstrated, fixatives containing acetic acid must be avoided and a fixative of choice is Zenker's fluid without acetic acid. Tissues to be stained for spirochetes must be fixed in formalin. In the selection of a fixative for bone marrow that will preserve all elements, including red blood cells, a good choice would be Helly's fluid, since the acetic acid in Zenker's fluid would destroy the red blood cells. The preferred fixation that preserves glycogen and permits it to be stained differentially is absolute alcohol or an alcoholic fixative such as Carnoy's fluid. The fixative of choice for fat is formalin, but since unsaturated fats form a black compound with osmium tetroxide, fat will be demonstrated in black after osmium tetroxide fixatives. Fixatives containing mercuric chloride must be avoided to preserve the iron component of hemosiderin. If all polysaccharides are to be adequately fixed, mercuric chloride fixatives must be avoided and cold alcohol-formalin, Gendre's fluid, and Rossman's fluid may be used.

FUNCTIONS OF FIXING AGENTS AND PRINCIPLES INVOLVED IN FIXATION

The five functions are the following:
1. To set organs or parts of organs so that the microanatomical arrangement of tissue elements will not be altered by subsequent processing
2. To set intracellular inclusion bodies so that the histologic and cytologic conditions of cells may be studied
3. To arrest autolysis and putrefaction and other changes
4. To bring out differences in the refractive index of tissues
5. To render cell constituents insoluble and make them resistant to subsequent processes necessary to make a histologic preparation

Since the removal of tissue by operative procedure initiates changes by autolysis and putrefaction, these must be inhibited by prompt fixation or immediate refrigeration, for a short time, prior to fixation. Putrefaction, the breakdown of tissue by bacterial action, is also called postmortem decomposition. It is common in the intestinal tract where we find a high bacterial content normally. Autolysis is the dissolving of cells by enzyme action from within. Enzymes, always present in living cells, synthesize various protoplasmic constituents, including proteins, during cell life. When cell activity stops, enzymes cease synthesizing amino acids into proteins. Other enzymes then act to split the proteins into amino acids, resulting in a general dissolution of the proteins, rendering them incapable of coagulation by heat or chemical agents. Since fixation is primarily the stabilization of proteins, and tissue must be subjected to a substance that renders proteins insoluble, autolysis must be inhibited to prepare good histologic sections.

To fix tissue and to prevent autolysis and putrefaction, a fixative fluid:
1. Must not shrink or swell tissue
2. Must not distort or dissolve tissue parts
3. Must render enzymes inactive
4. Must kill bacteria and molds
5. Must modify tissue constituents so that they retain their form when subjected to dehydrants, clearing agents, embedding media, cutting, staining, or mounting; any of which might distort or destroy tissue in its original state

In the early days of preparing microscopic slides, it was important to harden tissue for hand-razor sectioning; so our first great fixatives were formulated to make tissues hard and were known as hardening agents. Since that time, we have found means of supporting tissue with embedding agents and it is no longer necessary to create excessive hardening. We must, however, protect the tissue against the ravages of embedding, sectioning, and mounting. Dehydrants and clearing agents, involved in the processing, have a strong tendency to cause distortion. Embedding requires impregnation of tissue at a high temperature, and sectioning can mechanically damage tissue. Fixatives therefore must stabilize the tissue against these damaging processes.

Baker states that living cytoplasm has a refractive index of about 1.353, but when a fixative acts, a profound change occurs, and the evidence suggests that the protoplasm is now represented by interlacing submicroscopic fibers with a refractive index of dry protein at about 1.54. After fixation, dehydration, clearing, embedding and staining, when we mount the sections in a mounting medium close to that of dry protein, almost perfect transparency, modified by different types of staining, is obtained. Oil-immersion objectives may be used at their full aperture.

AGENTS USED IN FIXATION

Fixation agents are either physical or chemical. The only physical agents are dessication and heat. Dessication is effected by rapid drawing of a fresh piece of tissue across a slide to leave a thin film on the slide, which is then stained and mounted. A touch preparation is made when the slide is touched to the fresh tissue. Since fixation is primarily the stabilization of protein and since heat coagulates protein rapidly, it may be used but is not recommended because it produces extreme distortion. The substances therefore used for fixation are chemical agents, either solids in aqueous solution or liquids used with or without the addition of water.

Fixative ingredients

There are few fixative ingredients and they have been classified by Gray according to the role they play in fixation. The first group are mostly metallic salts that presumably denature to form compounds with the protoplasm, and one or more of these is found in almost all fixative mixtures. Gray lists the following as primary fixative agents:

Osmium tetroxide	Cupric chloride
Platinic chloride	Picric acid
Mercuric chloride	Chromium trioxide
Cupric sulfate	Potassium dichromate
Cupric nitrate	Sodium dichromate

Gray terms the following substances fixative modifiers and states that one, but never more than two, are used in fixative mixtures:

Formaldehyde
Acetaldehyde
Acetone

Acids compose the other additions to fixative mixtures, and no more than two are used in any fixing fluid. These are commonly used:

Acetic acid	Sulfuric acid
Trichloroacetic acid	Hydrochloric acid
	Oxalic acid
Formic acid	Trifluoroacetic acid
Nitric acid	

Osmium tetroxide

Osmium tetroxide is rarely used alone for fixation except in electron microscopy, because of high cost, poor penetration, and interference with staining methods. It occurs as pale yellow crystals, is soluble in water at 25° C at 7.24%, and is also soluble in liquid paraffin and certain lipids. The pH of the fixing solution is exactly that of the distilled water used to prepare it. The crystals and the aqueous solutions of osmium tetroxide give off a vapor that is damaging to the epithelium of the eyes, nose, and mouth. Because of the volatility of osmium tetroxide, it is extremely important to keep and use the solutions from tightly stoppered dark bottles. Most compounds of osmium are dark or black but are readily reduced when exposed to light, but this reduction by light is prevented by the strong oxidizers mercuric chloride, chromium trioxide, and potassium dichromate. Osmium tetroxide must be washed out by running water, and if any is left in the tissue, it could be gradually reduced by alcohol during processing, with resultant darkening. It penetrates poorly, is easily reduced in the presence of almost all organic material, leaves tissue soft and friable, and produces very poor paraffin sections. It is reduced by fats and lipids to form a black compound in tissue. It is a component of Fleming's solution,

which is known as the first great fixative and has been used for fixation since 1864. It is a noncoagulant of proteins.

Platinic chloride

Platinic chloride is considered by Gray to be a valuable and neglected fixative agent, with its main value in its mordanting power for after-staining. He states that it appears to interfere less with the staining properties of the tissues than any other reagent. He quotes Langeron as stating that it has all the advantages of chromic acid with none of the disadvantages resulting from the discoloration of the tissue and is particularly valuable in mixtures with chromic acid where it inhibits the production of chromic oxide, which causes such gross discoloration and prevents good afterstaining. Gray also states that the Bouin 1898 formula, which uses platinic chloride and mercuric chloride with formalin and formic acid, is a better general-purpose fixative than the picric acid–containing Bouin's fluid since it permits better and more brilliant afterstaining.

Mercuric chloride

Mercuric chloride dissolves in water from 6.6% to 7.1% and is also readily soluble in alcohol. There are three major disadvantages to its use even though many writers have, including Mallory, considered it one of the best fixative agents. The disadvantages are as follows:

1. It is a dangerous poison, which can be absorbed through the skin if one is sensitive to it and can produce chronic, cumulative mercury poisoning. Rubber gloves should be used when handling mercuric chloride. Even though not sensitive to it, utmost caution should be used to prevent contact of this dangerous material with the bare skin. When taken into the body in small quantities, it may cause acute nephritis, with the tubules and sometimes the glomeruli being affected (Baker).
2. The second disadvantage is that once a tissue has been placed in mercuric chloride solutions, it should not be handled with metal forceps or placed in metal containers, but may be handled with Teflon forceps or those coated with paraffin to prevent contact with the metal.
3. The third disadvantage is that it produces an artifact pigment that appears as small black, amorphous granules. This pigment is removed by the iodine–sodium thiosul-

fate sequence prior to staining. See p. 46.

Mercuric chloride has the tendency to render tissues brittle; they freeze poorly and cannot be used for routine frozen sections or cryostat sectioning.

Against these disadvantages, however, is the brilliant staining it produces since it acts as a permanent mordant. Nuclear and cytoplasmic structures are equally well stained. It is a protein coagulant, penetrates well, and is a particularly good fixative for mucin. Baker states: "Since mercuric chloride is readily soluble in ethanol, there is no purpose in washing in water if the tissue is going to be dehydrated."

Cupric salts

Cupric sulfate, nitrate, and chloride compounds are never used alone in fixation. Their chief value in fixative mixtures is their mordanting power for hematoxylin staining.

Picric acid

Picric acid is the only substance used in histopathology as both a fixative and a dye. It is soluble in water at room temperature at 1.18% and in alcohol at 9%. It should be dampened with distilled water for storage in the laboratory and must never be kept on the shelf in a dry form, since, in this stage, it is a highly dangerous explosive that for many years was used for military purposes. It is an excellent coagulant of proteins; lipids are not dissolved out by aqueous solutions of picric acid, and although it is not a fixative of carbohydrates, it has been strongly recommended as a constituent of fixatives for glycogen. The glycogen is apparently bound to the protein, and the picric acid acts on the protein in such a way that it inhibits the solution of the glycogen. Picric acid penetrates slowly and causes extreme shrinkage, which is frequently counteracted when used in solutions with acetic acid, since the swelling of the acetic acid counteracts the shrinking of the picric acid. It is not necessary to wash the picric acid out in water prior to processing, since the excess fixative is readily removed by alcohol. The yellow color remaining on the tissue on the slides may be removed during staining by washing of the slides in 50% to 70% alcohol or in a saturated solution of lithium carbonate in 70% alcohol during the staining sequence. Picric acid is tolerant of mixtures with ethanol, mercuric chloride, chromium trioxide, formaldehyde, osmium tetroxide, potassium dichromate, and acetic acid. Bouin's fluid is the most commonly used picric acid fixative. Lillie states that Lee recommended not more than 18 hours of fixation; Masson, up to 3 days; Cowdry, 24 hours; Lillie, 1 to 2 days; Gray condemns it; and we recommend 24 hours with storage of tissue after that time in 70% alcohol. Rossman's fluid and Gendre's fluid are picric acid fixatives recommended for the fixation of glycogen.

Chromium trioxide

Chromium trioxide as brownish red crystals, are extremely soluble in water, with a saturated solution having a concentration of 62.4%. Chromium trioxide in water forms chromic acid. Chromium trioxide was introduced into microtechnique by Hannover in 1840 (Baker). It is a powerful coagulant of proteins. It penetrates slowly and the excess fixative must be washed out in running water for 8 to 12 hours, since alcohol could reduce it to green chromic oxide, which is insoluble in ordinary solvents and resistant to acids and other reagents. Chromium trioxide oxidizes polysaccharides and converts them to aldehydes, which are then demonstrated by Schiff reagent. This is the basis of the Bauer technic for glycogen and the Gridley technic for fungus. "The reactions with lipids in general are similar to those of potassium dichromate, but quicker and apt to go too far. It may be for this reason that potassium dichromate is nearly always used when tissues are 'postchromed' to render lipids insoluble in lipidsolvents by partial oxidation" (Baker). It should not be mixed with formalin or alcohol, since these reduce it, but it is miscible with picric acid, mercuric chloride, osmium tetroxide, potassium dichromate and acetic acid.

Potassium dichromate

Potassium dichromate is soluble at about 10% in water at room temperature and insoluble in absolute alcohol. The pH of a 2.5% solution is 4.05 and differs only slightly from a 1% solution which is 4.10. Baker states that "if a solution of potassium dichromate is acidified to the same pH (0.85) as a solution of chromium trioxide containing the same weight of chromium, the ions present in the two solutions will be the same, except that the former will contain potassium ions and the anions of the added acid. If hydrochloric acid is used, one has a fluid almost identical with a solution of chromium trioxide to which potassium chloride has been added. Since potassium and chloride ions are inactive in fixation, it follows that an acidified potassium dichromate solution will act like a solution of chromium trioxide." Potassium dichromate was introduced as a fixative by Müller in 1860. It is a noncoagulant fixative but, if acidified, becomes a strong coagulant fixative. It attaches chromium to some lipids, which renders the lipids insoluble in lipid solvents. The chromium can then react with hematoxylin to form a black dye lake, which is demonstrated in Weigert's stain for myelin sheath. The Smith-Dietrich technic and the Baker technic for phospholipids are adaptations of this theory. It has been stated in the literature that a wide variety of unsaturated lipids can be rendered insoluble in lipid solvents by prolonged fixation in potassium dichromate but there is no action on saturated lipids. A valuable property of potassium dichromate is its ability to fix mitochondria by rendering their lipid components insoluble in lipid solvents. Storage fat is not preserved in paraffin sections of tissues fixed with potassium dichromate. An insoluble precipitate (chromic oxide) is formed if tissues are transferred from potassium dichromate fixatives directly to alcohol. They are, therefore, usually washed in running water overnight. Potassium dichromate is compatible with picric acid, mercuric chloride, and osmium tetroxide. It reacts rather slowly with formaldehyde, and in mixtures with this reagent the formaldehyde should not be added until the time of use. The most commonly used primary chromate fixatives are Orth's and Müller's (Regaud's) fluids. Lillie used Orth's extensively for routine work and considers it equal to formaldehyde for the study of early degenerative processes and necrosis and perhaps superior to formaldehyde for demonstrating rickettsias and bacteria. Fixation in a primary chromate fixative is critical in pheochromocytomas where even a 10-minute time in neutral buffered formalin (NBF) will destroy the cytoplasmic granules in the cells. Fixation time in Orth's fluid is 24 to 48 hours with overnight washing in running water prior to processing. Lillie states that glycogen is well shown by the Bauer method after fixation in Orth's fluid.

Formaldehyde

Formaldehyde, a colorless gas, is available commercially as an approximately saturated solution of the gas in water. Such solutions contain 37% to 40% by weight of formaldehyde gas and are commonly called formalin. It is the most widely used agent in anatomic pathology, since it may be used as a simple 10% or 20% solution

in water. One volume of formalin to nine volumes of water is a 10% solution (not 4%), and two volumes of formalin to eight volumes is a 20% solution (not 8%). Lillie states that the 10% solution contains 4.1% to 4.5% of formaldehyde gas and the 20% solution contains 8.2% to 9% of formaldehyde gas but should be designated as stated above. These solutions, prepared with distilled water, are acid because of oxidation to formic acid by atmospheric oxygen. If neutralized by the addition of an excess of calcium carbonate or magnesium carbonate, the solution remains neutral as long as it is in the storage jar but becomes acid when drawn off and used for fixation. This shift in pH may be avoided by the use of 4 gm of sodium phosphate, monobasic, monohydrate, and 6.5 gm of sodium phosphate, dibasic, anhydrous, to each liter of 10% formalin, giving a pH of 7.0.

Fixation in formalin is influenced by the concentration of the reagent and the temperature at which the fixative is used. Lillie states that 10% formalin fixes adequately in 48 hours at room temperature (20° to 25° C); 10% formalin fixes adequately at 35° C in 24 hours, and 20% formalin hardens in 3 hours at 55° C. Since autolysis is hastened at higher temperatures, it is better to fix tissues for a longer time at room temperature.

Formalin is a noncoagulant fixative. DNA and RNA are reduced by 10% to 35% by formalin fixation, and tissue for the demonstration of nucleic acids should be fixed in Carnoy's fluid. It is an excellent fixative of lipids for frozen sections, and although it does not fix soluble carbohydrates such as glycogen, it fixes proteins in a manner similar to that of picric acid, so that the escape of glycogen by solution in water is inhibited. Many authors have stated that formalin is a soft fixative, but Baker states that its hardening properties are exceeded only by alcohol or acetone. He further states that "there can scarcely be any doubt that formalin, with an indifferent salt, preserves the structure of the living cell better than any other primary fixative with the exception of osmium tetroxide."

If blood-rich tissues are fixed in nonbuffered 10% or 20% formalin for a long time, the tissue will contain an artifact pigment that lies over and on top of cells, but not within them. The pigment is removed by saturated alcoholic picric acid or a 1% solution of potassium hydroxide in 80% alcohol. NBF will prevent the formation of the pigment.

Cajal's formalin ammonium bromide is generally considered an excellent fixative for tissues from the central nervous system.

Acetic acid

Acetic acid is rarely used alone in fixation, since it swells the tissues and cells, and if they are not stabilized by the action of some other fixing agent, they will shrink strongly when dehydrated. It is, however, used extensively in combination with other fixative agents. It is a noncoagulant fixative, does not fix lipids, and neither fixes nor destroys carbohydrates. Fixatives containing acetic acid must be avoided in technics where it is important to demonstrate red blood cells, since it will destroy them. It also dissolves out the Golgi apparatus and mitochondria.

Other organic reagents

Other organic reagents used for fixation include ethanol, acetone, dioxane, pyridine, and chloral hydrate, which are all freely miscible with water. Chloroform is sometimes used, and although it is not miscible with water, it freely mixes with the alcohol and acetic acid to make up Carnoy's fluid. There is excessive shrinkage and distortion in tissues fixed in absolute alcohol and acetone, and these, sometimes used for fixing tissue enzymes, are not routinely used as fixatives in the histopathology laboratory. Unless the staining specifically requires fixation in one of these reagents, they should not be used alone but must be used in combinations.

Combinations of fixative agents to form fixation solutions

Combinations are much more commonly used than are single-solution substances, with the exception of formalin. In general, a combination should balance the swelling action of one reagent against the shrinking effect of another. Each component should compensate for the defect of another component. Baker analyzes Bouin's fluid as follows:

Formalin fixes cytoplasm and nuclear sap but hardens tissue and prevents paraffin from easily penetrating the tissue. It makes cytoplasm basophilic so that acid dyes do not work well and fixes chromosomes poorly. Picric acid compensates for most of these defects. It leaves tissues soft, coagulates cytoplasm in such a way that it readily admits paraffin, makes it strongly acidophilic and fixes chromosomes rather well. It has, however, two serious defects—it shrinks badly and makes chromatin acidophilic. Acetic acid compensates for both these defects.

Carnoy's fluid is another example. Alcohol is a poor fixative and acetic acid an indifferent fixative—with the alcohol producing shrinkage and the acetic acid producing swelling. In combination with chloroform, these reagents make an excellent fixative for glycogen and RNA.

Because of the effect of swelling and shrinking, it is possible by regulation of the proportions of each reagent, to adapt the fixative to the peculiarities of the tissue. For example, potassium dichromate, either as part of a fixative or as a postfixation mordant, is capable of making the lipid in the myelin sheath resistant to solution during processing and embedding in paraffin. However, one must not forget that the range of any one combination depends entirely on the constituent elements, some of which are capable of much wider application than are others.

FIXATIVE FORMULAS

Gray lists more than 650 fixatives in the 1954 edition of his book and is an excellent reference for practically any fixative called for by a technic. Those listed here are the routine fixatives commonly used in laboratories of pathologic anatomy.

Formalin fixatives

10% formalin solution
37% to 40% formalin	100 ml
Distilled water	900 ml

20% formalin solution
37% to 40% formalin	200 ml
Distilled water	800 ml

(The solutions listed above may produce formalin pigment in tissue.)

Formalin saline solution
37% to 40% formalin	100 ml
Sodium chloride	9 gm
Distilled water	900 ml

Neutral buffered formalin (NBF) solution
37% to 40% formalin	100 ml
Distilled water	900 ml
Sodium phosphate monobasic, monohydrate	4 gm
Sodium phosphate, dibasic, anhydrous	6.5 gm

Formalin with sodium acetate
37% to 40% formalin	100 ml
Sodium acetate	20 gm
Distilled water	900 ml

Formalin ammonium bromide solution
37% to 40% formalin	100 ml
Ammonium bromide	20 gm
Distilled water	850 ml

(This fixative is primarily used for fixing brain tissue.)

Alcoholic formalin

95% alcohol	906 ml
37% to 40% formalin	100 ml

Carson's modified Millonig's phosphate-buffered formalin*

37% to 40% formaldehyde solution technical grade	10 ml
Tap water†	90 ml
Sodium phosphate monobasic	1.86 gm
Sodium hydroxide	0.42 gm

This solution may be conveniently prepared in large quantities for routine use as follows:

1. Fill a 6½-gallon container (previously calibrated to 22 liters) approximately half full of water.
2. Add the contents of a 1-pound bottle of sodium phosphate monobasic and stir until dissolved.
3. Add 1000 ml of stock NaOH solution (411.2 gm per 4000 ml of water) and mix well.
4. Dilute to the 22-liter mark with water.
5. Add 2440 ml of technical grade 37% to 40% formaldehyde and mix well.

This volume is very convenient because only one weighing (stock NaOH solution) is required for every four times the solution is prepared.

The tissues fixed in this fixative routinely may also be used for electron microscopy.

Mercury fixatives

Zenker's fluid and Helly's fluid— stock solution

Distilled water	1 liter
Mercuric chloride	50 gm
Potassium dichromate	25 gm
Sodium sulfate	10 gm

Zenker's fluid. Add 5 ml of glacial acetic acid to 95 ml of stock solution just before use to prevent turbidity and a dark brown precipitate.

Helly's fluid. Add 5 ml of 37% to 40% formalin to 95 ml of stock solution just before use to prevent turbidity and a dark brown precipitate. When fixing tissues in either Zenker's or Helly's fluid, if the solution becomes brown and turbid, change it immediately.

Schaudinn's fluid (Lillie)

Saturated mercuric chloride in water (7% solution)	50 ml

---

*Freida L. Carson, Ph.D., Baylor University Medical Center, Dallas, Texas, personal correspondence, 1973.
†If the tap water in your area is extremely hard or contains a high percentage of total solids, deionized water is suggested for preparation of this solution.

Absolute alcohol	25 ml

Lillie considers the cytoplasmic fixation to be inferior to that of Zenker's fluid.

Ohlmacher's fluid (Lillie)

Absolute alcohol	32 ml
Chloroform	6 ml
Glacial acetic acid	2 ml

Add 8 gm of mercuric chloride to each 40 ml of solution.

Carnoy-Lebrun fluid (Lillie)

Absolute alcohol	15 ml
Chloroform	15 ml
Glacial acetic acid	15 ml

Saturate with 4 gm of mercuric chloride, just before use.

Lillie states that Ohlmacher's and Carnoy-Lebrun are rapid fixatives. If tissues are thin, Ohlmacher's will penetrate 2.5 mm in 2 to 3 hours.

Metal instruments and containers must be avoided when using fixatives containing mercuric chloride. Plastic-covered forceps may be coated with paraffin to avoid forming precipitate from the metal and the mercury.

B-5 fixative

Stock solution

Mercuric chloride	12 gm
Sodium acetate	2.5 gm
Distilled water	200 ml

Working solution

Stock B-5 solution	20 ml

Add 2 ml of 40% formalin immediately before use.

Mercury pigment and acid formaldehyde hematein are the two important artifact pigments that occur as the result of fixation. Mercury pigment may be removed by the iodine–sodium thiosulfate sequences. If you do not know whether tissue has been fixed in a fixative containing mercuric chloride, examine the sections microscopically after removing the paraffin and placing them in alcohol. Mercury pigment, if present, appears as a fine, brown granular deposit, which is more abundant at the center of the tissue since some of the deposit is removed during tissue dehydration because of the solubility of the salt in alcohol. The granules are usually larger than those of endogenous pigments and lie on top of cells and tissue, rather than within them. Treatment with iodine, by error, of tissue not fixed in mercuric chloride, will not harm it; it is merely a waste of time.

Removal of mercury pigment

1. Deparaffinize sections and bring them through graded alcohols to water.

2. Place in Weigert's iodine (1 iodine and 3 water) for 5 minutes.
3. Wash in distilled water.
4. Remove iodine with 5% sodium thiosulfate for 1 minute.
5. Wash in running tap water for 5 minutes.
6. Proceed with stain.

Weigert's iodine

Potassium iodide	2 gm
Iodine crystals	1 gm
Distilled water	100 ml

It is recommended, when the iodine solution is being made up, that the potassium iodide be first dissolved in a few milliliters of distilled water. When this is done, the iodine crystals go into solution immediately when added to the first solution. After they are completely dissolved, add the remaining water.

Sodium thiosulfate—5% solution

Sodium thiosulfate	5 gm
Distilled water	100 ml

Alcohol fixatives

Carnoy's fluid (Jones)

1.	Acetic acid	25 ml
	Absolute alcohol	75 ml
2.	Acetic acid	10 ml
	Absolute alcohol	60 ml
	Chloroform	30 ml

Carnoy's fluid is a rapid fixative that preserves ribonucleic acid and glycogen and dehydrates as it fixes. Remove the tissue into absolute alcohol, clear in cedarwood oil, followed by several 10- to 15-minute changes of xylene, impregnate, and embed in paraffin. This fixative causes excessive shrinkage if tissue remains in it more than 3 to 4 hours. Make pieces of tissue thin. Acetic acid destroys red blood cells.

Picric acid fixatives

Bouin's fluid is an excellent fixative for preserving soft and delicate structures. The shrinking of the picric acid is balanced by the swelling of the glacial acetic acid.

Bouin's fluid

Saturated picric acid (21 gm to 1 liter) in distilled water	1500 ml
Formalin	500 ml
Glacial acetic acid	100 ml

The yellow color may be removed during staining with 50% to 70% alcohol or 70% alcohol saturated with lithium carbonate.

Bouin's decalcifying fluid. Formic acid is used in the above fluid instead of acetic acid.

Bouin's fat fixative. We have used the following formula in our laboratory for many years, since unfixed fat frequently tears and produces a poor histologic slide.

Stock Bouin's fluid	75 ml
95% alcohol	25 ml

Lymph nodes are well fixed in 24 hours. Tissues solidly composed of fat, such as lipomas, require 48 to 72 hours.

Rossman's fluid (Lillie)

Absolute alcohol saturated with picric acid (4.9 gm to 100 ml)	90 ml
Neutralized commercial formalin	10 ml

Lillie states that the tissue should be fixed for 12 to 24 hours and washed for several days in 95% alcohol.

Gendre's fluid (Lillie)

95% alcohol saturated with picric acid	80 ml
37% to 40% formalin	15 ml
Glacial acetic acid	5 ml

Fix for 1 to 4 hours at room temperature (25° C). Wash and dehydrate in two changes each of 80%, 95%, and absolute alcohol. Lillie states that 4 hours at room temperature gives excellent fixation of tissue for glycogen.

Dichromate fixatives

Müller's fluid (Lillie)

Potassium dichromate	2.5 gm
Sodium sulfate	1 gm
Distilled water	100 ml

Möller's or Regaud's fluid

3% potassium dichromate	80 ml

Add 20 ml of 40% formalin at time of use.

Orth's fluid (Lillie)

Potassium dichromate	2.5 gm
Sodium sulfate	1 gm
Distilled water	100 ml
37% to 40% formalin	10 ml

Add formalin when ready to use.

This fixative must be used for the histochemical technics for the demonstration of chromaffin granules in the cytoplasm in cells of the adrenal medulla for the diagnosis of a pheochromocytoma. (See Sheehan, 1960.)

Other chromate fixatives are Romeis's and Ophuls' variants of Müller's fluid, Ciaccio's fluid, Kose's fluid, Tellyesniczky's acetic dichromate, Kolmer's fluid, and Held's fluid. The formulas for these may be found in Lillie's *Histopathologic Technic and Practical Histochemistry* (1965).

Lead fixatives

Lillie recommends the following fixative for the fixation of connective tissue mucins and umbilical cord:

Lillie's alcoholic lead nitrate formalin

Lead nitrate	8 gm
37% to 40% formalin	10 ml
Water	10 ml
Absolute alcohol	80 ml

Lillie suggests that tissues be fixed for 24 hours at 25° to 30° C, 2 to 3 days at −5° C, and 10 to 14 days at −25° C.

Osmic acid fixatives

Osmic acid fixatives were originally used for the fixation of fat. Since the advent of the clinical freezing microtome and the cryostat, these fixatives are rarely used in histopathology except for the fixation of tissue for electron microscopy.

Flemming's strong solution (all modern texts; Lillie)

2% osmium tetroxide	20 ml
1% chromic acid	75 ml
Glacial acetic acid	5 ml

Lillie states that the tissues should be fixed for 1 to 3 days and washed in running water for 6 to 24 hours. Tissues are stored in 80% alcohol.

Other osmic acid fixatives are Hermann's fluid, Marchi's fluid, and Mann's fluid. The formulas for these are found in Lillie's *Histopathologic Technic and Practical Histochemistry*, 1965.

Special fixatives
For metabolic bone disease, special fixative

$NaH_2PO_4 \cdot H_2O$	1.104 gm
Na_2HPO_4 (anhydrous)	4.675 gm

Solution is made up in 1 liter of water, and then 100 ml is discarded and 100 ml of formalin (37% to 40%) is added; pH 7.35 (check with pH meter). Volume of fixative should be 10 to 20 times the bone volume.

Paraformaldehyde

0.2 M s-collidine buffer

Solution A

s-collidine (2,4,6-trimethylpyridine)	2.64 ml
Distilled water	47.36 ml

Solution B

1 N HCl	9 ml
Distilled water	41 ml

Working solution

Equal parts of solutions A and B, pH 7.4 to 7.45

Paraformaldehyde solution

Paraformaldehyde	4 gm
Distilled water to make	66 ml

Add distilled water to the paraformaldehyde in a graduated cylinder until combined total is 66 ml. Warm in flask to 60° C. Depolymerize by adding 0.1 N NaOH, drop by drop; shake until solution is clear.

Working solution

Paraformaldehyde solution	66 ml
0.2 M s-collidine buffer	33 ml
0.5 M $CaCl_2$ (5.55 gm/100 ml)	1 ml

Adjust pH to 7.4 if necessary.

Zamboni's PAF fixative for light and electron microscopy

(PAF is picric acid and formaldehyde.)

20 gm of paraformaldehyde

150 ml of double-filtered, saturated aqueous solution of picric acid

Heat to 60° C to dissociate paraformaldehyde into formaldehyde. Add drops of a 2.52% NaOH (in water) to alkalize (solution should be clear). Filter and allow to cool. Make up to 1000 ml with *phosphate buffer.*

3.31 gm $NaH_2PO_4 \cdot H_2O$

33.77 gm $Na_2HPO_4 \cdot 7H_2O$ dissolve in 1 liter of water *or*

17.88 gm Na_2HPO_4

The PAF fixative should have a final pH of 7.3 and an osmolarity of 900 mOsm (Stefani, M., DeMartino, C. and Zamboni, L.: Nature **216:** 173, Oct. 14, 1976). PAF is very stable and not sensitive to light. Shelf life is 1 year at room temperature.

Characteristics

1. Fixation of large specimens by high-speed penetration
2. Stabilized cellular proteins
3. Not easily destroyed by tissue fluids
4. May be used without postosmication

Solutions for electron microscopy
Cacodylate buffer (0.2 M)

Dissolve 2.76 gm of cacodylic acid in 70 ml of distilled water. Cacodylic acid is an arsenic-containing compound and therefore poisonous. *Handle with care.*

Add 0.1 N HCl to adjust the pH to about 7.2 to 7.4.

Dilute to 100 ml with distilled water.

2% glutaraldehyde, pH 7.3

With 50% stock glutaraldehyde

0.2 M cacodylate buffer	50 ml
Stock glutaraldehyde	4 ml
Distilled water	46 ml

With 70% stock glutaraldehyde

Cacodylate buffer	35 ml
Stock glutaraldehyde	2 ml
Distilled water	33 ml

5% sucrose, pH 7.3

0.2 M cacodylate buffer	100 ml
Sucrose	10 gm

Dilute to 200 ml with distilled water.

TISSUE-HANDLING FIXATION CHART

General

1. *Quantity*—At least 15 to 20 volumes of fixative should be used for every volume of tissue.
2. *Penetration*—No fixative will penetrate more than 2 to 3 mm of solid tissue or 0.5 cm of porous tissue in a 24-hour period.
3. *Thickness*—Thickness would depend on the type of tissue, but no specimen should be more than *4mm* for good fixation; *3 mm* is preferable.
4. *Time*—Most tissues should remain in fixative for 24 hours and should then be stored in 70% alcohol.
5. *Temperature*—Most fixation is done at room temperature (25° C) but can be done for longer periods of time at 5° C.
6. *Primary purpose*—Fixation is primarily the stabilization of proteins, which must be rendered insoluble for satisfactory fixation.
7. *Heat*—Heat will coagulate protein but is not recommended for fixation since it also speeds autolysis.
8. *Special fixatives*—These are used to be sure the pathologic lesion is fixed and can be demonstrated in the finished slide.
9. Remember never to store picric acid in a dry form since it is highly explosive when dry.

Zenker's fluid

1. Use for exceptionally bloody specimens such as infarcts and congested spleen.
2. Use for unusual tumors such as rhabdomyosarcoma and malignant teratomas.
3. Use for viral inclusions such as Negri bodies.
4. Recommended for the preservation of tissue on which Feulgen plasma reaction is done.
5. Never use metal forceps or metal containers when handling any tissue fixed in mercurial fixatives.
6. Excellent trichromes after this fixative.
7. Omit the acetic acid and add it to the stock solution when ready to use.
8. An artifact pigment is formed with this mercuric fixative. Remove during staining sequence with the iodine–sodium thiosulfate sequence.
9. For excellent phosphotungstic acid–hematoxylin stains, tissues must be fixed in Zenker's fluid.

Helly's fluid

1. This fixative is known as Zenker's formol since it uses the same basic stock solution and formalin is not added to the stock until just before use to prevent a dark brown precipitate from forming.

2. Excellent for bone marrow including the preservation of red blood cells.
3. An artifact pigment is formed with this mercuric fixative, which must be removed during the staining sequence, with the iodine–sodium thiosulfate sequence.
4. Excellent for blood-forming organs.
5. Excellent for intercalated discs.

Carnoy's fluid

1. RNA (ribonucleic acid) must be fixed in this fixative if the methyl green pyronine technic is done.
2. *Never* use this fixative if acid-fast bacilli are to be demonstrated, since the bacilli are rendered non–acid fast.
3. Carnoy's fluid hemolyzes red cells and dissolves acid-soluble cell granules and pigments.
4. Nissl granules are well preserved in Carnoy's fluid.
5. Glycogen storage disease is preserved with fixation in Carnoy's fluid.

Formalin

1. The most widely used fixing agent for pathologic histology is formaldehyde (Lillie).
2. Formaldehyde is commercially available at 37% to 40% gas in water, sold as formalin. These fluids are regarded as 100% formalin and the 10% solution contains 4.1% to 4.5% of the formaldehyde gas and a 20% solution contains 8.2% to 9% of the formaldehyde gas.
3. Solutions of formalin diluted with distilled water are commonly acid from small amounts of formic acid as a manufacturing impurity or from oxidation of the gas.
4. NBF should not be prepared by storage over calcium carbonate or magnesium carbonate, since the fluid drawn off for fixation promptly becomes acid.
5. NBF should be prepared by the addition of a soluble buffer to prevent the formation of formalin pigment.
6. Fixation in formalin is influenced by the concentration of the reagent and by temperature. 10% fixes adequately in 48 hours at room temperature.
7. Many special stains are excellent after NBF fixation since it is compatible with most stains.
8. 10% formalin is the best fixative for tissues for fat stains since fewer artifacts are seen in the oil red O stains after this fixative.

Continued.

TISSUE-HANDLING FIXATION CHART—cont'd

9. Fixation in 10% formalin is a *must* for the Warthin-Starry technic for spirochetes.
10. Alcoholic formalin or alcoholic picroformalin is an excellent fixative for preserving glycogen.
11. For pH, best results are obtained if the pH of the formalin is 7.0. Formalin pigment is formed in solutions at pH levels below pH 5.6. An alkaline hematin is formed at pH levels above pH 8.0. Both pigments are dissolved either by alcoholic picric acid or by 1% potassium hydroxide in 80% alcohol.

Bouin's fluid

1. An excellent balanced fixative for routine surgical material.
2. Bouin's fat fixative should be used for grossly fatty tissue, especially fat containing lymph nodes, fatty breast tissue, and lipomas. Since this is a fat solvent, do not use for tissue on which fat stains may be required.
3. Remember to remove the yellow color with either 70% alcohol or saturated lithium carbonate in 70% alcohol during the staining sequence.
4. Excellent connective tissue stains after this fixative, particularly trichromes.

Special

1. *Metabolic bone disease*—Use special fixative (p. 48).
2. *Adrenal*—Fix in Orth's fluid which is a potassium dichromate fixative.
3. *Phospholipids*—Fix in Baker's formol-calcium.
4. *Tissue enzymes*, such as phosphatases and lipases—Fix in *acetone*.
5. *Central nervous system*—Fix in formalin ammonium bromide or in NBF, depending on staining technic.
6. *Uric acid* is destroyed by aqueous fixatives and must be fixed in absolute alcohol.
7. *Osmic acid fixatives* will blacken triglycerides and demonstrate them in this manner.

SPECIAL-STAINS FIXATION CHART

Technic	Recommended fixative(s)	Sections	Fixative(s) not recommended
Acid-fast technics			
Auramine and rhodamine	NBF*	Serial with Kinyoun's technic—sections 1 and 3 acid-fast and 2 and 4 auramine-rhodamine	
Fite's	AWFT*	5 μm par.*	
Fite's new fuchsin formaldehyde	AWFT		
Kinyoun's	AWFT		
Wade's modification of Fite's	AWFT		
Ziehl-Neelsen	AWFT		
Adrenal glands (chromaffin cells in medulla)			
Ferric ferricyanide reduction test	Orth's or Möller's (Regaud's) critical	5 μm par.	Do not use others
Gomori-Burtner methenamine silver	Orth's or Möller's critical	5 μm par.	Do not use others
Mallory's aniline blue collagen stain	Aqueous formalin, Bouin's fluid, Heidenhain's mercuric chloride, formalin	5 μm par.	Dichromates inferior, alcohol unsuitable
Periodic acid–Schiff	Orth's or Möller's critical	5 μm par.	Do not use others

*NBF, neutral buffered formalin; *AWFT*, any well-fixed tissue; *par.*, any paraffin-like substance.

SPECIAL-STAINS FIXATION CHART—cont'd

Technic	Recommended fixative(s)	Sections	Fixative(s) not recommended
Adrenal glands (chromaffin cells in medulla)—cont'd			
Sheehan technic for chromaffin	Primary chromate critical	5 µm par.	Do not use others
Gomori's chromaffin stain	10% NBF, Bouin's fluid, Heidenhain's mercuric chloride, formalin	5 µm par.	
Alpha cells of pancreas			
Grimelius	NBF or Bouin's	5 µm par.	
Bodian's method (islet alpha cells of pancreas)	Formalin	5 µm par.	
Ammoniacal silver methods (argyrophil technics for reticulin)			
Foot's modification of Bielschowski's method	AWFT		
Gridley's modification	AWFT, NBF preferred	5 µm par.	
Laidlaw's silver stain for reticulum	AWFT, Bouin's preferred	5 µm par.	
Snook's reticulum stain	AWFT	5 µm par.	
Wilder's reticulum stain	AWFT	5 µm par.	
Amyloid			
Congo red technics			
Puchtler's modification of Bennhold's Congo red	Carnoy's or absolute alcohol best; others may be used	10 µm par.	
Highman's modification of Bennhold's Congo red	Carnoy's or absolute alcohol best; others may be used	10 µm par.	
Metachromatic stains for amyloid (crystal violet, methyl violet)	10% NBF, absolute alcohol, Bouin's fluid	10 µm par.	
Argentaffin cells			
Fontana-Masson technic	10% NBF	5 µm par.	
Gomori-Burtner method	10% NBF	5 µm par.	
Bodian's method	10% NBF	5 µm par.	
Argyrophil cells (carcinoid tumors)			
Grimelius	NBF or Bouin's	5 µm par.	
Sevier-Munger	NBF or Bouin's	5 µm par.	
Australian antigen (hepatitis B surface antigen)			
Orcein	10% NBF	5 µm par.	Avoid chromates
Aldehyde fuchsin	10% NBF	5 µm par.	Avoid chromates
Bacteria			
Gram stain (Taylor modification of Brown-Brenn)	AWFT		
Gram stain (Hopps modification of Brown-Brenn)	AWFT	5 µm par.	
Spirochetes			
Giemsa stain	10% NBF	5 µm par.	Bouin's, Zenker's
Gram's technic	10% NBF	5 µm par.	Bouin's, Zenker's
Levaditi	10% NBF	5 µm par.	Bouin's, Zenker's
Warthin-Starry	10% NBF (critical)	5 µm par.	

Continued.

SPECIAL-STAINS FIXATION CHART—cont'd

Technic	Recommended fixative(s)	Sections	Fixative(s) not recommended
Bile pigment			
Hall's	10% NBF	5 μm par.	
Stein's	10% NBF	5 μm par.	
Blood dye stains			
Giemsa-Wolbach	Zenker's best, AWFT	5 μm par.	
Sheehan's modification of the Giemsa technic	Zenker's best, AWFT	5 μm par.	
Strumia universal blood stain	Zenker's	5 μm par.	
Calcium			
Von Kossa's silver test for calcium	Alcohol preferred, 10% formalin may be used	5 μm par.	
Alizarin red S for calcium	10% formalin	5 μm par.	
Carbohydrates			
Polysaccharides			
Periodic acid–Schiff	NBF, Zenker's, Bouin's (for some tissue components, remembering the main problem is that some carbohydrates are water soluble) (Quote Culling, Chapter 9, page 34)	5 μm par.	
Periodic acid–silver methenamine	NBF, Carnoy's fluid	5 μm par.	
Glycogen			
Bauer-Feulgen reaction for glycogen; PAS before and after diastase	Carnoy's fluid, Gendre's fluid / Acid alcoholic formalin	5 μm par. / 5 μm par.	Aqueous fixatives / Aqueous fixatives
Best's carmine stain for glycogen	Absolute alcohol or Carnoy's	5 μm par.	Aqueous fixatives
Mucoproteins and mucopolysaccharides			
Mayer's mucicarmine stain	AWFT	5 μm par.	
Metachromatic methods (toluidine blue, thionin)	Alcohol preferred; any general fixative may be used	5 μm par.	
Acid mucopolysaccharides			
Thionin stain for acid mucopolysaccharides	AWFT	5 μm par.	
Müller-Mowry colloidal iron–periodic acid–Schiff reaction	AWFT		
Mowry's alcian blue method for acid mucopolysaccharides, connective tissue mucin, and epithelial mucin	10% NBF or Bouin's	5 μm par.	
Alcian blue–PAS	10% NBF or Bouin's	5 μm par.	
Alcian blue–Feulgen	10% NBF or Bouin's	5 μm par.	
Cholesterol and its esters			
Schultz's method	10% NBF (frozen sections)	Frozen	Bouin's, Zenker's
Digitonin reaction	10% NBF or fresh (frozen sections)	Frozen	Bouin's, Zenker's
Connective tissue			
Collagen, reticulin, and basement membranes			

SPECIAL-STAINS FIXATION CHART—cont'd

Technic	Recommended fixative(s)	Sections	Fixative(s) not recommended
Connective tissue—cont'd			
Ammoniacal silver methods for reticulin			
Wilder's reticulum stain	Formalin, Zenker's, Helly's	5 μm par.	Picric acid fixatives not recommended
Foot's modification of Bielschowski's method	AWFT	5 μm par.	
Gridley's modification	NBF preferred; others may be used	5 μm par.	
Laidlaw's method	Bouin's or formalin	5 μm par.	
Snook's reticulum	10% formalin	5 μm par.	
Acid aniline dye mixtures with picric acid			
Van Gieson's picric acid–acid fuchsin stain	AWFT	5 μm par.	
Phosphotungstic and phosphomolybdic acid methods			
Masson's trichrome	Bouin's fluid preferred (Möller's, Regaud's, or mordanting in Bouin's)	5 μm par.	Do not use NBF without mordanting
Mallory's aniline blue collagen stain	Tissue must be Zenker-fixed	5 μm par.	Do not use other fixatives
Gomori's one-step trichrome	AWFT	5 μm par.	
Heidenhain's aniline blue or azan stain	Zenker's, Helly's, Bouin's, Carnoy's	5 μm par.	
Phosphomolybdic and phosphotungstic acid–hematoxylin methods			
Mallory's PTAH	Zenker's required; NBF may be mordanting in stock Zenker's	5 μm par.	
Mallory's PMAH	Zenker's required; NBF may be mordanting in stock Zenker's	5 μm par.	
Periodic acid oxidation methods			
Periodic acid–Schiff for collagen, reticulin, and basement membranes	NBF; Bouin's	5 μm par.	
Lillie's allochrome procedure	NBF, Bouin's	5 μm par.	
Copper (see under *Metals*)			
Elastic fibers			
Gomori's aldehyde fuchsin	10% NBF preferred; formalin and Bouin's give colorless background; mercury fixatives give lavender background	5 μm par.	Avoid chromates like Orth's or Möller's
Orcinol new fuchsin	AWFT	5 μm par.	
Verhoeff–Van Gieson	10% NBF or Zenker's preferred, AWFT	5 μm par.	
Weigert's resorcin fuchsin	10% NBF preferable; others give excellent results	5 μm par.	

Continued.

SPECIAL-STAINS FIXATION CHART—cont'd

Technic	Recommended fixative(s)	Sections	Fixative(s) not recommended
Fats and lipids			
In chemical methods			
Cholesterol and esters (see under letter *C*)			
Marchi's method for degenerating myelin	Fix 2 days in Orth's fluid or 10% formalin; follow special processing technic	5 μm par.	Do not use other fixatives
Nile blue sulfate technic	Formalin calcium solution	Frozen 8 μm	Do not use other fixatives
Osmic acid technics (frozen sections not permanent)	Formalin fixed	Frozen	Do not use other fixatives
Physical methods with dyes			
Oil red O in propylene glycol	10% formalin	Frozen	Zenker's, Helly's
Sudan black B in propylene glycol	10% formalin	Frozen	Zenker's, Helly's
Phospholipids			
Luxol fast blue for phospholipids	10% formalin	10 μm par.	
Smith-Dietrich method for phospholipids	Formol-calcium to prevent dissolution of the phospholipids	Embed in gelatin and cut frozen	No other fixatives
Baker's acid hematein method for phospholipids	Formol-calcium to prevent dissolution of the phospholipids	10 μm frozen	No other fixatives
Fischler's technic for fatty acids	10% formalin and cut frozen sections	10 μm frozen	No other fixatives
Fibrin			
Mallory's phosphotungstic acid hematoxylin	Zenker's	5 μm par.	Bouin's
Weigert's stain for fibrin	Absolute alcohol, Carnoy's or alcoholic formalin	5 μm par.	Bouin's
Fungi			
Brown-Brenn modified gram stain	NBF, Bouin's, Zenker's, Helly's	5 μm par.	
Gridley's technic	AWFT	5 μm par.	
Grocott's stain	10% NBF, Bouin's	5 μm par.	
PAS technic	10% NBF, Bouin's, Zenker's	5 μm par.	
Hotchkiss-McManus PAS technic	10% NBF, Bouin's, Zenker's	5 μm par.	
Hemoglobin pigment			
Lepehne's method	10% NBF; *caution:* results may be impaired if left too long in formalin	Frozen	Zenker's
Ralph's method	Absolute alcohol, Carnoy's, NBF	5 μm par.	Zenker's
Dunn-Thompson hemoglobin stain	10% NBF	5 μm par.	Bouin's, Zenker's, Helly's
Okajima's stain	10% NBF	5 μm par.	
Hepatitis B surface antigen (see *Australia antigen*)			
Inclusion bodies			
Lendrum's phloxine tartrazine method	9 parts saturated mercuric chloride–1 part formalin	5 μm par.	
Parson's stain for Negri bodies	10% formalin	5 μm par.	
Schleifstein's method for Negri bodies	Zenker's	5 μm par.	

SPECIAL-STAINS FIXATION CHART—cont'd

Technic	Recommended fixative(s)	Sections	Fixative(s) not recommended
Inclusion bodies—cont'd			
Ziehl-Neelsen method for acid-fast inclusion bodies	NBF	5 μm par.	
Lillie's safranin O–eriocyanine A (pale blue Negri bodies)	NBF, Orth's, Spuler's	5 μm par.	
Juxtaglomerular cells of kidney			
Bowie's stain for juxtaglomerular cells	Helly's fluid *critical*	5 μm par.	Other fixatives unsatisfactory
Harada's stain	NBF or B-5	5 μm par.	
Melanin pigment			
Argentaffin reactions for melanin			
Gomori's methenamine silver argentaffin reaction for melanin	NBF, Bouin's	5 μm par.	
Schmorl's ferric ferricyanide reduction test	NBF, Bouin's	5 μm par.	
Dopa oxidase	Definite procedure: follow all steps at stated times including fixation		Do not use others
Ferrous-ion uptake for melanin	NBF, Bouin's	5 μm par.	
Melanin bleaching reactions			
10% hydrogen peroxide for 1 to 2 days	Follow procedure		
Potassium permanganate, in 0.3% sulfuric acid for 10 minutes to several hours	Follow procedure		
Performic acid bleaching (p. 221)	Follow procedure		
Peracetic acid bleaching (p. 221)	Follow procedure		
Metals			
Calcium			
Alizarin red S	Formalin-fixed tissue	5 μm par.	
Von Kossa's silver stain	Alcohol preferred; formalin may be used	Frozen sections or 5 μm par.	
Copper			
Mallory-Parker stain	95% or absolute alcohol (formalin for copper)	5 μm par.	
Mallory's stain	Alcohol critical	5 μm par.	Do not use formalin
Rhodanine method	10% NBF	5 μm par.	
Rubeanic acid method	10% NBF	5 μm par.	
Gold (hydrogen peroxide method)	Formalin		
Iron			
Mallory's stain	Alcohol critical	5 μm par.	Do not use formalin
Prussian blue (ferric iron)	NBF	5 μm par.	

Continued.

SPECIAL-STAINS FIXATION CHART—cont'd

Technic	Recommended fixative(s)	Sections	Fixative(s) not recommended
Metals—cont'd			
Turnbull's blue (ferrous iron)	NBF	5 μm par.	
Lead (Mallory-Parker stain)	95% or absolute alcohol	5 μm par.	
Zinc (diphenylthiocarbazone or Dithizon technic)	Follow special procedure Cryostat sections postfixed for 1 hour in absolute alcohol or methanol		
Microincineration is the process employed to study mineral content in tissues and gives information on the amount and distribution of calcium, magnesium, silicon, and iron without the organic elements interfering	9 volumes of absolute alcohol to 1 volume of neutral commercial formalin	4 μm sections— quartz slides	Avoid chromates and mercuric salts
Nerve tissue			
Nerve cells and glia			
Cresyl violet stain	Formalin, or Bouin's, stains well	5 μm par.	
Holzer stain	10% formalin or formalin alcohol	5 μm par.	
Toluidine blue stain	Alcohol best; formalin serves well	5 μm par.	
Trichrome stain for astrocytes	10% formalin or Eloer's fixative	5 μm par.	
Myelin sheaths			
Luxol fast blue technic	NBF	10 to 15 μm par.	
Pal-Weigert method	AWFT	10 to 15 μm par.	
Weil's method	NBF	10 to 15 μm par.	
Peripheral nerve elements			
Bielschowski's method for neurofibrils and axis cylinders	3 to 6 weeks in formalin	Thin frozen sections	Use only stated fixatives
Bodian's method for myelinated and nonmyelinated fibers and neurofibrils	9 parts 95% alcohol and 1 part formalin	5 μm par.	Use only stated fixatives
Cajal's gold sublimate method for astrocytes	Formalin ammonium bromide	Frozen sections 20 to 30 μm	Use only stated fixatives
Gros-Bielschowski technic for axis cylinders, intracellular fibrils, and neurofibrils	Follow procedures carefully	Frozen sections	Use only stated fixatives
Nonidez's method for nerve endings, nerve fibers and axis cylinders	50% ethanol, 100 ml; chloral hydrate, 25 gm	5 μm par.	Use only stated fixatives
Rio-Hortega method for neurofibrils	10% formalin, formalin ammonium bromide, formalin uranium		Use only stated fixatives
Nissl substance			
Thionin stain for Nissl substance	Formalin		
Cresyl echt Violett Nissl substance	Formalin preferred		
Gallocyanine stain for Nissl substance	Zenker's, Helly's, or 10% formalin		

SPECIAL-STAINS FIXATION CHART—cont'd

Technic	Recommended fixative(s)	Sections	Fixative(s) not recommended
Pancreas			
Alpha cells of pancreas (argyrophil) with Grimelius's stain	10% NBF or Bouin's Zymogen granules destroyed by acetic acid, Carnoy's, and Bouin's; well preserved by NBF, Orth's, Kose's, Möller's	5 μm par.	
Combined Gomori methods for demonstrating pancreatic alpha and beta cells	10% NBF	5 μm par.	
Trichrome–PAS to demonstrate alpha, beta, and delta cells	Helly's preferred; 10% NBF may be used	5 μm par.	Zenker's and Bouin's unsatisfactory because of acetic acid
Sieracki's method for beta cells in pancreatic islets and their tumors	10% NBF, Bouin's	5 μm par.	
Scott's rapid staining of beta cell granules in pancreatic islets	Bouin's fluid	5 μm par.	
Gomori's chrome alum-hematoxylin-phloxine	10% NBF; Bouin's preferred	5 μm par.	
Paneth cells	NBF, Kose's, Möller's	5 μm par.	
Parasites			
Amebas			
Best's carmine technic	Alcohol or alcoholic formalin	5 μm par.	Aqueous fixatives
PAS technic	Alcohol or alcoholic formalin	5 μm par.	
Malarial Giema's technic	Alcohol or alcoholic formalin	5 μm par.	
Worms, PAS technic	Alcohol or alcoholic formalin	5 μm par.	
Pigments			
Artifact (fixation pigments)			
Formaldehyde	Results from acid formalin reaction on blood-rich tissue or prolonged fixation in acid formalin; avoid by using NBF as fixative; remove pigments with saturated alcoholic picric acid or 10% hydrogen peroxide		
Mercury	Results from fixation in fixatives containing mercury; remove from tissue with iodine–sodium thiosulfate sequence		
Endogenous—uric acid and sodium urate crystals			
Gomori's methenamine silver technic for urate crystal demonstration	Absolute alcohol (critical)	5 μm par.	Do not use aqueous fixatives
Endogenous of hematogenous origin			
Aposiderin		5 μm par.	May be prevented by use of NBF
Bile pigments (see bile pigment stains, p. 52)			

Continued.

SPECIAL-STAINS FIXATION CHART—cont'd

Technic	Recommended fixative(s)	Sections	Fixative(s) not recommended
Pigments—cont'd			
Hematins			
Acid hematin	10% NBF		
Formalin pigment (see artifact pigments, p. 130)			
Malarial pigment	10% NBF		
Hemoglobin (see *Hemoglobin pigment*)			
Hemosiderin (see *Metals, iron, Prussian blue*)			
Pigments of nonhematogenous origin			
Melanin (see melanin)			
Argentaffin (see argentaffin)			
Chromaffin (see chromaffin)			
Ceroid (see description on p. 225)			
Hemofuscin—Mallory's method	Zenker's, alcohol or 10% formalin	5 μm sections	
Pituitary (overfixation leads to granule depletion)	Try Elftman's chrome alum fixative		Destroyed by Bouin's, Gendre's, Carnoy's
Congo red for beta cells	10% NBF, 10% formalin	5 μm par.	
Gomori's aldehyde fuchsin for beta cells	Bouin's preferred, NBF	5 μm par.	If NBF is used, mordant with Bouin's; avoid chromates
Gomori's chrome alum hematoxylin phloxine	Bouin's preferred	5 μm par.	Avoid dichromates
Safranin O–eriocyanine A	Bouin's	3 μm par.	
PAS–orange G	Helly's, Zenker's, formal-saline	5 μm par.	
Polysaccharides (see under carbohydrates)			
Rickettsias			
Giemsa	10% NBF	5 μm par.	
Pinkerton's	10% NBF, Regaud's, Zenker's	5 μm par.	
Spirochetes (see under *Bacteria*)			

REFERENCES

Baker, J. R.: Principles of biological microtechnique: a study of fixation and dyeing, New York, 1958, Barnes & Noble, Inc.

Culling, C. F. A.: Handbook of histopathological and histochemical techniques, ed. 3, London, 1974, Butterworth & Co. (Pubs.) Ltd.

Gray, P.: The microtomist's formulary and guide, New York, 1954, The Blakiston Co. (McGraw-Hill Book Co.).

Jones, R. McClung: Basic microscopic technics, Chicago, 1966, The University of Chicago Press.

Lillie, R. D.: Histopathologic technic and practical histochemistry, New York, 1965, McGraw-Hill Book Co.

Sheehan, D. C.: A comparative study of the histologic techniques for demonstrating chromaffin cells, Am. J. Med. Technol. **26:**237-240, July-Aug. 1960.

CHAPTER 3

Processing of tissue

DEHYDRANTS, CLEARING AGENTS, AND EMBEDDING MEDIA

The most commonly used method of examining tissue microscopically is by sectioning. Since fixed tissues are not firm and cohesive enough to permit perfect thin sections to be cut on a microtome at 4 to 6 μm, it is necessary that they be completely impregnated with some supporting medium to furnish stability and to hold the cells and intercellular structures in proper relationship to each other. The commonly used sectioning methods require infiltration with various kinds of embedding masses.

The water-soluble masses are Carbowax, gelatin, agar, and OCT. Tissues embedded in these masses do not require dehydration.

To avoid distortion of soft and delicate structures and damage by heated paraffin, celloidin, a form of nitrocellulose, may be used. Tissues must be dehydrated, since this agent is not miscible with water, but since no heat is used in any step of the process, there is minimal shrinkage and distortion.

Tissues to be cut at 5 μm or thinner are usually embedded in a paraffin-like substance and must be dehydrated and cleared prior to impregnation. There are several such substances in the laboratory market today: Paraplast, Tissueprep,

and Bioloid.* These are purchased to be used at various melting points, require no filtration, and are well adapted for ribbon sectioning since they cohere and facilitate the cutting of thin sections.

DEHYDRATION

Before an embedding medium such as nitrocellulose or paraffin can enter tissue, fixed tissue that contains a high water content must be dehydrated and cleared.

Dehydration of tissue is usually carried out with ethyl alcohol, since other substitutes have made very little headway in their introduction to laboratory technic. Ethanol is supplied as absolute alcohol or rectified commercial spirits about 96% or 97% free from water. For all practical purposes this solution is considered 100% alcohol and should be used in this manner. Dehydrating agents, for the most part, must be water-miscible fluids, and it is generally believed that this process should be done in graded strengths of ethanol to gradually displace the water in the tissue with alcohol. The period of immersion in

---

*See p. 444.

59

the various-strength alcohols varies with the size and penetrability of the tissue. Additionally, alcohol has a hardening effect, which, to a certain point, is of considerable importance.

Dioxane has come into use in recent years in some laboratories. It mixes, in all proportions, with water, alcohol, and xylene and is a solvent of balsam and paraffin. It is unsuitable for laboratories where complete ventilation is a problem and the advantages of this reagent should not outweigh the possible effect it might have on the health of laboratory technologists.

Cellosolve, another of the newer methods of dehydration, will displace alcohol as well as water and is readily dissolved by all the commonly used clearing agents. Additionally, tissue may remain in it for months without injury. The cost, per gallon, is high for this material, but use of reduced quantities in dehydration compensates for this cost.

Acetone may be used as a dehydrant. When ethanol is difficult to obtain or expensive because of prohibitive taxes, this reagent will do a good job.

Isopropanol is cheaper than ethanol, is free of government restrictions, but has a limited use in the laboratory. It is a good dehydrant for paraffin embedding but cannot be used with nitrocellulose, since this reagent is insoluble in it. The limitation extends to staining, since stains are not soluble in isopropanol.

Universal solvents are those reagents that avoid the use of two solutions, a dehydrating and a clearing agent. Dioxane, tertiary butanol, and tetrahydrofuran are among this group. Most universal solvents are unsuitable for delicate tissue, which become distorted through heavy diffusion currents both in the original transfer from aqueous fixatives into the solvent and in the transfer from the solvent into paraffin. We have, however, found tetrahydrofuran a good universal solvent. It is miscible in all proportions with water and the solvents and infiltrating materials used in the processing of tissues; it dehydrates rapidly without creating artifacts and without causing excessive shrinkage or hardening of tissue. Under normal usage, it has a low toxicity and a low fire and explosion hazard and can be used for rapid processing of small pieces of tissue during the day. Standard precautions should be taken to avoid contact with the skin and eyes. All staining methods give good results with this dehydrant after the use of routine fixatives. The stained sections are indistinguishable from those done with the standard laboratory procedure of graded alcohols and chloroform clearing.

Table 3-1 lists the common dehydrants with their advantages and disadvantages.

CLEARING AGENTS

Alcohols and some of the other reagents used for dehydration and paraffin-like substances used for embedding are immiscible. Clearing

Table 3-1. Dehydrants—advantages and disadvantages

Dehydrant	Advantages	Disadvantages
Ethanol (ethyl alcohol) Boiling point 78.3° C	1. Nontoxic 2. Miscible in all proportions with water 3. Little shrinkage if graded alcohols are used 4. Can be used on eyes and embryos, if graded alcohols are used 5. Fast acting 6. Still considered best dehydrant 7. Reliable	1. Expensive 2. Avoid long periods in absolute ethanol to prevent excessive shrinkage and hardening 3. May be difficult to obtain 4. May have prohibitive taxes that necessitate troublesome bookkeeping 5. Extracts methylene blue and other thiazine dyes from sections
Butanol (butyl alcohol) Boiling point 117.7° C	1. Less shrinkage and hardening than with ethyl 2. Excellent for slow processing 3. Miscible with paraffin	1. Odorous 2. Long periods of infiltration necessary 3. Dehydrating power low
Tertiary butanol (butyl alcohol) Boiling point 82.8° C	1. Universal solvent—acts as dehydrant and clearing agent 2. May be used in staining series as a dehydrant 3. Mixes with water, ethanol, xylene, and paraffin in all proportions	1. Odorous 2. More expensive than butanol 3. Primary infiltration must be done in half tertiary butanol and half paraffin, prior to paraffin impregnation 4. Reagent tends to solidify at room temperature or below 25° C

Table 3-1. Dehydrants—advantages and disadvantages—cont'd

Dehydrant	Advantages	Disadvantages
Dioxane Refractive index 1.42 Boiling point 101.5° C	1. Universal solvent—dehydrates and clears 2. Miscible with water, alcohol, xylene, and paraffin 3. Does not harm tissue over long time periods 4. Produces less shrinkage than ethanol 5. Faster dehydrant than ethanol	1. Needs large volume for dehydration 2. Costs about four times more than does absolute alcohol 3. Must be used in well-ventilated rooms 4. Cumulatively toxic 5. Odorous 6. Distorts tissue-containing cavities
Acetone Boiling point 56° C	1. Rapid dehydrant 2. Less expensive than ethanol 3. Does not extract methylene blue and other dyes from stained sections	1. Requires a clearing agent 2. Volume must be 20 times that of the tissue 3. Best processing requires a graded series of a mixture of acetone and xylene before one can go into paraffin 4. Needs good ventilation; evaporates rapidly; flammable
Ethylene glycol monoethyl ether (Cellosolve) Boiling point 156.4° C	1. Rapid dehydrant 2. Tissue may remain in it for months without injury 3. Avoids distortion and does not require graded dilutions	1. Expensive 2. Rapidly absorbs water from the air 3. Requires clearing agent
Tetrahydrofuran Boiling point 65° C	1. Miscible in all proportions with water, ether, chloroform, acetone, and the hydrocarbons xylene, toluene, and benzene 2. Rapid without excessive shrinkage and hardening 3. Low toxicity; low fire and explosion hazard 4. Not toxic 5. Better results than most universal solvents 6. Solvents of mounting media	1. Odorous—should be used in well-ventilated room 2. Evaporates rapidly 3. Dyes are not soluble in tetrahydrofuran
Triethyl phosphate Boiling point 215° C	1. May be used in routine paraffin technic 2. Displaces water readily with slight distortion 3. Does not harden tissue excessively 4. May be used as a dehydrant in the staining sequence 5. Soluble in alcohols, benzene, toluene, xylene, ether, chloroform	None
Isopropanol (isopropyl alcohol) Boiling point 82.3° C	1. Excellent substitute for ethanol 2. Less shrinkage and hardening than ethanol 3. No government restrictions on its use 4. Sufficiently water-free to use in place of absolute ethanol 5. Lillie considers it "the best all-around substitute for ethyl alcohol" 6. Less expensive than tax-free ethanol	1. Cannot be used in the celloidin technic since nitrocellulose is insoluble in it 2. Cannot be used for preparing staining solutions, since dyes are not soluble in it
Pentanol (amyl alcohol) Boiling point 128° C	1. Miscible with 90% alcohol, toluene, and xylene 2. Dissolves paraffin wax	1. Toxic 2. Cannot be used in poorly ventilated rooms 3. Not miscible with water

Table 3-2. Advantages and disadvantages of common clearing agents

Clearing agent	Advantages	Disadvantages
Cedarwood oil Refractive index 1.50	1. Clears alcohol dehydrated tissue quickly without further shrinkage 2. Does not dissolve out aniline colors in the staining sequence 3. Clears celloidin without dissolving it 4. Little evaporation 5. Least harmful to cells of any known clearing agent 6. Gives least hardening to tissue 7. Excellent for hard tissues such as skin, uterus, muscle, and tendon 8. Clears from 95% alcohol 9. "One of the best" (Lillie)	1. Must be removed with xylene prior to impregnation with paraffin 2. Expensive 3. If the oil remains in the tissue, cutting is difficult with most tissue. The exception is uterus, where the retention of a small trace of the oil improves the cutting
Clove oil Refractive index 1.53	1. Rapid clearing 2. Clears from 74% alcohol 3. Good for minute dissections where some brittleness is advantageous	1. Dissolves celloidin 2. Extracts aniline dyes 3. Makes tissue brittle
Origanum oil Refractive index 1.483-1.510	1. Slow evaporation 2. Does not dissolve out aniline colors 3. Clears celloidin without dissolving it 4. Clears from 90% alcohol	1. Expensive 2. Odorous 3. Must be removed by several changes of xylene prior to paraffin impregnation
Sandalwood oil Refractive index 1.50-1.51	1. Slow evaporation 2. Clears celloidin without dissolving it 3. Clears from 90% alcohol	1. High cost of this oil makes its use prohibitive
Benzene Refractive index 1.50 Boiling point 80° C	1. Clears quickly 2. Makes tissue transparent so that end point of clearing is easily determined 3. Less shrinkage than with xylene and toluene	1. Considerable hardening of uterus, muscle, tendon, but not so excessive as xylene 2. Clears from absolute alcohol only 3. May be hazardous to health of laboratory technologists after long exposure 4. Should be used in well-ventilated rooms only
Toluene Refractive index 1.50 Boiling point 110.6° C	1. Considered, by many lab workers, best of the three hydrocarbons benzene, toluene, and xylene 2. Does not harden so excessively as xylene 3. Clears quickly and makes tissue transparent so that end point of clearing is easily determined 4. May be used for clearing in the staining sequence 5. "One of the best" (Lillie)	1. Tissues must be cleared from absolute alcohol 2. Fumes are toxic 3. Less volatile than benzene 4. More expensive than benzene 5. Flammable
Xylene Refractive index 1.50 Boiling point 138° C	1. "One of the best" (Lillie) 2. Clears quickly and makes tissue transparent so that end point of clearing is easily determined 3. May be used for clearing in staining sequence 4. Does not dissolve celloidin 5. Does not affect aniline colors	1. Tissue must be cleared from absolute alcohol 2. Hardens more than toluene, which is preferred for brain tissue 3. Not miscible with water. If solution becomes milky, change it immediately; solution contains water 4. Less expensive than benzene 5. Less volatile than benzene

Table 3-2. Advantages and disdvantages of common clearing agents—cont'd

Clearing agent	Adantages	Disadvantages
Chloroform Refractive index 1.45 Boiling point 61.5° C	1. Penetrates well 2. Produces some hardening, which is advantageous for sectioning. Does not harden excessively 3. Chloroform may be used to harden celloidin blocks 4. Better clearing agent for uterus, muscle and tendon—not so good as cedarwood oil, but better than the hydrocarbons 5. Makes tissue less brittle than xylene	1. Toxic 2. Must be used in well-ventilated room; fumes may be dangerous to health of technologist 3. Does not change the refractive index of tissue, which makes determination of end point of clearing difficult 4. Absorbs a good deal of moisture from the air; must be used in tightly covered containers 5. If used on Technicon in weekend processing, baskets should be filled to halfway mark with cassettes, because of rapid evaporation
Carbon bisulfide Refractive index 1.63 Boiling point 46.3° C	1. "One of the best" (Lillie)	1. Disagreeable odor 2. Fumes are toxic
Petroleum ether	1. "One of the best" (Lillie) 2. Does not render tissues brittle over long immersion periods 3. Gasoline and petroleum are in the same category as cedarwood oil in producing the least hardening of tissue 4. Excellent for clearing hard tissues such as uterus, tendon, muscle	1. Flammable 2. Lillie warns against the use of tetraethyl lead, which is dangerously toxic
Carbon tetrachloride Refractive index 1.46 Boiling point 76.7° C	1. "One of the best" (Lillie) 2. Cheaper than chloroform 3. Less toxic than chloroform	1. Flammable 2. Toxic

agents, therefore, which are miscible with both, are used between the alcohol and the paraffin. The phrase "clearing agent" is used because the high refractive index of these substances renders the tissue more or less transparent. Clearing agents are also used between alcohol and mounting with resinous mounting medium in the staining sequence.

Lillie lists the following as best paraffin solvents: "benzene, toluene, xylene, petroleum ether, carbon bisulfide, chloroform, carbon tetrachloride, cedarwood oil."

When using an essential oil for clearing, such as cedarwood oil, one must remove the oil by three 15-minute changes of xylene, prior to impregnation with paraffin. Small traces of oil destroys the cutting property of the tissue. Since oils, unlike the hydrocarbons xylene, toluene,

and benzene, are not volatile, the oil must be removed with the volatile hydrocarbon.

Table 3-2 lists the common clearing agents with their advantages and disadvantages.

PROCEDURES AND PROCESSING

See Table 3-3 for various tissue processes and Table 3-4 for a schedule for processing.

Rush sections

Rush sections, as a procedure, may be used on small fragments on an automatic tissue changer, when one with vacuum is not available. It takes approximately 6 hours to complete the processing, cutting, and staining of curettings or rectal biopsies.

Bouin's	15 min
Bouin's	30 min

Table 3-3. Various tissue processes for automatic tissue changers

Ethanol	Time	Dioxane	Time	Acetone	Time
1 basket 5 PM to 9 AM					
Bouin's	2 hr	Any fixative	2 hr	Any fixative	2 hr
Bouin's	2 hr	Any fixative	2 hr	Any fixative	2 hr
80% alcohol	1 hr	1st dioxane	1 hr	Acetone	40 min
80% alcohol	1 hr	2nd dioxane	1 hr	Acetone	40 min
95% alcohol	1 hr	3rd dioxane	1 hr	Acetone	40 min
95% alcohol	1 hr	4th dioxane	1 hr	Acetone	40 min
Absolute alcohol	1 hr	Dioxane-paraffin 1:1	1 hr	Tissueprep	30 min
Absolute alcohol	1 hr	Tissueprep	30 min	Tissueprep	1 hr
Chloroform	½ hr	Tissueprep	30 min	Tissueprep	1 hr
Chloroform	1 hr	Tissueprep			
Tissueprep	1 hr				
Tissueprep	2 hr				

Ethanol	Time	Collosolve	Time	Triethyl phosphate	Time
2 baskets 5 PM to 9 AM					
Bouin's	2½ hr	(Formalin fixation)		(Any fixative)	
Bouin's	1 hr	Normal saline	10 min	Triethyl phosphate	8 hr
80% alcohol	1 hr	Cellosolve	30 min	Triethyl phosphate	8 hr
80% alcohol	1 hr	Cellosolve	1 hr	Triethyl phosphate	8 hr
95% alcohol	1 hr	Cellosolve	1 hr	Benzene	½ hr
95% alcohol	1 hr	Cellosolve	1½ hr	Tissueprep (one change)	3 hr
Absolute alcohol	1 hr	Xylene	½ hr		
Absolute alcohol	1 hr	Tissueprep	½ hr		
Chloroform	½ hr	Tissueprep	1 hr		
Chloroform	1 hr	Tissueprep	1 hr		
Tissueprep	1 hr				
Tissueprep	3 hr				

Table 3-4. Schedule for processing with Autotechnicon at Hospital of the University of Pennsylvania

One basket	Time	Two baskets	Time
1. 80% alcohol	3:30 PM	1. Both baskets in 80%	3:30 PM
2. 80% alcohol	5:00	2. alcohol	
3. 95% alcohol	7:00	3. 95% alcohol	7:00
4. 95% alcohol	8:00	4. 95% alcohol	8:00
5. Absolute alcohol	9:00	5. Absolute alcohol	9:00
6. Absolute alcohol	10:00	6. Absolute alcohol	10:00
7. Absolute alcohol	11:00	7. Absolute alcohol	11:00
8. Chloroform	12:00	8. Chloroform	12:00
9. Chloroform	1:00 AM	9. Chloroform	1:00 AM
10. Tissueprep*	3:00	10. Tissueprep	3:00
11. Tissueprep	4:00	11. Tissueprep	4:00
12. Tissueprep	5:00	12. Tissueprep	5:00

Tissues are placed in vacuum embedding pots at 15 mm of mercury for 20 minutes prior to being embedded at 6:00 AM for final impregnation of the Tissueprep.

*Fisher Scientific Co., Fair Lawn, N.J.

80% alcohol	15 min
80% alcohol	15 min
95% alcohol	15 min
95% alcohol	15 min
Absolute alcohol	15 min
Absolute alcohol	30 min
Chloroform	15 min
Chloroform	15 min
Tissueprep	15 min
Tissueprep	1 hr

Suggested methods for tetrahydrofuran dehydration and clearing

Fisher Scientific Company has converted a Tissuematon to provide two series of six processing stations to process twice the quantity of tissue simultaneously. Tissues are fixed in 10% formalin before processing with tetrahydrofuran (THF).

Procedure by Fisher Scientific Company

1.	THF and water 1 : 1	1 hr
2.	3 changes of THF	1½ hr each
3.	THF-Tissueprep 1 : 1	2 hr
4.	Tissueprep at 60° C	2 hr (or until ready to embed)

Total time 9½ hr

Meyers' procedure (developed by Donald L. Meyers of Johns Hopkins Hospital)

1.	12% formalin at 37° C (see note 1)	1 hr
2.	12% formalin at room temperature	½ hr
3.	80% alcohol	½ hr
4.	95% alcohol	½ hr
5, 6, 7, 8.	THF with 1% celloidin (see note 2)	½ hr, ½ hr, 1 hr, ½ hr
9.	Xylene-toluene 1 : 1 (see note 3)	½ hr
10.	Tissueprep at 60° C	2 hr
11.	Tissueprep	2 hr
12.	Tissueprep	Until ready to embed

Total time 9½ hr

Note 1: The tissue processor used by Mr. Meyers has little insulation between containers. The first formalin container is warmed by heat transferred from the embedding pot, which is next to beaker no. 1 in the cycle.

Note 2: 1% nitrocellulose is used to "firm" tissue for easier cutting.

Note 3: Heat transfer from the paraffin bath prevented THF usage for clearing, because it would evaporate too quickly.

PRECAUTIONS IN USING AUTOMATIC TISSUE CHANGERS

1. Use small pieces of paper to identify the tissue. At the Hospital of the University of Pennsylvania, we have these printed in sheets holding 20 copies of each number. This expedites the work of preparing the cassettes and avoids numbering errors. For example, C 88795—the C indicates 400,000 and the tag might be smaller in a laboratory with a lower numbering system. If large pieces of paper are used in the cassettes, the preparation of fluid into tissue is inhibited.

2. Never place tissue on top of other tissue in the cassette. Any crowding will result in poor penetration of fluids for dehydration and clearing and of paraffin for impregnation.

3. Fluid levels must be at least 13 mm above the top of the cassettes. Do not crowd too many cassettes into one basket. The new square Autotechnicon baskets hold 26; the older round baskets held 18 to 22.

4. Unfixed tissue should be moistened with the fixative before it is placed into the cassette. Small pieces of tissue may be folded into small pieces of lens paper, moistened with fixative.

5. For routine pathologic purposes, the thickness of tissue for automatic processing should not exceed 3 or 4 mm, preferably 3 mm. Fluid cannot penetrate thick tissue.

6. If a basket of tissue on the automatic processor is in 95% alcohol in the morning instead of in paraffin, you should check to see whether the clock was set right; be sure that the clock was properly tightened and check the master switch.

7. When a large volume of work is done (two baskets on each instrument each night), the instruments should be cleaned and all fluids, including the paraffin baths, changed twice a week. The paraffin bath next to the last chloroform should be changed daily.

8. The temperature of all paraffin baths or paraffin dispensers should be checked and recorded, twice daily. This habits avoids the use of a bath with an erratic thermostat and avoids burning of tissue. The temperature of the paraffin for impregnation and embedding should be 2 to 4 degrees above the melting point of the embedding agent.

9. Always use clean tissue cassettes and baskets. Place them in a beaker of waste xylene immediately after embedding. After the xylene has removed the paraffin, put them in a receptacle of hot water and a detergent to cut the grease. Wash thoroughly and rinse thoroughly in hot water.

The drawn schedules work well in our laboratory where our technologists work from 7:30 to 4:00, with some of the staff starting the embedding at 6:00 AM. They can, however, be adjusted to fit any working schedule. (See Figs. 1-3 to 1-7.)

EMBEDDING METHODS AND MEDIUM
Embedding in paraffin

Embedding centers are conveniently used for paraffin embedding. Some are modular and some are singular units. Some of them are as follows:

1. Lab-Line's Timstation
2. Lab-Tek's Embedding Center
3. Lipshaw's Cryotherm Center
4. Thermolyne Embedding Center

All of these have wells for storing melted paraffin with dispensers, warm and cold plates, and cold storage. Two have forceps warmers. They are all aids in rapid embedding.

The literature contains many methods of embedding tissue in paraffin, multitissue embedding in large pans, multitissue embedding in paper boats, embedding with L-shaped metals, and embedding in metal molds. Suffice it to say that each laboratory must use the method that best protects the tissue of one patient from that of another. One cannot examine many of the printed methods without realizing that floaters, in multiple embedding, may result in false diagnosis. We safeguard against this danger by the use of Tissue-Tek.*

The molds and embedding rings for this method are pictured in Fig. 3-1. It is a convenient, simplified method for preparing tissue for cutting on a rotary microtome, as well as for filing. It eliminates the need for trimming blocks so that both edges are parallel to the cutting edge of the knife and provides a plastic framed block to fit into the microtome object clamp and remain on the block for permanent upright filing. The stainless steel base molds are reusable. They are thoroughly washed in hot water, coated with a solution of 95% alcohol and glycerol 1:1, and inverted on a towel to prevent dust collection on the inside of the mold. The molds come in various sizes: (1) ⅝ × ⅝ × ½ inch; (2) ⅞ × ⅞ × ½ inch; (3) 1¼ × 1 × ½ inch; (4) 1½ × 1 × ½ inch. The last three molds come in deeper depths and are good for embedding eyes.

The bottom of the mold is covered with paraffin and the tissue is oriented. Paraffin for embedding should be 2 to 4 degrees above the

*Ames Co., Inc., Elkhart, Ind.

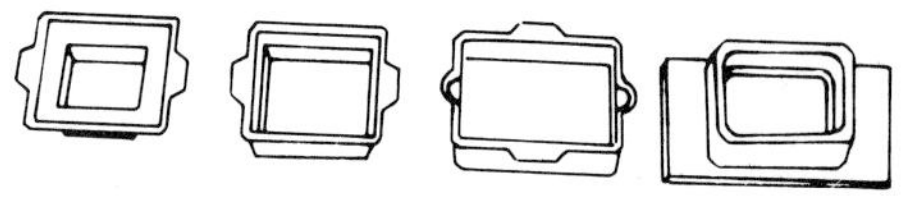

Embedding molds   Embedding ring (disposable)

Fig. 3-1. Tissue-Tek molds and embedding rings.

melting point of the medium and, to prevent dust collection, should be kept in a paraffin dispenser. The mold is then covered by the properly identified embedding ring and the ring is pressed firmly into place. The combined mold and ring are filled with paraffin and immediately cooled when the mold is placed on the bottom of a stainless steel pan containing ice cubes or a block of ice to keep the metal very cold. This method allows the block to harden from the surface of the mold to the top of the embedding ring. When a solid scum has formed on the top of the ring, turn the mold upside down in another stainless steel pan containing ice and water. Final cooling requires about 15 minutes. Slow hardening or too rapid hardening of paraffin causes crystallization. Paraffin that forms large crystals as it solidifies produces artifacts in tissue sections, whereas overheating the paraffin used in infiltrating and embedding tissue causes hardening of the tissue. The melting point of the paraffin used for embedding will depend on the climate in which you live. A ring of filter paper in the bottom of the paraffin dispenser will remove any particles of dust that may damage the cutting edge of the knife.

The paraffin dispenser

Several water-jacketed thermostatically controlled paraffin dispensers (Fig. 3-2) are sold on the laboratory market. These maintain a uniform temperature for up to 10 pounds of paraffin, ready for immediate delivery through the nonclogging, self-closing spigot.

Filing of blocks of tissue

A fiber utility storage case, 9¼ inches wide by 16½ inches deep by 13 inches high, with six removable plastic trays, for storing 1000 embedding rings is purchased with the embedding rings. The filing saves space and requires little time, and blocks are readily available for recutting.

We believe that the Tissue-Tek method is an extremely efficient one that avoids the danger of floaters and the errors by tags coming loose

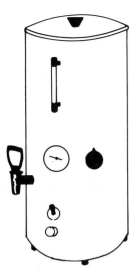

Fig. 3-2. The paraffin dispenser.

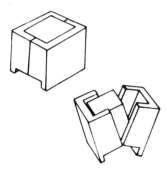

Fig. 3-3. Lipshaw Pop-Out embedding molds.

and provides a considerable saving of technical time.

Other methods of embedding in paraffin

The following method is used at the Armed Forces Institute of Pathology and can be found in Luna, L. G.: *Manual of Histologic and Special Staining Technics* (ed. 3, New York, 1963, McGraw-Hill Book Co.).

"Embedding can be accelerated by the use of shallow tin pans, which can be purchased or made by a tinsmith. For embedding of multiple blocks, pans with slightly sloping sides, ranging from 1 × 2 inches with a ¾-inch depth to 8 × 10 inches with a 1-inch depth is satisfactory.

"The pan is placed on a Masonite rack that holds it about 6 inches above the desk top. The pan is warmed gently with a Bunsen burner and filled with paraffin that has been melted and filtered. Each piece of tissue is placed in position

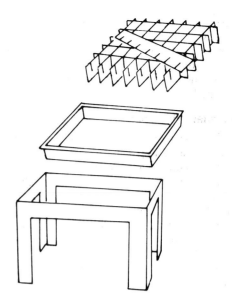

Fig. 3-4. Lipshaw Multi-Block embedding combination.

with the appropriate string tag beside it, and when all are in place, the lowest part of the paraffin is hardened when one rubs an ice cube across the bottom of the pan. When the paraffin has cooled sufficiently so that a heavy film forms across the top, the pan is floated on cold water. The paraffin, when hardened throughout, will contract from the sides of the pan and the mass can be lifted out and cut into blocks of appropriate size."

Pop-out embedding molds*

Pop-out embedding molds are made of precisely machined hard aluminum alloy in two sections and are hinged together to form the complete unit. The legs are designed to automatically hold the mold in a closed position ready for use. For removal of the paraffin, the mold is swung open and the block pops out (Fig. 3-3).

Lipshaw Multiblock Embedding Combination*

This combination (Fig. 3-4) consists of a stand, compound blocking forms with a base, and a tray. The blocking forms are made of precise, interlocking sections that are easily assembled and disassembled and available in two sizes. The tray prevents spillage of paraffin and the stand provides 5 inches of working

---

*Lipshaw Manufacturing Corp., Detroit, Mich.

space under the tray for the application of a Bunsen burner flame or ice cubes. The blocking forms are made of precisely hardened aluminum, interlocking sections fit together with ease, and they are easily assembled and easily cleaned.

Lipshaw Histo-molds*

The use of Histo-molds is a simple method of embedding. The perforated crown is easily and quickly removed from the embedded block. The frame adheres to the block to give rigidity for sectioning. The specimen number is permanently marked directly onto the form with a lead pencil to eliminate errors, and when sectioning is completed, the Histo-mold is ready for filing. The Histo-molds are sturdily fabricated of heavy-duty, white-coated fiberboard. The interior is coated with paraffin.

Lipshaw Peel-A-Way Molds

Peel-A-Way Molds (used in Winkler's method of processing needle biopsies) come in five sizes. To remove the paraffin block, peel off the mold and discard. Fingers are provided on the inside to hold the identification slip, which becomes a permanent record embedded in the paraffin.

Lab-Line Pre-Assembled Tims

Lab-Line Tims offers laboratories an excellent system for the processing and embedding of tissue. The Tims is preassembled and can be used in any automatic processor. Since the Idento-Frame carries the permanent identification of the tissue from fixation to filing, errors are mostly eliminated. (See Figs. 3-5 to 3-8.)

GENERAL NOTES ON PARAFFIN INFILTRATION AND EMBEDDING

1. Successful impregnation requires you to keep the tissue in the bath as long as necessary—neither more nor less.
   a. Clearing agent must be completely replaced by paraffin, or tissue will not section.
   b. Prolonged exposure causes shrinkage and hardening and prevents good sectioning. Shrinkage of tissue is greatest after paraffin embedding.
   c. Duration in paraffin bath depends on thickness and texture of tissue. The usual time for paraffin infiltration of tissue in a 16-hour processing schedule is 2 to 3 hours.

---

*Lipshaw Manufacturing Corp., Detroit, Mich.

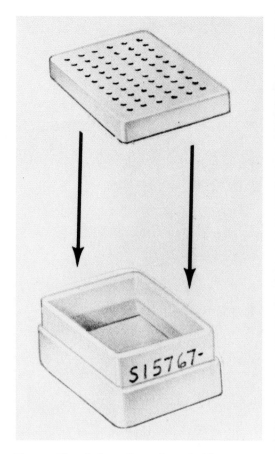

Fig. 3-5. Tims Indento-Frame for embedding tissue.

   (1) Medium-sized pieces of brain, spinal cord, and skin 5 to 10 mm in thickness require overnight impregnation.
   (2) Reduce time to a minimum for:
       (a) Nonstriated, striated, and cardiac muscle
       (b) Fibrous tissue
       (c) Spleen or other organs containing blood
       (d) Thrombi or emboli
       (e) Scar tissue
       (f) Fibromas
2. Keep a careful check on paraffin temperature. Never allow it to go more than 4 degrees above melting point of medium. (See Fig. 3-9.)

VACUUM EMBEDDING

Vacuum embedding is desirable for all tissue. The volatile clearing agent is more rapidly replaced by the paraffin, reducing the time in the paraffin bath considerably. It is an excellent method for air-containing tissue (such as lung),

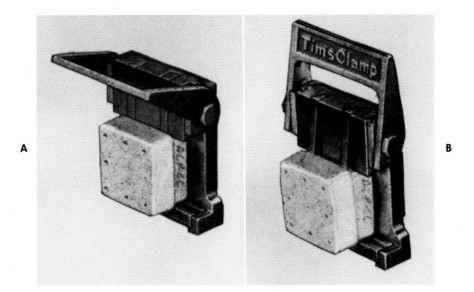

Fig. 3-6. A, Handle down—Tims positioned automatically. **B,** Handle up—Tims securely clamped and bottom removed automatically.

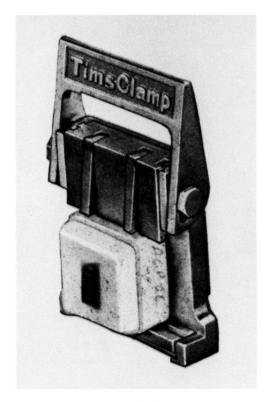

Fig. 3-7. Tims ready for sectioning.

large or dense pieces of brain, hard tissues such as muscle, fibrous tissue, scar tissue, fibromas, spleen, or other organs containing blood and thrombi or emboli.

NITROCELLULOSE EMBEDDING

If tissues are damaged by heated paraffin and a room temperature embedding medium must be used, the choice would be celloidin. The greatest advantage of this method is the lack of heat at any stage of the process, since the tissues are impregnated in solutions of increasing-strength celloidin at room temperature and are embedded in a 12% solution.

The greatest risk to successful embedding is water contamination. The requisite for successful infiltration of tissue is perfect dehydration with absolute alcohol that must be kept in airtight containers to avoid water from atmospheric conditions. The ether must be anhydrous, not commercial ether.

The dehydration must be done in airtight containers, starting at low-grade alcohols and ending with absolute alcohol–ether 1:1. Clearing agents are not used in this method.

The process may require weeks or even months. Infiltration is done in graded solutions of 4%, 8%, and 12% celloidin. The time will vary with the size and nature of the tissue. Complete impregnation must be ensured before one attempts to block and cut the sections.

The preparation of celloidin blocks may be done by evaporation of the alcohol-ether mix-

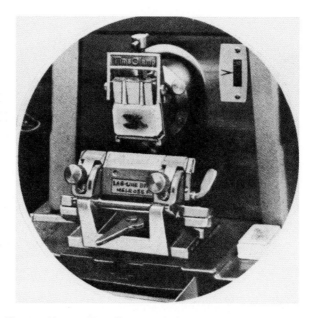

Fig. 3-8. Tims in TimsClamp ready for sectioning on microtome.

ture or removal of it with chloroform. Elsie Toms, chief histotechnologist in the Laboratory of Neurosurgical Pathology, Hospital of the University of Pennsylvania, uses the first method. She cuts the excess celloidin off the sides to make the block, coats the fiber block with a layer of thick celloidin, dips the bottom of the celloidin block in alcohol until it is tacky, and then firmly presses it onto the fiber block. The block is hardened in 70% alcohol and stored in 70% alcohol.

Another method involves making a paper collar from bond paper by tying it firmly around the edge of the wooden or fiber block to make a box, the floor of which is the wooden block and the sides the paper. Pour 6 mm of 12% celloidin into the box and place it in a desiccator until the alcohol-ether is evaporated and the block is firm when touched. Remove from desiccator, fill the box to the brim with the celloidin, place the tissue in the box, and orient it into position until it reaches the firm underneath layer. Fill the base of the desiccator with chloroform and place the block in the desiccator. The rapid vapor exchange between the alcohol-ether and the chloroform will harden the block.

With the method of Miss Toms, the sections are cut on a sliding microtome. The knife is kept moist with 70% alcohol and should be remoistened after cutting each section, which is individually removed from the knife and stored in 70% alcohol to avoid drying out before stain-ing. If sectioning must be interrupted, cover the block with absorbent cotton saturated with 70% alcohol. The knife for cutting celloidin sections is plano-concave, and the slice angle should be 10 to 40 degrees. The block is placed in the tissue holder so that the knife enters the block at an acute angle. If serial sections are being cut, the number may be stamped on the margin of the celloidin with a commercial numbering machine, and as each section is cut, it is placed on numbered filter paper or lens paper and stored in 70% alcohol.

Preparation of celloidin solution

Use thick celloidin at 12%. Dissolve 24 gm of celloidin or parlodion in 100 ml of absolute alcohol, stirring frequently with a heavy glass rod for 12 to 15 hours to ensure complete solution. When completely dissolved, add 100 ml of anhydrous ether. (The celloidin or parlodion goes into solution more quickly if dissolved in the absolute alcohol prior to the addition of the ether.) Dilutions may be made up from the 12% solution in the following manner:

Percent	Stock solution (ml)	Absolute alcohol and ether 1:1 (ml)
10	50	10
8	40	20
6	30	30
4	20	40
2	10	50

Attaching celloidin sections to slides before staining

Transfer the sections from 70% to 95% alcohol. Coat the slide with Mayer's egg albumin thinly and transfer the section from the 95% alcohol to the slide. Press it down between two layers of Whatman no. 4 filter paper and flood the slide with a thin coating of collodion, which is a pharmaceutical solution of pyroxylin. The collodion is prepared by the dissolving of 1 gm of commercial collodion in 10 ml of absolute alcohol–ether 1 : 1. Allow to dry and store in 70% alcohol until ready to stain.

Staining of celloidin sections

Celloidin sections are usually stained in small slender dishes or watch glasses and handled by being moved from one fluid to another with a section lifter. The celloidin protects the section against damage. Most staining methods may be done in this way, but the chief objection is that some stains are absorbed by the celloidin. This is particularly true of the basic aniline dyes. The stain is removed with 2% colophonium (or rosin) in 95% alcohol until the celloidin is colorless. Blot with fine filter paper and flood with xylene several times until the sections are clear.

Nuclear staining of celloidin sections is relatively easy, as are metal impregnations. After being stained, the loose sections are dehydrated through graded alcohols to 95% alcohol. They are cleared in Weigert's carbol-xylene mixture, which contains 100 ml of melted phenol crystals to 300 ml of xylene. Complete with several changes of xylene and mount in synthetic resin in xylene.

OTHER EMBEDDING AGENTS
Gelatin

Since the advent of the microtome cryostat, gelatin is not often used for frozen sections. This method may be used for the demonstration of fat:

1. Fix tissue in 10% formalin.
2. Wash in running water overnight.
3. Impregnate tissue in a 12.5% solution of gelatin in an incubator at 37° C for 24 hours.
4. Complete impregnation in a 25% gelatin solution in an incubator for 24 to 36 hours.
5. Embed in 25% gelatin and harden block in the refrigerator. A paper boat may be used for embedding.
6. Strip paper from hardened block and further harden in 5% formalin for 24 hours.

7. Cut sections on clinical freezing microtome. Remove section from knife with camel's hair brush and place briefly in a Petri dish of 50% alcohol. Remove from alcohol and dip briefly in 5% gelatin and place tissue in center of slide where the flexible tissue will flatten without difficulty. Drain off surplus fluid and stand slide upright in a Coplin jar contining 5 ml of 40% formalin. The formalin vapor will fix the section firmly to the slide. If storing is desirable after hardening, store in 5% formalin.

Solutions
25% gelatin—25 gm of gelatin in water until swollen and melted; dilute to 100 ml with distilled water.
2.5% gelatin—make fresh or dilute from 25% stock solution.

Carbowax

Carbowax is a water-soluble solid polyethylene glycol and is an embedding medium used to infiltrate tissue directly from aqueous fixatives. The method has been used successfully to demonstrate fat in pathologic conditions, but it will not impregnate adipose tissue, and the impregnation of brain or spinal cord is very slow.

Formula. The formula usually employs a mixture of Carbowax Compound 4000, which is hard, dry, and flaky, and Compound 1500, which is a blend of liquid polyethylene glycol and wax. The carbowaxes are combined, usually 9 parts of 4000 to 1 part of 1500, heated to 175° C for 30 seconds and then placed in an oven at 56° C. The solution should be kept in the oven. If it solidifies, it requires heating to 56° C to melt it.

Fixation. Any fixative may be used by following the rules for good fixation.

Infiltration. The mixture of the above formula may be varied to suit the climate in which you live. Pure 4000 may be used in very hot climates, or 85 gm of 4000 to 15 gm of 1500 may be used in cooler climates.

Infiltrate tissue in a small Stender dish in the oven at 56° C for 1 to 3 hours, agitating frequently to aid penetration. All tissue, including lung, must sink in the solution prior to embedding.

Embedding. After sufficient infiltration, remove tissue and embed in fresh solution in a Stender dish.

Hardening. Cover dish and harden at 5° C to avoid crystal formation.

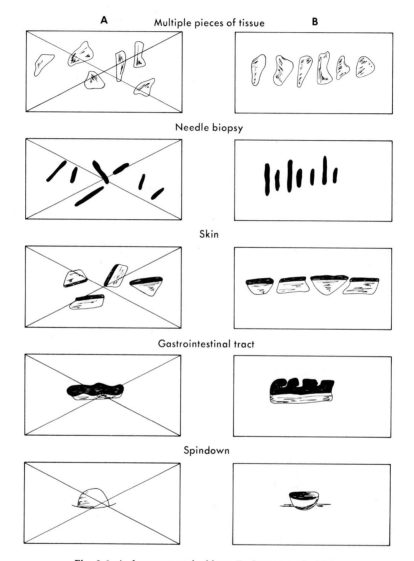

Fig. 3-9. A, Incorrect embedding. **B,** Correct embedding.

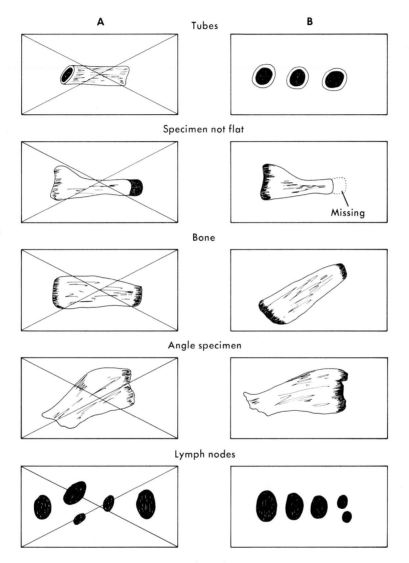

Fig. 3-9, cont'd. For legend see opposite page.

Trimming. Trim block with hot spatula and mount on fiber block.

Cutting. Tissues are cut at room temperature, but a cool, nonhumid room makes cutting easier. The sections are cut on a rotary microtome at 10 μm. The block edges must be parallel to the cutting edge of the knife. Wade (1952) suggests exposing the block to the air for several days if the sections do not ribbon or break up on handling. The moisture from placing a finger on the block briefly may make the sections ribbon.

Mounting sections. There are problems in mounting these sections to produce a wrinkle-free good histologic preparation, since the medium dissolves and the tissue disintegrates when placed in water. The literature contains various solutions to combat this problem:

Black and McCarthy method (1950)

Potassium dichromate	0.2 gm
Gelatin	0.2 gm
Distilled water	1 liter

Boil for 5 minutes and filter. Float the section on the solution, pick up on slide, and allow to dry.

Wade method (1952). Wade suggests using Tergitol 7 in distilled water to make a 0.005% solution and adds 10% of Carbowax 1540 to reduce shrinkage while the sections are drying.

Jones, Thomas, Wilbur, and O'Neal method (1959)

Diethylene glycol	100 ml
Formalin	7 ml
Carbowax	1 ml
Distilled water	400 ml

Float the sections on the solution. If greater spreading is desired, increase the water proportion.

Agar embedding

Tissues are infiltrated from water in melted 2% agar at 55° to 60° C for 2 to 4 hours. The mass becomes stiff on cooling and sections are cut on the clinical freezing microtome. It holds exudates and friable tissue in place and does not stain appreciably with commonly used stains.

OCT embedding

OCT is a water-soluble embedding medium, leaves no residue to discolor the section or slide, and freezes quickly in liquid nitrogen. A small amount of OCT is placed on the object holder and dipped in liquid nitrogen for slight freezing. It is removed from the liquid nitrogen and the tissue is carefully placed in the center of the compound. Additional OCT is placed around and over the tissue. The tissue is then frozen solidly in the liquid nitrogen, and the frozen sections are cut on the microtome cryostat. All tissues for rapid frozen section diagnosis and for histochemistry are frozen in OCT, with good success, in our laboratory.

WINKLER'S* METHOD OF PROCESSING NEEDLE BIOPSIES OF KIDNEY

All needle biopsies are hand processed. They are sent to the laboratory in 4% paraformaldehyde in 0.1 cacodylate, pH 7.3, and kept in this fixative overnight in the refrigerator.

The tissue is placed on a 1 × 2 inch strip of no. 237 Garland paper towel, folded, and put in a Lipshaw no. 331 Micro Tissue Capsule.

1.	50% alcohol	9 min
2.	80% alcohol	9 min
3.	95% alcohol	9 min
4.	Absolute alcohol	9 min
5.	Absolute alcohol	9 min
6.	Absolute alcohol	9 min
7.	Benzene	9 min
8.	Benzene	9 min
9.	Benzene	9 min
10.	Paraplast	10 min
11.	Paraplast	10 min
12.	Embed in filtered Paraplast in Peel-A-Way† disposable embedding molds (12 mm square truncated).	

Blocks are chilled on cooling plate and transferred to the Timsstation cooling unit.

Sections are cut at 2 μm by use of the Leitz Rotary Microtome and floated on a water bath and mounted on slides. For affixing sections to the slides, 0.25% plain agar adhesive is added to the heated water.

Plain agar adhesive‡

1. Prepare a solution of plain agar (0.25% in distilled water, with a few crystals of thymol.
2. Heat the solution in order to dissolve all the agar, and pour 45 ml of this into a 2750 ml Technicon water bath.

Preparation of fixative

1. Stock solution of 0.2 M sodium cacodylate acid, from its salt form $(CH_3)_2AsO_2Na \cdot 3H_2O$, 42.78 gm in 1 liter of deionized water.

*Rosemarie C. Winkler, Laboratory of Histopathology, Department of Pathology, University of Texas Medical Branch, Galveston, Texas.
†See p. 68.
‡Technical Bulletin of the Registry of Medical Technologists **38:**207, 1962.

Heat to dissolve and store in Pyrex bottle. May be kept at room temperature.

2. Stock solution of paraformaldehyde in 0.1 M cacodylate. Add 8 gm of paraformaldehyde to 100 ml of distilled water. Cover with watch glass or aluminum foil and heat on stirring plate. Add a few drops of NaOH to clear the solution. Cool and then add 100 ml of

0.2 M cacodylate stock and adjust the pH to 7.3. Yield is 200 ml of 4% paraformaldehyde in 0.1 M sodium cacodylate, which is conveniently kept in the refrigerator. Tissues may be kept in this solution for several weeks, as fixation time does not appear to be critical. See p. 444 for some products and the companies that manufacture them.

TISSUE-HANDLING CHART

How to ship tissue

1. *Important. Fresh tissue* should not be shipped because it would autolyze.
2. *Fixed tissue* remains in the fixative in a small glass vial sealed with paraffin *or* in a metal container sealed with paraffin *or* in a sealed polyethylene bag. Place the sealed bag in a second polyethylene bag, wrap securely in newspaper, and place in a box for mailing. Be sure the address and telephone number are on the inside as well as on the outside of the box. Mark box *fragile* and mail by safest method.
3. *Frozen tissue* is placed in a small polyethylene bag that is placed in a larger polyethylene bag tightly packed with large pieces of dry ice packed abundantly around the specimen. Wrap securely in newspaper. Place in a box and wrap securely with address and telephone number on the inside and outside of package. *Use fastest* delivery service to deliver package.

How to fix a specimen for electron microscopy

1. Zamboni's fluid (PAF) is the fixative of choice for electron microscopy. It contains PAF, that is, picric acid and paraformaldehyde, with a controlled pH and osmolarity. The fixative is very stable—up to a year at room temperature.
2. Pieces of tissue should be small, no more than 2 mm in any dimension, and should be placed in fixative very rapidly after the biopsy is taken. Fixation is done at room temperature and the tissue may remain in the fixative indefinitely without harm. One of the advantages of Zamboni's fixation is that the tissue may be used for both light as well as electron microscopy after this fixative. (See fixative solutions for electron microscopy, pp. 48, 328, and 329.)
3. Although Zamboni's is the preferred method, if it is not available, the tissue can be fixed in 2% glutaraldehyde in a cacodylate buffer. This is a more common fixative, can be pre-

pared more quickly, and may be more readily available. Fixation is done in the refrigerator; so the specimen is sent to the laboratory in ice (not Dry Ice). *Tissue cannot* remain in the glutaraldehyde fixative indefinitely, and if the specimen is not sent the same day, it should be removed from the fixative solution and placed in 5% sucrose in cacodylate buffer. (See fixative solutions, pp. 48 and 330.) This is a storage solution, and the remaining tissue can remain in it indefinitely. Tissue should *not remain in glutaraldehyde more than 5 hours*. Tissue in the sucrose solution should also be stored in the refrigerator and sent in ice (not Dry Ice).

How to handle lymph nodes

1. If the nodes are grossly normal, bisect and submit both halves after fixing the tissue in Bouin's fluid overnight.
2. If the nodes are grossly abnormal:
   a. Make a fresh cut through unfixed node to get a surface for touch preparations.
   b. *Rapidly fix* two or three touch preparations in acetone for H & E staining.
   c. Obtain five or six touch preparations of cut surface of node and air-dry them. Stain one with the Sheehan-Giemsa stain and refrigerate the remainder. Hold these latter slides until the case is signed out, if needed, for potential cytochemical procedures.
   d. If the node is small (less than 1 cm) submit both halves after overnight fixation in Bouin's fluid.
   e. If the node is larger than 1 cm, cut longitudinally or transversely at 2 mm intervals and submit the entire specimen (or at least three representative samples, if greater than 3 cm) after overnight fixation in Bouin's fluid.
   f. Obtain microbiologic cultures as indicated (suppuration, caseation, and so forth) if this has not been performed in the operating room.

Continued.

TISSUE-HANDLING CHART—cont'd

g. After overnight fixation process, embed in paraffin and cut sections at 3 μm.

How to handle a bone marrow biopsy

1. *The fixative used is very important.*
2. Submit entire needle biopsy after fixation in Bouin's fluid overnight, which is mildly acid and removes calcium.
3. Process and embed in Tissueprep.
4. Serially number eight slides and cut sections at 4 μm.
5. Stain slides 1 and 5 with H & E, slides 2 and 6 with Sheehan-Giemsa; 3 and 7 with iron; 4 and 8 with periodic acid–Schiff.

How to handle bone marrow for lymphoma staging or metastatic carcinoma

1. Cut 10 levels on numbered slides with one stained by H & E and one unstained at each level (for special histochemistry as required) plus Sheehan-Giemsa, periodic acid–Schiff, and iron at one random level.

How to handle a gastrointestinal biopsy

1. Fix in Bouin's fluid and process for embedding in Tissueprep.
2. Cut sections at 4 μm serially on slides numbered 1 to 9.
3. Stain sections 1, 3, 7, and 9 with H & E stain, but section 5 with alcian blue–periodic acid Schiff. The latter stain is a sensitive indicator of acid mucopolipaccharides, such as is produced in the presence of chronic gastritis and certain tumors.

How to handle plastic embedding of bone for metabolic bone disease

Use JB-4 Embedding Kit Cat. no. 0226B (Polyscience Inc.).
1. Tissue is undecalcified bone.
2. Maximum size 1 × 0.3 × 0.2 cm.
3. Fixation (see special fixative, p. 48) 20 times bone volume.
4. Store tissue in 70% alcohol.
5. *Process*
   2 changes of 95% alcohol for 30 minutes each.
   3 changes of absolute alcohol for 30 minutes each.
   If possible, use longer times for hard cortical bone.
6. *Infiltrate.* Use magnetic stirrer to dissolve 0.045 mg of catalyst in 5 ml of solution A.
7. *Embedding solution* (enough for two specimens):

Catalyst	0.045 mg
Solution A	5 ml
Solution B	7 drops

Keep solution B in refrigerator and warm with hand to dropping stage; embed tissue in embedding solution, pour liquid paraffin over the mold, and pivot to seal air out. Let stand overnight at room temperature.

Cutting

See cutting chart, pp. 83 to 85.

How to handle a kidney needle biopsy

1. Needle core biopsies are delivered to the laboratory immediately in a fresh state.
2. For any needle biopsy of reasonable length, that is, greater than 5 mm, cut with a single stroke approximately 15% off each end of the core for immunofluorescence. The longer, central portion of the core, that is, 70%, is put directly into Zamboni's solution for *3 hours.* This portion is cut in half longitudinally and both pieces are fixed overnight in Zamboni's fixative for light and electron microscopy. This longitudinal cut must be done after fixation because if it is done before fixation, the tissue will be crushed. If less than 5 mm, place the whole specimen in Zamboni's fixative.
3. For *immunofluorescence* the two end pieces are embedded in Lab Tek OCT (or similar) on a metal cryostat check. A sufficient amount of the embedding material should be used below, around, and above the specimen. The tissue should not be allowed to dry before freezing, and it should not be placed in any type of fixative.
4. For *light microscopy,* wrap one of the longitudinal pieces in lens paper next morning and process on a 4-hour cycle and embed in Tissueprep. Cut 15 sections at 2 μm on numbered slides and routinely do the following special stains:
   H & E nos. 1 and 15
   Periodic acid–Schiff nos. 2 and 14
   Periodic acid–silver methenamine
   Congo red and thioflavine T (Cut sections at 9 to 10 μm. Use of 2 μm sections for these stains would give a false negative or produce inconclusive results.)
   Trichrome
   Keep all other slides for further special stain requests.
5. For *electron microscopy* send second longitudinal piece of tissue to electron microscopy lab in Zamboni's fixative.

TISSUE-HANDLING CHART—cont'd

6. *OSU (Ohio State University) method for renal biopsies:* Place saline or Ringer's solution–moistened needle biopsy on an alcohol-cleaned glass slide, place on microscope, and examine using 10× objective. Check for tiny red dotlike areas; these are most likely glomeruli. Divide the biopsy according to the pathologist's desired priorities. This method gives a better chance to get glomeruli in all sections, that is, by light, immunofluorescence, and electron microscopies. It also eliminates the possibility of getting any fatty tissue that would be useless for diagnosis.

How to handle a liver needle biopsy

1. These should be wrapped in lens paper that is wet with fixative to prevent the tissue from sticking to the paper and fixed overnight in Bouin's fluid.
2. The tissue is processed on a 4-hour cycle on a vacuum processor or by the Winkler method if a vacuum processor is not available. Embed tissue in Tissueprep or similar paraffin-like substance. Cut 20 consecutively numbered sections at 4 μm for best demonstration of liver architecture.
3. The battery of special stains includes trichromes for detecting less obvious areas of fibrosis; iron, for iron storage, and reticulin, for general architecture. The aldehyde fuchsin and orcein are done for positivity on cells bearing hepatitis B and antigen. If the clinical information indicates a search for granulomatous hepatitis, multiple other levels are cut to save time since granulomas may be absent in one cut and obvious in another deeper cut in the same block.
   H & E nos. 1 and 15
   Special stains
       Periodic acid–Schiff nos. 2 and 14
       Trichrome
       Iron
       Reticulin
       Orcein
       Aldehyde fuchsin

How to handle a small intestine biopsy

1. These are received in the laboratory already oriented on plastic mesh in Bouin's fluid. Leave the specimen on the mesh where it remains to the embedding stage. The mesh, of course, must be removed prior to embedding and the tissue must be embedded on edge.
2. The tissue is looked at under the dissection microscope for the gross appearance of villi or lack thereof.
3. Nine serial sections are cut at 4 μm and placed on numbered slides well within the block.
4. H & E stains are done on sections 1, 3, 5, 7, and 9. Periodic acid–Schiff stains are done on sections 2 and 6. PAS is useful for general mucin secretion and to detect PAS-positive macrophages, including those of Whipple's disease, which may be in the lamina propria. Trichrome is done on sections 4 and 8. Trichrome, in addition to indicating the relation of collagen to the remainder of the biopsy, is useful in the search for *Giardia,* which stains better with Trichrome than it does with H & E.
5. *Alternate embedding suggestion for small intestine biopsy.* Tissue can also be embedded with villi parallel to the bottom of the block and 90 degrees to the vertical edge of the block. The block is then turned 90 degrees and placed in the chuck so that the knife-edge cuts from the base toward the free edge of the villi. This prevents excessive compression of the villi on the finished slide.

How to handle bone

1. To study undecalcified sections of bone biopsies of patients with various bone diseases, such as osteomalacia, osteoporosis, and renal osteodystrophy.
2. To study thin sections of tissue in which fine cellular detail is of special interest, such as *bone marrow biopsies* and *unusual tumors.*

Technical

1. *To avoid any decalcification of bone,* bone must be fixed in formalin to pH 7.35 (see fixation, p. 48). *This is critical in cases of metabolic bone disease.*
2. Bouin's fixation of bone marrow biopsies for *hemotologic* reasons will give better cytologic details and loss of bone calcium is useful.
3. Maximum specimen size is 1 × 0.3 × 0.2 cm.
4. For best sampling, bone biopsies for metabolic bone disease are longitudinally sectioned with a (Dremel) high-speed hard-bone hand saw before fixation is completed.
5. Specimens may remain in fixative indefinitely prior to processing. See processing and cutting plastics.

Continued.

TISSUE-HANDLING CHART—cont'd

How to handle a transbronchial lung biopsy

1. *Purpose*—diagnostic yield increased and diagnostic time decreased.

Technical

1. To provide levels through most of the block, since some lesions show up only in deeper cuts of the block.
2. To promptly provide those special stains likely to be useful in these biopsies.
3. To reserve some unsatined slides for other special stains or to repeat special stains when the initial ones are done at an inappropriate level.
   a. Fix tissue in Bouin's fluid several hours, process, and embed in Tissueprep.

b. Number 20 slides 1 to 20 and cut sections at 5 μm.
c. Stain as follows:
   Slides 2, 6, 11, 15, 20 with H & E
   Slides 7 and 13 with trichrome

If requested
Acid-fast and auramine-rhodamine

Slides 16 and 18   Slides 17 and 19
   (These must be serial.)
Grocott for *Pneumocystis*
   Slides 4 and 12
Brown-Brenn-Gram stain
   Slides 5 and 10
Unstained
   Slides 1, 8, 14

REFERENCES

Gray, P.: The microtomist's formulary and guide, New York, 1954, The Blakiston Co. (McGraw-Hill Book Co.).

Lillie, R. D.: Histopathologic technic and practical histochemistry, New York, 1965, McGraw-Hill Book Co.

Luna, L. G.: Manual of histologic and special staining technics, ed. 3, New York, 1963, McGraw-Hill Book Co.

References for Carbowax embedding

Blank, H., and McCarthy, P. A.: General method for preparing histologic sections with a water-soluble wax, J. Lab. Clin. Med. **36:**776, 1950.

Firminger, H. I.: Carbowax embedding for obtaining thin tissue sections and study of intracellular lipids, Stain Technol. **25:**121, 1950.

Jones, R. M., Thomas, W. A., Wilber, A., and O'Neal, R. M.: Embedding of tissues in Carbowax, Tech. Bull. Reg. Med. Tech. **29:**49, 1959.

McCormick, J. B.: Improved tissue embedding method for paraffin and Carbowax, Tech. Bull. Reg. Med. Tech. **29:**15, 1959.

Wade, H. W.: Notes on the Carbowax method of making tissue sections, Stain Technol. **27:**71, 1952.

CHAPTER 4

Sectioning

MICROTOMY

Microtomy is an art. All the pages printed cannot teach this very important art, since it must be learned by experience in the histopathology laboratory. It is here that the well-trained experienced histotechnologist stands out in sharp contrast against those with poor training, for she recognizes the difficulty, what caused it, and how it can be remedied.

Successful sectioning of tissue has four requirements:

1. *A skilled technologist.* Most of the problems of sectioning should be eliminated in the future when the histotechnologists, who are part of the laboratory team, have been trained in CAHEA approved schools. When on-the-job training is no longer the norm, students will be taught the why, when, where, and how of tissue technology and the importance of their work in the total care of the patient.

2. *A sharp microtome knife.* The microtome knife is an extremely important instrument in the histopathology laboratory. A well-sharpened, good-quality microtome knife may, at times, section poorly prepared material. A poor knife never produces good sections of perfectly prepared tissue.

3. *A proper microtome.* Different kinds of microtomes are available for different uses (see Chapter 1). These are precision instruments and require good care to give many years of service. Unless the microtome is abused, mistreated, rusty, caked with paraffin and dirt, and left unoiled, it is rarely, if ever, the cause of poor sections.

4. *Properly prepared material.* Specimens from surgery, for rapid diagnosis, section

better if frozen in OCT rather than in water. Other specimens require extensive fixation, dehydration, clearing, and embedding in a supporting medium that must match the physical characteristics of the specimen and have properties suitable for the cutting procedure to be used.

SECTIONING DIFFICULTIES

Tables 4-1 to 4-3 should help the technologist overcome many of the common difficulties. Since the microtome is rarely the cause of poor sections unless it is old, damaged, or obviously worn out, they should aid the technologist in overcoming difficulty in sectioning.

The process of sectioning paraffin-embedded material leads to distortion so that the sections are a little bit thicker and a little shorter than the block itself. The distortion results from the following:

1. Nature of the paraffin
2. Nature of the tissue
3. Action of the microtome knife

Different paraffins have different plastic points. The plastic point is the lowest temperature at which permanent deformation may be made without fracture. A paraffin with a low plastic point appears more translucent, is less brittle, but compresses more in sectioning than does one with a higher point. The hardness of the paraffin depends on its plastic point, which lies a few but variable number of degrees below the melting point. Large crystals are sectioned or pushed apart by the wedging of the knife, especially when the paraffin is brittle and has a high plastic point. This upsetting of crystals gives the smooth and velvety appearance to the topside of the sections as the ribbon is laid on the water. When the crystals are not of proper size to fit closely to the tissue, they cannot support it adequately and a section will be cut that cannot be completely flattened out. A fine crystalline paraffin gives adequate support, whereas a paraffin with large crystals produces artifacts in sections. Warm paraffin

79

Table 4-1. Difficulties common to all methods

Difficulty	Correction
Irregular sections, skipped sections, or thick and thin sections	These are usually the result of insufficient tilt of the knife, which compresses the block on the return stroke, or of too much tilt, which scrapes off the section instead of cutting it. Turn the knife holder to give the proper clearance angle between the cutting facet of the knife and the specimen.
Scored, grooved, smeared, and deformed sections	These are caused by a dull knife. Resharpen.
Regular, lengthwise scratches and splits in sections	These are caused by a defect in the knife edge or by dirt or hard material in the specimen. Moving the knife to an unused region, or replacing with a sharper knife, may restore good sectioning.
Sections fall out of matrix or show an amount of compression different from the embedding medium frame	Embedding medium is inadequate. Try different medium for embedding.
Mushy-appearing sections indicate insufficient dehydration or clearing	Sections of tissue that have not been dehydrated properly can rarely be salvaged. If the clearing agent has not been removed completely, return the tissue to several changes of paraffin and reembed. If sections are mushy in the celloidin technic, they can rarely, if ever, be salvaged, and new tissue must be processed.

Table 4-2. Difficulties common to paraffin-embedded material

Difficulty	Cause	Remedy
Ribbon fails to form	Room too cold or paraffin too hard.	Use lower melting point paraffin. Breath on knife and warm it slightly. Place a desk lamp so that light and heat fall on the knife and block.
	Knife tilt too great.	Tilt the knife less.
	Sections too thick.	Cut thinner sections.
	Knife is dull.	Resharpen. Unroll a section and hold it lightly against the knife with a camel's hair brush; if the first few sections can be held down, the ribbon will often form and follow.
Crooked ribbons	Blocks not trimmed parallel.	Trim blocks parallel or reembed in molds so that the edge of block is parallel to knife edge.
	Irregularity of knife edge.	Try another part of knife edge.
	Paraffin may be softer on one side of block.	Reembed the tissue and stir the melted paraffin.
	One side of block may be warmer than the other from a radiator, lamp, or draft.	Relocate microtome for uniform temperature. Cool block in ice water.
Sections vary in thickness or are skipped	Knife not tilted enough to clear facet or bevel, or tilted too much, and tissue is compressed until the inevitable expansion gives a thick section.	Retilt knife either more or less.
	Clamping set screws are loose.	Retighten.
	Knife block holder is loose.	Clamp firmly.
	Microtome worn through lack of lubrication, or not in adjustment.	Have microtome checked by manufacturer.

Table 4-2. Difficulties common to paraffin-embedded material—cont'd

Difficulty	Cause	Remedy
	Very large blocks, or blocks with hard regions, may spring knife edge while sectioning.	Soak in water or a solution of 9 parts of glycerin to 1 part of aniline oil for 30 minutes; if specimen is embedded in a plastic mold, be careful to keep the mold out of the solution.
Sections compressed, wrinkled, or jammed together	Knife too dull.	Resharpen.
	Room too warm.	Cool block in ice water.
	Knife tilt too slight.	Increase tilt.
	Knife edge gummed with paraffin.	Remove with facial tissue soaked with xylene and remove xylene with another facial tissue soaked with absolute alcohol.
	Cutting too rapidly.	Very thin sections should be cut slowly and evenly.
Sections crumble and specimen may tear out	Material incompletely dehydrated or not completely cleared.	Salvage rarely possible if material was incompletely dehydrated.
	Soft and mushy material incompletely infiltrated with embedding medium.	Reinfiltrate with paraffin and reembed.
	Object too long in paraffin bath or bath too hot.	Check thermostatically controlled paraffin baths daily and record temperatures.
	Subject hard and brittle because of clearing fluid.	Try chloroform or toluene instead of xylene for clearing, or a mixture of toluene and cedar oil.
	When the specimen shatters and falls out of the wax, it is too hard for paraffin.	Use a harder wax or wax mixture.
A split ribbon or lengthwise scratches in ribbon	Nicks in knife.	Resharpen.
	Too much tilt.	Use less tilt of knife so that it will cut rather than scrape.
	Knife edge dirty.	Clean as previously recommended.
	Object too hard for paraffin.	Use celloidin embedding.
	Hard particles in block may cause scratching.	Dirt in paraffin; refilter.
	Crystals from mercuric chloride fixation.	Washing was insufficient.
	Calcareous or silicious particles.	Decalcify or desilicify.
Knife rings on up stroke and sections are scratched	Knife tilt too great or too little.	Change knife tilt.
	Material is too hard.	Soak in water to soften.
	Material is too tough for paraffin method.	Try celloidin.
Sections lifted from knife on upstroke	Not enough knife tilt.	Increase knife tilt.
	Room too warm or paraffin too soft.	Try harder paraffin, cooler room, or cool block.
	Knife dull.	Resharpen.
Sections stick to knife	Knife edge dirty.	Clean with xylene and alcohol as previously described.
	Knife tilt too little.	Increase tilt.
	Knife dull.	Resharpen.
Undulations in the surface of the section	Set screws loose.	Tighten all screws.
	Knife holder loose.	Clamp tightly.
	Excessive knife tilt.	Decrease knife tilt.
Scratching noise during cutting	Material may be too hard.	Try celloidin embedding.
Sections fly and stick to parts of microtome or other nearby objects	Static electricity.	Boil water in open pan.
		Burn a Bunsen burner.
		Ground microtome to a water pipe with wire or chain.
		Ionize the air by an electrical method.

Table 4-3. Difficulties common to celloidin-embedded material

Difficulty	Correction
Improperly prepared material	Inadequate impregnation or inadequate dehydration prior to impregnation, as well as improperly hardened blocks, make it impossible to get good sections, start over with new tissue.
Lengthwise scratches or splits in the section	Nicks in the knife. Use a different portion of the knife or resharpen it. These may be caused by dirt in the stock solution; filter it. Or if too much calcium in the tissue, decalcify it.
Specimen falls out of the section	Dehydration was incomplete. Infiltration was incomplete. Hardening was incomplete. Tissue may be reinfiltrated and rehardened but never redehydrated.
Variation in thickness of section	Loose set screws or block holder on microtome; tighten all screws. Do not use pressure on the knife holder since this may depress the section and raise it while sectioning. Knife is not tilted enough to clear the facet of the cutting bevel. Knife is dull. Microtome is worn and out of adjustment. Material is not properly hardened; reharden. Do not let block dry out during sectioning. Slight drying will give this variation.

shrinks as it cools and compresses the tissue in the block. Tissue that is harder than the paraffin withstands this pressure, but soft or spongy tissue may be under considerable strain. When sectioned, the tissue tends to expand to the shape and size it had before compression, and if the tissue is confined by the paraffin around it, pleating or wrinkling results.

The melting point of paraffin therefore has to be adapted to the climate in which you live or the temperature at which sectioning is done. Additionally, it must be matched to the hardness of the tissue, which, for the most part, depends on the fixation, dehydration, and clearing of the tissue, as well as the temperature at which it is impregnated with the paraffin.

Unless the hardness of the paraffin is adapted to the temperature at which the cutting is done and to the nature of the tissue, good sections cannot be made, regardless of the excellence of the microtome and the microtome knife. If the tissue has been properly dehydrated and cleared, it is possible to reembed it in another paraffin, after several changes to wash out the old paraffin. If it has not been properly fixed, dehydrated, and cleared, salvage is rarely possible.

The microtome knife should be set and tilted to as little clearance angle as possible to give good sections. The clearance angle should be within 3 to 8 degrees. The knife edge should not show any definite serrations when examined with the microscope at 100 diameters.

A wooden cradle, available from American Optical Company, may be used for this, or the knife may be carefully laid on a piece of smooth white paper on the stage of the microscope. The only effective test is whether the knife cuts the tissue properly. Testing the knife by any other means merely dulls the edge in the process of testing.

March (1878) observed: "Of not less importance than the microtome is the section knife, to be used in conjunction with it. How perfect soever the former, and whatever the dexterity of the operator, unless he is provided with a suitable, well made knife, he will never succeed in obtaining satisfactory results." His statement is still true, and written direction cannot take the place of experience in learning to sharpen a knife. It is an art that must be learned if the knifes must be sharpened in the laboratory. With the high cost of technical time and the use of this time to its greatest advantage in the many technical procedures in the modern histopathology laboratory, we recommend commercial sharpening of microtome knives. (See section on microtome knives, p. 21.)

Routine paraffin sections are cut at 4 to 6 μm. A micrometer (formerly micron) is 1/1000 of a millimeter or 1/25,400 of an inch. Tissue to be stained for amyloid is cut at 10 μm, since small deposits of amyloid are demonstrated at this thickness. Tissues for the demonstration of myelin sheath are cut at 10 to 15 μm. Renal biopsies are cut at 2 to 4 μm.

FROZEN SECTIONS

Frozen sectioning of either fixed or fresh tissue may be accomplished by the use of either the clinical (standard) freezing microtome or the cryostat. The various planes for sectioning are shown in Fig. 4-1.

Refer to pp. 14 and 15 for sectioning and instrument information.

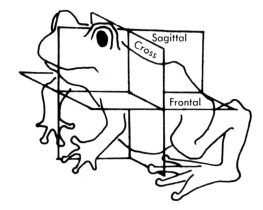

Fig. 4-1. Cross-section, sagittal-section, frontal-section embedding and sectioning.

TISSUE-HANDLING CHART FOR SECTIONING

Important points in cutting paraffin-embedded material

1. The block must be trimmed so that edges parallel to the knife are straight and parallel to each other. If this is not done, the ribbon will not be straight and distortion will be increased.
2. A camel's hair brush, a fine-eye forceps, or a dissecting needle, may be used to handle the ribbon as it comes off the microtome knife. We have found a fine-eye forceps excellent for this step, since it may also be used to remove bubbles when placed underneath the ribbon on the water bath to break the bubble. It is also excellent for removing fine wrinkles from the tissue on the water bath.
3. An intermediate step between the cutting of the ribbon and the water bath prevents wrinkling on the water bath. Fill a staining dish with distilled water and 95% alcohol (5 ml of 95% alcohol to 95 ml of distilled water). Float the ribbon on this solution prior to floating it on the warm water bath.
4. The temperature of the water bath should be 5 to 10 degrees below the melting point of the embedding medium, depending on the rapidity with which the technologist removes the tissue from the water bath. The bath is usually kept at 47° to 51° C, and a thermometer should be kept in the water bath while cutting is being done.
5. A thin coating of egg albumen glycerin is rubbed on the slide before the tissue is picked up. When the slides are dried, prior to staining, the albumen coagulates and sets the tissue firmly against the slide. Alternately, another method is to add ¼ teaspoon of U.S.P. gelatin to the warm water bath before the sections are floated on the water.
6. Avoid too much egg albumen. Thick albumen stains and makes a messy histologic preparation.
7. Tissues that cut well rarely come loose from the slides during staining. The exception is the tissue from the central nervous system and those for silver impregnation technics. The high alkalinity of the silver solutions will, at times, float the tissue off the slide. These may be coated with celloidin prior to staining.
   a. Remove the paraffin with xylene and place the slide in absolute alcohol for 2 minutes.
   b. Place the slide in 0.5% celloidin in ether alcohol 1:1 for 2 minutes.
   c. Drain off excess celloidin and place the slide in 80% alcohol for 5 minutes to harden the celloidin, prior to staining.
8. Be sure to tighten all set screws on the microtome to prevent undulations and thick and thin sections.
9. The water bath must be kept scrupulously clean and should be cleaned thoroughly after each block is cleaned. Kimwipes are excellent for this purpose. *Floaters are dangerous*—the result of carelessness.

Continued.

TISSUE-HANDLING CHART FOR SECTIONING—cont'd

10. Sections should be cut at a slow or moderately even pace. The rapid turning of the wheel cuts a ribbon of thick sections. A student may make a test by cutting a ribbon rapidly and laying it on the water bath with one cut at a slow even pace. The rapidly cut ribbon appears thick to the naked eye.

11. The technologist is frequently requested to cut a cross section, a sagittal section, or a frontal section of tissue. The embedding and cutting of cross, sagittal, and frontal sections is demonstrated in Fig. 4-1.

12. When ribbons fail to form, it may be the result of too slow a cutting speed, but too fast a cutting speed may cause the same defect or excessive wrinkling of the sections.

13. The crystalline structure of the wax will exert an influence on the quality of sections. Do not keep wax for prolonged periods in an oven or paraffin vat since it can lose its low melting point fractions and present difficulties in ribboning.

14. The quality of the sections you obtain is influenced by the degree of crystallinity of the wax in which you embed the tissue. A fine crystalline wax is preferred. Large and nonhomogeneous crystals in wax are detrimental to good sectioning. *Embedded blocks* must be cooled rapidly to prevent the formation of large crystals in the wax, and any trace of the clearing agent will result in large crystal formation.

15. When cutting bone sections, do not have the microtome knife enter the bone on the long axis. Embed the bone in the manner shown in Fig. 3-9, *B*, so that you enter the block at a small corner to cut better sections.

16. Be sure to remove the oil from your knife with xylene and remove the xylene with absolute alcohol before you start to cut sections.

17. If the problem is too hard a block, and softening is required to permit sectioning, then one of the following ways may be tried:
    a. The block may be faced off (paraffin removed) and placed in water for several hours to several days.
    b. Place the block in a solution of 9 parts of 60% ethanol and 1 part of glycerol for a few hours or days.
    c. Place the block in a solution of 9 parts of glycerol and 1 part of aniline. Be careful of using glycerol, since it could prevent the tissue from sticking to the slide flatly.
    d. The detergent "Joy" may be used in a 1% aqueous solution for a few hours or overnight.

18. To facilitate sectioning after the block has been faced off to the tissue level, hold a piece of cotton or facial tissue paper soaked in ice water against the face of the block, or directly apply an ice cube to the block surface. *Caution:* Crank the block back slightly or the first section will be too thick.

19. When cutting tissue like thyroid, use the alternate heat and cool method. Cool the block with the ice-cooled tissue paper and alternately heat it by dipping your thumb in warm water and and holding it against the block. Repeat several times until you get a good ribbon.

20. *Section levels*
    It is important when cutting small biopsies to cut them at several levels. The *first level* should be taken when you first reach the tissue. *Do not shave off the tissue.* Carefully cut into the block and take a ribbon of first-level sections. *Ribbon off 10* sections and take the second level ribbon. Carefully cut into the block (using the adjustment screws) until the ribbon matches the tissue in the block. When this happens, you have a full level for your third section.

21. *Serial sections*
    When preparing serial sections, slides are numbered, consecutively, and section ribbons are flattened and mounted on the slides from left to right. If the block is small enough, two ribbons are mounted on each slide from left to right. All sections are used after they are cut serially; so it is important to avoid wrinkles, if possible, since these cannot be eliminated from a serial section set. Remember to move the block back between ribbons to avoid losing any of the tissue.

22. *Affixing sections to slides with Mayer's albumen fixative*
    Prepared solution is economical to buy but may be made in the laboratory.
    a. Beat egg white until broken up but not stiff. Let stand overnight.
    b. Measure liquid from bottom of cylinder and add an equal volume of glycerin.
    c. Add a grain of thymol and filter through glass wool.

TISSUE-HANDLING CHART FOR SECTIONING—cont'd

When using Mayer's albumen fixative, you should rub a small amount over the surface of the slide. To avoid dead epithelial cells from the finger, use a small piece of plastic foam or a Lipshaw tissue capsule pad no. 845A.

23. *Gelatin in water bath*
    a. Drop ¼ teaspoon of U.S.P. gelatin into a clean hot water bath 47° C. The gelatin will dissolve in the water within a few minutes. Do not buy gelatin in large packets; buy it in small packets.
    b. Float sections on the water and pick them up on clean glass slides. Drain off water and dry.
       CAUTION:
       (1) Gelatin will pick up dyes if an excess of gelatin is used.
       (2) Gelatin may produce artifacts in some special stains.
       (3) When gelatin is used, the water bath must be kept scrupulously clean to avoid bacteria on tissue sections.

24. *How to section undecalcified bone*
    a. Use a Sorvall JB-4 Microtome with Micro-Macro Stage 45166 assembly and glass/diamond knife holder no. 45211.
    b. Insert the slide adaptor (45364) to hold the plastic block holder (45458).
    c. Put the glass knife in the knife holder and the block in the plastic block holder.
    d. Set the instrument to cut at 4 μm.
    e. Position magnifier-illuminator (No. 45314, DuPont Instruments–Sorvall, Newtown, Conn.) to view the cutting process.
    f. After cutting to desired level, take one section at a time using curved microdissecting forceps (Clay Adams, no. A1909; 6439). Hold the very tip of the plastic surrounding the section. Blow lightly and let the section fall to distilled water. Pick up on clean dry slide and place slide on hot surface at 50° C and let it dry. Use canned "Air It" (No. 11555-10, Matheson, Coleman & Belle, East Rutherford, N.J.) to clean away the excess sections and the debris on the knife. Be careful not to get forceps wet and do not touch the glass knife with the fingers since any moisture on plastic will cause it to stick.
    g. Place slides in 60° C oven overnight.
    h. Proceed with staining (p. 96). Eliminate xylene and hydration. Place slides directly into stains.
       Note: Glass knives may be made by using LKB knife maker style 7800 (LKB Instruments, Inc., Rockville, Md.) and following their instructions. Store glass knives in a dust-free container.

REFERENCE

Richards, O. W.: The effective use and proper care of the microtome, Buffalo, N.Y. 14215, 1959, American Optical Corporation, Scientific Instrument Division.

CHAPTER 5

Mounting media

General comments
Resinous mounting media
Aqueous mountants

GENERAL COMMENTS

The mounting of sections of stained tissue requires a medium:
1. To flow between the slide and the cover-slip
2. To fill the tissue and the tissue cavities
3. To release entrapped air bubbles
4. To dry to nonstickiness within a reasonably short period of time

The original resin mountants were natural resins such as Canada balsam and gum dammar, usually dissolved in xylene. These resins have the following detrimental characteristics:
1. Set slowly
2. Take months to dry to nonstickiness
3. Fade the eosin in hematoxylin and eosin stains within a few years
4. Are poor preservatives for basic aniline dyes
5. Fade Prussian blue preparations

Our experience and that of other histopathology laboratories during the past few years have led us to believe that the solvent of the resin is extremely important and that stained sections cleared in xylene prior to mounting should be mounted in a resin dissolved in xylene to avoid late aspiration of air bubbles. Lillie states that "it has been observed that highly volatile solvents, such as benzene and to a less extent toluene, are likely to produce air spaces under cover glasses because of their excessive evaporation. However, higher boiling solvents such as xylene, trimethylbenzene, and diethylbenzene are less likely to give rise to air bubbles."

In a surgical pathology laboratory, in a large teaching institution, it is not only important that slides be mounted without air bubbles, but that they remain so during the years in the files. Good technology requires this necessity in any size laboratory, since entrapped air bubbles dry out the tissue and spoil the histologic preparation.

The refractive index of the mountant is important and for stained sections should be close to that of the average refractive index of tissue (1.530 to 1.540) (Lillie). Lillie states that "the refractive index will lie between that of the solvent and the dry resin, and with the evaporation of the solvent, the refractive index of the mountant surrounding the tissue will gradually approach that of the dry resin." The natural resins such as Canada balsam and gum dammar are acid, whereas the synthetic resins, such as Permount,* Harleco synthetic resin, Bioloid synthetic resin, Technicon resin, Histoclad, and Namount are neutral.

RESINOUS MOUNTING MEDIA

Eukitt mounting medium has received laboratory approval for its hardening time of less than 20 minutes, its ability to spread quickly and evenly, and its unique technical characteristics.

Eukitt dissolves readily in the usual common lab solvents such as xylene, benzene, chloroform, propanol, and carbon tetrachloride. It spreads quickly and evenly without bubbles.

Eukitt is useful in Millipore filter preparations. As a solution it is slightly more viscous than most mountants; thus a higher percentage of resin and a predictably small degree of retraction is indicated. Its long molecules cause it to cohere within itself and to adhere to the slide and cover slip. Consequently, the final preparation is very stable, sets rapidly, and may be submitted to the cytotechnologist shortly after mounting without fear of dislocating the filter during screening and dotting.

The refractive index of Eukitt in the liquid state is 1.510.

It is useful in fluorescence dyes in bone (see Chapter 6).

The following chart gives the synthetic resins commonly used in histopathology laboratories.

---

*See p. 444 for obtaining this and following resins.

Table 5-1. Commonly used resins in histopathology laboratories

Resin	Refractive index		Advantages	Disadvantages
	Solution	**Dry**		
Harleco synthetic resin (HSR) (β-pinene polymer) 60% resin may be purchased dissolved in xylene or dissolved in toluene	1.5202	1.5390	**Excellent for** hematoxylin and eosin, Van Gieson's stain, Masson's trichrome, oxidative Schiff procedures **Very good for** azure in azure-eosin stains, fuchsin in Ziehl-Neelsen Cover glasses immovable in 1 hour; dries to nonstickiness in 1 day* This resin, dissolved in xylene, is excellent for routine work and most special stains	In our experience, if the resin is dissolved in toluene and slides are mounted from xylene, it gives rise to air bubbles, which are not a problem if the resin is dissolved in xylene "Appears to reduce Prussian blue to the greenish white ferrous ferrocyanide" (Lillie)
Fisher's Permount (β-pinene polymer) 60% resin in toluene	1.5144	1.5286	**Excellent for** H & E, Van Gieson's stains, Masson's trichrome, oxidative Schiff procedures Cover glasses immovable in 1 hour; dries to nonstickiness in 1 day* An excellent mountant for routine work and most special stains mounted from toluene	In our experience, if the resin is dissolved in toluene and slides are mounted from xylene, it gives rise to air bubbles "Appears to reduce Prussian blue to the greenish white ferrous ferrocyanide" (Lillie)
Willco Bioloid (β-pinene polymer) 60% resin in xylene	1.5272	1.5505	**Excellent for** hematoxylin, Masson's trichrome, hematoxylin–myelin sheath stains, oxidative Schiff procedures Dries to nonstickiness in 1 day except in high-humidity climates Does not form air bubbles in mounts	**Fair for** eosin **Poor for** fuchsin in Van Gieson's stain and fuchsin in Ziehl-Neelsen Takes 2 hours for cover-glass immovability
Technicon resin (coumarone-indene polymer) 60% resin in benzene:xylene 50:50	1.5649	1.6205	**Excellent for** H & E, azure-eosin stain, Nissl's thionin, Mann's methyl blue–eosin, fuchsin in Ziehl-Neelsen, fuchsin in Van Gieson's stain, hematoxylin–myelin sheath stains, oxidative Schiff procedures	**Fair for** methenamine silver **Complete fading** of ferric ferricyanide Tends to form air bubbles because of high volatility of benzene
Histoclad (a synthetic polymer) 60% resin in toluene	1.548	Not available	**Excellent for** routine H & E stains, Van Gieson, Masson's trichrome	In our experience, if resin is dissolved in toluene and slides are mounted from xylene, it gives rise to air bubbles
Namount (β-pinene polymer) 60% resin in xylene	1.53	1.5552	**Excellent for** H & E, azure-eosin, fuchsin in Ziehl-Neelsen, Masson's trichrome, oxidative Schiff procedures	**Fair for** eosin

*In high-humidity climate, slides should be dried for several weeks in drying file before permanent front-to-back filing.

Some of this material is from our own experience and some of it is from the "Final Report of the Committee on Histologic Mounting Media," *Stain Technology* (vol. 28, no. 2, March 1953). We refer you to this report for a complete listing, since only commonly used resins are charted.

AQUEOUS MOUNTANTS

Aqueous mountants are necessary to preserve tissue elements, such as fat, that are dissolved in alcohols and the hydrocarbons. They are also required for mounting of metachromatic stains such as crystal violet or methyl violet for amyloid. For many years we used the method recommended by Lieb (Am. J. Clin. Pathol. **17:** 413, 1947) and mounted the amyloid stains in Abopon. Since we are no longer able to purchase Abopon, our amyloid stains are mounted by the method of Miss Helen Futch.* The slides are

*Chief Histotechnologist, M. D. Anderson Hospital, Houston, Texas. (Personal correspondence, 1972.)

allowed to dry thoroughly, are briefly dipped in xylene, and mounted in HSR in xylene. There is no bleeding and the metachromasia of the amyloid is preserved.

Lillie (*Histopathologic Technic,* p. 103) gives an excellent chart on the composition and properties of water-miscible mounting media. In this chart he lists six mountants that are negative for bleeding of methyl violet.

Kaiser's glycerol gelatin may be purchased at a reasonable cost for mounting fat stains. These are ringed with clear fingernail polish to make a permanent mount.

REFERENCES

Gray, P.: The microtomist's formulary and guide, New York, 1954, The Blakiston Co. (McGraw-Hill Book Co.).

Lillie, R. D.: Histopathologic technic and practical histochemistry, ed. 3, New York, 1965, McGraw-Hill Book Co.

Bone

Part I. Decalcification

Before bone or any calcified tissue can be processed and sectioned with a routine microtome, the calcium salts must be removed by a process called "decalcification." Failure to decalcify tissue with large amounts of calcium salts will result in torn and ragged sectons and damage to the cutting edge of the microtome knife.

To ensure adequate fixation and decalcification, tissue selected should not exceed 4 or 5 mm in thickness. A fine-toothed hacksaw or the Buehler Isomet Low Speed Saw (Fig. 1-21) may be used to obtain thin slices of bone. At the completion of the decalcification process, the cut surfaces should be trimmed to remove the areas damaged by the saw in obtaining the specimen. When the marrow of cancellous bone is to be studied, time is saved and acid damage to the marrow cells reduced when the cortical bone is cut of as soon as the cancellous portion is soft enough.

Fixation is the next step after tissue selection and is usually performed before the actual decalcification process. Fixatives for bone and marrow should be chosen with the primary ob-

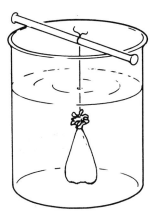

Fig. 6-1. Acid decalcification method. For best results, gauze-wrapped bone should be suspended in center of decalcifying fluid.

jective of study in mind and should have criteria similar to those used for soft-tissue fixatives. For routine diagnostic purposes, formalin is the fixative of choice. It is used unbuffered since the calcium phosphate present in the bone substance serves as an adequate buffer to keep the pH level of the fixative above 6.0 within the tissue and prevent the formation of formalin pigment. Nucleic acids are susceptible to ribonuclease digestion or digestion by mineral acids if formalin fixation is prolonged more than 2 days. Therefore formalin-fixed bone is best decalcified with 1 normal acetic or formic acid or with buffer mixtures of pH 2.0 or higher. Chromate fixatives such as Orth's, Kose's, and Möller's potassium dichromate formalin mixtures, and formalin-Zenker variants, are preferred by many for marrow cell study. These fixatives, or 1 normal hydrochloric or nitric acid, render nucleic acids less susceptible to hydrolysis either by ribonuclease or by acids and make the tissue moderately resistant.

Routine decalcification methods include those using (1) acids, (2) ion-exchange resins, and (3) electrical ionization. All these methods are greatly accelerated by heat. Heat, however, is not recommended since at 55° to 60° C the loss of calcium salts occurs rapidly, followed by swelling and hydrolysis of bone collagen, resulting in complete digestion of the tissue. This digestion will occur in about 24 hours with 8% hydrochloric acid, 24 hours with formic acid mixture, or 2 to 3 days with 5% formic acid. Decalcification at 37° C also causes undue swelling of tissue and may also impair subse-

quent staining processes. Alum hematoxylins, Weigert's iron hematoxylin, Feulgen reaction, and azure eosin stains are all impaired by decalcification at 37° C with formic-hydrochloric acid mixtures and by 5% formic acid. Five-percent formic acid may also impair Van Gieson and Masson trichrome staining results. Lillie states that when decalcification is performed at 15° to 20° C, satisfactory H & E, Van Gieson, Masson, and azure eosin stains are obtained with mineral acids, formic acid, and mixtures of both acids. Feulgen staining of nuclei is well preserved after formic acid decalcification at 24° C, but with mineral acids, even at a temperature of 3° C, this staining process is impaired.

DECALCIFICATION METHODS USING ACID SOLUTIONS

Acid solutions are most widely used for routine decalcification of large amounts of bone and calcified tissue. The principle underlying the action of acid decalcifying agents involves the solubilities of metallic salts. Calcium occurs in bones chiefly as the carbonate and phosphate salts, and these salts are only slightly soluble in water. An acid will act to release the calcium from its combination with the anions and effect an ion exchange to give a soluble calcium salt. For example, when hydrochloric acid is used as the decalcifying agent, the released calcium combines with the chloride ion to form calcium chloride, a soluble calcium salt. The calcium ions released will remain in the decalcifying solution itself and are effectively removed from the bone. The general technic to be followed when one employs acid decalcifying agents is as follows:

1. Selection of tissue (previously discussed).

2. Fixation (previously discussed). After fixation, the tissue is washed to remove excess fixative.

3. Decalcification. The selected tissue should be loosely wrapped in gauze and then suspended in the center of a large jar that is filled with the decalcifying fluid of choice (Fig. 6-1). About 100 times the volume of the tissue is a good approximate amount, and this large volume is necessary since the mineral content of a good-sized piece of bone will soon neutralize the small amount of acid present in the solution. Decalcifying fluids that may be used include aqueous or alcoholic solutions of the acids listed in Table 6-1. Although some authors claim that alcoholic solutions aid in preventing undue

Table 6-1. Acid decalcifying agents

Agent	Advantages	Disadvantages
Formic acid	5% formic acid is considered the best general decalcifying agent by Lillie. It is more economical than buffer mixtures and equally satisfactory and effective. It permits satisfactory nuclear and marrow cell staining when decalcification is performed at room temperature.	If decalcification is done at 37° C, alum hematoxylin staining and Weigert's iron hematoxylin staining of nuclei are impaired to some extent; Feulgen staining of nuclei is unsatisfactory and azure eosin stains give pink cytoplasm and nuclei. At 37° C, it also impairs Van Gieson and Masson staining of collagen and bone matrix.
Hydrochloric acid	Action is rapid, even in dilute solutions. This acid, when used at 37° C, preserves eosin stains of cytoplasm. When used at 15° to 25° C, satisfactory H & E, Van Gieson, Masson, and azure eosin stains may be done, if exposure is not prolonged. To remedy swelling of tissues, chromic acid or alcohol may be added to the solution. 15% NaCl may also be added to a 3% acid solution to counteract the swelling action.	Causes serious swelling of tissue. At 55° to 60° C loss of calcium salts occurs rapidly, followed by swelling and hydrolysis of bone matrix, which soon results in complete digestion. This occurs in as little as 24 hr in 8% hydrochloric acid. Decalcification at 37° C impairs alum hematoxylin staining and Weigert's iron hematoxylin staining of nuclei to some extent. Feulgen staining of nuclei is unsuccessful and azure eosin stains give pink cytoplasm and nuclei.
Sulfurous acid	Acts rapidly and preserves well. Best used after fixation in formalin.	If action is prolonged over 48 hours, nuclear staining is seriously impaired.
Nitric acid	Many writers highly recommend 5%, which causes no swelling and acts powerfully.	Even brief exposure to this acid renders unsatisfactory staining of bone marrow with Giemsa, Maximow's azure II-eosin or Lillie's azure eosin formula.
Trichloroacetic acid	4% solution gives energetic action, good preservation, and satisfactory nuclear and marrow staining.	Because of its high molecular weight, as compared with formic acid, much larger quantities are needed for efficient decalcification —it takes 3½ times more solution than formic acid.
Chromic acid		Weak decalcifying action and strong shrinking action. It should never be used in more than 1% solution.
Acetic, lactic, and picric acids		Usually unsatisfactory. Acetic and lactic acids have considerable decalcifying power, but cause great swelling. Picric acid has a very slow action and is suitable for very small structures.
Trifluoroacetic acid	A strong acid with powerful decalcifying properties, with a rapid action. Stains are good, bright, and sharp with little distortion of nuclear and cytoplasmic structure. Dense bone decalcified in 2 to 3 days in 10%, 5 to 6 days in 5%.	

swelling of the tissue, others believe that alcoholic solutions make inefficient decalcifying agents. Acids in 70% or 80% alcohol act slowly. A solution of 0.5 N hydrochloric acid in 70% or 80% alcohol decalcifies in 8 days at 25° C, compared with 4 days for the same concentration in 40% alcohol, and 2 days for the aqueous solution. Five-percent aqueous formic acid solutions will decalcify in 3 to 5 days; the same concentration in 30% alcohol will take 4 months; but the acid will not decalcify in several months in 80% alcohol. This delay occurs probably because the alcohol acts to suppress ionization, which in turn slows the ion-exchange reaction, rather than being caused by the insolubility of certain calcium salts in alcohol. Other formulas that may be used as acid decalcifying agents include those in Table 6-1.

Formulas for acid decalcifying agents

Von Ebner's hydrochloric acid–sodium chloride mixture

Concentrated hydrochloric acid (specific gravity 1.19)	15 ml
Sodium chloride	175 gm
Distilled water	1000 ml

During decalcification, add 1 ml of concentrated hydrochloric acid daily to each 200 ml of the above mixture, until decalcification is complete.

Richman-Gelfand-Hill formic-hydrochloric acid mixture

Concentrated formic acid (90%)	100 ml
Concentrated hydrochloric acid (specific gravity 1.19)	80 ml
Distilled water	820 ml

Kristensen's formula

1 N sodium formate (6.8%)	500 ml
8 N formic acid	500 ml

Evans and Krajian fluid

Sodium citrate crystals	10 gm
90% formic acid	25 ml
Distilled water	75 ml

Krajian's variant of Evans and Krajian fluid

85% formic acid	100 ml
95% ethanol (or 99% isopropanol)	100 ml
Sodium citrate crystals	20 gm
Trichloroacetic acid	1 gm
Distilled water	100 ml

For the rapid decalcification of bone, stronger solutions of nitric or hydrochloric acid may be used if employed in conjunction with phloroglucin. The phloroglucin acts, in a way not presently understood, to prevent organic constituents of bone from being injured by the swelling and macerating action of the strong acids. Some authors state that 40% nitric acid may be used with phloroglucin. A good mixture is the following:

Nitric acid	5 ml
Absolute alcohol	70 ml
Phloroglucin	1 gm
Distilled water	30 ml

Tissue should be removed from the decalcifying fluid as soon as the decalcification process is complete, otherwise the histologic and cytologic detail will be harmed. Testing for complete decalcification may be done by (1) flexibility of tissue, which is not recommended since it is not a completely reliable test of complete decalcification, (2) insertion of a needle to feel calcium deposits within the tissue, which is not recommended since it is injurious to tissue, (3) chemical testing, which is the most satisfactory test for determining the end point of decalcification and is performed as follows:

1. 5 ml of decalcifying fluid are nearly neutralized with 0.5 N NaOH (5 ml).
2. To the nearly neutralized decalcifying fluid, 1 ml of a 5% solution of sodium or ammonium oxalate is added. Turbidity in the fluid, caused by the formation of calcium oxalate, indicates the presence of calcium ions in the fluid and in the tissue. Absence of turbidity indicates a negative reaction, but several minutes should elapse before one should assume that the tissue is completely decalcified. If the solution turns turbid either immediately or in a few minutes, the solutions are changed and the test is repeated the next day. With tissues containing only small areas of calcium, the test should be repeated every hour while the tissues are in the decalcifying fluid.
3. It is important that the pH range of the nearly neutralized solution lie between 3.5 and 7.5. If the pH of the solution is less than 3.5, precipitation of the calcium ions with the oxalate will be incomplete, resulting in the possibility that a positive test will be read as negative and the tissue will be removed from the decalcifying fluid too soon. If the pH of the nearly neutralized solution is greater than 7.5, magnesium will be precipitated as $Mg(OH)_2$ and $MgNH_4PO_4$. This will also give a false end point, indicating that further decalcification is necessary when in fact it is not.

Most books on histologic procedures state that when the tissue is completely decalcified with mineral acid technics, the tissue should be neutralized before washing by treatment with alkali. This alkali treatment is optional, but it can be accomplished by placing the decalcified tissue in a 5% solution of lithium or sodium sulfate overnight. More important than a neutralization procedure, however, is a thorough washing of the tissue after decalcification before subsequent processing technics are done. This washing is easily accomplished when the tissue is left in running tap water for 24 hours. This is a necessary step to remove all traces of acid (or alkali if neutralization has been done). Failure to do so will impair a subsequent staining procedure.

ION-EXCHANGE METHODS FOR DECALCIFICATION

Before proceeding with this method for decalcification, one must fix and wash the selected

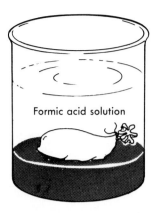

Fig. 6-2. Ion-exchange method. Gauze-wrapped bone is placed on top of resin.

tissue. Following these steps, the bone is decalcified with a mixture of formic acid and a commercially available ion-exchange resin. The calcium is rapidly removed from the solution of formic acid into the resin, and this eliminates solution changes that must be carried out to effect proper decalcification with the acid decalcification methods.

Tissue is placed (Fig. 6-2) in a bottle in a mixture of 10% or 20% resin and formic acid. Cancellous bone (2 to 3 mm in thickness) will decalcify in 2 to 3 hours in the solution and thicker pieces (5 to 6 mm in thickness) will take 4 to 8 hours to decalcify. A 40% resin and formic acid solution may be employed where speed is essential, but for good tissue preservation, the bone should not be left in this strength solution any longer than necessary (up to 8 days). If speed is not essential, tissue may be left in

the following solution up to 20 days without distortion of tissue:

WIN-3000 (ion-exchange resin)*	100 gm
10% formic acid (aqueous)	800 ml

The advantages of using the ion-exchange method for bone decalcification include well-preserved cellular detail, superior to that obtained with the acid decalcification methods; faster decalcification; and elimination of the daily solution change. In addition, the resin, once used, may be reclaimed for further use by washing to remove excess acid. The washing is followed by a 1% ammonia water wash, overnight treatment with saturated ammonium oxalate, and final water wash the next day.

ELECTROLYTIC DECALCIFICATION

This method employs electrolysis to shorten the time required for decalcification of bone sections. Materials used in the technic include a durable glass jar containing the acid decalcifying solution in which is immersed the electrode assembly and bone specimen, as shown in Fig. 6-3. The bone specimen is suspended by a platinum wire anode in the jar, and the insoluble calcium salts are changed to ionizable salts by the action of the acid in the solution. A recommended electrolytic decalcifying solution is as follows:

88% formic acid	100 ml
Hydrochloric acid	80 ml
Distilled water	820 ml

---

*Winthrop-Sterns, Inc., New York, N.Y.

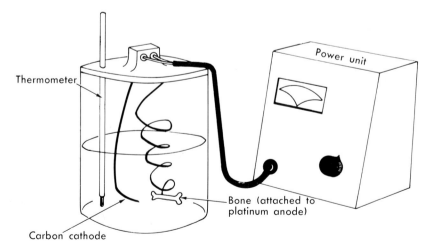

Fig. 6-3. Electrolytic decalcification apparatus.

Current, which is supplied by a power unit, causes an electric field between the electrodes, and this enables the calcium ions to migrate rapidly from the specimen (anode) to the carbon electrode (cathode). The acid radicals will migrate from the cathode to the anode. The temperature of the reaction is regulated between 30° to 45° C. Temperatures exceeding the upper limit of 45° C will cause the disintegration of the specimen. Solutions should be changed after 8 hours of use to ensure maximum speed of decalcification. Prolonged washing of the specimen after electrolysis is unnecessary; the tissues are rinsed well in alkaline water and the sections immersed in lithium carbonate before staining. The lithium carbonate treatment of a cut section will neutralize any remaining acid in the tissue so that the acid cannot interfere with any staining procedure. The chief advantage to the electrolytic method lies in the shortened time required for complete decalcification. This faster time will speed diagnosis and give better preservation of soft-tissue patterns. Staining reactions are usually better, since the method acts fast enough and the tissues have a relatively short time in the acid bath. Generally, cancellous bone 3 to 5 mm in thickness will decalcify in 45 minutes or less. More compact bone will take 16 hours or longer. A disadvantage to this method is that only a limited number of specimens may be processed at any one time. Maintaining contact between tissue and electrode may also create problems.

HISTOCHEMICAL METHODS FOR DECALCIFICATION

Standard methods of decalcification using nitric, hydrochloric, and other acids are unsatisfactory if histochemical technics are to be done on the tissue, since acid treatment will destroy the enzyme activity. Analytical methods for nucleic acids and polysaccharides should also be preceded by a histochemical, rather than routine, method for decalcification since these substances are largely destroyed by the acids employed in the routine technics. Histochemical decalcification methods include the use of chelating agents and buffer mixtures.

Buffer mixtures

Calcium salts may be removed from bone when it is placed into a buffered solution of citrate, pH 4.5. Calcium salts are soluble at this pH, and the zinc present in many buffered solutions of citrate will produce a reversible in-

activation of the alkaline phosphatases. (Subsequent reactivation will allow for their demonstration.) Daily changes of the buffer are necessary and the decalcification progress may be checked by use of the chemical oxalate test described in the section on acid decalcification methods.

Tissue should first be fixed in cold 80% alcohol for 24 to 48 hours. It is then placed in the buffer solution at refrigerator temperature (4° C) until decalcification is complete. Tissue is then washed in tap water, followed by distilled water, and then placed in a sodium barbital solution at 37° C for 6 hours to neutralize the tissue from the effects of acid citrate and to reactivate the enzyme activity. After the barbital treatment, the tissue is washed for 3 hours in running tap water, and processed for subsequent enzyme analysis. Solutions used are as follows:

Citric acid–citrate buffer (pH 4.5)

1 N citric acid (monohydrate, 7%)	50 ml
1 N ammonium citrate (anhydrous, 7.54%)	950 ml
1% zinc sulfate	2 ml
Chloroform	0.1 ml

Sodium barbital solution

Sodium barbital	100 ml
Glycine	75 mg

Other buffer mixtures

1. Molar hydrochloric acid–citrate buffer at pH 4.5

1 N hydrochloric acid	540 ml
1 M sodium citrate solution	460 ml

   (Use 29.4% of the dihydrate or 35.7% of the following compound: $Na(CO_2)_3C_3H_4OH \cdot 5\frac{1}{2}H_2O$.)

2. Lorch's citrate hydrochloric acid buffer at pH 4.4

Citric acid crystals	14.7 gm
0.2 N sodium hydroxide	700 ml
0.1 N hydrochloric acid	300 ml
1% zinc sulfate	2 ml
Chloroform	0.1 ml

3. Acetate buffer at pH 4.5

1 N acetic acid	520 ml
1 N sodium acetate (8.2% anhydrous or 13.6% crystalline)	480 ml
1% zinc sulfate	2 ml
Chloroform	0.1 ml

Chelating agents

General considerations. Chelating agents are organic compounds that have the power of binding certain metals. For decalcification, Sequestrene, or Versene (ethylenediaminetetraacetic acid, or EDTA), has the power of binding calcium ions according to the equation in Fig. 6-4.

Thin sections of bone are fixed for 24 hours in cold 80% alcohol, washed in running tap water, and transferred to a solution of EDTA, adjusted with sodium hydroxide to a pH of 6.0 to 6.5. The exact pH is not critical since satisfactory results can be obtained at values ranging from 5.0 to 7.2. A slightly acid pH is preferable, however, since alkaline phosphatase is more stable in an acid rather than alkaline solution. About 50 ml of a 5% solution is usually adequate, but the concentration is unimportant provided that a sufficient excess of the chelating agent is available to bind all the calcium and magnesium present in the bone. Decalcification by this method is slow and requires three changes of solution lasting 4 to 5 days each. The tissues also tend to harden, but tissues decalcified by this method also show a minimum of artifact and may be stained with most staining techniques with good results. The actual rate of decalcification varies with the size and density of the bone sample and can be hastened by occasional agitation or addition of fresh solution. Cancellous bone will usually be completely decalcified in about 3 days, whereas dense cortical bone requires as much as 2 weeks. Tissues that have been exposed to the chelating agent for as long as 6 weeks have yielded satisfactory preparations. When decalcification is complete, the tissue is washed thoroughly in running water and processed. Since the EDTA inactivates the alkaline phosphatase system in the process of decalcification, sections should be reactivated with a suitable activating ion, preferably magnesium. Placing the sections in a 1% solution of magnesium chloride for 2 to 6 hours or longer is usually sufficient to return them to maximal activity. During staining technics, a control section omitting the substrate is essential, as incomplete decalcification can produce areas of false reaction.

Demonstration of specific enzymes

1. For the demonstration of succinic dehydrogenase and NAD- and NADP-linked dehydrogenases and diaphorases, bone can be decalcified by a 3- to 5-day immersion at 4° to 10° C in 10% EDTA in a 0.1 M phosphate buffer of pH 7.0. The pH should be readjusted to 7.0 when both the buffer and EDTA are in the solution.

2. For the demonstration of acid phosphatase, tissues should be fixed for a maximum of 24 hours in a 10% to 20% solution of neutral formalin at 4° C. Since the use of chelating agents such as EDTA causes loss of acid phosphatase, a decalcifying solution composed of citrate and formic acid pH 4.2 is recommended. A pH below 3.8 will destroy the enzyme activity. The following solution may be used:

20% sodium citrate	50 ml
Formic acid	2.5 ml
Distilled water	47.5 ml
pH to 4.2	

After decalcification, frozen sections are prepared. Paraffin embedding will destroy the enzyme activity.

3. For the demonstration of alkaline phosphatase, tissues should be fixed in 70% ethanol or isopropanol at 20° to 25° C. Decalcification is carried out at 0° to 5° C in a buffer mixture of pH 4.5 or higher. Ammonium citrate and citric acid is effective, as well as normal acetate buffer. Both these mixtures will decalcify more rapidly than will Lorch's mixture or the 0.1 M citrate and citrate-hydrochloric acid mixtures. EDTA may also be used to decalcify. Solutions should be changed daily until the oxalate test is negative. If it becomes difficult to continue daily changes for decalcification, one may interrupt the process, washing briefly in water for 10 to 15 minutes, transferring to 80% alcohol, and storing at −20° to −25° C in a deep-freeze compartment until daily changes can be resumed. Tissues should be washed for 10 to 15 minutes in running tap water before being returned to the decalcifying solu-

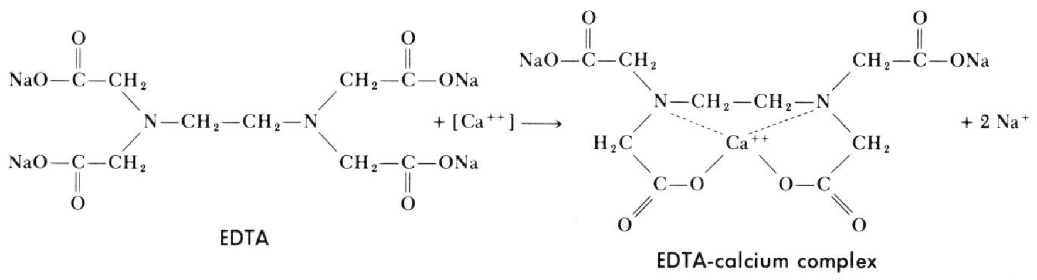

Fig. 6-4. Calcium chelation by EDTA.

tion. When the decalcification process is completed, tissues should be washed overnight in running water, incubated 6 hours in a 1% sodium barbital solution (containing 75 mg/dl glycine) to reactivate the enzyme, washed 2 to 4 hours to remove the glycine, dehydrated, cleared in gasoline or petroleum ether, and infiltrated 10 to 15 minutes in paraffin at 58° C in a vacuum.

Demonstration of glycogen in decalcified tissues

Total or partial losses of glycogen result when tissues are decalcified with acids or EDTA. Glycogen in muscle and marrow cells will withstand decalcification best when fixed in aqueous formalin acidified with acetic or formic acid. Thorough fixation of protein surrounding glycogen and embedding in celloidin before paraffin will create semipermeable membranes surrounding the glycogen and thus hinder diffusion and re-solution. Lillie uses the following technics for decalcification to subsequently demonstrate glycogen:

Technics
1. Celloidin
    a. Tissue should be fixed in acetic alcohol formalin 24 hours at room temperature (25° C) or 3 to 4 days at 5° C. Dehydrate with alcohols and infiltrate for 3 days with 1% celloidin in equal volumes of alcohol and ether.
    b. Transfer to 80% alcohol to harden celloidin.
    c. Decalcify with 5% formic acid (aqueous); solution should be changed daily until a negative chemical test is obtained.
    d. Wash 6 to 8 hours in running water, dehydrate, clear, and embed in paraffin.
2. Hard protein fixative
    a. Fix tissues as described above.
    b. Transfer to Bouin's fluid for 3 days at 25° C.
    c. Decalcify in daily changes of 10% formalin with 5% formic acid.
    d. Wash 8 hours in running water; dehydrate, clear, and embed in paraffin.

REFERENCES

Dotti, L., Paparo, G. P., and Clarke, B. E.: The use of ion exchange resin in decalcification of bone, Am. J. Clin. Pathol. **21:**475-479, 1951.

Lillie, R. D.: Histopathologic technic and practical histochemistry, ed. 3, New York, 1965, McGraw-Hill Book Co.

Pearse, A. G. E.: Histochemistry, theoretical and applied, ed. 2, Boston, 1960, Little, Brown & Co.

Preece, A.: A manual for histologic technicians, ed. 2, Boston, 1965, Little, Brown & Co.

Richman, I., Gelfand, M., and Hill, J. M.: A method for decalcifying bone for histologic section, Arch. Pathol. **44:**92-95, 1947.

Sobel, A. E., and Hanok, A.: Rapid method for determination of ultramicro quantities of calcium and magnesium, Proc. Soc. Exp. Biol. Med. **77:**737-740, 1951.

Part II. Basic preparation and staining of undecalcified bone

Antonio R. Villanueva

The primary objective of using undecalcified bone in histopathology is to gain insight into the histologic diagnosis and investigation of certain metabolic bone diseases, particularly the osteomalacias.[1,6,11,19] It is also an essential prerequisite for distinguishing mineralized from nonmineralized areas, for contact microradiography, and for histomorphometric analysis of bone remodeling. Mineralized sections of bone suitable for microscopy have been used by several investigators,[2,3,10,14,15,17] but such sections were rarely employed in the routine histopathology laboratory.

During the last few years, many biopsies from suspected cases of metabolic bone diseases have been reported routinely from decalcified sections. The use of decalcified sections, however, have not proved as reliable as undecalcified sections in distinguishing between mineralized bone and osteoid. Therefore, for routine histologic and pathologic study of certain metabolic bone diseases, the ideal histologic technic is the use of undecalcified bone, a condition where the tissue deviates minimally from the living state thus permitting maximum resolution of the components.

MINERALIZED BONE TECHNIC

(In this text, "mineralized" is interchangeable with "undecalcified.")

Preparation of undecalcified sections of bone

There are four methods of preparing and sectioning mineralized bone. First, there is the use of electrically powered machines that have a diamond cutting wheel and can do thin sectioning; second, there is the use of plastic embedding procedures, followed by cutting with one of the thin-sectioning machines, Jung "K" microtome or other heavy duty microtomes; third, there is the use of double embedding techniques with low-viscosity nitrocellulose or celloidin in combination with paraffin wax after impregnation with the celloidin, followed by cutting in a heavy-duty base sledge microtome; and fourth, there is the method of Frost's for preparing mineralized, fresh, ground, thin sections of bone.[8,9]

In general, procedures of preparing undecalcified bone for histopathology have very much in common with routine paraffin sections. Except for a little modification, the sequence is the following: (1) fixation, (2) dehydration, (3) clearing, (4) infiltration, (5) embedding (plastic), (6) sectioning (grinding), (7) staining.

Sectioning machines

The increasing use of mineralized bone work resulted in the development of various thin-sectioning machines. Currently there are several on the market, but the most common ones used today are the following: Gillings-Hamco Thin Sectioning Machine, Buehler Isomet, The H/I Bright 5030 Universal Rotary Retracting Microtome, Sorval Porter Blum JB 4 Microtome, Jung-K Microtome, and Leitz Sledge Microtome.* The first two are excellent for cutting bone sections at 50 to 100 μm thick, and the other four are for celloidin or plastic embedded sections at 5 to 10 μm thick.

Ground sectioning

There is another method developed as a technic for manual grinding of fresh, unembedded bone specimens. It is a very simple method for preparing sections of undecalcified bone

*Companies making thin-sectioning machines: *Gillings-Hamco,* Bronwill Scientific, Rochester, N.Y.; *Buehler Isomet,* Buehler Ltd., Evanston, Ill.; *H/I Bright 5030,* Hacker Instruments, Inc., Fairfield, N.J.; *JB-4,* DuPont Instruments–Sorvall, Newtown, Conn.; *Jung-K,* American Optical Corp., Buffalo, N.Y.; *Leitz Sledge,* Scientific Products Div., American Hospital Supply Corp., McGaw Park, Ill.

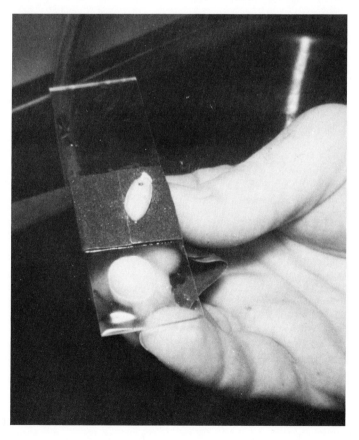

Fig. 6-5. Abrasive paper is wrapped around a microslide and held as indicated in this figure. Bone section will adhere to this strip of paper when placed upon it.

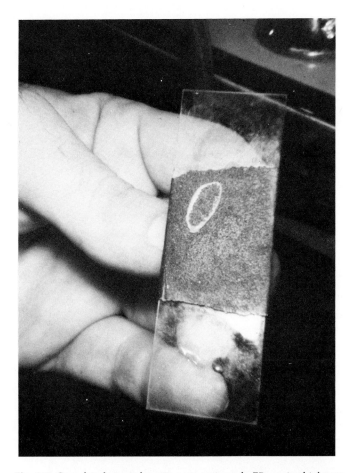

Fig. 6-6. Completed ground section approximately 75 μm in thickness.

with use of abrasive sandpaper of various grades (wet or dry waterproof adhesive) on a flat, plastic or glass sheet where the sections are ground by hand under gently running water.

Method of preparing ground sections

1. Bone specimens are sawed to 2 or 3 mm thick with a very fine toothed jewelers' saw or coping saw. The material may be held in a small vise, or in a conventional wooden V-block during the sawing process. While cutting, moisten the specimen with water intermittently in order to minimize friction. Finally bone slabs are placed in a beaker of saline or alcohol (or acetone) depending on the substance under study.

2. The slab of bony tissue is then ground to approximately 75 to 100 μm thick. Abrasive waterproof Carborundum sandpaper is employed for this purpose. This abrasive material is a sandpaper found in most paint and hardware stores and known as "wet-or-dry" sandpaper because the adhesive is waterproof.

   Section grinding is simple. The sandpaper should be placed on a flat, smooth surface of acrylic plastic (Plexiglas) while the sections are ground by hand in a circular motion under gently running tap water. The trick to the procedure is illustrated in Figs. 6-5 and 6-6. A strip of the same abrasive paper wrapped around a microslide as indicated in Fig. 6-5 is used to attach the section intact during grinding. The specimen will adhere to this strip when placed upon it. Should the sections fail to adhere to the strip of paper, a fresh one must be substituted. Accordingly, when the hand ground section is finished, as in Fig. 6-6, the section of bone adheres to the paper beneath.

   Each finished ground section is placed into a beaker of distilled water until ready for washing in a detergent solution (0.01% mild detergent or 0.1% Zephiran Chloride solution). The process removes grinding debris and bone dust and prepares the bone section for staining. The average time required to grind a section such as a rib, is approximately 2 minutes, whereas larger ones such as the tibia and femur would take at least 15 minutes or longer.

PLASTIC EMBEDDING

Several types of plastic materials used differ chiefly in the hardness of the final product and the ease of impregnation and polymerization. Some of these plastics used today are the following: methyl (or butyl) methacrylate embedding, Araldite embedding, Bio-Plastic, and Poly/Bed 812 embedding media. In our laboratory polymethyl methacrylate is used because it is relatively simple and can be used either for Jung K microtome sectioning or can be sawn for ground preparations.

The number of methods for plastic embedding are legion, but all of them have the same thing in common, which is they all go through the process of fixation, dehydration, infiltration in the plastic monomer, embedding with polymer, and polymerization or hardening of the plastic.

Procedure for routine processing and methacrylate embedding of bone tissue

When bone specimens are received, such as by iliac bone trephination or by needle or rib biopsies, they are placed immediately in one of the fixatives conducive to such study. Examples of these fixatives are alcohol, 10% buffered formalin, and formol-calcium. *Heavy-metal fixatives, dichromate, regular 10% formalin, and fixatives containing acid interfere with the staining and should not be employed.*

If tetracycline has been given, or if bone-seeking radionuclides such as plutonium are used and radioautography is the main objective, alcohol fixations should be employed to minimize bleaching of the tetracycline or isotope.

Preparation of bone specimen for simultaneous tetracycline-osteoid seam assessment and histomorphometric quantitative analysis[13]
Preparation of polymethyl methacrylate embedding medium

Add the following ingredients (do not make more than 250 ml at a time): 250 ml of methyl methacrylate monomer; 2.5 gm of benzoyl peroxide. Stir and dissolve thoroughly for 2 minutes; then add 100 gm of polymethyl methacrylate beads. Stir the mixture in a closed container on a magnetic stirrer. Frequently, at hourly intervals, mix beads manually into the mixture. Total stirring time may require up to 2 full working days. *Note: Do not let mixture be stirred overnight.* When all the beads are dissolved, the medium is ready for embedding.

Store in the refrigerator in a tightly closed container. *Note: If catalyzed monomer has been stored in the refrigerator, it should be allowed to warm gradually to room temperature before use. This is necessary to prevent condensation of water, which will interfere with polymerization.*

Processing and embedding procedure

1. Fresh or fixed bone specimens are stained in Villanueva's bone stain for 72 hours.
2. Dehydrate in vacuum desiccator according to the following:
   a. 1 change of 70% ethanol for 1 hour
   b. 2 changes of 95% ethanol, 1½ hours each
   c. 2 changes of 100% ethanol, 1½ hours each
   d. Acetone, 1½ hours
3. Infiltrate in the following:
   a. Equal parts of acetone and methyl methacrylate monomer, for overnight
   b. Methyl methacrylate monomer, for 24 hours
   c. Embedding medium for 24 hours; place in the refrigerator. *Note: These are the standard times used for iliac bone specimens. For larger or denser bones, doubly increase staining time and dehydration and infiltration times to those given above.*
4. Using Peel-A-Way embedding molds,* embed specimens in the embedding medium.
5. Polymerize in a vacuum oven at 37° to 40° C at a pressure of 15 to 20 pounds of mercury. *Note: If there is a shrinkage of plastic while polymerizing, add more embedding medium to compensate for this phenomenon. Repeat as necessary.*
6. Polymerization takes approximately 3 to 5 days. Plastic must be completely hardened before cutting.

Sectioning

There are two methods used for cutting sections: (1) dry method and (2) wet method. In the dry method, sections are cut without application of alcohol on the block and may be used for qualitative as well as quantitative analysis. They are most suitable for observation of tetracycline labels. The wet method involves the application of alcohol on the block during cut-

---

*Peel-A-Way Scientific, 1800 Floradale Ave., South El Monte, CA 91733.

ting and are used for future staining to suit individual requirements.

Procedure for dry sections

1. Cut sections at 5 or 10 μm thick.
2. Do not use ethanol in cutting these sections.
3. Trim away excess plastic from each section, handling as carefully as possible to minimize shattering.
4. Mount with Eukitt's mounting medium.

Procedure for wet sections

1. Apply 35% ethanol to the cutting surface of the specimen block.
2. Cut sections 5 to 10 μm thick.
3. Trim excess plastic from each section, handling as carefully as possible to minimize shattering.
4. Place a liberal amount of Haupt's gelatin affixative on a slide.
5. Place bone section on top of affixative and cover with bibulous paper.
6. Flatten gently with a roller and allow to set for several minutes.
7. Lift bibulous paper and place several drops of 2% formalin on the section and blot again with fresh bibulous paper.
8. After 5 minutes remove bibulous paper and place slides on a slide-warming plate set at 50° to 60° C for 1 hour.
9. Dissolve plastic off these sections by immersing slides in fresh xylene and then place in the oven at 50° to 60° C for 3 to 5 hours.
10. Remove slides from xylene and allow to air-dry for at least 1 hour. Stain as desired.

Comments

In our laboratory most of the bone specimens received are prestained with the Villanueva bone stain for 72 hours before dehydration and embedding because it gives a better differentiation of osteoid seams and tetracycline fluorescence when studied with the light and fluorescence microscope respectively. Fixation of bone specimen prior to staining with the bone stain is not necessary; the bone stain itself acts as a fixative, since it contains 70% alcohol.

METHODS OF STAINING

Methods of staining mineralized, thin sections of bone have changed little in recent years. The many attempts to stain fresh, hydrated, unembedded, and plastic-embedded mineralized bone sections have resulted in few successes.

The following staining methods have proved to be excellent in the approach to mineralized or undecalcified bone staining.

Frost's basic fuchsin stain[9] (for staining fresh or fixed, unembedded sections of bone)

Fixation. 70% alcohol.

Solution

Basic fuchsin solution	1 gm
Ethanol, 80%	100 ml

Dissolve the basic fuchsin thoroughly in the alcohol and then filter.

Note: For the bone of infants, young children, or very immature animals, reduce the stain concentration to 0.3%, since such bones contain large volumes of incompletely mineralized matrix, which will be deeply, often opaquely stained.

Procedure

1. Grind sections to approximately 50 to 100 μm thick.
2. Rinse in distilled water.
3. Stain in the basic fuchsin solution for 48 hours.
4. After staining, place sections in tap water then lightly grind surface stains.
5. Wash sections in 0.1% Zephiran Chloride or in 0.1% mild household detergent, such as Lux or Ivory.
6. Again wash sections in tap water and then rinse in distilled water.
7. Place sections between two slides with one slide surface covered with filter paper trimmed to the length and width of the slide. Clamp the slides gently with a Hoffman clamp and allow to dry in a 45° C oven overnight.
8. Mount in Eukitt's mounting medium.

Results

Fully mineralized bone—unstained

Early stages of mineralization and new bone formation—fuchsin stain

Halo volumes (perilacunar red density of appreciable numbers around the osteocytes)[7]

Villanueva's bone stain[20] (for staining fresh, or fixed, unembedded, or plastic-embedded sections of bone)

Fixation. 70% ethanol.

Solutions

Villanueva's bone stain*

0.01% glacial acetic acid in 70% methanol

0.1% Zephiran Chloride (or 0.01% mild household detergent)

Procedure

1. Cut bone into slabs to approximately 2 to 3 mm thick.
2. Grind sections to 50 to 100 μm thick under gently running water. (This method may be

---

*Either from Histo-Cyto-Prep Inc., Box 524, Bloomfield Hills, MI 48013, or from Polysciences, Inc., Paul Valley Industrial Park, Warrington, PA 18976.

omitted if thin-sectioning machine is used to cut sections at desired thickness prior to staining.)

3. Rinse sections in distilled water.
4. Stain in the Villanueva bone stain:
   a. 1 or 2 sections for 90 minutes.
   b. 2 to 4 sections for 48 hours.
      Note: The 90-minute staining yields fast stains of diagnostic usefulness but with incomplete permeation of the section by the stain; the 48-hour staining is for complete permeation of bone and tissue elements.
5. Transfer sections into tap water and then grind surface stains. (Optional if sections are cut to desired thickness with thin-sectioning machine.)
6. Wash sections with 0.1% Zephiran Chloride or in 0.01% mild household detergent.
7. Again wash sections with tap water and then rinse with distilled water.
8. Differentiate in 0.01% glacial acetic acid in 95% methanol:
   a. For the 90-minute staining, differentiate for 3 to 5 minutes.
   b. For the 24-hour staining, differentiate for 10 minutes.
   c. For the 48-hour staining, differentiate for 20 to 25 minutes.
9. Dehydrate in the following:
   a. 95% alcohol   15 min
   b. 100% alcohol   15 min
10. Clear in the following:
    a. Equal parts of alcohol, 100%,   10 min
       plus xylene
    b. 1 part of 100% alcohol and   5 min
       3 parts of xylene
    c. 1 part of 100% alcohol and   5 min
       9 parts of xylene
    d. Xylene   10 min
    e. Xylene   5 min
    f. Xylene   5 min
11. Mount in Eukitt's mounting medium.

Results

Osteoid seams—transparent green to jade green or homogeneous red
Zone of demarcation—orange-red
Low-density bone—red
Moderately permeable bone—orange
Osteocytes, canaliculi, halo volumes—red
Nuclei of osteoclasts, osteoblasts—greenish blue to dark purple
Cytoplasm—green or light green

Villanueva's tetrachrome bone stain[18]
(for staining fresh or fixed unembedded mineralized sections of bone)

Fixation. 70% alcohol.

Solutions
A. Fast green FCF   0.1 gm

Orange G   2 gm
Distilled water   100 ml
Note: The mixture is adjusted between pH 6.5 and 6.8 with 3 N acetic acid. Add a few crystals of thymol.
B. Azure II   0.25 gm
   Ethanol, 50%   100 ml
C. Basic fuchsin   1 gm
   Ethanol, 50%   100 ml
D. For staining, mix 1 ml of solution B and 9 ml of solution C.

Procedure

1. Prepare sections about 75 to 100 μm thick by Frost's[1] method. Before making sections, rehydrate any alcoholated material by soaking it in a large volume of distilled (or tap) water for an hour to decrease its brittleness. Even 5% alcohol may make the bone unworkably brittle.
2. By manual or mechanical agitation wash in 0.1% invert soap (Zephiran Chloride) in tap water and then rinse in distilled water for 1 minute each.
3. Stain in solution A for 12 to 15 hours. (In biopsy material, 1 hour yields fast stains of diagnostic usefulness but with incomplete permeation of the section.)
4. Remove surface stain by regrinding lightly under tap water. Rinse in distilled water.
5. Counterstain in solution B for 1 to 2 hours. (In biopsy material, 15 to 30 minutes will permit quick reading but incomplete permeation of the section.)
6. Repeat step 4.
7. Repeat step 2.
8. Differentiate in 0.01% acetic acid in 95% methanol, 3 to 5 minutes. At 1-minute intervals, examine the section under a microscope to determine the staining of osteoid seams, taking care that the sections are not allowed to dry. Differentiate until the osteoid seams have acquired the maximum green tint.
9. Dehydrate in:
   95% alcohol   9 min
   100% alcohol   8 min
10. Clear in the following:
    Equal parts of 100% alcohol   7 min
       plus xylene
    1 part of 100% alcohol and   6 min
       3 parts of xylene
    1 part of 100% alcohol and   5 min
       9 parts of xylene
    Xylene, 2 changes   4 and 3 min
                                    respectively
11. Mount in Eukitt's mounting medium.

Results
See results in the bone stain method.

Modified Villanueva-Gomori trichrome[21]
(for plastic-embedded sections of bone)

Fixation. 70% ethanol, 10% buffered formalin.

Solutions
Weigert's hematoxylin—modified
Solution A

Hematoxylin crystals	2 gm
Ethanol, 95%	200 ml

Solution B

Ferric chloride, FeCl$_3$ · H$_2$O, 62%	8 ml
Distilled water	190 ml
Hydrochloric acid	2 ml

Solution C
Equal parts of solutions A and B. (Make up fresh working solution for each new batch of slides, and prepare stain immediately before use.)

Trichrome stain mixture—modified

Chromotrope 2R C.I. 16570	0.2 gm
Light green C.I. 42095	0.1 gm
Glacial acetic acid	1.0 ml
Phosphotungstic acid	0.8 gm
Distilled water	100 ml

Filter solution before using.

Procedure
1. Deplasticize to distilled water.
2. Stain in Weigert's hematoxylin solution for 5 minutes.
3. Rinse under running water, differentiate in 1% aqueous hydrochloric acid, rinse in water, blue with saturated aqueous solution of lithium carbonate, and wash under running water for 3 to 5 minutes.
4. Transfer to the modified trichrome mixture for 5 minutes.
5. Differentiate in aqueous 0.5% or 1.0% acetic acid for 1 minute.
6. Rinse in distilled water. Check microscopically and repeat steps 4 and 5 until proper differentiation of bone matrix is reached.
7. Dehydrate:

95% alcohol	10 dips
100% alcohol	15 dips
100% alcohol	20 dips

8. Clear in:

Xylene	25 dips
Xylene	1 min
Xylene	5 min

9. Mount in Eukitt's mounting medium.

Results
Bone matrix and collagen—bluish green
Nuclei—dark purple to black
Osteoid seam—bright red
Muscle—red

Modified Villanueva-Goldner trichrome[21]
(for plastic-embedded sections of bone)

Fixation. 70% ethanol, 10% buffered formalin.

Solutions
Weigert's hematoxylin (see solution C in preceding column)
Masson's Ponceau-fuchsin stock solution

Ponceau de xylidine, C.I. 16150, 1% aqueous solution	3 parts
Acid fuchsin C.I. 42685, 1% aqueous solution	1 part

Dilute 1 : 10 with 0.2% acetic acid for staining.

Phosphotungstic-phosphomolybdic solution

Phosphotungstic acid	2.5 gm
Phosphomolybdic acid	2.5 gm
Distilled water	100 ml

Dissolve thoroughly.

Naphthol green B solution, 1%

Naphthol green B, C.I. 10200	1 gm
Distilled water	100 ml
Acetic acid	1 ml

Alcohol saffron solution

Safran du Gâtinais Chroma* 5A-394	1 gm
Absolute ethanol	100 ml

Place in stoppered flask in 55° to 60° C oven for 2 days. Agitate from time to time. Cool and filter.

Procedure
1. Deplasticize to distilled water.
2. Stain in modified Weigert's iron hematoxylin for 20 minutes. Rinse under running water, differentiate with 1% aqueous hydrochloric acid, rinse with water, blue with saturated aqueous solution of lithium carbonate, and wash under running water for 3 to 5 minutes.
3. Transfer to Masson's Ponceau-fuchsin (dilute formula) for 1 hour. Rinse in 1% acetic acid.
4. Place in phosphotungstic-phosphomolybdic acid for 5 minutes. Rinse with 1% acetic acid, and place in fresh 1% acetic acid for 5 minutes.
5. Transfer to naphthol green B solution for 15 minutes.
6. Rinse in the following:

Distilled water	8 dips
95% alcohol	20 dips
100% alcohol	20 dips
100% alcohol	20 dips

7. Place in the alcoholic saffron solution for 15 minutes.
8. Transfer to

100% alcohol	15 dips
100% alcohol	15 dips
Xylene	15 dips
Xylene	15 dips
Xylene	1 min

9. Mount in Eukitt's mounting medium.

Results
Nuclei—dark purple to black
Cytoplasm—bright pink

---

*Roboz Surgical Instrument Co., Inc., Washington, DC 20006.

Bone matrix and collagen—bright greenish yellow
Muscle—scarlet
Osteoid seams—bright red

Villanueva's blood stain[22]

(for plastic-embedded sections of bone)

Fixation. 70% ethanol, 10% buffered formalin, B-5.

Solutions

Stock Villanueva's blood stain I*
Stock Villanueva's blood stain II*
Working phosphate buffer

Solution C	2 ml
Solution D	2 ml
Distilled water	96 ml

Working staining mixture I

Solution A	10 ml
Distilled water (or solution E)	30 ml

Working staining mixture II

Solution B	5 ml
Distilled water (or solution E)	45 ml

0.5% glacial acetic acid, aqueous

Procedure

1. Cut sections to approximately 5 μm.
2. Decalcify plastic embedded section of bone in one of the decalcifying solutions for 2 to 5 minutes.
3. Wash in water for 5 minutes and then rinse in distilled water.
4. Stain in working staining mixture I for 10 minutes. Discard after use.
5. Transfer directly to working staining mixture II for 45 minutes. (It may be left in this solution longer to suit individual requirements.) *Note: Carry one slide at a time in the next remaining steps.* Discard mixture after each use.
6. Differentiate in 0.5% glacial acetic acid solution, 5 to 10 dips. Immerse slide in distilled water and then check differentiation under a microscope to ascertain the depth of staining but take care that the preparation is *not* allowed to dry. If the desired degree of staining has not been attained, return the slide to the differentiating solution and rinse again with distilled water before further examination. This process may be repeated several times until differentiation is complete. *The landmarks are pink eosinophil granules and sharp, brilliant purple nuclei.*
7. Dehydrate and clear in the following:

95% ethanol	5 to 10 dips
100% ethanol	5 to 10 dips
Equal parts:	
Xylene plus 100% ethanol	10 to 20 dips
Xylene	10 to 20 dips
Xylene	1 to 5 min

8. Mount in Eukitt's mounting medium.

---

*Polysciences, Inc., Paul Valley Industrial Park, Warrington, PA 18976.

Results

Nuclei of bone marrow cells—dark bluish purple
Cytoplasm—light blue to gray
Nuclei of osteocytes, osteoblasts, osteoclasts—dark purple
Cytoplasm—light blue to gray
Eosinophil granules—bright pink
Mast cell and basophil granules—dark purple

A modification of Movat's pentachrome stain [16]

(for plastic-embedded sections of bone)

Fixation. 5% phosphate-buffered formalin, 40% ethanol, Carnoy's fluid.

Solutions

Weigert's iron hematoxylin

Solution A

Hematoxylin	1 gm
Ethanol, 95%	100 ml

Solution B

Ferric chloride ($FeCl_3 \cdot 7H_2O$)	1.19 gm
Distilled water	98 ml
Hydrochloric acid, 25%	1 ml

Working solution

Mix equal parts of solution A and solution B. The mixture is stable for approximately 8 days.

Brilliant crocein–acid fuchsin

Solution A

Brilliant crocein (C.I. 27290)	0.1 gm
Distilled water	99.5 ml
Glacial acetic acid	0.5 ml

Solution B

Acid fuchsin (C.I. 42685)	0.1 gm
Distilled water	99.5 ml
Glacial acetic acid	0.5 ml

Working solution

Mix 8 parts of solution A with 2 parts of solution B. The mixture is stable for several months, but it should be replaced when it begins to stain weakly.

Alcoholic saffron

Safran du Gâtinais (C.I. 75100)	3 gm
Ethanol, 100%	100 ml

Place the solution in a tightly plugged bottle in an incubator at 50° C for 48 hours before use. This is done to extract the saffron. Keep the solution in a fully filled air-tight dark bottle to prevent hydration, which will make the solution useless. The stability of the solution is largely dependent on the adherence to these precautions.

Alcian blue

Alcian blue 8 GS (C.I. 74240)	1 gm
Distilled water	100 ml
Glacial acetic acid	1 ml

The solution is stable for 2 to 4 weeks.

Procedure

1. Remove methyl methacrylate with 2 changes of methyl Cellosolve acetate followed by 2

changes of methyl Cellosolve acetate containing 1% celloidin, 15 minutes each.
2. Hydrate to water through 70% and 40% ethanol, 5 minutes each.
3. Rinse in distilled water.
4. Wash in running tap water for 6 minutes.
5. Transfer to alkaline ethanol (pH over 8) for 1 hour. Prepare by adding 10 ml of concentrated ammonium hydroxide to 90 ml of 95% ethanol. This converts the alcian blue into the insoluble nonfading pigment monastral fast blue.
6. Wash in running tap water for 10 minutes.
7. Immerse sections in Weigert's iron hematoxylin for 10 minutes.
8. Rinse in distilled water.
9. Wash in running tap water for 10 minutes.
10. Rinse again in distilled water.
11. Immerse sections in brilliant crocein–acid fuchsin for 8 minutes.
12. Rinse in 0.5% acetic acid.
13. Differentiate in 5% aqueous phosphotungstic acid until mineralized bone matrix is merely pale pink; this usually requires 15 to 20 minutes.
14. Wash in 0.5% acetic acid under continuous agitation for 2 minutes.
15. Rinse thoroughly in 3 changes of 100% ethanol for 5 minutes each. (It is essential not to use less concentrated ethanol, which will dissolve away the cytoplasmic stain and prevent the tissue from taking the collagen stain.)
16. Immerse sections in alcoholic saffron solution for 30 to 40 minutes.
17. Rinse thoroughly again in 3 changes of 100% ethanol for 3 minutes each.
18. Transfer into methyl Cellosolve acetate for 2 minutes.
19. Clear in 2 changes of xylene and mount in Eukitt's mounting medium.

Results
Nuclei—black to bluish gray
Cytoplasm—red
Elastic fibers—yellow (coarse fibers—red)
Cartilage—red or yellow
Calcified cartilage—sea green
Osteoid—red
Mineralized bone—yellow

Gordon and Sweet's method for cement lines [5]
(for plastic-embedded sections of bone)

Fixation. 70% ethanol, 10% buffered formalin.

Solutions
Acidified permanganate solution
Potassium permanganate, 0.5%	48 ml
Sulfuric acid, 3.0%	2 ml

This solution is stable for 48 hours.
Oxalic acid, 1%

Iron alum (ferric ammonium sulfate), 2.5%
Diamine silver hydroxide solution

To 10 ml of 10% solution of silver nitrate, add 28% ammonium hydroxide drop by drop. A precipitate will form. Continue to add ammonium hydroxide, shaking vigorously until the precipitate disappears. Then add 10 ml of 8% sodium hydroxide. Again add ammonium hydroxide and dissolve the precipitate, which forms in the same manner. Add distilled water to make 100 ml. Filter into brown bottle. Solution remains stable when refrigerated.
Formalin, 10%
Gold chloride, 0.2% (Solution is very stable, may be used repeatedly; keep refrigerated.)
Sodium thiosulfate, 5%
Mayer's hematoxylin or Gill II hematoxylin

Procedure
1. Deplasticize for 4 hours in 55° C xylene.
2. Bring to 100% ethanol.
3. Dip in 1% celloidin and then air-dry for 5 to 10 seconds.
4. Hydrate with:
95% ethanol	2 changes
70% ethanol	1 change
Distilled water	1 change
5. Oxidize in acidified permanganate solution for 1 minute.
6. Wash in distilled water for 2 minutes.
7. Bleach in 1% oxalic acid for 1 minute.
8. Wash in tap water for 2 minutes.
9. Wash in 2 changes of distilled water, 1 minute each.
10. Mordant in 2.5% iron alum for 1 minute.
11. Wash in tap water for 2 minutes, followed with with 2 changes of distilled water for 30 seconds each.
12. Permeate with the diamino silver solution 1 minute.
13. Rinse in distilled water for 20 seconds.
14. Reduce in 10% formalin for 3 minutes.
15. Wash in water for 3 minutes.
16. Tone in 0.2% gold chloride for 10 minutes.
17. Wash in tap water and then for 5 minutes in 5% $Na_2S_2O_5$ (sodium thiosulfate), and again wash in tap water for 3 minutes.
18. Stain in Mayer's hematoxylin for 1 minute; wash in water and then rinse in distilled water.
19. Dehydrate:
95% ethanol	2 changes
100% ethanol	1 change
20. Rinse in 100% ethanol.
21. Clear in 2 changes of xylene.
22. Mount in Eukitt's mounting medium.

Results
Bone—bluish gray with well-defined unstained, cement lines
Reticulum fibers—black

Phosphotungstic acid hematoxylin[5]
(for plastic-embedded sections of bone)

Fixation. 70% alcohol, 10% buffered formalin.

Solutions

Phosphotungstic acid hematoxylin (PTAH)

Hematoxylin	0.5 gm
Phosphotungstic acid	10 gm
Distilled water	500 ml
Potassium permanganate	0.09 gm

Dissolve the hematoxylin with half of the water by heating it moderately. In the remaining water, dissolve the phosphotungstic acid. Cool and then combine the solutions. Next add the potassium permanganate. When combined, store in the refrigerator. The solution remains stable for about 4 weeks.

Eosin Y

Eosin Y	0.5 gm
Ethanol, 95%	50 ml
Glacial acetic acid	1 drop

This solution is very stable.

Procedure

1. Deplasticize slides in 55° C xylene for 4 hours.
2. Air-dry completely then transfer to
   100% ethanol
   100% ethanol
   95% ethanol
   95% ethanol
   70% ethanol
   Distilled water
3. Incubate in PTAH either overnight or 2 hours at 60° C. Although the use of heat intensifies the colors, it also loosens the sections from the slides.
4. Differentiate in 95% ethanol (3 quick dips is usually optimum). Check with microscope. Osteoid seams should be clearly differentiated, being stained a medium purple.
5. Counterstain with the eosin Y for 1 minute.
6. Dehydrate rapidly:
100% ethanol	10 dips
100% ethanol	10 dips
7. Clear in 2 changes of xylene and mount in Eukitt's mounting medium.

Results

Osteoid—light to dark purple
Nuclei, bone matrix—reddish pink
Cytoplasm—light pink

Modified Von Kossa's method[23] *(for calcium deposits modified for plastic-embedded sections of bone)*

Fixation. 70% alcohol, 10% buffered formalin.

Solutions

Aqueous silver nitrate, 5%
Aqueous sodium thiosulfate, 5%

Mayer's hematoxylin
Basic fuchsin in 70% ethanol, 0.1%

Procedure

1. Deplasticize in xylene for 4 hours at 55° C.
2. Transfer to
   100% ethanol
   100% ethanol
   95% ethanol
   95% ethanol
   70% ethanol
   Distilled water
3. Incubate in silver nitrate solution at room temperature under ultraviolet light for a minimum of 6 hours.
4. Wash thoroughly in distilled water for 3 to 5 minutes.
5. Rinse in the sodium thiosulfate solution for 2 to 3 minutes.
6. Wash thoroughly in distilled water for 3 to 5 minutes.
7. Stain in Mayer's hematoxylin for 15 minutes.
8. Wash in distilled water for 5 minutes.
9. Transfer to 70% alcohol for 1 minute.
10. Stain in 0.1% basic fuchsin for 15 to 30 seconds.
11. Dehydrate and clear in the following:
95% alcohol	10 dips
100% alcohol	15 dips
100% alcohol	15 dips
Xylene	20 dips
Xylene	20 dips
Xylene	1 min
12. Mount in Eukitt's mounting medium.

Result

Calcium deposits—dark brown to black
Osteoid seams—bright pink
Nuclei—purple
Cytoplasm—pink

Solochrome cyanin R[12] *(for plastic-embedded sections of bone)*

Fixation. 70% alcohol, 10% buffered formalin.

Solutions

Solochrome cyanin R solution

Solochrome cyanin R	1 gm
2% acetic acid, aqueous	100 ml

Note: A pH of approximately 2 is obtained by the acetic acid.

Procedure

1. Deplasticize slide for 4 hours in 55° C xylene.
2. Transfer to
   100% ethanol
   100% ethanol
   95% ethanol
   95% ethanol
   70% ethanol
   Distilled water
3. Stain for 10 minutes in the 1% Solochrome cyanin R solution.

4. Wash in warm water approximately 30° C until the sections become bluish and the water is no longer colored red. (Check the differentiation under the microscope: calcified bone should be blue and osteoid seams, red.)
5. Dehydrate and clear:
   95% ethanol
   95% ethanol
   100% ethanol
   100% ethanol
   Xylene
   Xylene
6. Mount with Eukitt's mounting medium.

Results
Osteoid—bright orange
New bone—light purple
Old bone—dark purple

Toluidine blue stain for calcification front, cement line, and osteoid seams[24]
(for plastic-embedded sections of bone)

Fixation. 70% ethanol, 10% buffered formalin.

Solution
Stock solution
   Toluidine blue O staining solution, 1% aqueous
Working solution

Toluidine blue O stock solution	0.75 ml
Distilled water	100 ml
Certified buffer tablet* (pH 8.0)	1 tablet

Dissolve the buffer tablet in distilled water. Add toluidine blue O and dissolve thoroughly. *Note:* The staining solution must be prepared fresh for each batch of slides. *Do not prepare stain until ready to use.*

Procedure
1. Deplasticize sections in xylene at approximately 6 to 12 hours.
2. Allow sections to dry.
3. Stain sections in working solution for 24 hours.
4. Dehydrate sections in the following way:
   a. 2 changes of 95% ethanol   20 dips each
   b. 2 changes of 100% ethanol   20 dips each
   c. Clear in 2 changes of xylene: 20 dips for the first and 1 minute or longer in the second.
5. Mount in Eukitt's mounting medium.

Results
Osteoid seams—light blue
Mineralized bone—dark purple
Cement line—scalloped, bright purple
Calcification front—dark, granular, bluish-purple
Nuclei of osteoclasts, osteoblasts, osteocytes—dark blue or dark purple

---

*Lot no. 13, Formula no. 30, Catalog no. 001-0060, The Perkin-Elmer Corp., Coleman Instruments Division, Oak Brook, IL 60521.

Cytoplasm of osteoclasts, osteoblasts, osteocytes—light blue or light purple

Modified methyl green pyronine Y stain[4] *(for plastic-embedded sections of bone)*

Fixation. Absolute alcohol, cold acetone.

Solutions
Stock solution
Make 2% aqueous solutions of each dye and then extract each solution in a separatory funnel separately with equal volume of chloroform. Methyl green should be extracted at least six times. After this washing, check for contaminant methyl violet by exposing filter paper with a drop of methyl green on it to ammonia fumes. After a few seconds, the blue color will fade away. If any violet at all is apparent, repeat the washing process until the paper comes white with the test. Pyronine Y should be washed at least 10 times. Both solutions will remain quite stable if stored over chloroform. The chloroform wash can be cleaned and reused for washing by being filtered through activated charcoal.
Working staining solution
Prepare just before use:

Aqueous methyl green, 2%	9 ml
Aqueous pyronine Y, 2%	5 ml
Distilled water	20 ml

Procedure
1. Deplasticize for 4 hours in xylene at 55° C.
2. Transfer to:
   a. 100% ethanol
   b. 100% ethanol
   c. 95% ethanol
   d. 95% ethanol
   e. 70% ethanol
   f. Distilled water
3. Incubate 12 to 24 hours in refrigerator in methyl green–pyronine Y solution.
4. Blot carefully with paper towel or filter paper.
5. Dehydrate *rapidly* (3 dips) in each of the solutions below:
   a. 50% acetone in distilled water
   b. 95% acetone in distilled water
   c. 100% acetone
   d. Equal parts of acetone and xylene
   e. 100% xylene
   f. 100% xylene
6. Mount in Eukitt's mounting medium.

Results
DNA—green
RNA—red
Nuclei—blue-green
Bacteria, osteoblasts, basophilic cytoplasm—red
Background—colorless to pale pink

Control for RNA in methyl green pyronine Y. Because pyronine Y is not specific for ribo-

nucleic acid, it is important to run controls. It is best to use two control systems. *First,* with each run, include a section known to contain significant amounts of RNA. (In our laboratory, we use a section from a patient with Paget's disease because of its significant amounts of RNA in the osteoblast's cytoplasm.) *Second,* since pyronine Y is not specific for RNA, run a second set of slides from which the RNA has been removed. Although other methods which showed promise were less expensive, we received best results using ribonuclease.

Incubation medium. Weigh 0.5 to 1 mg of ribonuclease dissolved in 1 ml of 0.21% sodium bicarbonate (M/40). (According to Chayen,[4] optimal pH is 7.7. Others use various buffers and distilled water, but the M/40 sodium bicarbonate at pH 8.2 works well.)

Method. Incubate one slide at 37° C in ribonuclease solution for 2 hours. Incubate a second slide just like the first, but omit the ribonuclease. Just use sodium bicarbonate solution.

REFERENCES (Basic preparation and staining of undecalcified bone)

1. Arnstein, R. R., Frame, B., and Frost, H. M.: Recent progress in osteomalacia and rickets, Ann. Intern. Med. **67**:1296-1330, 1967.
2. Baylink, D. J., Stauffer, M., Wergedal, J., and Rich, C.: Formation, mineralization, and resorption of bone in vitamin D–deficient rats, J. Clin. Invest. **49**:1122-1134, 1970.
3. Bordier, P. J., and Tun-Chot, S.: Quantitative histology of metabolic bone disease, J. Clin. Endocrinol. Metab. **1**:197-215, 1972.
4. Chayen, H.: The methyl green pyronine method, Exp. Cell Res. **3**:652, 1952.
5. Clayden, F. C.: Practical section cutting and staining, ed. 5, Edinburgh, 1971, Churchill Livingston.
6. Frame, B., Arnstein, A. R., Frost, H. M., and Smith, R. W., Jr.: Osteomalacia: studies with tetracycline bone labeling and metabolic balance, Am. J. Med. **38**:134-144, 1965.
7. Frost, H. M.: Some observations on bone mineral in a case of vitamin-D resistant rickets, Henry Ford Hosp. Med. Bull. **6**(4):300-310, 1958.
8. Frost, H. M.: Preparation of thin, undecalcified bone sections by rapid manual method, Stain Technol. **33**:273-277, 1958.
9. Frost, H. M.: Staining of fresh, undecalcified thin bone sections, Stain Technol. **34**:135-146, 1959.
10. Frost, H. M., Villanueva, A. R., and Roth, H.: Tetracycline staining of newly forming bone and mineralizing cartilage "in vivo," Stain Technol. **35**:135-138, 1960.
11. Frost, H. M., Frame, B., Ormond, R. S., and Hunter, R. B.: Atypical axial osteomalacia: a report of three cases: Clin. Orthop. **23**:285-295, 1962.
12. Martajt, H., and Hioco, D.: Solochrome cyanin R as an indicator dye of morphology, Stain Technol. **41**:97-99, 1966.
13. Mathews, C. H. E., and Mehr, L.: Staining and processing bone specimens for simultaneous tetracycline—osteoid seam assessment and histomorphometric quantitative analysis, J. Histotechnol. **2**:23-24, 1979.
14. Meunier, P., and Edward C.: Quantification of osteoid tissue in trabecular bone methodology and results in normal iliac bone. In Jaworski, Z. F. G., editor: Proceedings of the First International Workshop on Bone Morphometry, Ottawa, 1976, Ottawa University Press.
15. Melseen, F.: Histomorphometric and dynamic studies of osteoporosis, Univ. of Utah Workshop on Osteoporosis, Sun Valley, Utah, Aug. 1977.
16. Olah, A. J., Simon, A., Gaudy, M., Herrmann, W., and Schenk, R. K.: Differential staining of calcified tissue in plastic embedded microtome sections by modification of Movat's pentachrome stain, Stain Technol. **52**:331-337, 1977.
17. Schenk, R. K., Merz, W. A., and Muller, J.: A quantitative histological study on bone resorption in human cancellous bone, Acts Anat. **74**:44-53, 1969.
18. Villanueva, A. R., Hattner, R. S., and Frost, H. M.: A tetrachrome stain for fresh mineralized bone sections: useful in the diagnosis of bone diseases, Stain Technol. **39**:87-94, 1964.
19. Villanueva, A. R., Ilnicki, L., Frost, H. M., and Arnstein, A. R.: Measurement of the bone formation rate in a case of familial hypophosphatemic vitamin-D resistant rickets, J. La. Clin. Med. **67**:973-982, 1966.
20. Villanueva, A. R.: A bone stain for osteoid seams in fresh unembedded, mineralized bone, Stain Technol. **49**:1-8, 1974.
21. Villanueva, A. R., and Mehr, L.: Modifications of the Goldner and Gomori one-step trichrome stains for plastic-embedded thin sections of bone, Am. J. Med. Technol. **43**:536-538, 1977.
22. Villanueva, A. R.: A modified blood stain useful in the diagnosis and evaluation of hematologic elements, J. Histotechnol. **1**:19-22, 1977.
23. Villanueva, A. R.: A Von Kossa variant modification. (Unpublished data, 1977.)
24. Villanueva, A. R.: A toluidine blue stain for calcification front, cement line and osteoid seams in plastic embedded undecalcified sections of bone, J. Histotechnol. **2**:139, 1979.

Part III. Histomorphometric quantitative analysis of bone

Antonio R. Villanueva

Microscopic histomorphometric analysis of mineralized bone is rarely applied in a pathology laboratory. Most of the work on morphometry is done in specialized research laboratories[4,16,18,24,28-30] where analytic techniques are available for quantitating dynamics of tetracycline-labeled bone. But the methods of demonstrating and measuring bone kinetics histomorphometrically have never attracted many pathologists. Because of this oversight undecalcified bone is one of the most neglected types of tissue in the pathology laboratory.

Today undecalcified bone has assumed a firm role in pathology and in medicine—a situation that was not true 20 years ago. Probably the first investigator who contributed to the improvement of quantitative bone histomorphometry is Frost.[10,11,13] He developed and pioneered one of the most important areas of potential study of patients—the quantitative histologic methods for the study of bone dynamics.[5-8] His pioneering techniques yielded large amounts of valid information essential to the pathologic interpretation of bone biopsies, particularly in the field of metabolic bone diseases.[3,9,12,14,21,29,31]

The following section is devoted to the quantitative measurements of various structures and their estimation. For the purpose of those interested in the histomorphometric quantitative analysis, only two kinds of bone surfaces will be discussed: (1) cortical and (2) trabecular surfaces.

METHODOLOGY

Bone specimens suitable for this kind of measurement are obtained from the iliac crest by trephine biopsy[1,17] or from the eleventh rib.[27]

Complete measurement of at least one iliac crest (or rib) section is adequate if the measured values must be significant. The iliac crest must be a complete section cut transversely from cortex to cortex, or a complete cross section of a rib.

For microscopic identification of cells and other related structures, Villanueva's bone stain[32] is most satisfactory, particularly if simultaneous assessment of osteoid seams and tetracycline is determined.

LABELING TECHNICS

The labeling technic is basically Frost's concept[10] but modified by Dr. A. M. Parfitt (Director of the Bone Mineral Research Laboratory, Henry Ford Hospital, Detroit, Michigan).

The following instructions for bone labeling and biopsy protocol are described below:

1. Schedule biopsy first and then initiate protocol exactly 21 days earlier.
2. First label—oxytetracycline, 250 mg every 8 hours for 3 days.
   Second label—after an interval of 11 days, demeclocycline HCl (Declomycin), 300 mg every 8 hours for 3 days.
3. Do not vary the labeling schedule even if osteomalacia is suspected.
4. The following precautions should be adhered to as closely as possible:
   a. The time of administration should be 7 AM, 3 PM, and 11 PM or as close to this as possible with the patient's schedule.
   b. No milk or dairy products should be consumed by the patient from 1 hour before to 2 hours after medication, which should be taken with water only. Nondairy foods do not affect absorption.
   c. No aluminum-containing antacids should be taken from 1 hour before to 2 hours after medication.

With the above schedule of time, the periods available for ingestion of dairy products and aluminum-containing antacids are 9 AM to 2 PM and 5 PM to 10 PM.

Basically the labeling protocol calls for oxytetracycline, 250 mg every 8 hours for 3 days, followed by an 11-day gap, followed by Declomycin, 250 mg every 8 hours for 3 days. The biopsy will be performed on the fourth day after the completion of the second label. If the first day of the label is counted as day 1, the biopsy should be performed on day 21.

RECOGNITION OF HISTOLOGIC STRUCTURES
Osteoid seams

Bone is a highly specialized tissue consisting of specialized cells and organic and inorganic substances. One of these specialized cells is called an "osteoblast." These cells are often called "bone builders." They are responsible in laying down new unmineralized organic matrix, commonly known as osteoid seams. Some time after 14 days this matrix begins to mineralize and the mineralized matrix is now called "bone." An osteoid seam therefore constitutes a layer of unmineralized organic matrix of bone. After mineralization, the convention is to term the bone matrix simply the matrix—a highly calcified tissue. See Figs. 6-7 and 6-8.

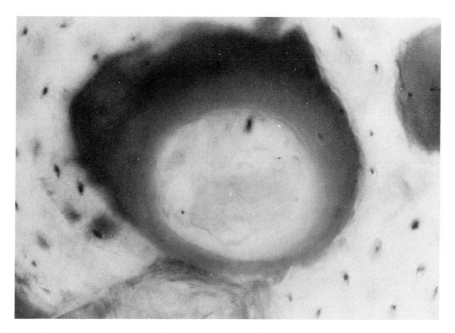

Fig. 6-7. Photomicrograph of osteoid seam, *gray* (originally green), taken from a mineralized unembedded, ground cross section of bone. At periphery of seam is a *dark* (originally reddish orange) staining area of incompletely mineralized bone. Dark-staining cells in bone matrix are osteocytes. (Villanueva bone stain, 250×.)

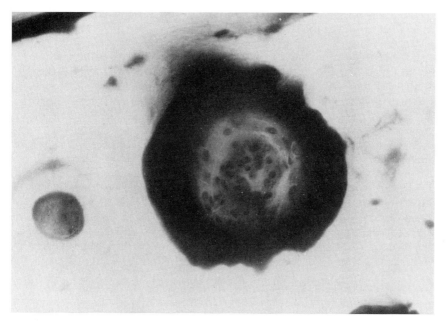

Fig. 6-8. Same case as in Fig. 6-7 but this figure shows histologic feature of a red osteoid seam. It is indicated by dark circular band lining the intima of haversian canal. Just around seam is a highly mineralized bone matrix, and osteoid itself is densely stained. (Villanueva bone stain, 250×.)

Trabecular surface

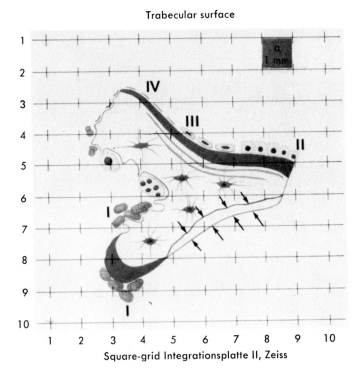

Square-grid Integrationsplatte II, Zeiss

Fig. 6-9. Diagram of trabecular surface. Area and perimeter measurements by point (hits) and line (intersects). Square grid is comprised of 100 possible hits, 10 series of parallel-horizontal, and 10 series of superimposed parallel-vertical test lines. Each square represents an area equal to 1% as indicated above, and *a* represents spacing between parallel lines. Dark bands lining the upper and lower trabecular surfaces are osteoid seams. Two lighter bands, peripheral to upper osteoid seam, are two tetracycline labels. Lining the intima of these seams are the four types of osteoblasts (*I* to *IV*). Note also two osteoclasts—one mononucleated and the other multinucleated.

If a stained, undecalcified section of bone is examined with a high dry objective of the microscope and moved about on the stage, a field somewhat similar to that illustrated in Figs. 6-9 and 6-10 should be found easily. Osteoid seams appear in two major colors, red and green, lining the haversian or trabecular spaces in fresh unembedded ground sections stained with the Villanueva bone stain but red when embedded in plastic. On the average, the thickness measured on over 5000 osteoid seams in normal individuals is 11.6 ± 1.25 μm.[25,26] Seams are hyaline and clear and contain canaliculi and lacunae, which in turn contain osteocytes. Special stains or phase-contrast microscopy will reveal these features. At the junction between osteoid and bone lies a zone of demarcation measuring about 2.5 μm in width.[33] Under high power, the zone of demarcation reveals a highly granular structure advancing upon the osteoid seam.

Osteoid seams possess the following properties, which one may need to measure: (1) a perimeter, (2) a thickness, (3) the rate of apposition and of mineralization, (4) the number in a unit amount of bone tissue, and (5) the location or distribution throughout a given bone in the whole skeleton.

Osteoid seams normally occur in the following sites: (1) actively forming haversian systems, (2) actively forming endosteal new bone, (3) actively forming trabeculae or portions of trabeculae in cancellous bone.

Frost's basic fuchsin, Goldner's trichrome, Villanueva's bone stain, and Von Kossa's readily differentiate such osteoid seams.

Trabecular surface (Fig. 6-9)

The trabeculae are thin and average approximately 125 μm in thickness.[17] The spaces between the trabeculae are filled with marrow. The trabeculae also has the properties of shape, width, volume, and length. Similarly, they undergo a progressive, net loss in thickness and

Haversian surface

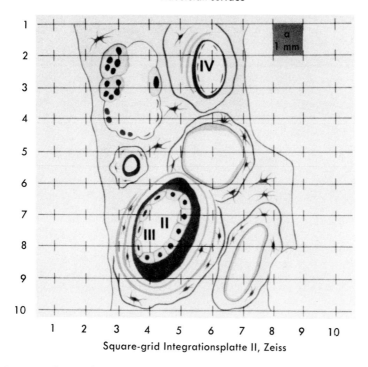

Square-grid Integrationsplatte II, Zeiss

Fig. 6-10. Diagram of cortical surface. Areas, porosity, and circumference measurements by point (hits) and line (intersects). Square grid is comprised of 100 possible hits and 10 series of superimposed parallel-vertical test lines. Each square represents an area equal to 1% as indicated above, and *a* represents spacing between parallel lines. Dark bands lining the intima of three haversian canals are osteoid seams. Smaller seam is unlabeled but larger ones are labeled, as indicated by double lighter bands peripheral to osteoid seams. Note the three types of osteoblasts (*II* to *IV*) without type I. A single resorption surface is also observed at upper left. Note also two multinucleated and one mononucleated osteoclasts enclosed in Howship's lacunae.

number with age. This loss in trabecular bone mass begins soon after longitudinal growth stops and continues for the remainder of life.[25] The amount of surface trabecular bone exposed to histologic remodeling activity (that is, the surface-to-volume ratio for trabeculae) varies depending on age and sampling site in comparison to that exposed by equivalent amounts of compact bone.[20]

Haversian surface (Fig. 6-10)

The space enclosed by the walls of all the haversian canals in bone constitutes the haversian surface. Its changes with normal aging are relatively small compared with those of the other surfaces, and in normal adults its volume may be considered as approximately constant.[25] Included in the haversian surface are cylindric structures, or canals, running longitudinally with the axes of long bones. Communicating with the haversian canals are narrow channels,

Volkmann's canals, originating from the periosteal and endosteal surfaces, which make a way through the bone obliquely or at right angles through the bone's long axis. These canals contain blood vessels and nerves. In cross sections of bone, haversian canals are seen to be surrounded by concentric lamellae and sometimes by osteoid seams or by resorption spaces. The inner surface of the normal haversian canal is lined with endothelium-like cells. Haversian canals in stained sections are easy to identify and count.

Primary osteons

Primary osteons are produced by enfolding of the periosteal circumference around longitudinally coursing vessels during growth. Such osteons are not considered in Frost's methods but are included in Parfitt's fractional cortical calculations.[22]

Secondary osteons

Secondary osteons are haversian systems that have been formed after formation of the cortex. Most of Frost's data are measured from these systems.

Osteocytic lacunae

Osteocytic lacunae are small holes in bone. Branching out from these lacunar walls are several canaliculi. These are small tubular holes in bone, anastomosing with one another and then connecting to a vascular channel.

Bone resorption

In eroding a bone surface, osteoclasts produce shallow indentations called "Howship's lacunae." Osteoclasts are active, motile cells, and once having performed their function, they disappear. When osteoclasts resorb bone, they remove both mineral and organic phases simultaneously. Bone resorption in the whole skeleton therefore constitutes all the destructive activity of osteoclasts. The evidence of the previous existence of Howship's lacunae after they have been covered by bone matrix remains as scalloped irregularities in the cement lines of osteons or trabeculae. At the light-microscope resolution these shallow, scalloped excavations on the surface of the bone, which are Howship's lacunae, can be seen prominently. A good example of this type of cement line is those seen in Paget's disease.

MICROSCOPIC MEASUREMENTS[2,15,23]

A standard binocular medical microscope with a Zeiss Integrationsplatte II Micrometer at $160\times$ with a 0.4 N.A. objective is used for these measurements. This eyepiece micrometer contains 10 series parallel-horizontal and ten series superimposed parallel-vertical test lines and 100 possible hits (Figs. 6-9 and 6-10). During measurement of the sections, the micrometer eyepiece is optically superimposed upon the image of the section being evaluated in increments of one field. When a reticule line crosses the image of the bone surface, it is recorded as an "intersect" with respect to (1) which of the four types of osteoblasts adjacent to an osteoid seam it crossed, (2) which of the four types of osteoblasts corresponds to a labeled or unlabeled osteoid seam, (3) which inert surface it crossed, (4) which of the five kinds of cell types it crossed adjacent to Howship's lacunae, and (5) the time that two reticule lines intersect immediately upon the image of a bone surface, whereby the intersects record a "hit" with respect to all points hitting upon an osteoid seam, haversian or Volkmann's canals (cortex only), bone, and marrow cavity. Proceed to the next field, recording all the information observed, until every section area is scanned (see Table 6-2). Cover the section systematically so that about 400 to 500 intersects and 2000 to 5000 hits (for bone and Volkmann's and haversian canals) accumulate at the haversian surface and 500 to 1000 inter-

Table 6-2. Tabulated data from Figs. 6-9 and 6-10

	Haversian surface	Trabecular surface
Intersects		
Cell types of osteoid seams		
I—Mesenchymal pre-osteoblasts		
Tetracycline label	0	0
No tetracycline label	0	4
II—Cuboid osteoblasts		
Tetracycline label	5	2
No tetracycline label	0	0
III—Intermediate osteoblasts		
Tetracycline label	3	3
No tetracycline label	0	0
IV—Flat, elongated lining cells		
Tetracycline label	3	1
No tetracycline label	3	2
Unidentifiable cells or absence of osteoblasts		
Tetracycline label	0	0
No tetracycline label	0	1
Inert surface	14	6
Cell types of Howship's lacunae		
Multinucleated osteoclasts	3	2
Mononuclear osteoclasts	1	2
Flat, elongated lining cells	2	2
Mesenchymal pre-osteoblasts	0	3
Unidentifiable cells	2	1
Absence of cells	2	1
Hits		
Porosity (Haversian or Volkmann's canals)	16	
Bone	36	14
Osteoid	3	4

sects and 3000 to 5000 hits (for bone, osteoid seams, and marrow) accumulate at the trabecular surface per section.

Convert all raw data to percent, micrometers, millimeters, days, micrometers per day, mm³/mm³/year, and so forth, of a given surface according to the formulas and examples described in this text.

Trabecular surface
Circumference formula (Fig. 6-9)

$$\frac{H + V}{\text{No. of throws}} \times \frac{3.1416}{2} \times a = \text{Circumference, or perimeter (Zeiss Intergrationsplatte II)}$$

H, Total horizontal intersects; V, total vertical intersects; a, width between parallel spacing test lines.

Example (Fig. 6-9)
Given:

Horizontal intersects	12	Number of throws = 2	
Vertical intersects	18	a = 1 mm	
TOTAL INTERSECTS	30		

Substituting from above formula:

$$\frac{H + V}{\text{No. of throws}} \times \frac{3.1416}{2} \times a, \text{ or } \frac{30}{2} \times \frac{3.1416}{2} \times 1 = 23.6 \text{ mm}$$

Surface measurements of trabecula

1. % of osteoid seams of total surface = $\dfrac{\text{Total intersects of osteoid seam}}{\text{Total intersects}} \times 100 = \dfrac{13}{30} = 43.3\%$

2. % of label of total surface = $\dfrac{\text{Total intersects of label}}{\text{Total intersects}} \times 100 = \dfrac{6}{30} = 20\%$

3. % of fractional label of total surface = $\dfrac{\text{\% of label of total surface}}{\text{\% of osteoid seams of total surface}} \times 100 = \dfrac{20}{43.3\%} = 46.2\%$

4. % that is inert of total surface = $\dfrac{\text{Total intersects of inert surface}}{\text{Total intersects}} \times 100 = \dfrac{6}{30} = 20\%$

5. % of Howship's lacunae of total surface = $\dfrac{\text{Total intersects of Howship's lacunae}}{\text{Total intersects}} \times 100 = \dfrac{11}{30} = 36.6\%$

6. % of osteoblastic activity = $\dfrac{\text{Total intersects of cuboid + intermediate osteoblasts}}{\text{Total intersects of osteoid seams}} \times 100 = \dfrac{5}{12} = 41.7\%$

7. % of osteoclastic activity = $\dfrac{\text{Total intersects of multinucleated osteoclasts}}{\text{Total intersects}} \times 100 = \dfrac{2}{30} = 6.67\%$

8. % of relative osteoid volume = $\dfrac{\text{Total osteoid hits}}{\text{Total bone + Osteoid hits}} \times 100 = \dfrac{4}{18} = 14.3\%$

9. % of fractional osteoid volume = $\dfrac{\text{Total osteoid hits}}{\text{Total hits}} \times 100 = \dfrac{4}{100} = 4\%$

10. % of fractional bone volume = $\dfrac{\text{Total bone hits}}{\text{Total hits}} \times 100 = \dfrac{14}{100} = 14\%$

11. % of total bone volume = % of fractional bone volume + % of fractional osteoid volume = 14% + 4% = 18%

12. Mean trabecular thickness = $\dfrac{2 \times a \times (\text{Total bone hits + Osteoid hits})}{\text{Total intersects}} = \dfrac{2 \times 1 \times 18}{30} = 1.2 \text{ mm}$

Rates involved with bone remodeling

1. *Assuming measured mean width between two tetracycline labels is 9.1 μm and number of days between two labeling episodes is 14 days, one may calculate the appositional rate, μm/day (M), according to the formula below:*

$$M (\mu\text{m/day}) = \frac{\text{Mean width between two tetracycline labels}}{\text{Number of days between labeling episodes}} = \frac{9.1}{14} = 0.65 \ \mu\text{m/day (uncorrected)}$$

Corrected M_f (μm/day) = Uncorrected M × % of fractional label of total surface = 0.65 × 0.462 = 0.3 μm/day

2. Assuming mean wall thickness of inert surface's cementing line is 50 μm (Fig. 6-9, *arrows*), one can calculate formation time, σ_f, as follows:

$$\sigma_f \text{(day)} = \frac{\text{Mean wall thickness}}{\text{Corrected } M_f} = \frac{50 \ \mu\text{m}}{0.30 \ \mu\text{m day}} = 167 \text{ days}$$

3. Assuming mean width of osteoid seam as 10 μm, one may now calculate mineralization lag time, M_{Lt}, as follows:

$$M_{Lt} = \frac{\text{Width of osteoid seam}}{\text{Uncorrected } M} = \frac{10 \ \mu\text{m}}{0.65 \ \mu\text{m/day}} = 15.4 \text{ days (} M \text{ based)}$$

$$M_{Lt} = \frac{\text{Width of osteoid seam}}{\text{Corrected } M_f} = \frac{10 \ \mu\text{m}}{0.30 \ \mu\text{m/day}} = 33.3 \text{ days (} M_f \text{ based)}$$

4. Bone formation rate (volume based, mm³/mm³/year) =

$$\frac{\text{Appositional rate} (M) \times \dfrac{365}{1000} \times \text{Total tetracycline intersects}}{\text{Bone hits} + \text{Osteoid hits} \times a} = \frac{0.65 \times 0.365 \times 6}{18 \times 1} = 0.079 \text{ mm}^3/\text{mm}^3/\text{year}$$

Haversian surface (Fig. 6-10)
Cortical area, mm² (A_c)

1. The number of hits within the cortical matrix is 55. To calculate the area, the formula is given below:

$$A_c(\text{mm}^2) = \frac{\text{No. of cortical hits} \times \text{Area of grid (mm}^2\text{)}}{\text{No. of possible hits} \times \text{No. of throws}}$$

$$\text{Substituting} = \frac{55 \times 100}{100 \times 1}$$

$$A_c = 55 \text{ mm}^2$$

2. No. of osteoid seams/mm² = (A_f)
   No. of osteoid seams = 3
   Cortical area (A_c) = 55 mm²
   $A_f = \dfrac{3}{55} = 0.054/\text{mm}^2$

3. Mean circumference of osteoid seams, mm (S_f)
   Two osteoid seams with a total horizontal and vertical intersects of 14. To calculate S_f, the equation is similar to the formula used at the trabecular surface:

$$S_f(\text{mm}) = \frac{H + V \text{ (intersects)}}{\text{No. of throws} \times \text{No. of osteoid seams}} \times \frac{3.1416}{2} \times a$$

$$= \frac{14}{2 \times 2} \times \frac{3.1416}{2} \times 1$$

$$= 5.50 \text{ mm}$$

4. Appositional rate, μm/day, uncorrected. If 0.75 μm/day is the uncorrected calculated appositional rate (M), the corrected appositional rate (M_f) using Parfitt's formula[22] would be as follows:

$$M \times \text{Fractional labeled seams} = M_f (\mu\text{m/day})$$
$$0.75 \times 0.785 = 0.59 \ \mu\text{m/day}$$

using Frost's formula[11]

$$M (\mu\text{m/day}) \times \frac{\text{No. of osteoid seams labeled}}{\text{Total no. of osteoid seams}} = M_f (\mu\text{m/day})$$

$$0.75 \times \frac{2}{3} = 0.50 \ \mu\text{m/day (} M_f \text{ based in } \mu\text{m/day)}$$

$$0.50 \times \frac{365}{1000} = 0.18 \text{ mm/year} \,(M_f \text{ based in mm/year})$$

5. Mineralization lag time, days (M_{Lt}). If the mean width of osteoid seams is 9 μm, the mineralization lag time may now be calculated:

$$M_{Lt} = \frac{\text{Width of osteoid seam } (\mu m)}{M \, (\mu m/day)} = \frac{9}{0.75} = 12 \text{ days } (M \text{ based})$$

$$M_{Lt} = \frac{\text{Width of osteoid seam } (\mu m)}{M_f \, (\mu m/day)} = \frac{9}{0.59} = 15.2 \text{ days } (M_f \text{ based})$$

6. Formation time, days (σ_f). If mean osteon wall thickness, MWT, is 68 μm, this can be calculated according to the equation below:

$$\sigma_f = \frac{MWT}{M_f} = \frac{68 \, \mu m}{0.59 \, \mu m/day} = 115.2 \text{ days, or } 0.32 \text{ years}$$

7. Activation frequency, foci/year (μ_f)

$$\mu_f = \frac{A_f}{\sigma_f (\text{years})} = \frac{0.054}{0.32}$$

$$\mu_f = 0.17$$

8. Bone formation rate, mm³/mm³/year (V_f)[22]

$$V_f = \frac{M \times 0.365 \times \text{No. of tetracycline intersects}}{\text{Total no. of cortical hits} \times a}$$

$$V_f = \frac{0.75 \times 0.365 \times 11}{55 \times 1}$$

$$V_f = 0.0548 \text{ mm}^3/\text{mm}^3/\text{year}$$

Using Frostian[11] dynamics (V_f), one can also calculate according to the formula:

V_f = No. of osteoid seams/mm² (A_f) × Circumference of osteoid seams (S_f) (mm) × Radial closure rate (M_f) mm/year

$$= 0.054 \times 5.50 \times 0.18$$

$$V_f = 0.0535 \text{ mm}^3/\text{mm}^3/\text{year}$$

9. Porosity, %

$$P = \frac{\text{Total no. of haversian + Volkmann's canal hits}}{\text{Total cortical hits}} \times 100$$

$$P = \frac{16}{55}$$

$$P = 29.1\%$$

Measurements of haversian surface

1. % of osteoid seams of total surface $= \dfrac{\text{Total intersects of osteoid seams}}{\text{Total intersects}} \times 100 = \dfrac{14}{38} = 36.8\%$

2. % of label of total surface $= \dfrac{\text{Total intersects of label}}{\text{Total intersects}} \times 100 = \dfrac{11}{38} = 28.9\%$

3. % of fractional label of total surface $= \dfrac{\text{\% of label of total surface}}{\text{\% of osteoid seams of total surface}} \times 100 = \dfrac{28.9}{36.8} = 78.5\%$

4. % that is inert of total surface $= \dfrac{\text{Total intersects of inert surface}}{\text{Total intersects}} \times 100 = \dfrac{14}{38} = 36.8\%$

5. % of Howship's lacunae of total surface $= \dfrac{\text{Total intersects of Howship's lacunae}}{\text{Total intersects}} \times 100 = \dfrac{10}{38} = 26.3\%$

6. % of osteoblastic activity $= \dfrac{\text{Total intersects of cuboid + intermediate osteoblasts}}{\text{Total intersects of osteoid seams}} \times 100 = \dfrac{8}{14} = 57.1\%$

7. $\% \text{ of osteoclastic activity} = \dfrac{\text{Total intersects of multinucleated osteoclasts}}{\text{Total intersects}} \times 100 = \dfrac{3}{38} = 7.90\%$

8. $\% \text{ of relative osteoid volume} = \dfrac{\text{Total osteoid hits}}{\text{Total bone hits + osteoid hits}} \times 100 = \dfrac{3}{39} = 7.69\%$

9. $\% \text{ of fractional osteoid volume} = \dfrac{\text{Total osteoid hits}}{\text{Total hits}} \times 100 = \dfrac{3}{55} = 5.46\%$

10. $\% \text{ of fractional bone volume} = \dfrac{\text{Total bone hits}}{\text{Total hits}} \times 100 = \dfrac{36}{55} = 65.4\%$

11. $\% \text{ of total bone volume} = \% \text{ of fractional bone volume} +$

$$\% \text{ of fractional osteoid volume} = 65.4 + 5.46 = 70.9\%$$

REFERENCES (Histomorphometric quantitative analysis of bone)

1. Bordier, P. J., and Tun-Chot, S.: Quantitative histology of metabolic bone disease, J. Clin. Endocrinol. Metab. **1:**197-215, 1972.
2. Chalkley, H. W., Cornfield, J., and Park, H.: A method for estimating volume-surface ratios. Science **110:**295-297, 1949.
3. Duncan, H., Frost, H. M., Villanueva, A. R., and Sigler, J.: The osteoporosis of rheumatoid arthritis, Arthritis Rheum. **8:**843-954, 1965.
4. Epker, B. N., and Frost, H. M.: A histological study of remodelling at the periosteal, haversian canal, cortical endosteal, and trabecular endosteal surfaces in human rib, Anat. Rec. **152:**129-136, 1965.
5. Frost, H. M., Villanueva, A. R., and Roth, H.: Measurement of bone formation in a 57 year old man by means of tetracycline, Henry Ford Hosp. Med. Bull. **8**(2):230-254, 1960.
6. Frost, H. M., and Villanueva, A. R.: Measurement of osteoblastic activity in diaphyseal bone, Stain Technol. **35:**179-189, 1960.
7. Frost, H. M., Villanueva, A. R., and Roth, H.: Qualitative method for measuring osteoclastic activity, Henry Ford Hosp. Med. Bull. **10:**217-228, March, 1962.
8. Frost, H. M., and Villanueva, A. R.: Human osteoclastic activity: qualitative histological measurement, Henry Ford Hosp. Med. Bull. **10:**229-236, March 1962.
9. Frost, H. M.: Bone dynamics in metabolic bone diseases, J. Bone Joint Surg. **48-A:**1192-1203, 1966.
10. Frost, H. M.: Tetracycline-based histologic and analysis of bone remodelling, Calcif. Tis. Res. **3:** 211-217, 1969.
11. Frost, H. M.: Mathematical elements in lamellar bone remodelling, Springfield, Ill., 1973, Charles C Thomas, Publisher.
12. Frost, H. M.: Orthopedic lecture series, vol. III: Bone remodelling and its relationship to metabolic bone diseases, Springfield, Ill., 1973, Charles C Thomas, Publisher.
13. Frost, H. M.: Bone remodelling dynamics, Springfield, Ill., 1963, Charles C Thomas, Publisher.
14. Heaney, R. P., and Recker, R. R.: Estrogen effects on bone remodelling at menopause, Clin. Res. **23:**535A, 1975.
15. Henning, A.: A critical survey of volume and surface measurement in microscopy, Zeiss Werkzeitschrift **20:**3-12, 1958.
16. Jaworski, Z. F., Meunier, P., and Frost, H. M.: Observations on two types of resorption in human lamellar cortical bone, Clin. Orthop. **83:**279-285, 1972.
17. Jowsey, J.: The bone biopsy, New York, 1977, Plenum Medical Book Co.
18. Jowsey, J.: Microradiography. A morphologic approach to quantitative bone turnover. In Frame, B., Parfitt, A. M., and Duncan, H., editors: Clinical aspects of metabolic bone disease, Amsterdam, 1973, Excerpta Medica Foundation.
19. Jett, S., Ramser, J. R., Frost, H. M., and Villanueva, A. R.: Bone turnover and osteogenesis imperfecta, Arch. Pathol. **81:**112-116, 1966.
20. Meunier, P., and Edward, C.: Quantification of osteoid tissue in trabecular bone methodology and results in normal iliac bone. In Jaworski, Z. F. G., editor: Proceedings of the First International Workshop on Bone Morphometry, Ottawa, 1976, Ottawa Press.
21. Morgan, B.: Osteomalacia, renal osteodystrophy and osteoporosis, Springfield, Ill., 1973, Charles C Thomas, Publisher.
22. Parfitt, A. M.: The physiologic and clinical significance of bone histomorphometric data. In Recker, R., editor: Bone histomorphometry, techniques and interpretations, Boca Raton, Florida, C.R.C. Press. (In press.)
23. Parfitt, A. M.: The stereologic basis of bone histomorphometry, theory of quantitative microscopy and reconstruction of the third dimension. In Recker, R., editor: Bone histomorphometry, techniques and interpretations, Boca Raton, Florida, C.R.C. Press. (In press.)
24. Parfitt, A. M., Villanueva, A. R., Crouch, M. M., Mathews, C. H. E., and Duncan, H.: Classification of osteoid seams by combined use of cell morphology and tetracycline labeling. Evidence for intermittency of mineralization. In Meunier, P. J.: Proceedings of Second Workshop on Bone Morphometry, Paris, 1977, Armour Montagu.

25. Pirok, D., Ramser, J. R., Takahashi, H., Villanueva, A. R., and Frost, H. M.: Normal histologic, tetracycline, and dynamic parameters in human mineralized bone sections, Henry Ford Hosp. Med. Bull. **14:**195-218, 1966.

26. Schulz, A., and Delling, G.: Age-related changes of new bone formation—determination of histomorphometric parameters of the iliac crest trabecular bone. In Jaworski, Z. F. G., editor: Proceedings of the First International Workshop on Bone Morphometry, Ottawa, 1976, Ottawa University Press.

27. Sedlin, E. D., Frost, H. M., and Villanueva, A. R.: The eleventh rib biopsy in the study of metabolic bone disease, Henry Ford Hosp. Med. Bull. **11:** 217-219, June 1963.

28. Takahashi, H., and Frost, H. M.: A tetracycline based comparison of the number of cortical bone forming sites in normal diabetic persons, J. Jpn. Orthop. Assoc. **39:**13-23, 1966.

29. Teitelbaum, S. L., Rosenberg, E. M., Richardson, C. A., and Avioli, L. V.: Histological studies of bone from normocalcemic postmenopausal patients with increased circulating parathyroid hormone, J. Clin. Endocrinol. **42:**537-543, 1976.

30. Villanueva, A. R., Frost, H. M., Ilnicki, L., Frame, B., Smith, R., and Arnstein, A. R.: Cortical bone dynamics in 21 cases of osteoporosis measured by means of tetracycline labeling, J. Lab. Clin. Med. **68:**599-616, 1966.

31. Villanueva, A. R.: Quantitative histology of bone remodelling dynamics. In Frame, B., Parfitt, A. M., and Duncan, H., editors: Clinical aspects of metabolic bone disease, Amsterdam, 1973, Excerpta Medica Foundation, ICS ser. no. 270.

32. Villanueva, A. R.: A bone stain for osteoid seams in fresh unembedded, mineralized bone, Stain Technol. **49:**1-8, 1974.

33. Villanueva, A. R.: Unpublished data, 1978.

CHAPTER 7

General staining considerations

Part I. Theoretical aspects

The constituent parts of cells and intercellular material are usually transparent, and unless there exist appreciable differences in refractive index, they are not distinguishable from one another. Leeuwenhoek, in 1719, was the first to attempt the use of a coloring agent to overcome this difficulty, but it was not until 1848 that the use of dyes in microscopic work became common. Dyes adapted for microscopic use are termed "biologic stains" and possess a high degree of purity. There are three broad classes of biologic stains. The first category is the general tissue stains, which use one, two, and occasionally three dyes to differentiate the nucleus from the cytoplasm of cells and permit the differentiation between the different types of tissue. The second category involves the use of special staining procedures, for example, connective tissue stains, which demonstrate collagen and elastin in detail. The third classification includes heavy metal impregnation methods. These are not actual staining technics, but rather depend on the use of metal salts that are deposited on the tissue, and the tissues are visualized where the metal salts are converted to their metallic form.

CLASSIFICATION

Dyes themselves can be classified into two groups—the natural dyes (those not produced by artificial means) and the artificial dyes (produced from chemical transformations from substances found in coal tar). There are only a few dyes that can be classified as natural, and the chemistry of these is less well known than that of the artificial dyes. The most important of the natural dyes are hematoxylin, indigo, cochineal and its derivatives, orcein, and brazilin.

Natural dyes

Indigo was formerly manufactured only from a plant of the genus *Indigofera*, but can now be synthesized artificially. A glucoside known as indican is present in the plants, and this indican is converted by a fermentation process into the indigo dye. See Fig. 7-1 for the generally accepted formula.

Another member of the indigo dye family is the sodium salt of indigo disulfonic acid. The dye, known as indigo carmine, is colored blue, has acid properties, and is sometimes used as a plasma stain. Petragnani used an indigo carmine and acid fuchsin mixture as a special stain

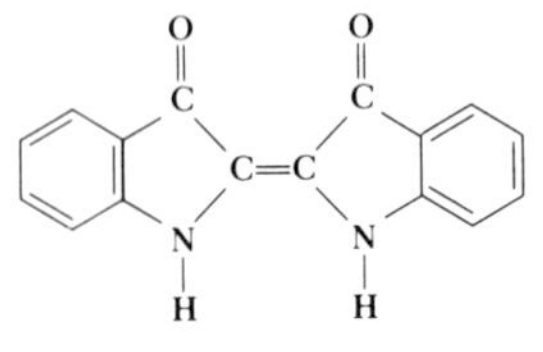

Fig. 7-1. Indigo. Based on artificial manufacture, the generally accepted formula is $C_{16}H_{10}N_2O_2$. Molecular weight 262.272.

for Negri inclusion bodies. See Fig. 7-2 for the generally accepted formula.

Cochineal and its derivatives form another class of natural dyes. Cochineal is obtained by a process of grinding and extracting the dried bodies of the female tropical cochineal insect. The deep red dye (cochineal) obtained from this process has little affinity for tissues unless the tissues contain some metal such as aluminum or iron. It is usually used with an alum mordant in aqueous solution for staining in bulk and gives a red-violet color to the nuclei, orange color to blood and muscle cells, and pale coloring to cytoplasm. Cochineal is little used in today's microtechnic, and recent methods will call for carmine (the purer coloring matter extracted from cochineal) or carminic acid (the nearly pure dye component). Carmine itself is less expensive than the purer carminic acid and is used for staining in bulk. In the form of acetocarmine it can be used as a chromatin stain for fresh material in smear preparations. Carmine and aluminum chloride combine to form mucicarmine, which is used to stain mucin with Mayer's mucicarmine technic. The dye is also used in Best's carmine stain for glycogen where the glycogen stains intensely with the solution. The carminic acid mentioned is the actual dye principle of both the cochineal and carmine. This substance is a strong dibasic acid and forms soluble salts with the alkali metals, and insoluble salts with the heavy metals. See Fig. 7-3 for the generally accepted formula.

Orcein is another natural dye that has begun to be synthesized artificially. Orcein is obtained principally from certain types of lichens (*Lecanora tinctoria* and *Rocella tinctoria*).

These colorless lichens, when treated with boiling water, have the lecanoric acid component split to yield orcinol, which is resorcinol with a methyl group attached (Fig. 7-4). This orcinol, when treated with air and ammonia, becomes orcein. The exact formula for orcein is unknown, but it is a weak acid, soluble in alkalis, and violet colored. Artificially produced orcein is synthesized from orcinol by the already indicated processes. The compound is used in a number of staining methods including Unna's orcein stain for elastic tissue, Mollier's quadruple stain, and Fullmer's orcinol new fuchsin for elastic tissue.

Brazilin is a natural dye that is rarely used in routine histotechnology. It is obtained by an extraction process from the bark of the brazilwood (redwood) tree. See Fig. 7-5, *A*, for the formula of the colorless brazilin. A colorless solution of brazilin may be converted to the red dye brazilein (Fig. 7-5, *B*) on exposure to air. This oxidized substance may be used as a nuclear stain (Mayer's brazalum stain) or to stain plant chromosomes.

Hematoxylin (Fig. 7-6), one of the most valu-

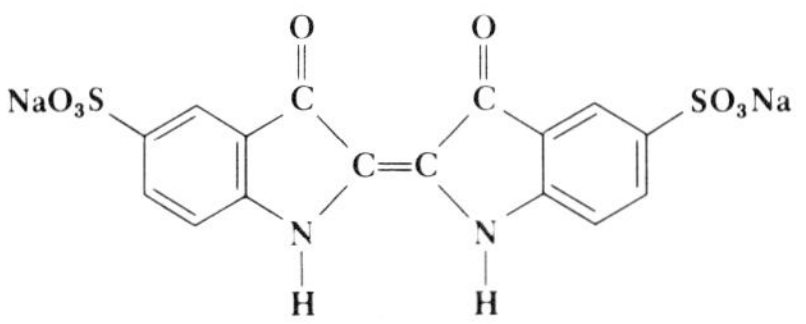

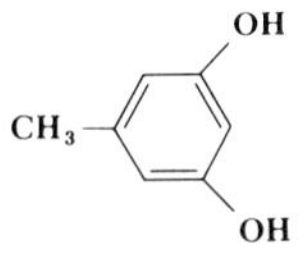

Fig. 7-4. Orcinol.

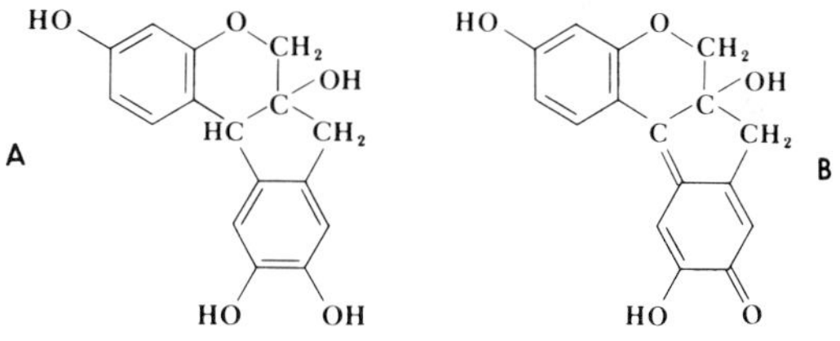

Fig. 7-5. Brazilin. **A,** Colorless. $C_{16}H_{14}O_5$. Molecular weight 286.288. **B,** Red dye, brazilein. $C_{16}H_{12}O_5$. Molecular weight 284.272.

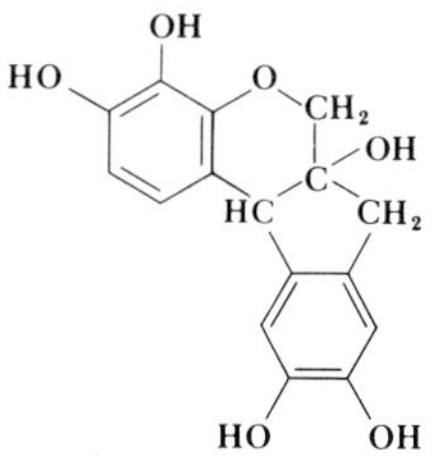

Fig. 7-2. Indigo carmine. $C_{16}H_8N_2O_8S_2Na_2$. Molecular weight 466.370.

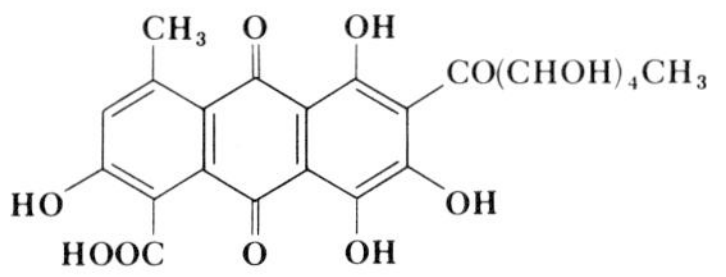

Fig. 7-3. Carminic acid. $C_{22}H_{20}O_{13}$. Molecular weight 492.402.

Fig. 7-6. Hematoxylin. $C_{16}H_{14}O_6$. Molecular weight 302.288.

able dyes in microtechnic, is obtained by an extraction process from the bark of the logwood tree. Hematoxylin and brazilin are similar compounds, but hematoxylin possesses one more hydroxyl group. On standing, this hematoxylin is converted into its oxidation product, hematein (Fig. 7-7), which is responsible for staining when combined with a mordant. Staining with hematoxylin solutions is further discussed under the section on nuclear staining.

Artificial dyes

Dyes classified as artificial far outnumber the natural dyes. The first artificial dyes were synthesized from aniline and all artificial dyes are sometimes referred to as aniline dye derivatives. Of the great variety of artificial dyes used in today's microtechnic, not all can be properly classified as aniline derivatives. The expression "coal-tar dyes" is more accurate to denote artificially produced dyes, as all artificial dyes are ultimately derivatives of the ingredients found in coal tar, especially benzene.

Benzene, empirical formula C_6H_6, has the structural fromula shown in Fig. 7-8. Benzene, being a member of the aromatic series of organic compounds, undergoes substitution reactions to combine with other radicals and form new compounds. Some of these radicals can combine in certain ways to give a colored product, which with further changes in the molecule, will become a dye.

There is still much to be understood regarding the structural formula of a compound and its relation to color. It is known that certain definite atomic groupings are associated with color. These are called chromophores, and the most

important are $C=C$, $C=O$, $C=S$, $C=N$, $N=N$, $N=O$, and NO_2. The more chromophores that occur in a compound, the deeper the color of that compound. Some of the chromophores mentioned have an acid character, such as the nitro group (NO_2), which occurs in picric acid and the quinoid benzene ring (Fig. 7-9). Basic chromophores include the azo grouping ($N=N$) and azin group (Fig. 7-10).

Benzene compounds containing chromophore radicals are called chromogens. Although colored by the presence of the chromophore radical, the compound itself possesses no affinity for tissue cells or fibers and is easily removed from tissue by simple mechanical processes. For a compound to be called a dye and possess affinity for tissue, it must have in the molecule not only the chromophore grouping, but also an additional auxiliary group known as an auxochrome. The auxochrome gives the compound the property of electrolytic dissociation, and it is this salt-forming property that gives the dye an affinity to attach itself to tissue. Auxochromes, one may note, may alter the shade of the color of the compound to a certain extent, but are not themselves the actual cause of color. A well-known example that illustrates the difference between a chromogen and a dye is that of trinitrobenzene and picric acid (Fig. 7-11).

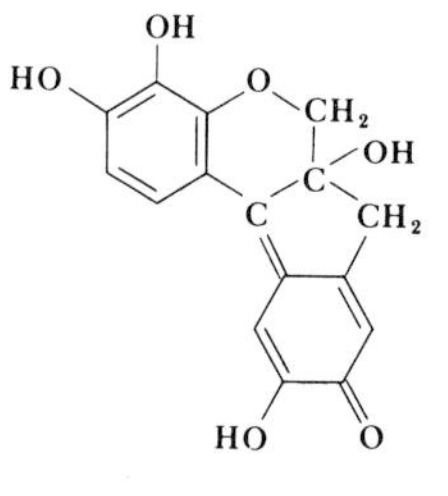

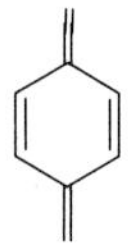

Fig. 7-9. Quinoid benzene ring.

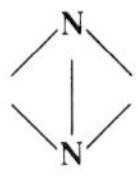

Fig. 7-10. Azin grouping.

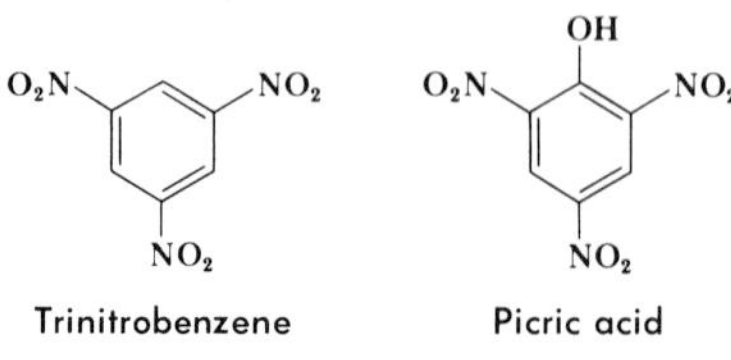

Fig. 7-7. Hematein. $C_{16}H_{12}O_6$. Molecular weight 300.272.

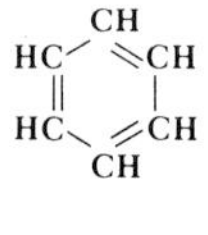

Fig. 7-8. Benzene.

Trinitrobenzene   Picric acid

Fig. 7-11. Trinitrobenzene (a chromogen) versus picric acid (a dye).

Table 7-1. Classification of synthetic dyes

Dye	Identifying structure	Example
Nitroso	Quinone oxime (nitrosophenol)	Fast green G
Nitro	$-NO_2$ group	Picric acid
Azo	Azo group ($-N=N-$) joining benzene or naphthalene rings 1. Monoazo	Orange G, Ponceau 2R, tartrazine, Metanil yellow
	2. Diazo	Oil red O, Congo red, Suden black B, Biebrich scarlet
Quinone-imine	Indamin group ($-N=$) and quinone benzene ring 1. Indamin	Toluylene blue
	2. Indophenol	Indophenol blue
	3. Azins	Safranin O
	4. Oxazins	Gallocyanin, Nile blue A, celestin blue
	5. Thiazins	Thionin; azure A,B,C; methylene blue; toluidine blue

Xanthene	Xanthene derivatives
	1. Fluorenes (aminoxanthenes)
	  a. Pyronins
	  b. Succineins
	  c. Rosamines
	  d. Rhodamines
		
		Pyronin Y
		Rhodamine S
		Sulforhodamine B
		Rhodamine B

	2. Rhodols (aminohydroxyxanthenes)	Rhodamine 12GM
	3. Fluorones (hydroxyxanthenes)	Fluorescein, eosin B, eosin Y, phloxine
Arylmeth-ane	Methane nucleus (CH_4) with phenyl groups substituting for hydrogen groups 1. Diphenylmethanes	Auramine O
	2. Diaminotriphenylmethanes	Light green SF
	3. Triaminotriphenylmethanes	Basic fuchsin, acid fuchsin, methyl violet 2B, crystal violet, aniline blue
	4. Hydroxytriphenylmethanes	Chrome violet CG *Note:* Phenolphthaleins and phenolsulfon-phthaleins are now grouped in this class
	5. Mono- and di-phenylnaphthyl-methanes	Victoria blue R
Anthra-quinone	Anthraquinone ring	Alizarin red S
Thiazole	Thiazole ring	Thioflavine B
Phthalo-cyanine	Complex compounds, similar in structure to chlorophyll with $C_6H_4 \cdot C_2N_2$ radicals surrounding a central metal atom, usually copper	Alcian blue Luxol fast blue

Trinitrobenzene contains three nitro groups, and these chromophores impart a yellow color to the compound as a whole. The compound, however, will not dissociate electrolytically and will not form salts with acids or alkalis. If the hydrogen group is replaced by a hydroxyl group as it is in picric acid, the compound becomes a dye because the hydroxyl group functions as an auxochrome and enables the picric acid to form salts with alkalis and dissociate electrolytically to attach itself to tissue. A dye, therefore, is an organic compound containing chomophoric and auxochromic groups attached to a benzene ring. The color is caused by the presence of the chromophoric groups and the dyeing properties from the salt-forming properties of the auxochromic groups.

Classification of synthetic dyes

On the basis of the chromophore present, the simple synthetic dyes may be classified into several groups (Table 7-1). Grouping them like this does not classify them in relation to color, as a single chromophore may occur in dyes of all colors, and it is difficult to determine from a chemical formula just what the color should be. Classification is based only on similar chemical structure. As far as color is concerned, the most general rule is that the more hydrogen atoms that are replaced by other radicals, the deeper the color of a given compound. In any group of similar dyes, the simplest dyes are yellow, and as more substituting groups are introduced into the molecule, the colors deepen through red to violet to blues to greens.

Acid and basic dyes

The terms "acid" and "basic" dyes do not refer to the hydrogen-ion concentration of the dye solution. Nor do the terms mean the commercial products are acids or bases as the products sold are usually salts. An acid dye is the salt (usually the sodium salt) of a color acid, that is, the chromophoric groups are located in the anionic part of the molecule; the basic dye is a salt (usually a chloride, sulfate, or acetate) of a color base, that is, the chromophoric groups are located in the cationic part of the molecule. It is the auxochromes, the salt-forming groups of dyes, which ordinarily determine whether a dye is classified as acidic or basic. The most common basic auxochrome encountered in dye chemistry is the amino group ($-NH_2$). The amino group is classified as basic because of the ability of the nitrogen atom to become pentavalent by the addition of the elements of water or of an acid. The compound then ionizes to yield hydroxyl ions and acts as a cation in forming salts. This would classify the entire molecule as a basic dye. A common acidic auxochrome is the carboxyl group ($-COOH$). This group ionizes to yield hydrogen ions by electrolytic dissociation and is found in most of the important acid dyes. The hydroxyl ($-OH$) group is a weaker acidic auxochrome that can also dissociate to give hydrogen ions in solution. How strongly acidic or basic a dye compound is will depend on the relative amount of the acidic and basic groups in the molecule as a whole. Other groups in the compound will affect the strength of the compound as a whole. The nitro grouping, an acid chromophore, makes hydroxyl groups in a compound more dissociated electrolytically and hence would give a more strongly acidic compound as a whole.

The sulfonic group ($-SO_3 \cdot H$) is frequently encountered in dyes. This salt-forming group dissociates electrolytically but is only weakly auxochromic as far as increasing the dyeing property of the compound as a whole. The chief function of this group is to make a dye water soluble or to change a basic dye into an acid dye. Basic fuchsin, for example, is changed into acid fuchsin by introducing sulfonic groupings into the basic fuchsin molecule. It should be noted that a compound with chromophoric and sulfonic groupings will have color but will not possess true dyeing properties unless there is also present a true auxochromic group.

Leuco compounds

Although the different chromophores differ considerably from one another in many ways, they all possess the common property of being easily reducible, that is, they will combine easily with hydrogen. On reduction, the nitro group would, for example, be reduced to an amino group; the azin bond could break to allow two hydrogen atoms to attach to the nitrogens; double bonds in a compound could be reduced to single bonds, with the simultaneous addition of the hydrogen atoms. The reduction process will destroy the chromophoric grouping, and the dye compound will lose its color. Colorless compounds produced this way are called leuco compounds. The reduction reaction is reversible under oxidizing conditions, and this property enables the dyes to be used as redox indicators. Fig. 7-12 is an example of the addition of hydrogen to fuchsin.

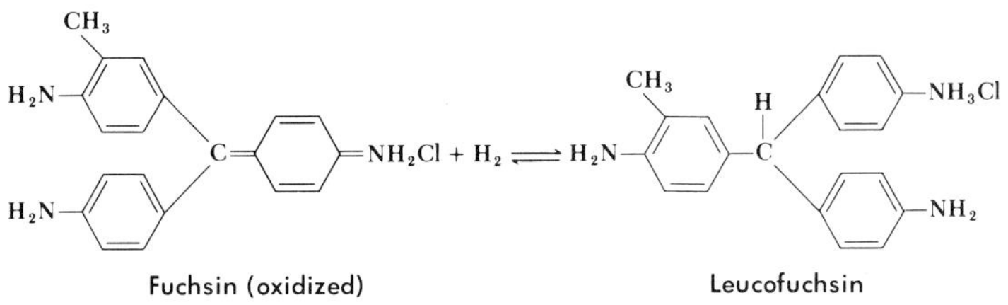

Fig. 7-12. Leuco compound formation.

Other types of leuco compounds, called leuco bases, may be formed, usually with the triphenyl methanes and xanthenes. Basic dyes usually occur as the salt of a colorless acid, and with the above dyes, when the acid radical is removed, the compound becomes colorless. Atoms in the molecule rearrange to give not a true dye base but a compound known as a carbinol. The chromophore is absent; so the compound as a whole is colorless. Carbinols are important as intermediates in the preparation of dyes. Chromophoric groupings may be similarly broken in the case of acid dyes.

APPLICATION OF STAINS

Stains may be used to color both living and fixed tissue and the purpose of staining is to make various tissue and cell constituents more evident.

Vital staining

Staining living tissue with vital dyes has become less frequent with the advent of phase-contrast and interference microscopy. However, vital techniques are useful for distinguishing certain cellular and tissue components that possess nearly identical refractive indices.

Vital stains may be employed in one of two ways. The first, also called intravital staining, depends on dye uptake by phagocytic cells. Dyes used for this purpose are colloidal solutions of nontoxic coloring matter suspended in sterile water and injected into the living animal by use of one of a number of routes. After a prescribed period of time, the animal is killed and appropriate tissues are excised for fixation, processing, sectioning, and staining. Trypan blue and trypan red (1% aqueous solutions) are commonly used dyes in intravital work, as is india ink. These dyes withstand formalin fixation and routine paraffin processing. Theoretically, any dye used in intravital work must have particles sufficiently small for uptake by single cells, and a strong tendency to flocculate into particles of colloidal dimension. A dye that does not possess this flocculating ability, that is, a dye that exists simply as small ions, can diffuse in and out of a cell very easily and cannot be used in intravital work for this reason. The actual coloring action itself may be caused by the dye's flocculating outside the cell and then being engulfed or first penetrating the cell in a somewhat dispersed state and then aggregating into microscopically visible particles within the cell.

The second use of vital technics, also called supravital staining, involves the application of specific dyes that penetrate all cells and color certain cellular or tissue components. Methylene blue (0.025% to 0.25%) has been used to demonstrate nerve endings in dissociated muscle tissue. In hematology, supravital staining with solutions of Janus green B and neutral red has been employed to assist in distinguishing myeloblastic from lymphoblastic leukemia. A dye used for supravital work should be able not only to enter the cell, but also to diffuse through the protoplasm without killing the cell and to color preexistent cell inclusions distinctively or color the whole of the cytoplasm of particular cells strongly enough that those cells stand out from surrounding intercellular material and other cells.

The appearance of cells after supravital dyeing is different from a routine fixed section. With vital dyeing the nucleus and ground cytoplasm are little affected as a rule, but cytoplasmic inclusions such as vacuoles, lipid globules, mitochondria, and so forth, are colored. The fact that chromatin is usually not colored may be caused partly by the difficulty of the dye entering the nuclear membrane and partly by the fact that the phosphoric groups of the DNA are still combined with protein and not free to react with the basic dye before a fixative has acted. One should keep in mind that fixation and embedding dissolve out certain colorable cell inclusions and change the reaction in others, and this fact would explain many of the differences seen with a vital section versus a fixed section. In fixed preparations, the dye penetrates most of the tissue and the end point can be determined, and excess dye can be removed from the tissue by differentiation. In vital dyeing, the concentration at which the dye will act cannot be controlled, and a state of equilibrium is built up between the dye and the fluid of the cell.

Postmortem application

The majority of staining processes are done on tissue that has been fixed and this is a postmortem application of stains. There are four main ways in which a color may diffuse throughout and adhere to a particular structure. The first phenomenon is surface adsorption, a physical reaction dependent both on the charge of the ionized dye and the charge upon the materials on which the dye is precipitated. The second involves direct staining that employs a weak solution of a stain on the assumption that it will be differentially absorbed by various structures and tissues. Density of the tissue is a factor in controlling the absorption of the dye. The third way color may adhere involves indirect staining where the dye is applied from a relatively strong solution and is subsequently extracted from the unwanted structures either by a solvent or by some additional chemical reagent. The fourth type of staining employs mordants. A mordant is a salt or hydroxide of a divalent or trivalent metal and serves to strongly attach dye to a tissue. The compound formed by a dye radical with the mordant is called a lake, and these lakes may be unstable or insoluble depending on the exact nature of the combination and the solvents subsequently employed. There are three ways in which mordants may be used: mordant preceding dye; mordant and dye used together; mordant following dye. The use of mordants in dyeing technics has the advantage of making the dye relatively permanent in tissue (once the mordant-dye has combined with the tissue). It renders the dye insoluble in neutral solutions, enables other forms of staining to follow the mordant-dye technic, and will not decolorize on dehydration.

The practical application of stains is influenced by the character of the material, that is, whether the staining is to be done on a whole organism, a whole organ, tissue only (histologic), or cells (cytologic). If the organism is small, it is more desirable to stain it entirely, as then all parts are seen in their normal rela-

tion to each other and, by the selection of proper staining agents, may be well differentiated from each other. Generally, the best stains to use for such a purpose are the carmine mixtures, either alone or combined with picric acid. It is sometimes desirable to study single organs entirely, and these may be treated in the same manner as the whole organism.

Most staining takes place using tissue sections or cells. Differentiation among the four primary tissue types may be done, for example, with the Mallory connective tissue stains or the various neurologic methods. Parts of cells may be distinguished by specific staining reactions, and the most general differential effect is that obtained by the use of nuclear stains, which distinguish these cellular elements by their specific reaction with basic dyes.

Besides entire organisms or organs, tissue section, or cells, there are several other types of material that one may encounter in staining. These include stretched material, which is essentially the same as sectioned material except that there are no cut surfaces through which the stain can easily penetrate, and tissue imprints, made by holding a slide firmly against a piece of freshly cut tissue. These are fixed prior to staining.

In action, stains may be classified as substantive, adjective, or impregnation stains. A substantive stain is one that acts immediately and directly upon the tissue without the intervention of any other substance. An adjective stain is one in which the tissue is first treated with some agent, which in turn attaches the stain to the tissue, such as is done in mordant staining. Impregnation stains involve the deposition of sensitive metallic substances over selected cells and tissue structures that are rendered visible by a subsequent reduction of the metal. Many neurologic methods employ impregnation. Actually this method is not staining in the true sense of the word, and it differs in that structures demonstrated are usually rendered opaque or black, the coloring matter is particulate, and the deposit is on or around, but not in, the element demonstrated.

In time, stains may be classified as progressive or regressive. Progressive staining is done by watching the degree of staining in sections under the microscope at various points during the staining process and stopping the process when the selective action of the stain has differentiated the desired parts. Regressive staining is employed when the most extreme sharpness of differentiation is desired. By use of this method, the whole tissue is completely stained and then differentiated to remove excess dye from the parts desired unstained. For further information, see the section on differentiation.

In the degree of their action upon tissue, stains may be classified as general or selective. A general stain is one that attacks all parts of the tissue with approximately equal vigor and thus produces no significant differentiation. Using regressive action methods, one may make a general stain exhibit more selective action. A selective stain will differentiate between classes of tissue or between parts of cells.

DIFFERENTIATION

When regressive staining technics are employed, all the stainable tissue components are completely saturated with dye. To have any value as a readable slide, some of this excess stain must be removed, and this process is called differentiation. Differentiation usually gives sharp staining contrasts because the hydronium and hydroxide ions in the solvents used to differentiate diffuse more rapidly than does any dye ion, and this accounts for the more even results obtained. The differentiation step is a relative one and removes the dye from certain tissue components more easily and rapidly than from others. A properly destained section will have the desired features retaining sufficient stain to make them clearly visible, and the other tissue components will be completely cleared from the dye. Some of the ways in which a section may be differentiated include the use of acidic or basic mediums, excess mordant, buffers, or oxidizers.

It is generally known that basic dyes are differentiated by a weakly acid medium, and acid dyes are differentiated by a weakly basic one. For example, when staining in alum hematoxylin, one may use a solution of acid alcohol to differentiate the section. If a section has been overstained in eosin (an acid dye), it can be differentiated in a basic medium composed of alcohol containing 0.1% to 0.5% concentrated ammonium hydroxide. Many of the acid and basic differentiators use alcoholic solutions rather than aqueous, since the alcoholic solutions usually give a better control of the differentiation process itself than do the aqueous ones. The reason is that the majority of dyes used in staining tissue are more soluble in water than in alcohol, and although staining should be done in a more soluble medium (aqueous),

better differentiation is always obtained if this step is done in a less soluble medium for the dye (alcoholic). The alcoholic solution would also permit less ionization of the differentiator compared to the aqueous, and this would also be a factor in giving better controlled differentiation.

The general rule that the acid dyes are differentiated by the weakly basic medium and vice versa, does not state at which pH a given tissue component will be destained. Staining and differentiation are influenced to a great extent by fixation and any additional treatment given tissues prior to the actual staining process. Much research remains to be done on the pH of dye solutions, differentiators, and their relationship to the isoelectric point (IEP) of the tissue components. (Isoelectric point is usually defined as that pH point at which the protein molecule behaves neither as an acid nor as a base, with the positive and negative charges being equal in number.) Fixation gives precipitated protein aggregates, and the IEP of these aggregates may be similarly defined. If the aggregate at IEP is placed in a solution whose pH is above the IEP, the aggregate will behave as an acid. If placed in a solution whose pH is below IEP, it will behave as a base. Each fixative tends to give an aggregate of differing IEP. Formalin, for example, shifts the IEP toward a lower pH value because it combines with the basic radicals and leaves the carboxyl acid radicals of the protein free. Fixation in solutions of the heavy metals, such as the mercuric chloride fixatives, shifts the IEP to a higher value, as these fixatives combine with the carboxyl groups and leave the amino groups free. Differences in IEP caused by the fixing solutions will influence how differently fixed sections will be stained and differentated. It is not just a simple acid-base equilibrium that determines whether a section will be stained by a certain solution or destained by another. The pH of dye, differentiating agent, and IEP of tissue components all influence uptake of dye by tissue and its subsequent removal.

Sections can also be differentiated by the use of excess mordant. With an excess of mordant present around the tissue, the mordant-dye complex in the tissue is broken up and the dye moves out of the tissue into the differentiating fluid. Certain tissue components hold more of the mordant-dye complex than others, and it is the components that hold the lesser amount that lose their dye first into the differentiating fluid. At the proper extraction point, the slides are taken out of the differentiating fluid and thoroughly washed to remove any excess fluid, which if left in the tissue would cause the stain to fade in time.

A buffer solution is sometimes used as a differentiator. In Wright's stain, for example, a weak solution of dihydrogen potassium phosphate and disodium hydrogen phosphate pH 6.0 to 6.5, can be used as the differentiating agent. The hydrogen-ion concentration of the buffer is intermediate between the ranges of maximum staining of the dye components (eosin and methylene blue). The buffer acts as a basic differentiator toward the eosin and as an acid differentiator toward the methylene blue.

The use of oxidizers is the fourth method of differentiating an overstained section, and by this method the dye is oxidized to a colorless condition. Oxidizers are rather slow in action, and the parts of the cell holding only small amounts of dye will be bleached before those holding a greater quantity of the dye. With hematoxylin stains, two methods of differentiation are possible. The first uses the effects of pH in an acid alcohol medium. The second method uses oxidizers such as ferricyanide, bisulfite, and permanganate. With the first method, the nuclei of cells retain the stain better than do other tissue components; with the oxidizers, staining reveals myelin sheaths and red blood cells.

Regardless of the method used for differentiation, the differentiating action must be slow enough to permit it to be stopped by the next alcohol bath or dehydration series. If carried into the next fluid, strong differentiating solutions may cause continued fading of the stain. A thorough water wash may eliminate the possibility of fading, as it would remove the excess differentiating fluid. Acetone, tertiary butyl alcohol, clove oil, and an absolute alcohol–xylene mixture may be used to stop differentiation in some technics.

STAINING MECHANISMS

Today most biochemists agree that there are both physical and chemical phenomena involved in staining action.

Strictly physical theories that influence staining include the forces of capillarity and osmosis, absorption, and adsorption. The first two mentioned can account for the penetration of the dye into the interior of the tissue. The *absorption or solution theory* postulates a passing of the dye molecule from the dye bath solution to the solution in the substance being dyed. The dye supposedly distributes itself between the actual staining solution and tissue in the same manner in which it would between any two immiscible solvents in each of which it is soluble. This theory is supported by the fact that staining a tissue with a dye causes the tissue to become the same color as the solution of the dye, not the color of the dye as it appears in dry form. For example, dry fuchsin is green but in solution it is red. Tissue stained with fuchsin is also red. All staining phenomena cannot be explained by this physical theory, however.

The *adsorption theory,* which has both physical and chemical overtones, postulates a deposition of dye on the surface of the dyed material. Aqueous solutions of acid and basic dyes are moderately colloidal in some instances (that is, they are more of a true ionic solution, with a tendency toward moderate colloidal properties). Other dyes are decidedly colloidal. Dyes can probably be adsorbed in either the ionic or colloidal form, depending on the influencing factors. These are physical aspects. Chemically speaking, certain ions are adsorbed by certain substances much more readily than by others, and the rate of adsorption of any ion is strongly influenced by the presence of other ions in solution. For example, a greater concentration of hydroxyl ions in the solution (giving a higher pH) influences the adsorption of basic dyes; a greater concentration of hydrogen ions (giving a lower pH) influences greater acid dye uptake. Certain studies have shown that adsorption itself may take place only at specific sites as with the carboxyl or amino groups of the protein chain. Cells in which the carboxyl (acid) groups are blocked by the formation of methyl esters do not stain well with basic dyes. This implies not just pure physical surface adsorption, but also the possibility of salt linkages of dye to the protein chain, and this further implies chemical action. The charged groups that would form salts with acid dyes are those free basic groups of the amino acids such as lysine, histidine, and arginine. Basic dyes would tend to be bound to the free carboxyl groups of aspartic and glutamic acids, to the hydroxy groups of certain other amino acids, and to the free acidic groups of phosphoproteins and mucoproteins.

Consideration of *metachromatic staining* is pertinent to the discussion of the adsorption theory. Certain single dyes may react with tissue components to stain these components a different color from that of the dilute dye solution. For example, if a preparation of mesentery tissue is stained with toluidine blue, mast cells will color red-purple (metachromatic staining) and the rest of the preparation will be colored blue (orthochromatic staining). The actual color change in one dye is called *metachromasia* (or metachromasy), and this phenomenon is generally attributed to the cationic or basic dyes. These dyes include methylene blue; new methylene blue; azure A,B,C; thionin; toluidine blue; celestine blue; Bismarck brown; safranin; crystal violet; methyl violet; and pinacyanol. The blue or violet dyes will show a color shift toward red; the red dyes will show a color shift toward yellow.

Substances that stain metachromatically are sometimes called chromotropes and a high molecular weight seems to be a common property of these chromotropes. Sulfated mucopolysaccharides are the most active naturally occurring substances that will stain metachromatically. Amyloid, cartilage, mast cells, nucleic acid compounds, and hyaluronic acid also show metachromasia.

Although the exact mechanism of metachromasia is not known, some theories are available. Studies have shown that the absorption spectra of aqueous solutions of metachromatic dyes change with variations in concentration, pH, temperature, and so forth. One peak, called alpha, is observed in dilute dye solution, and as the concentration of dye increases, there is seen a beta peak, followed by a gamma peak. The first peak is believed to correspond to the monomer dye molecules in the dilute dye solution. The beta peak shows a color shift because of formation of dimer molecules as the concentration of dye increases. A further color change, represented by the gamma peak, is attributable to the formation of polymer dye molecules. The color change in the solutions is analogous to that observed in metachromasia; thus metachromasia is believed to be caused by polymerization of the dye molecules in the tissue.

Just how these dye molecules form polymers is believed to be dependent on the presence in tissue of macromolecules with electronegative radicals with a periodic negative surface charge. These macromolecules will bind dye molecules in such a way that interaction between them can occur, with a resultant color change as the polymer forms. The polymerization probably depends on hydrogen bonding and van der Waals forces. In addition, water molecules intercalate between the dye molecules and have an important influence on the metachromatic reaction. In a *labile metachromatic reaction*, treatment of the sections with a dehydrating agent will destroy the metachromatic reaction entirely. A *stable metachromatic reaction* resists the dehydrant's action, and sufficient metachromasia is maintained to be recognized as such. The degree of metachromasia seen will depend primarily on the nature of the negative radicals and increases in the following order: carboxymethyl < carboxyl < phosphate < sulfate. Concentration of these radicals, pH of solution, temperature, and time of staining are other factors that affect the metachromatic effect. Overstaining can even cause certain metachromatic structures to appear orthochromatic.

When a metachromatic dye is used, it is important that it be pure. If contaminants are present, they may give a result similar to that of the pure metachromatic dye. Certain fixatives that contain strong oxidants may produce a false metachromasia in tissue sections; formalin or alcohol are best for fixing tissue for these stains. When there is a background of strong orthochromatic staining, an acidic pH (3 to 4) of the staining solution will tend to reduce the orthochromatic effect. Examples of metachromatic staining methods are given in the section on carbohydrates.

In some instances the chemical aspects of the adsorption theory may predominate. In others, the physical aspects such as surface area and density of the adsorbing medium and the size of the adsorbed particles may have a greater influencing effect. The theory itself may be used to explain differential staining that occurs with dyes of the same general type. Selective action of one dye for one part of a tissue may be accounted for by predominately chemical factors; a second dye for another part may be accounted for by physical factors. Some authors also believe that adsorption may also account for metachromatic staining of tissue and that metachromatic agents may be tautomeric forms of the same dye (that is, differ considerably in arrangement of dye atoms, but existing in equilibrium in the same dye solution). These tautomers may have different chemical and physical properties that cause them to be adsorbed either "chemically" or "physically." The ease with which differentiation is effected may also aid in determination of whether a dye is combined to tissue in more of a chemical sense or more of a physical sense. Water and alcohol, the two most widely used differentiators, are not inert chemically speaking, but the ease with which they act to remove certain dyes from tissue points to a great deal of pure physical action uniting dye to tissue, and it may be that where dyes are readily removed by the action of differentiators they were only combined in a physical sense to the tissue. Where they are not so readily removed may point to a firmer chemical combination between dye and tissue.

Chemical factors of staining center around the fact that certain cell parts are assumed to be acid in character and other parts are alkaline. The acid parts would tend to combine with basic dye, whose color exists in the cations; whereas the alkaline parts would combine with the acid dyes, whose color exists in the anions. Cell nuclei, for example, are acid in character because of nucleic acid components and will stain with basic dyes such as crystal violet or methylene blue; cytoplasm is comparatively basic in character and will stain with acid dyes such as eosin. pH studies for acid and basic dyes show a definite reaction between dye ions and oppositely charged ions of protein and nucleic acid. The reaction is one of chemical equilibrium, rather than the type to go to completion.

The chemical theory assumes that acids and bases that are found in the cell are amphoteric in character; that is, they act as bases in acid solution and acids in basic solution. The hydrogen-ion concentration at which any compound is at minimum electrolytic dissociation and can change from acid to base depending on the nature of the solution in which it is placed is known as the isoelectric point. Dissociation of the protein molecule would give acidic and basic groups, which are the free side groups of certain amino acids, the terminal groups, and the charged substances, which may be conjugated to the protein. Free basic groups may be more abundant in one protein than in another, and the same holds true for acidic groups. According to the relative number of acidic and basic groups

and their degree of dissociation, the net charge on the protein molecule at a particular time may be negative, positive, or zero. At IEP, charges do exist, but are equal in number and give a net charge of zero, as shown in Fig. 7-13.

The degree of ionization of the free acid or basic groups of proteins depends on the pH of the solution (Fig. 7-13). When acid is added to the solution, the dissociation of the free acidic (carboxyl) groups is decreased; the pH of the solution is below IEP of the tissue. In other words, since the pH stands in an inverse relationship to the hydrogen-ion concentration, the hydrogen-ion concentration of the dye solution is above the hydrogen-ion concentration of the IEP. The free amino groups are increased and the protein becomes less negatively and more positively charged, according to the above equation. The greater positive charge makes the tissue more receptive to acid dyes, whose color portion exists in the anion, or negatively charged part of the dye salt. If the pH of the solution is above the IEP of the protein (that is, the hydrogen-ion concentration of the solution is below that of the IEP), the dissociation of the free carboxyl groups is increased. Protein is left with a net negative charge, which makes it more susceptible to combine with basic dye, whose color exists in the cation of the dye salt.

Studies have shown, as mentioned, that there is this tendency for the cationic or basic dyes to combine with the amionic elements of tissue and vice versa. Most of this work tests tissue with very acid staining solutions and, in a staining series, increases the pH of the solution until the tissue is being stained at a very alkaline pH. With the very acid solutions even the nucleus takes the acid dye, and with the very basic solutions, even the cytoplasm takes the basic dyes. At solutions of pH 7, the nucleus takes the basic dyes, and the cytoplasm takes acid dyes, and this is interpreted to mean that the actual IEP of the nucleus is considerably on the acid side of neutrality and the IEP of the cytoplasm in general lies on the basic side of neutrality. One

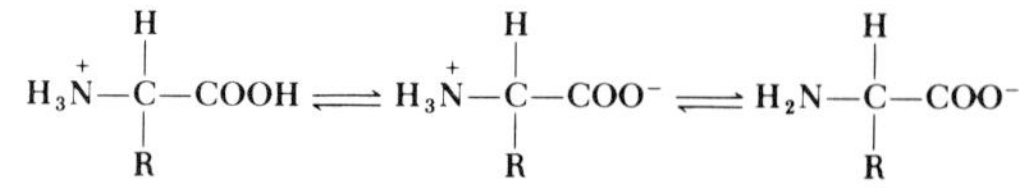

$$\underset{\substack{\text{Net charge }+1 \\ \text{Structure in a solution} \\ \text{acid to IEP}}}{\overset{\overset{\displaystyle H}{|}}{H_3\overset{+}{N}-C-COOH}} \underset{R}{\rightleftharpoons} \underset{\substack{\text{Net charge 0} \\ \text{IEP}}}{\overset{\overset{\displaystyle H}{|}}{H_3\overset{+}{N}-C-COO^-}} \underset{R}{\rightleftharpoons} \underset{\substack{\text{Net charge }-1 \\ \text{Structure in a solution} \\ \text{basic to IEP}}}{\overset{\overset{\displaystyle H}{|}}{H_2N-C-COO^-}}$$

Fig. 7-13. Amphoteric property of an amino acid.

must note, however, that staining is done on fixed tissue, not fresh, and that fixation alters the IEP of proteins. Even in consideration of this, though, these facts indicate a definite chemical reaction of an acid-base type taking place in some types of staining.

The preceding discussion limits chemical aspects of staining to those relating to the electrostatic bond between dye and tissue. The salt linkage may operate in many cases, especially where only small ions are involved. There are, however, additional forces of hydrogen bonding, hydrophobic bonding, and van der Waals forces to be considered. (Refer to p. 351 for a more complete discussion of these forces.) These short-range forces may operate in actual dye binding, whereas the electrostatic may assist or oppose diffusion of dye to dye-binding sites.

ADDITIONAL FACTORS INFLUENCING DYE BINDING

Other factors that influence staining include ionic strength of the dye solution, dye concentration, fixation of tissue, temperature, and staining equilibrium.

Dissolved salt, either neutral or buffered, in the dye solution influences the interaction of dye and tissue. The activity of salt ions in solution is best expressed by ionic strength, and increasing ionic strength of the dye solution may either decrease or increase the staining intensities of certain tissue components. It may be that the salt ion competes with the color ion for the binding site on the protein molecule and therefore limits the actual amount of dye that can be bound to the tissue. Increased staining could result from the salt's increasing the activity coefficient of the dye. More recently, it has been proposed[1] that the various effects of inorganic salts on staining could be explained by the Donnan membrane equilibrium.

Dye concentration influences staining, in that greater amounts of dye are bound with increasing concentrations of the dye. The amount of dye bound by a tissue is limited by the number of available binding sites and by the number of already bound dye molecules on the incoming dye molecules.

In the living state, dyes may readily penetrate cells, but binding capacity is slight. When the cell is fixed, there is a pronounced affinity for stains observed. The reorganization of the protein molecule to render the chemical groups more available to the dye is the general characteristic action, as regards staining, that is shared by all fixatives. Further specific action by certain fixatives alters permeability of the protein for certain molecules, that is, the fixatives will bind certain end groups and simultaneously leave other end groups receptive to the dye. The increase in acid and basic dye binding capacity is not equal and varies according to the actual fixation treatment. As mentioned previously, there is a relatively greater increase in basic dye uptake after formalin fixation, and more acid dye is taken up after fixation with mercuric chloride fixatives. This is probably because formaldehyde tends to combine with the basic amino groups leaving less of these to combine with the acid dye; heavy metals would form linkages with the acid carboxyl groups and decrease basic dye affinity because there would be more amino groups for the acid dye to bind and relatively less carboxyl groups for the basic dyes to bind.

Temperature may influence staining in a number of ways. Increase in temperature increases the diffusion rate of the dye molecule in a physical sense and therefore increases the rate of staining. Temperature also causes the protein molecule to swell the fiber and render it more open to the penetration of the dye. Dyes of low dispersive powers require increased temperature to operate, as with fat staining with oil red O.

Staining is a reversible reaction and when the solution environment is changed, there is an alteration in the equilibrium concentration within the tissue. Dye may then be lost to the solution or removed from it. pH changes may favor dissociation of the dye-protein complex, for example, increased pH favors dissociation of acid dyes from tissue and vice versa. The rate of dye removal varies with the tissue, dye, and actual removal conditions.

Chemical action does not fully explain the action of solvents employed during differentiation, nor does it explain all staining phenomena. (For example, it does not explain why certain basic dyes have stronger affinities for certain parts of the nuclei than for other parts. We can only speculate as to the amounts of RNA and DNA that would account for such staining results.) Physical theories do not adequately explain all staining action either. The two processes act simultaneously to give the finished result of specifically stained tissue.

Part II. Practical aspects

PROCEDURES FOR PARAFFIN SECTIONS

After sectioning and drying of paraffin sections, the general procedures outlined next are performed for most routine and special staining methods:

Deparaffinization
Hydration
Staining
Dehydration
Clearing
Coverslipping

Deparaffinization

The deparaffinization process functions to remove the paraffin wax from the tissue and surrounding area on the slide. *Xylene* is the usual reagent used for this purpose and *three changes over a 10-minute period* are desirable for complete removal of the paraffin wax. Sections should appear clear at this stage of the process. If white patches are seen, it most likely means that the slide has not been dried sufficiently and that water has been trapped under the paraffin. Put such sections in absolute alcohol for a few minutes; the water is soluble in this reagent. Then return the slide to xylene for completion of the deparaffinization process, and follow with the regular hydration sequence.

Slides that have just been removed from the drying oven should be allowed to cool to room temperature before being placed in the xylene. Slides should *not* be allowed to dry from the time hydration is begun until coverslipping is completed in most cases. An exception would be if celloidin-coating proved to be necessary, and this procedure is described in the hydration section, p. 131. All solutions used should adequately cover the tissue and slide itself during the deparaffinization and subsequent processes. Slides should be placed in the staining rack, basket, or other container, so that the side on which the tissue is mounted is facing the same direction for all the slides. This facilitates the coverslipping process.

Hydration

After deparaffinization, slides are hydrated. Hydration is a gradual process that uses a series of graded alcohols until water is used. The purpose of this process is to prepare the tissue to stain with a dye that has been dissolved in an aqueous solvent. The following procedure is suggested as a good guideline to proper hydration:

Reagent	Approximate time of immersion
Absolute (100%) ethanol	3 to 5 min
Absolute (100%) ethanol	3 to 5 min
95% ethanol	3 to 5 min
95% ethanol	3 to 5 min
80% ethanol	3 to 5 min
70% ethanol	3 to 5 min
60% ethanol	3 to 5 min
Tap water	until sections are clear

Comments on hydration process

1. Sections will turn from clear to slightly opaque when they are immersed in the absolute alcohol. If clear patches are visible after the tissue is immersed in the absolute alcohol, it means that all the paraffin has not been removed, and if this is the case, the section or sections should be returned to xylene.
2. Drain sections as completely as possible before transferring to the next reagent.
3. Reagents used in the deparaffinization and hydration process should be changed at regular intervals depending on laboratory use. To economize, it is helpful to make the second change of each reagent (where applicable) the first change, and use fresh solutions to comprise the second change.

Any of the following additional procedures may have to be done during the hydration process:

1. Tissue stored for long periods in nonbuffered or in acetate-buffered formalin may show formalin-pigment formation.[2] If the section is known to contain *formalin pigment,* hydrate the section to water, rinse in distilled water, and then treat sections with a saturated (6% to 8%) alcoholic solution of picric acid for 10 minutes or until the artifact pigment is removed. Rinse sections well in tap water to remove all traces of the picric acid before proceeding with staining.

   An alternate method to the preceding requires a 2% to 3% (volume per volume) solution of 28% ammonium hydroxide in 70% alcohol. Sections may need anywhere from 10 minutes to several hours of treatment for removal of formalin pig-

Table 7-2. Commonly used iodine solutions

Name	Potassium iodide (gm)	Iodine (gm)	Distilled water (ml)
Weigert's (Gram-Weigert)	2	1	100
Gram's	2	1	300
Langeron's	2	1	200
Lugol's	2	1	12

In all cases, it is advisable to dissolve the potassium iodide in one to two times its weight of distilled water (that is, if the directions require 2 gm of KI, dissolve this in 2 to 4 ml of distilled water). After the KI is dissolved, dissolve the iodine in the concentrated KI solution. After the iodine is dissolved, dilute to final volume by adding the rest of the distilled water.

ment. After this treatment, wash sections well in water to ensure complete removal of all traces of the ammonia and then proceed with staining. *Both formalin and malarial pigment* are removed by the following procedure:

Sections are hydrated to water and immersed for 1 hour in a solution containing 50 ml of 95% ethanol and 15 ml of 28% ammonium hydroxide. After the immersion, sections are washed well in running tap water, rinsed in distilled water, and stained.

2. If the sections are known to contain *mercury pigment*, hydrate sections to water and then (a) place in a solution of Gram's iodine for 15 minutes, or Weigert's iodine for 5 minutes; (b) rinse in tap water; (c) treat in 5% sodium thiosulfate for 3 to 5 minutes; (d) wash in tap water for 10 minutes and proceed with staining. Table 7-2 gives the amounts and directions for the preparation of commonly used iodine solutions.

3. If Bouin's fixed tissue is being stained and the yellow color of the *picric acid* is not removed as part of the processing procedure, it will have to be removed during the hydration sequence. Treat the sections with a filtered saturated solution of lithium carbonate in 70% alcohol. Alternatively the use of longer periods of time in 50% or 70% alcohol will also serve to remove the yellow color.

4. Sometimes the gelatin or egg-albumin adhesive applied when sectioning is being done proves inadequate to keep a tissue on the slide. It may be helpful to *celloidin-coat* the section, and the procedure for this follows:

a. Deparaffinize and bring sections through two changes of absolute alcohol.

b. Immerse sections in 0.5% to 1% celloidin solution for 1 to 2 minutes.

c. Drain off the excess celloidin for 1 to 2 minutes. Sections may be air-dried for 30 minutes at this stage, or you may proceed with step d.

d. Immerse sections in 80% or 70% ethanol for 2 minutes to harden the celloidin.

e. Rinse in distilled water and proceed with staining.

Note: Celloidin has an affinity for the following staining solutions: Schiff's reagent, mucicarmine, alcian blue, and aldehyde fuchsin. Enzyme-demonstration methods cannot be performed on celloidin-coated material, since the celloidin prevents the substrate from gaining access to the enzyme present in the tissue. Celloidin-coating is advantageous for maintaining tissue adherence in many of the long alkaline silver procedures.

Dehydration and clearing

After staining, sections are commonly dehydrated by successive changes of graded alcohols and cleared in several changes of xylene. The following outline is a guide to proper dehydration and clearing, using ethanol and xylene as the principal reagents:

95% ethanol	15 sec to 1 min
95% ethanol	15 sec to 1 min
Absolute ethanol	15 sec to 1 min
Absolute ethanol	15 sec to 1 min
Xylene	15 sec to 1 min
Xylene	15 sec to 1 min
Xylene	15 sec to 1 min

Comments on dehydration and clearing. Ethanol also functions to differentiate certain stains, notably eosin in the H & E technique. Besides ethanol, the following reagents may be used to dehydrate tissue: isopropanol, acetone, and *tert*-butanol. These other three dehydrants give better preservation of thiazin dye staining than does ethanol and are used in certain special staining technics. After the xylene treatment, sections should appear clear. If sections appear opaque either completely or in spots, it means that the dehydration process was inadequate and that water remains in the tissue. The inadequacy of the dehydration process is commonly caused by (1) insufficient time in the dehydrating fluids and (2) water-contamination of the dehydrating fluids. If reason 1 is the cause, sections should be re-treated with absolute alcohol for several minutes and then cleared again in xylene. If reason 2 is the cause, the contaminated alcohols should be changed and the sections dehydrated in the fresh absolute alcohol, followed by xylene clearing.

Xylene that is water-contaminated appears somewhat milky. Such xylene should be properly discarded in accordance with safety precautions. If the same dish has to be reused, make sure it is *well-dried* prior to filling it with fresh xylene. It is preferable to fill a clean *dry* dish with fresh xylene.

A solution of carbol-xylene may be used in the dehydrating process to assist in removal of all water traces. This solution has the following composition: melted phenol crystals (carbolic acid), 1 part; xylene, 3 parts. Two quick dips are usually sufficient for 5 μm paraffin sections.

Xylene that has been used for deparaffinizing slides should *not* be used for clearing after dehydration, since it contains paraffin in solution that will subsequently interfere with the proper hardening of the mounting medium.

Coverslipping

The purpose of coverslipping is to preserve the stained-tissue section for subsequent handling and microscopic examination. The cover slip (cover glass) is attached to the slide by a reagent called a mounting medium. There are numerous kinds of mounting media available and the indications for use of these is given in Chapter 5.

Cover slips are purchased from laboratory supply companies in various sizes and are commonly used in laboratories in three different thicknesses.

Thickness number	Average thickness of cover slip
1	150 μm
1½	180 μm
2	210 μm

The cover slip that provides an ideal range for photomicrography is number 1½.

Coverslipping should be done in a clean, well-lighted area. Have a flat surface available for placing slides while the mounting medium dries. Have the necessary materials ready:

1. The mounting medium needed (the medium should be of a good consistency for rapid and even spreading)
2. Coverslipping forceps
3. Gauze or some lint-free cloth
4. Cover slips of various sizes

Methods

1. Drain the excess xylene from the slide to be coverslipped, and wipe the back of the slide using the lint-free cloth. Extraneous tissue or nonspecific stain may also be wiped off at this time. This wiping should be done quickly. *Do not allow the tissue to dry* or it will appear opaque when viewed microscopically. Reimmerse the tissue section in xylene if the section appears to be drying out.

2. The amount of mounting medium needed will vary depending on the size of the area to be coverslipped and the nature of the medium itself. Too much mounting medium will result in a messy slide and will cause the section to appear cloudy when viewed microscopically. Too little mounting medium will cause air bubbles that can later enlarge and impair the quality of the section.

3. The correct amount of medium may be placed either on the slide or on the cover slip.
   Slide method: Place the correct amount of medium over the section and angle the slide so that the medium flows down to the bottom edge of the slide. Then place the cover slip against the bottom edge of the slide at about a 45-degree angle and allow the medium to run along the bottom edge of the cover slip. *Gently lower* the cover slip, and the medium should spread over the section and slide. Allow the medium to harden.
   Cover-slip method: Place the correct amount of medium in the center of the lower edge of the cover slip. Bring the slide up to the edge of the cover slip, position the slide so that the tissue will be adequately covered by the cover slip, and invert the slide over the cover slip. The medium should spread quickly under the cover slip and the slide is inverted again and allowed to dry.

Either of the above methods should take only 5 to 10 seconds to complete. When coverslipping by use of a synthetic resinous mounting medium and the coverslipped section shows that there are a few air bubbles present, gently remove them by applying pressure with the coverslipping forceps. If there are numerous air bubbles present, it is a waste of time to try to chase them out and, in addition, the tissue itself can be harmed. Instead, reimmerse the section with the cover slip in the xylene until the cover slip is removed. After the cover slip is removed, gently slosh the slide to remove traces of mounting medium, and remount the section. Never leave the removed cover slips in a jar of xylene. Cover slips become almost invisible in xylene (and other liquids) and can cause cuts. In addition, cover slips can break easily and will cut a finger even through heavy dishwashing gloves.

If there is excess *synthetic resinous* mounting medium present, it may be cleaned off immediately by gentle wiping of it with some xylene-moistened gauze. Do not disturb the cover slip during this process. Excess *aqueous* mounting medium may be cleaned off the slide using water-moistened gauze.

Removal of cover slips mounted with synthetic mounting medium: On occasion, it is necessary to remove a cover slip that has become well adhered to the slide. One may do this as follows: (1) Place the slide in a covered Coplin jar containing xylene and leave the slide immersed until the cover slip detaches. Do not force the cover slip off, since this can damage the tissue. (2) The removal process can be facilitated when the covered Coplin jar (screw-cap variety) containing the slide immersed in xylene is placed into the paraffin oven (56° to 58° C). Usually the cover slip detaches in about 30 minutes with this process. CAUTION: This process is best done in a hood. There is a fire and explosion hazard if an improperly calibrated oven is used and the solution becomes too warm. (3) If liquid nitrogen is available, put the slide in a metal dish or hold the slide with long forceps. Dip in the liquid nitrogen and the cover slip will pop off. Dispose of all removed cover slips properly.

Destaining and restaining

If it is necessary to destain and restain a slide, first remove the cover slip with one of the methods described above and hydrate the slide to 70% alcohol. The section may then be treated with a 1% solution of hydrochloric acid in 70% alcohol until it is fairly colorless. It is then washed well in tap water to remove traces of acid and rinsed in distilled water, and the new staining procedure is begun. Alternatively, weak ammonia alcohol or 5% oxalic acid may assist in removing color from any previously stained slide. Sections previously stained with an iron hematoxylin stain should not be restained with the conventional Prussian blue reaction, since the iron-lake still present will react with the potassium ferrocyanide. The iron lake may be removed by treatment of the sections for 1 to 2 hours in 5% sodium dithionite ($Na_2S_2O_4$).[2]

GLASSWARE AND RELATED MATERIALS USED IN STAINING
Glassware items in common use

Stock stains and reagents should be kept in glass-stoppered or screw-cap glass containers. These containers may be made of clear or brown glass. Any reagent that should not be exposed to the light (for example, silver solutions) should be kept in a brown-glass container. Various sizes of glass-dropper bottles are also available and are useful for a variety of purposes.

Different sizes of dishes and racks adaptable for sequence staining of large numbers of slides are available commercially. These are used most frequently in the conventional H & E setup, with separate dishes for each reagent needed. Washing trays are also helpful, especially in the H & E technic.

For special stains there are available slotted staining dishes (100 ml capacity) that hold up to 19 slides if slides are staggered, glass Coplin jars (50 ml capacity) that hold up to 16 slides if slides are placed back to back, and glass Coplin jars (50 ml capacity) that hold up to 9 slides if the slides are staggered. The Coplin jars may be of the glass-lid or screw-cap variety. There are also various kinds of polyethylene Coplin jars available commercially. (Some polyethylene Coplin jars tend to be slippery and hard to handle in a water bath. In addition, the lids tend to pop off if they are grasped by the lid or just below the lid, and this can result in spillage of the solution contents.)

For enzyme staining (or any procedure requiring staining on cover slips) there are 10 ml-capacity Columbia staining dishes, with either a screw cap or a glass lid, that hold up to 14 cover slips when the cover slips are placed back to back and staggered. Glass stender dishes and racks for holding coverslips make it possible to stain cover slips in a fashion similar to that used for staining slides in the H & E method.

For free-floating sections, such as celloidin and unmounted fats or silvers, various kinds of glass stender and staining dishes are available. In addition, bent glass rods are also necessary for section carryover from one dish to the next.

Glassware cleaning

In many cases, glassware is adequately cleaned when it is washed in hot water with a laboratory detergent recommended for lab glassware. One should remove stain precipitates, traces of metallic solutions, and insoluble organic residues by soaking the glassware in a cleaning solution composed of potassium dichromate–sulfuric acid for a variable period of time, from a few minutes to 24 hours. It is important that all traces of soap or acid cleaning reagent be removed from the glassware by thorough rinsing of the glassware in several changes of tap water. A final rinse of cleaned glassware should be made with distilled deionized water. Glassware should then be dried and stored.

Potassium dichromate–sulfuric acid cleaning mixture for glassware

Potassium dichromate	200 gm
Distilled water	1 liter
Concentrated sulfuric acid (cheapest grade)	750 ml

Use a heat-resistant glass container to prepare this solution! Dissolve the potassium dichromate in the water. While stirring this mixture with a glass rod, slowly pour in the sulfuric acid. Heat will be generated. When the solution has cooled, it may be stored in a glass-stoppered bottle. The solution is a dark red-brown and the mixture may be reused for soaking until it becomes dark green in color. *Caution: Use this solution with extreme care—it is highly corrosive!*

Staining reagents and procedures

Supplies used in staining should be procured from reliable sources. Whenever possible, use dyes that have been certified by the Biological Stain Commission. Such certification means that a particular batch of dye has met the various physical, chemical, and staining requirements required by the Commission, in collaboration with various other laboratories and manufacturers. Only dry biologic stains are certified; if solutions of dyes are purchased, they should be prepared from dry dyes that have been Commission-certified. Since certification is given on a batch basis, each new batch of stain must be submitted to the Stain Commission for certification to be granted.

Solutions should be prepared accurately according to technic specifications. (Pages 384 to 392 describe various kinds of solution preparations.) Bottles with solutions prepared in the laboratory should be clearly labeled with the following information:

Contents
Concentration of contents and specific solvent
Stock solution or working solution (if applicable)
Whether solution is reusable or to be discarded after use
Date of preparation
Expiration date (or a date when solution usability should be reverified, for example, pH check)
Initials of person who prepared the solution

Solutions should be stored properly. Some reagents need storage in brown bottles for protection against the light; others should be stored in clear glass. In addition, check the procedure to see if the reagent in question should be stored at room temperature (about 25° C), at refrigerator temperature (about 4° C), at freezer temperature (below 0° C), or in the deep freeze ($-40°$ to $-60°$ C). Most stains are stored at room temperature; however, Schiff's reagent, aldehyde fuchsin, and Gomori's methenamine silver should be refrigerated.

Some reagents are used only once and then discarded. Others may be reused as stock solutions for varying periods of time. All stock solutions of dyes should be filtered into their storage bottles and, if they are the reusable variety, filtered back after use. Still other reagents are stored as stock solutions and diluted to make working solutions when needed. The working solutions are usually discarded after use. The term "counterstain" refers to a dye solution that is applied after the primary stain has acted; for example, eosin is the counterstain used after hematoxylin; metanil yellow is the counterstain used after the mucicarmine primary stain. Counterstaining should enhance the slide's value by coloring additional components that have not been demonstrated with the primary stain. Obviously, counterstains should not obscure the primary stain.

All stains should be kept covered when not in use. During use, covering the staining solution is optional and related to time factors. If the slide has to remain in a particular fluid for some time, it is wiser to cover the Coplin jar or staining vessel and protect the solution from foreign particles. The tissue section itself should be completely covered with the dye solution while the stain is acting; otherwise part of the section will be unstained. Using sufficient staining solution to "just cover" the tissue section is *not* a good practice if the procedure requires prolonged incubation with heat (for example, Luxol blue for myelin demonstration). Some staining solution can be lost through evaporation and a partially stained section results. In such cases, it is wiser to fill the Coplin jar with some extra staining solution to allow for possible evaporation.

Alcohols used in staining and processing should be checked periodically with a hydrometer. The specific gravity of absolute ethanol is 0.794; the specific gravity of 95% ethanol is 0.816.

In many cases the terms "rinsing slides" and "washing slides" are used synonymously. Unless a time is specified, usually two to three changes of the rinsing agent are sufficient. "Quick rinses" should be performed once and the slide moved rapidly to the next solution. If the rinsing agent is not specified, then distilled water should be used.

Some general troubleshooting guidelines

If a staining procedure does not give the anticipated result, the following reasons may apply:

1. The material was not fixed in the proper fixative. Postmordanting a hydrated tissue section in the fixative that should have been used initially and repeating the stain may assist in correcting this problem.
2. There may be insufficient color.
   a. Check that the dye solution is correctly prepared for weight of dye.
   b. Check that the proper dilution has been made to the required volume.
   c. Check that the proper solvent has been used for the dilution process.
   d. Correct pH, if applicable.
   e. If a new batch of dye is being used, the percent dye content may differ from the old batch that was previously used. If this is the case, the solution preparation can be changed according to the change in percent dye content. (See the lab math section on dye content adjustment, p. 386.)
   f. Check that the material was stained for sufficient time. Sometimes simply pro-

longing time in a given solution will give the desired staining effect.
   g. A prolonged differentiation may result in insufficient staining, and it may be necessary to shorten the differentiation time or dilute the strength of the differentiator.
   h. Check that the proper dehydrating agent was employed. Ethanol, the commonly used dehydrating agent, may extract certain dyes, and an alternate solvent may be necessary.
   i. Uneven staining (or lack of staining) can at times be attributable to the fact that the staining solution or solutions have not gained access to the tissue. Common causes for this include (a) slides becoming attached together (loose slide slots or incorrect placement in slots) and (b) tissue side of slide adheres to the front of a Coplin jar or staining dish. (It may help to turn the first slide in these vessels toward the opposite direction.)
3. Staining results are also affected by temperature. The warmer the stain, the faster the reaction. Use of a cold solution may require a longer staining time for proper color results to be achieved.
4. In the case when too much color is seen, it may help to shorten the time in the reagent that is responsible for the excess color. It is possible that the solution may need further dilution. The strength of the differentiating agent may be insufficient and need a fresh preparation.

The instructions in many methods list variable periods of time to allow staining to occur. It is important to realize that in many cases the instructions are guidelines and not absolutes. Staining times are affected by the variable strength of dye lots. Also, fixatives used vary and staining qualities of the tissue are thereby altered. Most laboratories make modifications in staining procedures to adjust for their particular cases. However, if a new method is being tried for the first time, it is recommended that the technic be carried out exactly to the specifications listed for that method. If results are not satisfactory, modifications should be attempted.

USE OF CONTROL TISSUES

Control sections are used by the technologist to check the staining reactions prior to giving

Table 7-3. Control tissues for use in special staining procedures*

Substance	Control tissue	A suggested stain (example)
Acid-fast bacteria	Tissue with acid-fast bacilli	Kinyoun's
Amyloid	Tissue with amyloid	Congo red
Argentaffin granules	Small intestine	Fontana-Masson
Basement membrane	Kidney	Jones
Bile	Obstructed bile duct	Fouchet's (Hall's)
Calcium	Calcified lesions	Von Kossa; alizarin red S
Chromaffin granules	Orth's fixed adrenal	Sheehan; PAS
Cholesterol	Gallbladder with cholesterolosis; adrenal cortex (formalin-fixed frozen sections)	Schultz
Collagen	Kidney; liver	Trichrome methods
Copper	Wilson's disease (tissue from patient); fetal liver	Rubeanic acid; rhodanine
DNA and RNA	Lymph node (Carnoy-fixed)	Methyl green–pyronin
Elastic fibers	Aorta; kidney; skin	Verhoeff–van Gieson; aldehyde fuchsin; resorcin fuchsin
Fibrin	Blood clot (less than 72 hours old)	Weigert's fibrin, PTAH, or immunofluorescence
Fats	Adrenal cortex; fatty liver	Oil red O
Fungi	Tissue with fungus	Grocott's modification of Gomori's methenamine silver (GMS)
Gram + and gram − bacteria	Infected appendix (or other)	Brown-Brenn
Glycogen	Carnoy's fixed liver	PAS with diastase
Hyaluronic acid	Umbilical cord; skin	Colloidal iron with hyaluronidase
Iron	Liver or spleen with hemochromatosis	Prussian blue
Mast cells	Skin	Luna
Melanin	Skin	Ferrous ion uptake
Mucin	Small intestine	PAS and mucicarmine
Reticulum	Lymph node; liver	Wilder's
Uric acid	Gouty tophi (alcohol-fixed)	Gomori's methenamine silver

*From Hrapchak, B. B.: Self-assessment in histology, Bellaire, Texas, 1977, American Society of Medical Technology. For further information, see Judge, M. S.: Am. J. Med. Technol. **36:**49-63, 1970, and Luna, L. G.: Stain technology control (an editorial), Histo-Logic **VI:**77, 1976.

the slides to the pathologist. If a known good control does not show the proper reaction, the technical procedures must be reviewed and the patient's slides redone when the source or sources of error are determined.

No single tissue will serve all control needs. A list of commonly used control tissues is given in Table 7-3.

REFERENCES

Baker, J. R.: Principles of biological microtechnique, New York, 1958, Barnes & Noble, Inc.

Barka, T., and Anderson, P.: Histochemistry, New York, 1965, Harper & Row Publishers.

Culling, C. F. A.: Handbook of histopathological and histochemical techniques, ed. 3, London, 1974, Butterworth & Co. (Pubs.), Ltd.

Davenport, H. A.: Histological and histochemical technics, Philadelphia, 1964, W. B. Saunders Co.

Galigher, A. E., and Kozloff, E. N.: Essentials of practical microtechnique, ed. 2, Philadelphia, 1971, Lea & Febiger.

Lillie, R. D.: Conn's biological stains, ed. 8, Baltimore, 1969, The Williams & Wilkins Co.

Lillie, R. D., and Fullmer, H. M.: Histopathologic technic and practical histochemistry, ed. 4, New York, 1976, McGraw-Hill Book Co.

Luna, L. G., editor: Manual of histologic staining methods of the Armed Forces Institute of Pathology, ed. 3, New York, 1968, McGraw-Hill Book Co.

Pearse, A. G. E.: Histochemistry, theoretical and applied, ed. 3, vol. 1, London, 1968, vol. 2, Edinburgh, London, 1972, Churchill Livingstone.

Thompson, S. W.: Selected histochemical and histopathological methods, Springfield, Ill., 1966, Charles C Thomas, Publisher.

Thompson, S. W., and Luna, L. G.: An atlas of artifacts, Springfield, Ill., 1978, Charles C Thomas, Publisher.

Specific citations

1. Bennion, P. J., and Horobin, R. W.: Some effects of salts on staining: use of Donnan equilibrium to describe staining of tissue sections with acid and basic dyes, Histochemistry **39:**71-82, 1974.

2. Lillie, R. D., and Fullmer, H. M.: Histopathologic technic and practical histochemistry, ed. 4, New York, 1976, McGraw-Hill Book Co.

CHAPTER 8

Nuclear and cytoplasmic stains

Cell nuclei can be stained with basic (cationic) dyes or sequence procedures employing a metal mordant and dye. The former process depends on the presence of DNA and RNA to form dye-salt unions with the basic dye, and the latter depends on a chelate complex of dye and mordant that is bound in turn to tissue groups not necessarily acid in nature. This second method is more widely used in routine pathology because the mordanted stains also demonstrate the nucleus in material from which the nucleic acids have been extracted, as in decalcified tissue, whereas for the dye-salt linkages the nucleic acids themselves must be present.

Nuclear staining technics are classified on the basis of the reagents employed and the manner of their employment. Dyes used may be either natural or synthetic in origin.

CARMINE[1-3]

Cochineal and its derivatives, carmine and carminic acid, have already been mentioned in the section for natural dyes. Cochineal is the deep red dye extracted from the dried bodies of the female cochineal insect, and it is from this substance that carmine is manufactured. Carminic acid is the active staining principle of the two substances, and there is a relatively greater proportion of this principle in the purer carmine. Carmine was widely employed in the dyeing trade prior to its introduction into microtechnic.

Four general classes are recognized for nuclear staining purposes; however, it should be noted that the carmine solutions do not bring out nuclear detail so sharply as do the hematoxylin formulas. The four classes are as follows:

Simple extract of cochineal
Alkaline carmine stains
Alum cochineal and alum carmine stains
Acid carmine stains

The first two varieties are little used. With the alkaline carmine stains, the dye molecules carry a negative charge and, because many cell structures bear positive charges, the alkaline carmines stain diffusely. The use of an acid differentiating solution after the carmine stain can assist in nuclear demonstration.

In the alum cochineal and alum carmine stains, the dye molecules are positively charged and therefore stain the nuclei and other structures that are negatively charged. Some of the formulas that have been used include the following:

Grenacher's alum cochineal

Powdered cochineal	6 gm
Ammonium alum (mordant)	6 gm
Distilled water	100 ml
Thymol (preservative)	1 gm

Boil cochineal, alum, and water for 30 minutes. Add water to bring volume to 100 ml. Filter and add thymol.

Grenacher's alum carmine

Carmine	2 gm
Ammonium alum	3 to 5 gm
Distilled water	100 ml
Thymol	1 gm

Combine the carmine, alum, and water and boil for 1 hour. Add enough water to bring solution back to volume. Cool, filter, and add the thymol. According to Mallory, this stain is good for sections as well as bulk work.

Mayer's carmalum

Carminic acid	1 gm
Ammonium or potassium alum	10 gm
Distilled water	200 ml
Salicylic acid (preservative)	0.2 gm

Combine the carminic acid, alum, and water. Dissolve, using heat if necessary. Cool and add salicylic acid.

Method

1. Fix tissues in alcohol or formalin.
2. Stain paraffin or celloidin sections for 5 to 20 minutes.
3. Wash thoroughly in water. If nuclei are not sharply outlined, differentiate in a 0.5% to 1% aqueous solution of alum. For sections, this differentiation should take a few seconds to a few minutes. For bulk work, 12 to 24 hours are necessary. Differentiation should be followed by a thorough water wash.
4. Dehydrate paraffin sections in 95% and absolute alcohol and clear in xylene. For celloidin sec-

tions, dehydrate in 95% alcohol and clear in terpineol or oil of origanum.
5. Coverslip, using a synthetic mounting medium. When the above solutions for staining bulk work are used, staining time is 24 to 48 hours. Overstaining will not occur, and nuclei are stained bright red by these methods.

Meyer's alcoholic carmine (paracarmine)

Carminic acid	1 gm
Aluminum chloride (mordant)	0.5 gm
Calcium chloride (mordant)	4 gm
70% alcohol	100 ml

Dissolve, using gentle heat if necessary. Allow solution to settle and then filter. Section staining requires 15 to 30 minutes. Differentiation is accomplished with 70% alcohol. If a sharper nuclear stain is desired, 2.5% glacial acetic acid may be added to the 70% alcohol used for differentiation. Bulk staining requires 24 to 48 hours.

In acid carmine stains, the dye molecules are positively charged and therefore stain nuclei and other negatively charged substances. Acetocarmine is the most widely used acid carmine solution and has been used to stain chromosomes in squash preparations. Details on chromosome staining with acetocarmine and other solutions follow.

CHROMOSOME STAINING[1,4]

Staining of chromosomes has been done with acetocarmine, aceto-orcein, and acetolacmoid. Small tissue pieces, cell suspensions, and impression smears may be immersed fresh in one of the following solutions:

Acetocarmine
Stock solution
Boil 1 gm of carmine in 200 ml of 45% aqueous acetic acid for 5 minutes. Allow solution to cool and filter.
Working solution
Use equal parts of the stock solution and 45% acetic acid.

Aceto-orcein
Add 1 to 2 gm of orcein (synthetic orcein is satisfactory) to 45 ml of hot acetic acid. Dissolve the dye. When solution has cooled, add 55 ml of distilled water. Filter before use.

Acetolacmoid
Dissolve 1 gm of lacmoid in 100 ml of 45% acetic acid. Filter before use.

The technique used will vary depending on the type of sample to be stained. With cell suspensions, place a drop of suspension on a clean slide, add a few drops of either of the above stains, lower a cover slip on top of the slide, and apply gentle firm pressure. Stain for 5 minutes, and then remove excess stain by applying filter paper to the edge of the cover slip. Temporary slides may be made by sealing the cover slip with wax.

Alternatively, slides may be briefly counterstained in 0.02% fast green FCF, dehydrated, cleared, and coverslipped using a synthetic mounting medium.

If tissue pieces are being stained, they may be soaked in a small volume of any of the stains mentioned for 5 minutes or longer (up to 48 hours, according to Lillie). Tissue pieces are then crushed under a cover slip so that a single cell layer can be examined. Either temporary or permanent mounts may be made by the methods previously described.

Results
Chromosomes are red with the acetocarmine solution, but purple with the orcein and lacmoid solutions.

HEMATOXYLIN
BACKGROUND INFORMATION

Hematoxylin, the most widely used natural dye, is extracted from the heartwood of the logwood tree, *Haemotoxylon campechianum,* a species native to Central America. Extracts of logwood were used for dyeing purposes in America prior to A.D. 1520, and after that date, the substance became important in textile dyeing in Europe. Some 300 years ago, scientist Robert Hooke mentioned using logwood as a coloring matter for fluids, but it was not until the 1860s that hematoxylin solutions began to be used to any extent for histologic staining.

Solutions of the dye have been used for the demonstration of a variety of tissue components including nuclei and mitotic structures, mitochondria, mucin, hemoglobin, elastic fibers, muscle, collagen, axons, phospholipids, protozoa, fatty acids, myelin sheaths, alpha cells of the pituitary, beta cells of the pituitary and pancreatic islets, and certain metals.

OXIDANTS AND MORDANTS

Most histotechnologists are aware that hematoxylin (Fig. 7-6) has little affinity for tissues; hence the phrase "stain with hematoxylin" is a bit misleading. With few exceptions, hematoxylin solutions should contain hematein and a metal mordant.

Hematein is the oxidation product of hematoxylin, and its formula is similar to hematoxylin

(Fig. 7-7). The conversion of hematoxylin to hematein (a process known as ripening) may be achieved naturally through air exposure as is the case with Delafield's solution. This natural ripening process takes time; however, there are also available a variety of chemical oxidants to hasten the ripening process. Examples of well-known oxidizing agents include mercuric oxide, sodium iodate, and potassium permanganate.

The pH of the solvent used in the hematoxylin solutions will have some effect on the rate of oxidation.[1] Neutral aqueous solutions will form hematein in a few hours; alkaline solutions will also effect a more rapid oxidizing process; acid solutions will form the oxidation product more slowly.

There are continuous chemical changes occurring in a hematoxylin solution as it is being oxidized to hematein. The first is the simple oxidation to hematein; the second is the continuous formation of a precipitate caused by the further oxidation of the hematein, and for this reason it is necessary to filter alum hematoxylin solutions before use. Hematoxylin is used, though, rather than solutions of hematein, since hematein solutions lose strength rather quickly by flocculation of the products of further oxidation, and it is better to have some hematoxylin present to replenish the dye lost gradually by overoxidation.

The second solution component that a good hematoxylin stain will require is a mordant. It is traditionally considered that the primary function of the mordant is to serve as a link attaching the dye to the tissue. This traditional view has been questioned recently by those who state that the substantivity for tissue shown by the metal complex dyes could be explained by the large molecular size of these complexes and not by the presence of the metal mordant per se.[7]

In certain cases the mordant may incidently function as an oxidizer and facilitate the conversion of hematoxylin to hematein. To prepare comparatively stable solutions of combined mordant and dye, one should select the mordants that cause little or no oxidizing action. In this category may be listed ammonium alum, potassium alum, phosphotungstic acid, and phosphomolybdic acid. Mordants with vigorous oxidizing action can be used for solutions that would be used and then discarded in a matter of hours. For example, Weigert's iron hematoxylin, with the strong oxidizer ferric chloride being used as mordant, is prepared immediately before use and discarded within 3 to 4 hours.

Other mordants besides ferric chloride that possess this strong oxidizing capacity are ferric acetate and ferric alum.

The combination of mordant and dye is called a "lake," and for hematein-mordant combinations, this lake carries a positive charge and functions as a cationic or basic dye.[8,9] Tissue components that stain with such a lake are sometimes called "basophilic"; however, Lillie[1] points out that this term is misleading when mordant-dye solutions are used for staining. Some tissue components that do not possess acid groups and would not stain with conventional basic dyes can, in fact, be colored with mordant-dye combinations. Metals used as mordants in hematoxylin solutions include aluminum, iron, lead, copper, tungsten, molybdenum, and chromium. Aluminum and iron are the most commonly used mordants in today's microtechnic.

Aluminum mordanted hematoxylin solutions
Staining theory and uses

Hematoxylin solutions mordanted with aluminum are routinely used in the histopathology laboratory for nuclear staining (Fig. 8-1). The location and appearance of the nucleus will vary somewhat depending on the type of cell, but in all cases it is critical to distinguish a normal nucleus from an abnormal one. In malignancy, the nucleus undergoes changes; increased size, hyperchromatic staining pattern, mitotic figures, enlarged nucleolus, and irregular nuclear contour may all be seen. Indications of injury or cell death are also judged by the nuclear appearance: irregular shrinkage and wrinkling (pyknosis), fragmentation (karyorrhexis), or decrease in basophilia. Since the nucleus reflects so many of the dynamic processes occurring within the cell, it follows that the adequate demonstration of this structure is invaluable to the pathologist for diagnostic purposes.

In an unextracted tissue section, DNA is the major chemical component of the nucleus. The DNA exists in two states: heterochromatin (metabolically inactive and stainable with basic dyes) and euchromatin (metabolically active and not demonstrable with basic dyes). DNA is composed of units of deoxyribose sugar condensed with the purine or pyrimidine bases. Phosphoric acid residues unite these units, and these residues are believed to serve as binding sites for cationic dyes (Fig. 8-2). In the case of both the simple cationic dyes (class I dyes, according to Scott[10]) and the mordant-dye complexes (class II dyes, according to Scott), the initial attraction for the negatively charged tissue groups is electrostatic.[8] Tissue-affinity studies have shown the class I dyes have a higher affinity for tissue polysulfates; the class II dyes, a higher affinity for polyphosphates.[11]

Electrostatic bonding is influenced by the pH of the solution. The pH of most alum hematoxylin solutions ranges from 2.2 to 2.9. This pH lies above the isoelectric point (IEP) of nucleic acids, since the IEP of nucleic acids occurs in the pH range of 1.5 to 2.0.[12] The nucleic acid will therefore dissociate to give a greater number of negative charges to increase

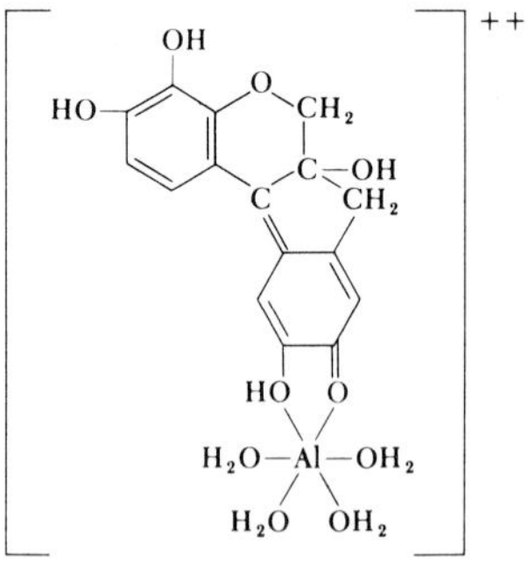

Fig. 8-1. Aluminum-hematein dye-lake. Probable structural formula. (After Baker, J. R.: Principles of biological microtechnique, New York, 1958, Barnes & Noble, Inc.)

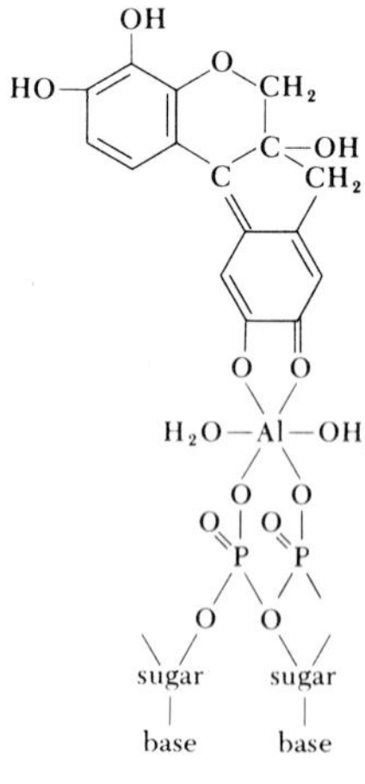

Fig. 8-2. Binding of aluminum-hematein complex with DNA phosphoryl groups. Possible structural formula. (After Baker, J. R.: Principles of biological microtechnique, New York, 1958, Barnes & Noble, Inc.)

staining with the positively charged dye lake.

In the case of the mordant-dye complexes, it has been postulated that the initial electrostatic attraction is replaced by covalent bonds.[8] The basis for this claim is that the simple basic dyes (which bind electrostatically) may be removed from tissue with alcohol treatment, whereas the mordant-dye complexes remain in tissue even after alcohol treatment. A stable covalent linkage is believed to account for the alcohol insolubility of the latter. Other researchers state that the differential alcohol solubility of the mordant-complex dyes is sufficient explanation, and no special linkages need to be postulated.[7]

In the natural state, DNA is bound by the phosphoric acid residues to nuclear proteins called "histones." In a tissue section from which the DNA is extracted, the positive staining is believed to be caused by the reaction of the histone fraction with the dye. Possible binding of arginine residues of the histone fraction with the hematoxylin dye is shown in Fig. 8-3.

The traditional formulas for nuclear demonstration using an aluminum mordant are those of Delafield, Harris, Ehrlich, and Mayer. All use aluminum alum (ammonium aluminum sulfate) as the mordant salt. Since the aluminum salts are not in themselves oxidizers, it is necessary to expose the hematoxylin solution to air or chemicals to effect the conversion of hematoxylin to hematein. The above-mentioned formulas are also used in special staining procedures as counterstains for nuclear demonstration. These procedures include periodic acid–Schiff (PAS) with Harris's hematoxylin, Congo red for amyloid, Best's carmine for glycogen, Lendrum's stain for inclusion bodies, and oil red O for fats.

In 1974, Gill et al.[13] developed a formula for a "half-oxidized" hematoxylin. The half-oxidation is achieved by use of one half the amount of sodium iodate needed to oxidize 1 gm of hematoxylin; natural ripening completes the oxidation process. The mordant used is aluminum sulfate.

General comments on aluminum hematoxylin solutions[1,14]

Purpose of reagents used

1. The selectivity for nuclei is traditionally believed to be increased by the presence of an excess of aluminum salts in the solution. However, Thompson and Luna[14] caution that if the alum mordant is not properly dissolved, or if excessive quantities are used, the alum can precipitate on top of the tissue, resulting in a crystalline artifact.
2. Alcohol functions principally as a preservative to inhibit the growth of mold.
3. Glycerol tends to stabilize the system against overoxidation and aids in preventing rapid evaporation.
4. The addition of acid to alum hematoxylin solutions is believed to increase the selectivity of the stain for the nuclei and to counteract the rapid oxidizing effects of chemical oxidizing agents. This latter function enables the solution to maintain some hematoxylin in equilibrium with the hematein to ensure a better stain.
5. The degree of blueness of the solution depends largely on the freshness of the alum mordant, and as the solution becomes older, free sulfuric acid is gradually formed from the alum, causing the solution to lose its bluish or purplish tint and become reddish.
6. On standing, traditional alum hematoxylin solutions develop a sheen of oxidized dye; hence they should be filtered before use. If filtering is not done, a blue-black precipitate will result on the stained section.

Testing alum hematoxylin solution. There

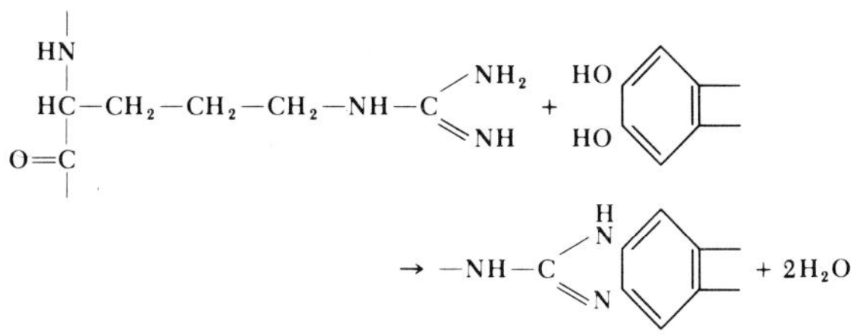

Fig. 8-3. Proposed binding of arginine residues with hematoxylin. (From Lillie, R. D., et al.: Acta Histochem. **49S:**204-219, 1974.)

are a number of *empirical tests* to aid in determining if the alum and acid alum hematoxylins are ready for use. The first is odor, and a good stain should have a winy smell. The color of the solution should be a deep purple-red. If ready for use, a few drops of hematoxylin solution should turn bluish black when dropped into a beaker of tap water. An insufficiently ripened stain, or an aged stain, will keep the red color. In addition to the tap water test, a few drops of hematoxylin should be placed on a piece of filter paper. If there is a good stain, the pattern produced by the diffusion of the hematoxylin drops on the filter paper will be maroon color ending in a dark purple edge. The purple border is absent in a solution that is not yet ready for use. The final test for any hematoxylin and mordant combination is staining. The cell nucleus should be precisely outlined, and the nuclear detail brought out sharply.

Differentiation. When aluminum-hematein solutions are employed as regressive stains, subsequent differentiation is necessary. Theoretically, the differentiating agent can attack linkages at two points: between the tissue and the mordant or between the mordant and the dye. Acid solutions are commonly used to differentiate alum hematoxylins and, though the mechanism is not fully understood, Baker[9] proposes that the acids attack the tissue-mordant links. One theory why tissues turn a reddish color when placed in the acid differentiator is that the freed dye-mordant complex is predominately reddish at an acid pH. Another possibility is that the acids attack the mordant-dye linkages. In this case, hematein would dissociate. Hematein has an IEP of 6.5 and becomes red when placed in a solution that is acid to its IEP. The differentiating agent commonly used, acid alcohol, would give this effect.

Bluing. Alkaline solutions (of ammonia water, lithium carbonate, Scott's tap water substitute, p. 143) are used for bluing hematoxylin stains. At an alkaline pH, the mordant-dye lake, which is itself blue, re-forms in those tissue sites that were most intensely stained in the first place and therefore more resistant to the differentiation action of the acid alcohol.

Preparation of aluminum-mordanted hematoxylin solutions

Delafield's formula

Saturated solution of ammonium aluminum sulfate

Dissolve 180 gm of ammonium aluminum sul-

fate in 1 liter of distilled water. Heat until dissolved. When cool, some of the alum will crystallize and settle to the bottom of the flask. The supernatant will be saturated.

Hematoxylin solution

Hematoxylin crystals	4 gm
95% alcohol	25 ml
Saturated solution of ammonium alum	400 ml

Dissolve the hematoxylin in the alcohol and add this to the alum solution. Expose solution to sunlight and air in a clear, cotton-plugged bottle for 3 to 4 days. Filter and add the following:

Glycerol	100 ml
95% ethanol	100 ml

Age for 3 to 6 months in the light and then test solution to see if it is ready to use.

Ehrlich's formula

Hematoxylin	2 gm
95% alcohol	100 ml
Distilled water	100 ml
Glycerol	100 ml
Ammonium or potassium alum	3 gm
Glacial acetic acid	10 ml

Dissolve the hematoxylin in the alcohol and add other ingredients. Ripen by exposure to air in a cotton-plugged bottle for 2 weeks or longer, mixing frequently. It may be ripened instantly by adding 0.4 gm of sodium iodate to the mixture. This hematoxylin will give a sharp nuclear stain, but sections must be washed thoroughly in tap water after staining to remove all traces of acetic acid and to bring out a clear blue color. Staining methods and results are similar to Delafield's. Solution keeps for years in tightly stoppered bottle.

Mayer's formula

Hematoxylin	1 gm
Distilled water	1 liter
Sodium iodate	0.2 gm
Ammonium or potassium alum	50 gm
Citric acid	1 gm
Chloral hydrate	50 gm

Dissolve the hematoxylin in the water, using gentle heat if necessary. Add sodium iodate and alum. Shake until alum is dissolved, and then add the citric acid and chloral hydrate. The solution should turn a red-violet color. This formula will keep a long time without overripening.

Harris's formula

Solution A

Hematoxylin	6 gm
Absolute alcohol	60 ml

Combine these two ingredients.

Solution B

Ammonium or potassium alum	120 gm
Double distilled water	1200 ml

Combine these two ingredients and bring solution to a boil.

1. When solution B is boiling, add solution A to it and bring these to a boil quickly and remove from heat.
2. Place flask in cold water and add 3 gm of mercuric oxide. Do not add the mercuric oxide all at once; otherwise the solution will splash and could result in injury.
3. Keep in cold water until mixture develops a dark purple color.
4. When it is cold, add 48 ml of glacial acetic acid to increase selectivity of stain for the nucleus (optional).
5. Allow stain to ripen for 1 week and test for use. Solution keeps well for 1 to 2 months.

Gill's formula[13]

Distilled water	730 ml
Ethylene glycol	250 ml
Hematoxylin, anhydrous powder (C.I. 75290)	2 gm
Sodium iodate	0.2 gm
Aluminum sulfate, $Al_2 (SO_4)_3 \cdot 18H_2O$	17.6 gm
Glacial acetic acid	20 ml

Combine the above reagents in the order given and stir for 1 hour at room temperature using a magnetic stirrer. Gill et al.[13] make the following comments:

1. If crystalline hematoxylin is purchased, substitute 2.36 gm in the above directions. (Hematoxylin is purchased from Roboz Instrument Co., 810-18th St., N.W., Washington, D.C. 20006.)
2. Accurately weigh the sodium iodate to ±0.01 gm.
3. Adjust the weight of aluminum sulfate according to the formula being used, if different from the formula given above.
4. One gram of citric acid can be substituted for the 20 ml of glacial acetic acid.
5. Stain may be used immediately; however, initially a slightly longer staining time may be needed.
6. Filter stain before use even though there will be no visible precipitate.

The above formula is used for cytologic specimens. Cytologic material that has been fixed with commercial spray fixatives containing carbowax should be treated with 95% ethanol for 10 minutes prior to staining; otherwise, the nuclear stain will be unsatisfactory. Stain cytologic smears for 2 minutes.

For use in paraffin section staining, stain at least 10 minutes in the above formula. To make a progressive stain that will selectively color nuclei in 3 minutes, double the amounts of hematoxylin and sodium iodate in the above directions, and quadruple the amount of aluminum sulfate.

Gill's hematoxylin is commercially available (Fisher Scientific Co., Pittsburgh, Pa.) in three strengths. Gill 1 is regular strength for cytology; Gill 2 is double the strength of Gill 1 and may be used for cytology and histology; Gill 3 is triple strength and used primarily for staining tissue sections.

General procedure for regressive hematoxylin and eosin stain using either Delafield's, Ehrlich's or Harris's formula

Most laboratories have a regular setup for the H & E stain consisting of large staining dishes each containing the separate reagents needed at each step. Wash pans containing continuously running water facilitate the rinsing and washing requirements. Tissue slides are placed in staining baskets, and the basket is transferred to the next reagent when the immersion time in the preceding reagent is complete.

1. Hydrate slides (p. 130).
2. Suitably remove, if necessary, any mercury precipitate, formalin pigment, or yellow color caused by fixation in a picric acid–containing fixative such as Bouin's fluid (pp. 47 and 50).
3. Stain in *either* Delafield's, Ehrlich's, or Harris's formula for 8 to 15 minutes. (Experience will determine the best timing for a particular laboratory situation.)
4. Rinse slides in tap water to remove excess hematoxylin.
5. Differentiate using a 1% hydrochloric acid mixture in 70% ethanol. Usually 5 to 10 seconds is a sufficient time; however this may have to be changed depending on the results of the subsequent microscopic examination.
6. Rinse well in tap water to remove excess differentiator, otherwise the differentiating action will continue and result in a poor nuclear stain.
7. Blue the sections for 30 to 90 seconds in *either* a weak ammonia solution or a dilute lithium carbonate solution.
   Ammonia solution
   To 1 liter of tap water, add 3 ml of 28% ammonium hydroxide and mix.
   Lithium carbonate solution
   Equal parts mixture of filtered saturated aqueous lithium carbonate and distilled water.
8. Wash well in running tap water for 5 to 10

minutes. Inadequate washing after the bluing step will result in uneven eosin staining. Check microscopically. Sections should show blue nuclei with a well-defined chromatin pattern and nuclear membrane; cytoplasm should be almost colorless. *Note:* In some areas, prolonging the tap water rinse after bluing for more than 3 minutes can result in sections that are colored a brown-purple with poor nuclear detail.

9. Counterstain in the eosin solution of choice. (See p. 153 for various formulas.) Timing of the counterstain will vary from 15 seconds to 3 minutes depending on the freshness of the eosin solution and the depth of stain desired. Slight agitation of the slides may promote more even staining.

10. Dehydrate in two changes of 95% ethanol for 1 to 2 minutes each change. All excess eosin should be removed.

11. Dehydrate in two changes of absolute ethanol for 1 to 2 minutes each change.

12. Clear in an equal-parts mixture of absolute ethanol and xylene; follow this with two changes of xylene; coverslip, using a synthetic mounting medium.

Results

Nuclei—blue
Cartilage and calcium deposits—dark blue
Cytoplasm and other tissue constituents—varying shades of red
Blood—bright red

Progressive hematoxylin and eosin procedure using Mayer's hematoxylin

1. Hydrate slides and remove any artifact pigments if necessary (pp. 130 and 131).

2. Stain in Mayer's hematoxylin for 15 to 20 minutes.

3. Rinse slides. If they show a grayish or bluish tint after step 2, they may be immersed in a bath of 0.5% acetic acid in 80% alcohol. This tinting is usually caused by excess egg albumin or gelatin adhesive on the slide.

4. Wash slides in running tap water for a minimum of 15 minutes. This develops bright blue nuclei and will prevent the stain from fading in the future.

5. Continue with steps 9 to 12 described in the regressive H & E procedure.

Results. See previous method.

Comments on staining tissue sections with H & E stains

1. A phloxine-saffron counterstain may be desired instead of eosin. (See p. 154 for details.)

2. If sections appear too blue when viewed microscopically at step 8, reimmerse them in acid alcohol for a few seconds; repeat steps 6 to 8 and recheck microscopically.

3. If sections show pale nuclei when viewed microscopically at step 8, reimmerse them in the hematoxylin for further staining. When this second immersion is complete, repeat steps 4 to 8. It may be necessary to shorten the time in the acid differentiator.

4. As alum hematoxylins become older, they stain more quickly but also more diffusely. This diffusion may be counteracted when enough alum is added to make the stain precise again, or the solution may be replaced completely.

5. The alcohol used at steps 11 and 12 serves a twofold purpose: one is dehydration of the tissue; the other, equally important, is the removal of excess eosin. By passing rapidly through these alcohols, excess eosin will remain in the section and overshadow many diagnostic features such as pigments and inclusion bodies. Proper differentiation of counterstain is as important as proper differentiation of hematoxylin.

6. Zenker's and Helly's fixed tissues generally require a longer staining time in the hematoxylin and a shorter staining time in the eosin.

7. Occasionally, the reagents used in the H & E are known to be working satisfactorily, yet some sections show a lack of nuclear staining. This can be attributable to (a) autolysis of that tissue section, (b) prolonged storage of the wet tissue in nonbuffered formalin, (c) overexposure to decalcifying fluids, (d) insufficient washing of the tissue after decalcification, and (e) dried or burned tissue. Basophilic staining properties may sometimes be restored by treatment of the hydrated section with one of the following solutions: 5% aqueous sodium bicarbonate overnight followed by a 5-minute wash in tap water prior to staining or 5% aqueous periodic acid overnight, followed by three changes of distilled water prior to staining.[5]

Stains for cytologic material
PAPANICOLAOU METHOD FOR STAINING CYTOLOGIC SMEARS[15]

Fixation. Fix smears immediately while they

are still wet with either 95% ethanol for 15 minutes or a commercial spray fixative. Viscous specimens may be smeared onto clean glass slides and fixed. Body fluids and serous exudates are usually centrifuged; the sediment is smeared onto a slide that has been coated with Mayer's egg albumin and then fixed. Extra sediment may be sent to the histology laboratory for processing and sectioning as a "cell block."

Solutions

1. Harris's hematoxylin without acetic acid. (See formula, p. 142; do not include the acetic acid.) Alternatively, commercially prepared hematoxylin may be used.
2. 0.25% hydrochloric acid
3. Orange G6 (OG 6), commercial grade
4. Eosin-azure 50 (EA 50), commercial grade

Method

1. After fixation, transfer the still-wet slides from 95% ethanol through graded alcohols to distilled water.
2. Stain in hematoxylin solution for 2 to 3 minutes.
3. Rinse in tap water.
4. Differentiate in 0.25% hydrochloric acid for 1 to 2 seconds.
5. Wash in gently running tap water for 5 minutes. Nuclei should be blue at this step.
6. Rinse in distilled water and dehydrate to 95% ethanol using graded alcohols.
7. Orange G6 counterstain for 2 minutes.
8. Rinse in 3 changes of 95% ethanol.
9. Eosin-azure 50 counterstain for 2 minutes.
10. Rinse in 3 changes of 95% ethanol, 2 changes of absolute ethanol, and several xylenes. Coverslip using a synthetic mounting medium.

Results

Nuclei—blue
Cell cytoplasm—varying shades of pink, yellow, green, blue, and gray

STAINING OF CYTOLOGIC MATERIAL USING GILL'S HEMATOXYLIN[13] (gynecologic and nongynecologic cell spreads, Nucleopore filters, Millipore and Gelman filters)

Reagents

1. Gill's hematoxylin (formula on p. 143)
2. Scott's tap water substitute
   a. Tap water — 1 liter
   b. Magnesium sulfate, $MgSO_4$ or — 10 gm
   $MgSO_4 \cdot 7H_2O$ — 20 gm
   c. Sodium bicarbonate — 2 gm
3. Eosin-azure 50 counterstain (commercially available)
4. Orange G6 counterstain (commercially available)
5. Absolute 2-propanol

Method for gynecologic and nongynecologic cell spreads and Nucleopore filters

1. Fix samples in 2 changes of 95% ethanol over a minimum of 10 minutes. Carbowax-coated fixed air-dried specimens will display poor nuclear staining unless this step is performed.
2. 2 changes of tap water — 10 dips each change
3. Gill's hematoxylin — 2 min
4. 2 changes of tap water — 10 dips each change
5. Scott's tap water substitute for bluing slides — 1 min
6. 2 changes of tap water — 10 dips each change
7. 2 changes of 95% ethanol — 10 dips each change
8. Orange G6 counterstain — 1 min
9. 3 changes of 95% ethanol — 10 dips each change
10. Eosin-azure 50 counterstain — 10 min
11. 3 changes of 95% ethanol — 20 dips each change
12. 3 changes of absolute ethanol — 10 dips each change
13. 3 changes of xylene — 10 dips each change
14. Coverslip, using a synthetic mounting medium.

Results

Similar to those for the Papanicolaou stain.

The method for staining Millipore and Gelman filters is similar with minor alterations including the following:

After step 4 of the preceding method, treat these filters with 0.05% hydrochloric acid for 30 seconds. This is to remove the hematoxylin from the background of the filter. Follow the hydrochloric acid treatment with 2 changes of tap water, 10 dips each change. Proceed with steps 5 to 7 of the preceding method. Then counterstain the Millipore and Gelman filters as follows:

8. Orange G6 counterstain — 2 min
9. 3 changes of 95% ethanol — 1 min each change
10. Eosin-azure 50 counterstain — 8 min
11. 95% ethanol — 4 min
12. 95% ethanol — 2 min
13. 95% ethanol — 1 min
14. 3 changes of absolute 2-propanol (isopropanol) — 1 min each change (This alcohol is used because absolute ethanol can soften and possibly dissolve these filters.)
15. 3 changes of xylene — 1 min each change
16. Coverslip slides, using a synthetic mounting medium.

Iron mordanted hematoxylin solutions
Uses and general considerations

The second most commonly used mordant is iron. Iron exists in two oxidation states, the 2+, or ferrous, form and the 3+, or ferric, form. Both states have been used as mordants. Ferrous chloride or ferrous sulfate are compounds used to provide ferrous iron; ferric chloride or ferric alum are commonly used to provide ferric iron. Iron hematoxylins are used to demonstrate nuclei and mitotic figures, muscle striations, protozoa, cell organelles, cell inclusions, and myelin sheaths. Of course, not all these structures are seen when one uses a single technic. The common factor is the iron mordant, but variations exist in procedure (pH of solution, time of staining, temperature of staining, single solution of mordant and dye versus separate solutions of each, and differentiation technics—excess mordant versus acid solutions versus alkaline solutions of oxidizers).

Single solution mixtures of iron mordant and hematoxylin are frequently used in special staining procedures. Generally, an iron hematoxylin solution should always be used when the succeeding stains are very lengthy or quite acidic, since an aluminum-mordanted hematoxylin stain would tend to decolorize with those conditions. Formulas that may be used include those of Janssen, Weigert-Lillie, and Weigert. The last formula is frequently used in selective stain procedures such as the allochrome method, trichrome methods for demonstration of muscle and connective tissue, Van Gieson procedure, mucicarmine methods, and pentachrome procedures. The mordant is taken up both by the phosphoric acid groups of the nucleic acids and by the carboxyl groups of the nucleoprotein as previously described; hence nuclei will be demonstrated in both extracted and unextracted tissue sections.

Single-solution iron hematoxylin formulas
Lillie and Earle's hematoxylin
Solution A

Ferric alum, $Fe_2(SO_4)_3(NH_4)_2SO_4 \cdot 24H_2O$	20 gm
Distilled water	200 ml

Solution B

Hematoxylin	2 gm
Absolute methanol	60 ml
Glycerol	60 ml

For use, mix equal amounts of solutions A and B.

Janssen's hematoxylin
Solution A

Ferric alum (formula given in preceding method)	15 gm
Ferrous sulfate, $FeSO_4 \cdot H_2O$	15 gm
Distilled water	100 ml

Solution B

Hematoxylin	1 gm
95% ethanol	50 ml
Glycerol	50 ml

For use, mix equal amounts of solutions A and B. It is usable for about 3 months. Color should be blue-black to purplish. When color turns brown, discard solution.

Weigert's iron hematoxylin
Solution A

29% ferric chloride	4 ml
Distilled water	95 ml
Concentrated hydrochloric acid	1 ml

Solution B

Hematoxylin	1 gm
95% ethanol	100 ml

For use, mix equal parts of solutions A and B. Best results are obtained when used fresh each time.

General staining method for use with single-solution iron hematoxylin formulas

When the above solutions are used, the following general procedure may be followed. Tissue may be fixed in any general fixative, routinely processed, and paraffin embedded.

1. Deparaffinize and hydrate slides to water.
2. Where applicable, remove mercury precipitates caused by fixation in Zenker's or Helly's solutions.
3. Stain in Weigert's hematoxylin (or Lillie and Earle's variation; Janssen's) for 10 minutes. Rinse in tap water and check microscopically for good nuclear detail.
4. Wash in running water 5 to 10 minutes.
5. Counterstain as desired.
6. Dehydrate through 95% ethanol and absolute ethanol, clear in xylene, and coverslip, using a synthetic mounting medium.

Results
Nuclei—black
Other tissue constituents—color of counterstain used

HEMATOXYLIN STAINING CLASSIFICATION

Hematoxylin staining is sometimes classified to be one of two types: "mordant hematoxylin staining" and "direct hematoxylin staining". These terms are confusing since both classifications use both mordant and dye. The distinction is *how* each is used. "Mordant hematoxylin staining" employs *separate* solutions of mordant and of dye during the staining process. "Direct hematoxylin staining," on the other hand, has both the dye and the mordant combined together in a *single* solution during the staining process. Most of the hematoxylin solutions used in microtechnique may be classified as direct-staining hematoxylins; all those considered thus far in this chapter have been direct-staining formulas.

When two separate solutions are used, as is the case with mordant hematoxylin staining, a mordant of either little or vigorous oxidizing action can be used if followed by a well-ripened hematoxylin solution. If the hematoxylin solution is insufficiently ripened, the mordant should be one possessing vigorous oxidizing power, for example, the ferric or chromium salts, because this will facilitate the conversion of hematoxylin to hematein. One advantage of mordant hematoxylin methods is that the dye itself can be preceded by a mordant salt that would not be able to be used in the same solution in a direct staining method. For example, ferric chloride may be used as a mordant in a mordant hematoxylin method and be followed by a hematoxylin solution containing an ammonium salt as one of its components. If used in combination, however, the two would form undesirable precipitates of ferric hydroxide.

A mordant followed by a solution of a hematoxylin containing the same mordant will also give good results. Mordants for separate use in the first solution include ammonium or potassium alum, ferric ammonium alum (2 to 3 drops of hydrochloric acid will increase contrast), and ferric chloride. Used together with hematoxylin, they give the following colors:

Ammonium alum—bright blue nuclei
Potassium alum—lilac or violet
Chrome alum—gray-blue
Iron alum—blue to blue-black

Iron is usually employed in mordant hematoxylin staining procedures. Two mordant hematoxylin methods use Heidenhain's iron hematoxylin and Mallory's iron chloride hematoxylin. Any fixative may be used, and tissues may be embedded in paraffin or celloidin. Cut sections at 5 μm.

Heidenhain's iron hematoxylin procedure

Solutions

Ferric ammonium sulfate (mordanting solution)
    Ferric ammonium sulfate   2.5 gm
    Distilled water   100 ml
Alcoholic hematoxylin
    Hematoxylin   0.5 gm
    95% alcohol   10 ml
    Distilled water   90 ml

Dissolve hematoxylin in the alcohol and add water. Place in bottle with cotton plug and allow to ripen for 4 to 5 weeks. Dilute with equal parts of distilled water for use. Solution may be reused.

Method

1. Mordant sections in ferric alum for 3 to 12 hours at room temperature or for 30 to 45 minutes at 56° C.
2. Wash quickly in water.
3. Stain for 1 to 36 hours in the alcoholic hematoxylin solution. A higher temperature will result in faster staining.
4. Rinse in water.
5. Differentiate with the ferric alum solution (this is differentiation by use of excess mordant). Sections should have differentiation controlled by microscopic observation. Rinse sections in tap water to stop the differentiation before examining under microscope.
6. Thoroughly wash in running water (15 minutes).
7. Counterstain, if desired, in any of the following:
   a. 0.1% aqueous acid fuchsin
   b. 0.1% aqueous orange G
   c. 0.1% aqueous light green
   Time of counterstaining ranges from 5 to 15 minutes. Since this is an iron hematoxylin method, Van Gieson's stain may also be used as a counterstaining method. Aqueous eosin may also provide good contrast.
8. Rinse in 50% alcohol.
9. Dehydrate in 95% alcohol, 2 changes minimum, followed by absolute alcohol, 2 changes.
10. Clear in xylene and coverslip using a synthetic mounting medium.

Result

Chromatin, nucleoli, mitochondria, and certain parts of striated muscle are stained black with the hematoxylin-ferric mordant lake.
Other tissue constituents are colored according to the counterstain used.

Mallory's iron chloride hematoxylin procedure

Solutions

Iron chloride (mordanting solution)
    Ferric chloride   5 gm
    Distilled water   100 ml
Hematoxylin
    Hematoxylin   0.5 gm
    Distilled water   100 ml
Prepare solutions fresh each time they are used.

Method

1. Mordant sections for at least 1 hour in the ferric chloride solution.
2. Rinse sections in 2 or 3 changes of tap water.
3. Stain in the hematoxylin solution until sections are a deep blue-black. Minimum time 1 hour.
4. Rinse in water.
5. Differentiate and decolorize in a 0.25% solution

of aqueous ferric chloride. Differentiation process should be controlled with a microscope.

6. Wash thoroughly in tap water to remove excess mordant that might cause continued decolorization of sections.

7. Counterstain at this point, as desired. Refer to preceding method for suggestions.

8. Dehydrate in 95% alcohol, followed by absolute alcohol, several changes in each.

9. Clear in xylene and coverslip using a synthetic mounting medium.

If celloidin sections are used, they should not be dehydrated with absolute alcohol because this will tend to dissolve the celloidin. Instead, after the 95% alcohol, clear in terpineol, or oil of origanum; blot and then coverslip, using a synthetic mounting medium.

Results

Nuclei—deep blue to blue-black

Other tissue constituents—colorless or colored according to counterstain used

Mallory notes that liver hyalin, if not too old, can be stained with this method.

RECOMMENDED HEMATOXYLIN SUBSTITUTES

The hematoxylin shortage that occurred a few years ago stimulated research to produce satisfactory substitutes for the hematoxylin dye. The results of this research are as follows:

1. For *routine use* in the H & E technics, as a substitute in the Papanicolaou stain, and as a counterstain for simple lipid dyes such as oil red O, use the following solution[16,17]:

Celestine blue	1 gm
Iron alum (ferric ammonium sulfate)	4 gm
Distilled water	200 ml

   The dye and the iron alum are dissolved separately, each in half the amount of water. (It may be necessary to allow the iron alum to dissolve overnight.) Mix the two solutions. The staining solution is dark blue and ready for use. Filter before use.

   To substitute for hematoxylin in the H & E technic, stain the tissue in the above solution for 5 to 30 minutes. Follow this by several water rinses; dehydrate sections in 95% ethanol; counterstain for 30 to 60 seconds in 0.1% eosin Y in 95% alcohol, dehydrate with absolute alcohol, clear in xylene, and coverslip, using a synthetic mounting medium.

   When using the above *as a substitute in the Papanicolaou technic,* stain nuclei for 1 to 2 minutes. There is little effect on cytoplasmic coloration with this timing.

Staining for approximately 1 minute will demonstrate nuclear detail if one follows simple fat-demonstration methods.

2. *As a substitute for Weigert's iron hematoxylin* in the Van Gieson methods, use an iron gallein (C.I. 45445) solution. This solution is modeled on Weigert's iron chloride hematoxylin, with a modification in acid content and substituting the iron alum of Weil's myelin methods. The iron gallein is prepared as follows[18]:

   Stock solution A
   Dissolve 1 gm of gallein in 20 ml of ethylene glycol.
   Add 80 ml of absolute ethanol. Shake until dissolved.

   Stock solution B
   To approximately 90 ml of distilled water, add 1.6 to 2 ml of concentrated hydrochloric acid. Mix well. To this, add 4 gm of iron alum (ferric ammonium sulfate).
   Dissolve the iron alum and dilute to a final volume of 100 ml.
   The pH of the solution should be between 1.4 and 1.6.

   Working solution
   Mix equal parts of solution A and solution B. This mixture should turn a blue-black color.

Stain nuclei for 20 minutes, followed by a thorough water wash.

Note: Decreasing the hydrochloric acid content obscures intranuclear detail and results in a gray coloration of muscle and cytoplasm.

SYNTHETIC NUCLEAR STAINS[1]
Classification, uses, and general staining method

The term "synthetic nuclear stains" is used here in contrast to those stains extracted from natural sources, such as hematoxylin and carmine. These synthetic dyes are derivatives of the substances found in coal tar. They are valuable nuclear stains and may be subdivided into several groups, including oxazines, safranin, and thiazins. Most synthetic nuclear stains are soluble in both water and alcohol, and differentiation of the stains may be accomplished by use of either of these substances. Although they may be employed as either progressive or regressive stains, they are generally used regressively. It is recommended to make the stock solutions to some strength just short of saturation because strictly saturated solutions are of unknown strength. The colors are most effective after chromic or osmic acid fixatives, but sections fixed in a picric acid–formalin–acetic acid mixture (such as Bouin's) may be mordanted in Flemming's solution before staining and similar results will be achieved. The following general method may be used to demonstrate nuclei using these synthetic dyes:

1. Hydrate slides.
2. Stain sections in a strong aqueous solution of the dye or weaker alcoholic solution for 5 to 30 minutes.
3. Wash in water.
4. Differentiate in 95% alcohol.
5. Dehydrate in absolute alcohol.
6. Clear in xylene.
7. Coverslip, using a synthetic mounting medium.

The above can be followed exactly for paraffin sections. If celloidin sections are used, after differentiation the sections should be blotted with filter paper and then covered with xylene; blotting is repeated; xylene is repeated until specimen is cleared. Absolute alcohol is not used as the dehydrating agent because it will dissolve the celloidin. Coverslip sections, using a synthetic mounting medium. The nuclear stain may be made even sharper if the water wash is done with slightly acidulated water, or if the first alcohol differentiation is done with a few drops of acetic or hydrochloric acid added.

Subdivisions of synthetic nuclear dyes

The first group of synthetic nuclear dyes includes the *oxazine dyes,* such as gallocyanine, gallamine blue, and celestine blue. These form metallic lakes in the course of the preparation of the staining solutions; with a chrome mordant they will give a blue nuclear color, and with an iron mordant they will give a blue-black nuclear color. The o-diphenol group that all possess serves as a metal chelation site for the mordant.

The iron lakes of the oxazines are recommended as the more selective of the nuclear stains, and these lakes may be prepared by being boiled for 3 to 5 minutes as either a 0.5% solution of celestine blue B (C.I. 51050) or gallamine blue (C.I. 51045) or gallocyanine (C.I. 51030) in a 5% ferric ammonium alum solution.

Safranin is a widely used synthetic nuclear stain, and a safranin–light green combination may be used as a substitute for an H & E stain. Tissues to be stained in safranin may be fixed in alcohol, Flemming's, or Zenker's. Recom-

mended solutions (according to Mallory) include a saturated aqueous solution (about 5.45%) made with the aid of heat, and a saturated solution (Babes' aniline safranin 1887) in aniline water. The latter is made up by the addition of excess safranin O to 100 ml of 2% aniline water, with the solution being heated in a flask set in hot water at 60° to 80° C, and being filtered when cool. This powerful stain will act instantly on nuclei and will keep about 2 months.

Magenta (basic fuchsin) is less widely employed as a single nuclear stain than it is in combination with plasma stains in complex technics. The formula of Ziehl (1882) is just as good a nuclear stain as it is for microorganisms (see p. 237 for formula).

The *thiazins* comprise another class of synthetics and include thionin and its mono-, di-, tri-, and tetra-methyl derivatives as azure A, azure B, azure C, methylene blue, toluidine blue, and new methylene blue. Methylene blue may be oxidized to azures and methylene violets in a process known as "polychroming," and mixtures of methylene blue with these products are called "polychrome methylene blue." Polychroming occurs freely in alkaline solutions without oxidants and is expedited by a rise in pH level above 8 and heat.

All the thiazins mentioned are excellent and specific nuclear stains, but tend to be extracted by alcohols, and must be mounted in neutral mounting media. They may also exhibit metachromasia to a greater or lesser extent.

Several of the solutions of the thiazins that may be used are the following:

Thionin. 0.5% solution of thionin in 20% alcohol is preferred to a simple aqueous solution, since an aqueous solution does not preserve well.

Toluidine blue O. May be used in a 0.3% to 1% aqueous solution. A 0.5% solution in 20% alcohol is recommended for staining of frozen sections of unfixed tissue.

Methylene blue. A saturated solution (about 1.48%) in 95% or absolute alcohol may be used as a stock solution. It can be diluted for use when 1 part of the stock is added to 9 parts of water.

Other solutions of methylene blue are the following[1,3,19]:

Löffler's methylene blue solution. 30 ml saturated methylene blue solution in 95% alcohol; 100 ml of 1:10,000 aqueous solution of sodium hydroxide. This is a very useful stain and will keep for a long time without losing staining power.

Terry's acid polychrome methylene blue (for fresh unfixed frozen sections)

1% aqueous methylene blue	6 ml
1% potassium carbonate	6 ml
Distilled water	18 ml

Combine the above three reagents and boil over a flame for exactly 2½ minutes. Cool solution in running tap water. When it is cooled, dilute remaining solution to a 30 ml volume with distilled water. Filter before use.

Terry's acid polychrome methylene blue (for fixed frozen sections)

1% aqueous methylene blue	20 ml
1% potassium carbonate	20 ml
Distilled water	60 ml

Combine the above three reagents and boil gently for 2½ minutes. Cool rapidly under running tap water. To the cooled solution, add 10 ml of 10% aqueous acetic acid. Shake this mixture for 1 minute. Dilute to a final volume of 100 ml with distilled water. Filter before use.

Unna's alkaline methylene blue solution

Methylene blue	1 gm
Potassium carbonate	1 gm
Distilled water	100 ml

The above is useful as a general stain in combination with phloxine or eosin, and also as a stain for plasma cells. Stain should be ripened for 1 to 2 weeks and diluted 1:10 or 1:5 for use.

Unna's polychrome methylene blue solution

This solution is merely an old solution of alkaline methylene blue, described above. Over time, the oxidation process forms methyl violet and methylene red in the solution. The months-long oxidation process at normal temperature may be shortened by means of heat.

The *crystal violets* and *gentian violets* are the final class, and although very specific for nuclei, their chief use has been in the gram-positive stains of Brown-Brenn and Gram-Weigert. About 1.68 gm in 100 ml will give a saturated aqueous solution; 13.87 gm in 100 ml of absolute alcohol will give a saturated alcoholic solution. Gentian violet is not a definite chemical substance but a mixture of methyl violet, dextrin, and crystal violet. Solutions calling for gentian violet as an ingredient should have it replaced with crystal violet, as this will give more consistent staining results.

NUCLEIC ACIDS

The substance in the nucleus that stains strongly with the nuclear dyes is called nuclear chromatin. This chromatin is composed of nucleoproteins—a combination of protein and nucleic acid. The two types of nucleic acid are deoxyribonucleic acid (DNA), found chiefly in the nucleus, and ribonucleic acid (RNA), present in the nucleolus and cytoplasm (in free ribosomes and ribosomes on rough endoplasmic reticulum). DNA functions principally in cell heredity by carrying the code for future cell replication and in the synthesis of RNA. RNA itself functions principally in protein synthesis.

Feulgen reaction

Principle. The purpose of this technic is to demonstrate DNA in tissue sections. Tissues are first treated with a mild acid—a hydrolytic step that splits off the purine bases (adenine and guanine) and then the pyrimidines (thymine and cytosine) from the sugar-phosphate groupings and releases aldehyde groups from the deoxypentose sugar. Longer hydrolysis gives a more intense reaction; however, if carried out too long, the hydrolysis will destroy the reaction entirely. Uncovered aldehyde groups then form a stable-colored compound with the Schiff reagent. See PAS reaction for further information on the aldehyde combination with the Schiff reagent.

Solutions

Schiff's reagent (See PAS reaction, p. 165.)
1 N hydrochloric acid (HCl)
  To 916.5 ml distilled water, add 83.5 ml concentrated HCl.
Sulfurous rinse (See PAS reaction, p. 166.)
Working solution of light green (p. 187)

Method

1. Hydrate sections.
2. Rinse sections in 1 N HCl and transfer to 1 N HCl that has been prewarmed for 45 minutes at 60° C.
3. Allow sections to hydrolyze in the 1 N HCl for 8 to 12 minutes. Keep sections at 60° C for this hydrolytic procedure.
4. Place sections in Schiff reagent for 40 to 60 minutes.
5. Rinse sections in 3 changes of sulfurous rinse—2 minutes each change.
6. Wash in tap water for 10 minutes.
7. Counterstain in working light green solution for 1 to 2 minutes.
8. Dehydrate, clear, and mount in a synthetic mounting medium.

Results

Nuclei—magenta
Background—green

Methyl green–pyronin methods

Principle. This technic is used to demonstrate

DNA and RNA in tissue sections. The DNA stains with the methyl green, while the RNA is colored red with the pyronin. There is no purely chemical explanation, as yet, for the staining phenomenon, but there have been a few theories offered as to why two basic dyes combine differently with two different nucleic acids. Studies suggest evidence that the differential staining may be caused by the differing degrees of polymerization of the two molecules. Methyl green is bound by the more highly polymerized DNA, whereas RNA, a lower polymer, is bound by pyronin. Studies supporting the polymerization theory show that if DNA undergoes depolymerization with exposure to acids, ultraviolet irradiation, or certain fixatives, the ability to bind the methyl green is lost, and the DNA then stains with the pyronin.

Method 1[20]

Fixation. Carnoy's at 4° C is best.
Embedding. Cut paraffin sections at 5 μm.

Solutions and materials

Walpole's acetate buffer, pH 4.1
Stock solution A: 0.1 N acetic acid
Stock solution B: 0.1 N sodium acetate
For 100 ml of pH 4.1 buffer, use 80 ml of solution A and 20 ml of solution B. Mix well.
Dyes needed (purchase from Roboz Surgical Instrument Co., 810-18th St., N.W., Washington, DC 20006):
  1. Chroma-Gesellschaft Methylgrün GA (purified and free of methyl violet)
  2. Chroma-Gesellschaft Pyronin GS
Ice-cold distilled water
tert-Butanol

Procedure

1. Prepare the staining solution. For 100 ml of the staining solution:
   a. Weigh 0.5 gm of the methyl green dye and dissolve it in 100 ml of the mixed buffer.
   b. Adjust pH of the above mixture to 4.1.
   c. Add 0.2 gm of pyronin to the pH-adjusted solution of methyl green and mix well.
2. Stain hydrated slides in the above mixture for 1 hour at 37° C.
3. Rinse sections for 1 to 2 seconds in *ice-cold distilled water*. This is a critical step!
4. Blot sections evenly.
5. Rinse sections with vigorous agitation in *tert*-butanol.
6. Dehydrate sections with 2 changes of *tert*-butanol for 5 minutes in each change.
7. Clear sections in several changes of xylene and coverslip using a synthetic mounting medium.

Results

DNA—green
RNA—red

Method 2[21]

Fixation. Carnoy's or another alcoholic fixative is preferred. Satisfactory results can be obtained after fixation in 10% NBF.
Embedding. Paraffin or frozen sections; also smears or imprints.

Solutions

0.2 M acetic acid
  Glacial acetic acid   11.55 ml
  Distilled water   to make 1 liter
0.2 M sodium acetate
  Sodium acetate ($C_2H_3O_2Na$)   16.4 gm
  or
  Sodium acetate ($C_2H_3O_2Na \cdot 3H_2O$) 27.2 gm
  Distilled water   to make 1 liter
Acetate buffer, pH 4.7—store in refrigerator
  0.2 M acetic acid   44 ml
  0.2 M sodium acetate   54 ml
0.4% methyl green–pyronin solution
  Purified methyl green–pyronin*   0.4 gm
  95% ethanol   2.5 ml
  Dissolve powder in the alcohol and add:
  Acetate buffer, pH 4.7   97.5 ml
  Stir the solution until all the particles are dissolved. Store the prepared solution in the 56° to 60° C oven. Solution is stable for approximately 3 to 4 weeks.

Method

1. Deparaffinize and hydrate sections to distilled water.
2. Stain in filtered 0.4% methyl green–pyronin solution for 5 to 30 minutes (better if 30 minutes) in oven 56° to 60° C.
3. Rinse slides briefly in distilled water.
4. Blot dry.
5. Dehydrate quickly in acetone and then acetone-xylene. Use individual beakers and dehydrate the slides one at a time. (A slight rinse in tetrahydrafuran may be used before the acetone.)
6. Clear the slides in 2 changes of xylene. Coverslip, using a synthetic mounting medium.

Results

Nuclear chromatin (DNA)—blue-green
Nucleoli and cytoplasmic granules (RNA)—rose red
Remainder of tissue components—pale pink to colorless

Nucleic acid extraction methods[1,4,5]

Extraction procedures should require a minimum of two slides per case. One of the tissue sections should be given the complete extraction treatment. The second slide should receive treatment identical to that given the first, except

---

*Michrome 421, Edward Gurr, Ltd., 42 Richmond Road West, London, SW 14, England.

that the second is not exposed to the actual extracting agent.

Extracting agents that have been employed for nucleic acid identification include the following:

Deoxyribonuclease (DNAse)—digests deoxyribonucleic acid (DNA)

Ribonuclease (RNAse)—digests ribonucleic acid (RNA)

Trichloroacetic acid (TCA)—digests DNA and RNA

Perchloric acid—extracts either RNA, or DNA and RNA depending on time and temperature of exposure

Deoxyribonuclease digestion procedure

Fixation. Carnoy's, Bouin's, or 10% neutral buffered formalin.

Embedding. Cut paraffin sections at 5 μm.

Solutions

TRIS buffer, pH 7.3

0.2 M tris(hydroxymethyl)-aminomethane	10 ml
0.1 N hydrochloric acid	17 ml
Distilled water	13 ml

Mix the above reagents and adjust pH to 7.3.

Digestion solution

Crystalline deoxyribonuclease	0.001 gm
0.2 M magnesium chloride	22.5 ml
0.2 M calcium chloride	2.5 ml
0.1 M TRIS buffer, pH 7.3	20 ml
Distilled water	55 ml

Method

1. Hydrate slides and treat one with the digestion solution and one with the buffer only for 2 hours at 37° C.
2. Rinse both sections in running tap water for 10 minutes, rinse in distilled water, and stain using Feulgen or methyl green–pyronin methods.

Results

DNA should stain in the section treated with the buffer only. Staining should be absent in the section treated with the digestion solution.

Comments. Tissue should not be fixed in a heavy metal fixative. If 10% formalin or Bouin's has been used, stain with the Feulgen method. If Carnoy's fixative has been used, either the Feulgen or the methyl green–pyronin method may be used after digestion is complete.

Ribonuclease digestion procedure

Fixation. Carnoy's best. See previous technic for additional comments.

Embedding. See preceding technic.

Solutions

Various dilutions of crystalline ribonuclease have been employed for digestion, usually in a 0.2 to 0.5 mg/ml amount. Adjust pH of distilled water to 6.8.

Crystalline ribonuclease	0.2 to 0.5 gm
Distilled water pH 6.8	100 ml

Method

1. Hydrate sections and treat one with the digestion solution and the second with the distilled water only for 1 to 3 hours at 37° C. Timing should be the same for both the control and the test slide.
2. Wash sections in running tap water for 10 minutes and stain both with methyl green–pyronin. (The Feulgen method should not be used as a follow-up stain, since the Feulgen technic demonstrates DNA, not RNA.)

Results

After the methyl green–pyronin stain, RNA should stain red in the section that was pretreated with the distilled water only. RNA staining should be absent in the slide that was exposed to the digestion solution.

Trichloroacetic acid (TCA) extraction

Treating a section for 15 minutes with a 4% TCA solution at a temperature of 90° C should effectively remove both DNA and RNA. Test sections should be washed well in tap water to remove all acid traces, rinsed in distilled water, and stained with the methyl green–pyronin method.

For the unextracted section, staining results for DNA and RNA should be as previously described. Staining should be abolished in the extracted section.

Perchloric acid extraction

To remove RNA alone, treat test sections with 10% aqueous perchloric acid for 12 to 18 hours at 4° C. The control section should remain in distilled water for the same time and at the same temperature as the test slide.

To remove both DNA and RNA, treat sections with 5% perchloric acid at 60° C for 20 to 30 minutes. The control should remain in distilled water for the same time and at the same temperature as the test slide.

Either of these procedures may be followed by staining using the methyl green–pyronin method.

ACRIDINE ORANGE FLUORESCENT METHOD FOR DNA AND RNA[4]

Fixation. Fresh frozen sections, or Carnoy's fixed tissue, or other alcoholic fixative. Smears should be fixed for 30 minutes in ether-alcohol. Formalin and Bouin's fixed material should not be used, since the results are inferior.

Table 8-1. Commonly used plasma stains

Name	Color index		Solubility gm/dl	
	Number	Color	Water	Alcohol
Picric acid	10305	Yellow	1.18	8.96
Orange G	16230	Orange	10.86	0.22
Ponceau 2R	16150	Red	Soluble	Very slight
Metanil yellow	13065	Yellow	5.36	1.45
Tartrazine	19140	Yellow	Very soluble	Slight
Biebrich scarlet	26905	Red	Soluble	Slight
Eriocyanine A	42576	Blue-violet	Soluble	Soluble
Eosin Y	45380	Orange-red	44.2	2.18
Eosin B	45400	Red	39.11	0.75
Erythrosin B	45430	Red	11.1	1.87
Phloxine B	45410	Red-red purple	Soluble	Soluble

For further listing of plasma stains, see Lillie, R. D., and Fullmer, H. M.: Histopathologic technic and practical histochemistry, ed. 4, New York, 1976, McGraw-Hill Book Co.

Solutions

0.067 M phosphate buffer, pH 6.0
    0.067 M sodium phosphate, dibasic   15 ml
    Na_2HPO_4 (9.465 gm/liter)
    0.067 M potassium acid phosphate   85 ml
    KH_2PO_4 (9.07 gm/liter)
Acridine orange solution: 0.1% acridine orange (C.I. 46005) in phosphate buffer, pH 6
0.1 M calcium chloride
1% acetic acid

Technic

1. Hydrate material through graded alcohols to distilled water.
2. Rinse in 1% acetic acid for 6 seconds.
3. Rinse in 2 changes of distilled water.
4. Treat with acridine orange solution for 3 minutes.
5. Wash with phosphate buffer, pH 6, for 1 minute.
6. Differentiate in 0.1 M calcium chloride for 30 seconds.
7. Coverslip using a drop of the 0.1 M phosphate buffer and examine with the fluorescent microscope.

Results

DNA should fluoresce green.
RNA should fluoresce red.

Comment. Control sections employing the enzyme digestions previously described for deoxyribonuclease and ribonuclease should be used.

PLASMA STAINS[1,5]

Plasma stains are usually acid dyes that contain sulfonic and carboxylic acids that combine with tissue bases, especially those proteins with an excess of the basic amino acids such as arginine, lysine, hydroxylysine, histidine. The two most frequently used are picric acid and eosin. Other counterstains are listed in Table 8-1.

Picric acid is a nitro dye and is used as a yellow contrast stain in collagen methods as well as a simple plasma stain with hematoxylin. With the hematoxylin methods, either the acid itself or ammonium salt may be used; with the Van Gieson type of collagen stains, the ammonium salt is not effective.

Eosin as a counterstain for hematoxylin may be used in either an aqueous or alcoholic solution, and the strength of the solution used varies with the tissue and the fixative used but generally lies between 0.5% to 2% after a hematoxylin stain. When eosin is used before an aniline dye such as methylene blue, a 5% or saturated solution should be used. Eosin will demonstrate red blood cells and muscle fibers clearly. After Zenker's fixation these substances stain intensely; so after Zenker's a dilute eosin solution should be used. Alternatively, a shorter staining time may be employed for the usual strength solution.

Solutions

2% Aqueous eosin solution
    Eosin Y, water soluble   25 gm
    Distilled water   1250 ml
    Glacial acetic acid   2 to 4 ml
Alcoholic eosin solution
    3% aqueous eosin Y   100 ml
    Absolute alcohol   125 ml
    Distilled water   375 ml
    Optional: few drops of acetic acid
Eosin-phloxine solution
    Eosin stock solution
        1% aqueous solution of eosin Y, water soluble

Phloxine stock solution
  1% aqueous solution of phloxine B
Working solution of eosin-phloxine

Stock eosin	100 ml
Stock phloxine	10 ml
95% ethanol	780 ml
Glacial acetic acid	4 ml

The eosin-phloxine combination is an excellent counterstain for routine H & E stains. Working solution should be changed at least once a week.

Another useful counterstain for hematoxylin preparations involves the use of a *phloxine-saffron counterstain.*[5] Although the type of fixation is not critical, color shades seen in the final result will vary somewhat depending on the fixative solution employed. Solutions used are 1.5% aqueous phloxine B and 2% safran du Gâtinais in absolute ethanol. (The safran du Gâtinais is available from Roboz Surgical Instrument Co., 810-18th St., N.W., Washington, DC 20006.) The saffron solution should not be left open to the air for any length of time, otherwise the solution will evaporate. The counterstaining method is as follows:

1. After the hematoxylin-stained slides have been blued and washed, stain in 1.5% phloxine B for 2 minutes.
2. Wash slides in tap water for 5 minutes.
3. Dehydrate slides in 3 changes of absolute alcohol.
4. Stain in the alcoholic safran du Gâtinais for 5 minutes.
5. Rinse with 2 changes of absolute alcohol; clear in 2 changes of xylene for 2 minutes each change; coverslip, using a synthetic mounting medium.

Results of phloxine-saffron counterstain
Collagen—yellow
Muscle and cell cytoplasm—red
Red cells—bright red-pink
Bone—yellow
Cartilage—yellow to yellow-green
Nuclei (if previously stained with an aluminum-mordanted hematoxylin)—blue

POLYCHROMATIC STAINS[1,22,23]
Theory

The concept of blood dyes evolved to an extent from Ehrlich's idea of a "neutral dye." Ehrlich allowed a basic dye (methyl green) to react with an acid dye (orange G) and found this combination gave a different product, which he called a neutral dye. He believed that this was formed from the simultaneous decomposition of the two original dyes and also discovered that a small amount of extra acid dye would allow the neutral dye to dissolve. On staining a blood smear, Ehrlich found that using a neutral dye would permit differentiation among the leukocytes: acidophilic granules would stain with the acid dye component; basophilic granules would stain with the basic dye component; and neutrophilic granules would stain with both components to a certain extent.

Romanowsky, using Ehrlich's idea of a neutral dye, tried another dye combination, with methylene blue as the basic dye component and eosin as the acid dye component. It is these two dyes that are used today in staining blood films, parasites, bone marrow, and so forth, and the two commonly used azure-eosin formulas are those of Wright and Giemsa. The azures (basic) consist of mono-, di-, tri-, and tetra-methyl thionin. Tetramethyl thionin is commonly known as methylene blue. The eosins (acidic) that may be used comprise eosin Y, eosin B, erythrosin B (an iodine derivative of eosin), and phloxine B. Using these, one can see a wide color range when staining parasites and blood. This is sometimes referred to as the Romanowsky color range and is seen with all mixtures or compounds of eosin and methylene blue (and allied dyes as the azures). The range is exemplified in the following manner:

Chromatin of white blood cells	Purple
Nuclei of parasitic protozoa	Red
Basophilic cytoplasm of lymphocytes, monocytes, and parasitic protozoa	Blue
Eosinophilic granules	Pink
Neutrophilic granules	Purple
Red blood cells	Pink (to bluish)
Bacteria	Deep blue

Researchers wondered why the color range was so unusual. The basophilic cytoplasm naturally stained with the basic dye methylene blue, and the acidophilic granules naturally had an affinity for the acidic eosin. The colors seen demonstrating the parasitic nucleus and acidic chromatin of white blood cells remained to be explained.

Further work showed that it was not the neutral dye concept that was responsible for the color range, but rather impurities present in the actual dye solution. On standing in solution, particularly in an alkaline pH, methylene blue gives rise to new substances, metachromatic in nature, and these are azure A, azure B, and methylene violet. This dye complex of methylene blue and derivatives is known as polychrome methylene blue and may be made up when an aqueous solution of methylene blue is boiled and a mild alkali (sodium bicarbonate) is added to the solution. The final staining solution therefore contains methylene blue, methylene violet, azure A, and azure B. These impurities are the ones responsible for the color range. One theory suggests that the nucleus of parasitic protozoa is red because the chromatin is not stained in it, but rather the highly basic protein, protamine. This protamine combines with eosin and also with the basic dye azure A. This results in the formation of an imino base, and imino bases of the azures are red. Metachromasia may also be responsible for the red staining; the problem is not completely solved.

To ensure uniform staining results, it is better to use a solution of known composition with weighed amounts of the azures. This not only gives better staining results, but eliminates the necessity to polychrome the methylene blue. One may make a stock solution by dissolving the above substances in methanol or a mixture of methanol and glycerol. Before actual staining, the stock solution should be diluted with water or aqueous buffer to permit ionization of dyes.

General comments for polychromatic procedures[1,24]

1. The following blood dye methods list directions for dehydrating tissue and smear samples, clearing them in xylene, and coverslipping them using a synthetic mounting medium. However, it is also possible to examine air-dried, stained peripheral blood smears by use of immersion oil. If the smear has been made on a slide, place a small amount of immersion oil over the smear and examine. No cover slip is necessary. If the smear has been made on a cover slip, first place a small drop of oil on a slide; mount the cover-slip smear side up on the slide using the oil as an adhesive; finally, place another drop of immersion oil on the top of the smear and examine microscopically.
2. Blood dyes, especially Wright's stain, tend to be somewhat hygroscopic and can absorb water if the container is left uncapped. Staining with such a solution then causes the hemoglobin to leach out of the red cells, and this results in the appearance of small artifact defects in the red cells.
3. All neutral stains are greatly influenced by the pH of the solution, and the major cause

of unsatisfactory staining when these solutions are used can be attributed to incorrect pH. Optimal staining results are seen only when the pH of the solution lies between 6.4 and 6.9. If the red corpuscles stain blue-gray and the white cells stain only blue, the stain is most likely too alkaline. If examination shows that the red corpuscles are bright pink and the white cells unstained or very slightly stained, the solution is too acid. Be sure all recommended buffers are correctly prepared.
4. Working solutions of the blood dyes should be freshly prepared just before use and discarded after use.

Wright's stain for blood smears[1]

Solutions
Wright's stain (commercial)
Buffer solution

Sodium phosphate, dibasic	0.3 gm
Sodium phosphate, monobasic	0.7 gm
Distilled water	100 ml

Method
1. Lay thin blood smears face up on a horizontal staining rack.
2. Cover smear with Wright's staining solution (about 15 drops).
3. Let sit for 1 minute and then add twice the volume of distilled water, or instead of water, a 1:6 dilution of the above buffer stock solution. You should see a metallic sheen on the solution before proceeding with step 4. Allow the water or buffer and dye mixture to remain on the slide for at least 2 minutes.
4. Drain off and rinse with diluted buffer or distilled water until the thinner portions of the blood film are pink.
5. Blot dry, and mount in synthetic mounting medium.

Results
Given in previous discussion section.

Sheehan's modification of Giemsa technic[25]

Fixation. Zenker fixation gives the best results. Other well-fixed tissue may be used.
Embedding. Cut paraffin sections at 5 μm.

Solutions
Giemsa stain

Phosphate buffer, pH 6.8	100 ml
Giemsa stain (Wolbach)	5 ml
Methanol (*acetone free*)	5 ml

Acetic water

Acetic acid	1 ml
Distilled water	400 ml

Technic

1. Remove paraffin with 3 changes of xylene.
2. Take sections through 2 changes of absolute alcohol.
3. Take sections through 3 changes of methanol (acetone free).
4. Place slide on rack and cover with Wright's stain for 5 minutes.
5. Add an equal amount of distilled water until a metallic gleam appears on the surface of the Wright stain–water combination. Leave for 5 minutes.
6. Pour off stain and place slides (without washing) into Coplin jar containing Giemsa staining solution for 45 minutes.
7. Differentiate and dehydrate in the following manner:

Acetic water	1 dip
Acetic water	2 dips
Distilled water	2 dips
95% alcohol	3 dips
Absolute alcohol	3 dips
Absolute alcohol	3 dips
Xylene–absolute alcohol	3 dips
Xylene	2 changes

8. Coverslip, using a synthetic mounting medium.

Results (Plate 2, *M*)

Nuclei—blue
Cytoplasm—pale blue
Rickettsias—reddish purple
Erythrocytes—yellowish pink

In our laboratory, we found the above modification gave a better color range for routinely fixed tissue than that found when using Wright stain or Giemsa stain alone.

Giemsa stain—Wolbach's modification[1]

Fixation. Zenker-fixed tissue gives the best results. Other well-fixed tissues may be used.

Embedding. Cut paraffin sections at 5 to 6 μm.

Solutions

Giemsa stock solution—One should purchase Giemsa stain from a reputable dye manufacturer, insisting on certification by the Biological Stain Commission.

Working solution—Giemsa stain

Stock Giemsa	2.5 ml
Methanol	3 ml
Distilled water (to which has been added 2 to 4 drops of 0.5% aqueous solution of sodium bicarbonate)	100 ml

Colophonium stock solution

Colophonium	10 gm
Absolute alcohol	100 ml

Working solution—colophonium

Colophonium stock solution	10 ml
95% alcohol	40 ml

Note: The colophonium in the differentiating fluid is believed to function as a weak acid and gives sharper, better controlled differentiation than that obtained with regular alcohol.

Technic

1. Hydrate slides.

Plate 1. **A,** Kinyoun's acid-fast stain for tubercle bacillus (red). **B,** Berg's technic for spermatozoa (red). **C,** Auramine rhodamine fluorescent technic for tubercle bacillus (yellow fluorescence). **D,** Warthin-Starry technic for spirochetes (black). **E,** Periodic acid–silver methenamine technic for *Pneumocystis carinii* (black). **F,** Tissue touch preparation, Mallory's variant of Weigert's fibrin stain for *Pneumocystis carinii* (blue-purple). **G,** Grocott technic for fungus (*Coccidioides immitis*) (black). **H,** Gridley technic for fungus (*Candida albicans*) (purple). **I,** MacCallum-Goodpasture technic for gram-positive (blue) and gram-negative (red) bacteria. **J,** Taylor's modified Brown-Brenn technic (gram-negative organisms, red). **K,** Taylor's modified Brown-Brenn technic (gram-positive organisms, blue). **L,** Pearse periodic acid–orange G technic in the pituitary (basophils, red; acidophils, yellow). **M,** Gomori's chrome alum–hematoxylin–phloxine in an islet of Langerhans in the pancreas (beta cells, bright blue; alpha cells, red). **N,** Bowie's technic for juxtaglomerular granules (purple) in the kidney. **O,** Fontana-Masson technic for argentaffin granules (black). **P,** Kereny's Congo red technic for beta cells in the pituitary (granules of beta cells, orange; granules of alpha cells, yellow). **Q,** Sieracki, Michael, and Clark technic for beta cells (deep purple) in pancreatic islets. **R,** Mallory's phosphotungstic acid–hematoxylin (muscle fibers, purple; collagen, orange). **S,** Masson trichrome stain in myometrium (muscle, red; collagen, blue). **T,** Gomori's aldehyde fuchsin technic (elastic fibers, purple). **U,** Snook's technic for reticulum (reticulin fibers, black). **V,** Lillie's allochrome procedure in the kidney (collagen, blue; glomerular basement membranes, red-purple). **W,** Verhoeff–Van Gieson technic (elastic fibers, black; collagen, red). **X,** Gomori's modified iron reaction (Prussian blue) (hemosiderin, blue, in Kupffer cells in the liver).

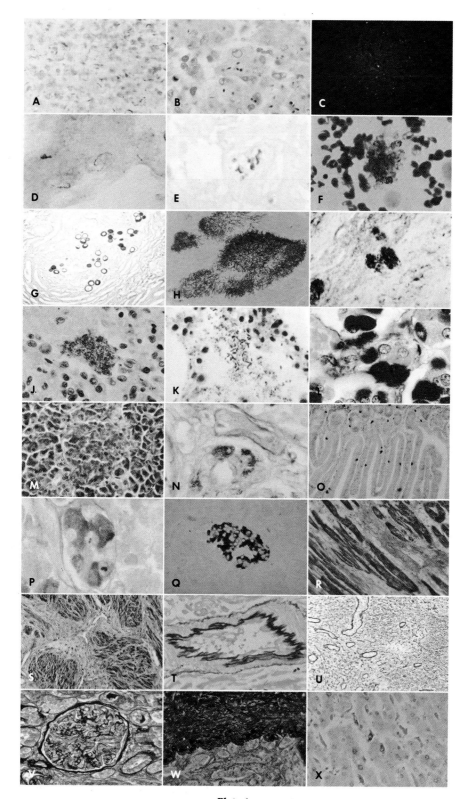

Plate 1

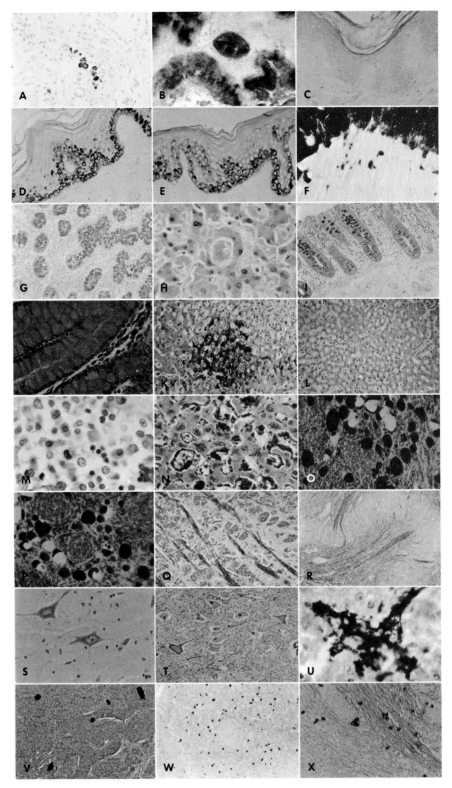

Plate 2

2. Iodine and 5% sodium thiosulfate if Zenker-fixed.
3. Wash well in running water.
4. Rinse in distilled water, 3 changes.
5. Make a working Giemsa solution and pour it over the slides immediately after mixing.
6. Change to *fresh stain, freshly prepared,* twice during the first hour.
7. Leave sections overnight in third change of staining solution.
8. Differentiate in working colophonium solution until sections assume a purplish pink color. *Check with microscope.*
9. Dehydrate in 2 changes of absolute alcohol.
10. Clear, 2 changes of xylene; coverslip, using a synthetic mounting medium.

Results

Nuclei—blue to violet
Rickettsias—intense reddish purple
Cytoplasm—varying lighter blue shades
Collagen and muscle—pale pink
Erythrocytes—gray to yellow or pink

May-Grünwald Giemsa stain[5]

Fixation. Zenker's or other well-fixed tissue.
Embedding. Cut paraffin sections at 5 μm.

Solutions

Jenner stock solution
Jenner stain (dry powder)	1 gm
Absolute methanol	400 ml

Jenner working solution (prepare fresh before use)
Use equal parts of Jenner stock and distilled water.

Giemsa stock solution
Giemsa powder	1 gm
Glycerol	66 ml

Mix these two materials and place in a 60° C oven for 2 hours. After the incubation, add 66 ml of absolute methanol. Mix well.

Giemsa working solution (prepare fresh before use)
Stock Giemsa solution	2.5 ml
Distilled water	50 ml

1% aqueous acetic acid

Technic

1. Hydrate slides.
2. Rinse in 2 changes of methanol, 3 minutes each change.
3. Stain in working Jenner solution for 6 minutes.
4. Stain in working Giemsa solution for 45 minutes. Do not rinse between steps 3 and 4.
5. Quickly rinse in distilled water.
6. Differentiate in 1% acetic acid until nuclei are well differentiated.
7. Quickly rinse in distilled water.
8. Dehydrate, clear, and coverslip, using a synthetic mounting medium.

Results

See previous technic.

Plate 2. A, Von Kossa technic for calcium (black). **B,** Gomori's methenamine silver technic for urate crystal demonstration (urate crystals, black). **C,** Potassium permanganate bleaching reaction of melanin. **D,** Gomori's methenamine silver argentaffin reaction for melanin (black). **E,** Schmorl's ferric ferricyanide reduction test for melanin (blue). **F,** Alizarin red S technic for calcium (red). **G,** Müller-Mowry colloidal iron technic (acidic mucin, blue). **H,** Puchtler's modification of Bennhold's Congo red for amyloid (pink to red). **I,** Mayer's mucicarmine technic (mucin, red). **J,** Rapid mucin stain (rose to red). **K,** Periodic acid–Schiff technic for glycogen (red). **L,** Periodic acid–Schiff technic for glycogen (glycogen removed by diastase digestion). **M,** Sheehan's modification of the Giemsa technic. Bone marrow after formic acid decalcification. **N,** Highman's crystal violet technic for amyloid (red-purple). **O,** Oil red O in propylene glycol for fat (red). **P,** Chiffelle-Putt Sudan black B in propylene glycol for fat (black). **Q,** Klüver's Luxol fast blue for myelin sheath (myelin sheath, blue; nerve cells, lavender). **R,** Weil's method for myelin sheath (blue). **S,** Cresyl violet stain for nerve cells (nucleus and Nissl bodies, blue). **T,** Bodian technic (anterior horn cells in the spinal cord). **U,** Chrome artifact (red-brown) resists all solvents. Results from incomplete washing of tissue in running water (12 to 16 hours) after fixation in a potassium dichromate fixative prior to alcohol dehydration. **V,** Precipitated silver (black) in a reticulum technic is usually the result of dirty glassware. Clean all glassware chemically for silver technics. **W,** Mercury artifact (granular black precipitate) is always present in tissue after fixation in a fixative containing mercuric chloride. It must be removed by the iodine–sodium thiosulfate sequence prior to staining slides. **X,** Red staining artifacts, sometimes seen in Masson trichrome or Heidenhain's azan technic. May be alleviated by rinsing the slides in 1% aqueous acetic acid after the Biebrich scarlet–acid fuchsin in the Masson trichrome or the azocarmine B solution in Heidenhain's azan technic.

REFERENCES

1. Lillie, R. D., and Fullmer, H. M.: Histopathological technic and practical histochemistry, ed. 4, New York, 1976, McGraw-Hill Book Co.
2. Galigher, A. E., and Kozloff, E. N.: Essentials of practical microtechnique, ed. 2, Philadelphia, 1971, Lea & Febiger.
3. Mallory, F. B.: Pathological technique, New York, 1961, Hafner Publishing Co.
4. Culling, C. F. A.: Handbook of histopathological and histochemical techniques, ed. 3, London, 1974, Butterworth & Co. (Pubs.), Ltd.
5. Luna, L. G., editor: Manual of histologic staining methods of the Armed Forces Institute of Pathology, ed. 3, New York, 1968, McGraw-Hill Book Co.
6. Hrapchak, B. B.: Selective staining with hematoxylin, applications and theory: a review, Am. J. Med. Technol. **42:**371-379, 1976.
7. Marshall, P. N., and Horobin, R. W.: The mechanism of the action of "mordant" dyes—a study using preformed metal complexes, Histochemie **35:**361-371, 1973.
8. Baker, J. R.: Experiments on the actions of mordants, I. Single-bath mordant dyeing, Q. J. Micro. Sci. **101:**255-272, 1960.
9. Baker, J. R.: Experiments on the action of mordants, II. Aluminum-haematein, Q. J. Micro. Sci. **103:**493-517, 1962.
10. Scott, J. E.: Binding of cationic dyes to nucleic acids and other biological polyanions, Nature **209:** 985-987, 1966.
11. Marshall, P. N., and Horobin, R. W.: Measurements of the affinities of basic and "mordant" dyes for various tissue substrates, Histochemie **36:**302-312, 1973.
12. Elias, J. M.: Chemistry of H & E staining, Am. J. Med. Technol. **40:**513-514, 1974.
13. Gill, G. W., Frost, J. K., and Miller, K. A.: A new formula for a half-oxidized hematoxylin that neither overstains nor requires differentiation, Acta Cytol. **18**(4):300-311, 1974, International Academy of Cytology, The Williams & Wilkins Co.
14. Thompson, S. W., and Luna, L. G.: An atlas of artifacts, Springfield, Ill., 1978, Charles C Thomas, Publisher.
15. Papanicolaou, G. N.: Atlas of exfoliative cytology, Cambridge, Mass., 1954, Harvard University Press; AFIP modification, from Luna, L. G., editor: Manual of histologic staining methods of the Armed Forces Institute of Pathology, ed. 3, New York, 1968, McGraw-Hill Book Co.
16. Lillie, R. D., Pizzolato, P., Welsh, R. A., Holmquist, N. D., Donaldson, P. T., and Berger, C.: A consideration of substitutes for alum hematoxylin in routine histologic and cytologic diagnostic procedures, Am. J. Clin. Pathol. **60:**817-819, 1973.
17. Catalano, R. A., and Lillie, R. D.: Iron alum celestine blue B substitution for hematoxylin in fat stain, Stain Technol. **48:**354, 1973, The Williams & Wilkins Co.
18. Lillie, R. D., Pizzolato, P., and Donaldson, P. T.: Iron gallein in Van Gieson technics replacing iron hematoxylin, Stain Technol. **48:**348-349, 1973, The Williams & Wilkins Co.
19. Terry, P. T.: The rapid preparation of polychrome methylene blue stains for frozen sections of fresh and fixed tissue, J. Lab. Clin. Med. **8**(3): 159-164, 1922.
20. Elias, J.: Effects of temperature, poststaining rinses and ethanol-butanol dehydrating mixtures on methyl green–pyronin staining, Stain Technol. **44:**201-204, 1969, The Williams & Wilkins Co.
21. Personal communication, Helen N. Futch, M. D. Anderson Hospital and Tumor Institute, Houston, Texas.
22. Baker, J. R.: Principles of biological microtechnique, New York, 1958, Barnes & Noble, Inc.
23. Davenport, H. A.: Histological and histochemical technics, Philadelphia, 1964, W. B. Saunders Co.
24. Personal communication, Dr. R. D. Hamstra, University of Colorado Medical Center, Denver, Colorado.
25. Modification used at Laboratory of Surgical Pathology at Hospital of the University of Pennsylvania, Philadelphia, Pennsylvania.
26. Strumia, M. M.: A rapid universal blood stain, J. Lab. Clin. Med. **21:**930-934, 1935-1936.
27. Lillie, R. D., Pizzolato, P., and Donaldson, P. T.: The Clara hematoxylin reaction, Acta Histochem. **49S:**204-219, 1974.

CHAPTER 9

Carbohydrates

Carbohydrates, widely distributed in both plants and animals, are defined chemically as aldehydes or ketone derivatives of the higher polyhydric (containing more than one OH group) alcohols, or as compounds that yield these compounds on hydrolysis. Often termed "starches" or "sugars" they may be further divided biochemically as monosaccharides, which cannot be hydrolyzed into a simpler form; disaccharides, which give two molecules of either the same or different monosaccharides when hydrolyzed; and polysaccharides, which yield more than two molecules of monosaccharides on hydrolysis. On the basis of chemical structure, polysaccharides (glycans) may be further subdivided—those yielding only one product on hydrolysis as "homoglycans" and those yielding a mixture of products as "heteroglycans."

CLASSIFICATION OF CARBOHYDRATES IN TISSUE

Classification of carbohydrates is a complex subject because terminology varies, frequently there are several terms for the same substance, and not all terms used are considered to be totally accurate. In addition, the results of histochemical methods cannot in all cases be compared to those from biochemical assay technics. This is primarily because carbohydrates occur in the body as a mixture of carbohydrate with protein, carbohydrate with lipid, or carbohydrate with lipid and protein. Carbohydrates that have been identified in tissues are described in Table 9-1. This classification is essentially that of Spicer.[25]

Table 9-1. Carbohydrate classification

Substance and chemical characterization	Location	Staining reactions
A. *Polysaccharides (homoglycans)*, glycogen (starch and cellulose are examples in plants) Glycogen—branched polymer of D-glucose units bound in 1,4 linkages except at branching points where the linkage is 1,6	Hepatocytes, parathyroid cells, skeletal and cardiac muscle	PAS-positive, diastase-sensitive, Best's carmine–positive, Bauer-Fuelgen–positive
B. *Neutral mucosubstances* Contain sugars but no free acidic groups or sulfate esters; includes neutral glycoproteins, immunoglobulins, fucomucins, mannose-rich mucosubstances in epithelial and connective tissue	Gastric surface epithelia and thyroid colloid of humans, guinea pigs, and rabbit; coagulating gland fluid in mouse and rat	PAS-positive, diastase-resistant, negative for other mucosubstance stains
C. *Acid mucosubstances (anionic heteroglycans)* 1. Sulfated mucosubstances a. Connective tissue mucopolysaccharides (strongly sulfated)		Weak or negative reaction with alcian blue (AlBl) at pH 2.5; moderate reaction at pH 0.5; metachromatic with azure A and toluidine blue at pH 2.0; negative at pH 3.0 and above; PAS-negative
(1) Resistant to testicular hyaluronidase (a) Keratosulfate (keratan sulfate), heparin	Cornea, mast cells, cartilage, arterial walls	
(b) Dermatan sulfate (chondroitin sulfate B)	Skin, aorta, heart valves (biochemically)	Digestion procedures and critical electrolyte concentration (CEC) provide additional information
(c) ? Heparitin sulfate (heparan sulfate)	Aorta, cerebral and coronary arteries and skin*	
(2) Sensitive to testicular hyaluronidase (a) Chondroitin sulfates in cartilage (chondroitin-4-sulfate [chondroitin sulfate A] and chondroitin-6-sulfate [chondroitin sulfate C])	Cartilage, ovarian follicular fluid	
(b) Chondroitin sulfates in vascular tissues	Aorta, heart valves, renal papilla, some areas of cartilage	
b. Epithelial sulfomucins or epithelial mucosubstances (weakly sulfated; resistant to testicular hyaluronidase) (1) Negative to oxidation with periodic acid		PAS reaction variable; positive AlBl staining at pH 2.5; weak at pH 0.5; strongly metachromatic with azure A and toluidine blue at pH 2.0; weak at pH 3 and above
(a) Sulfate esters on vicinal-glycols (vic-glycols)	Sublingual glands of Chinese hamsters; glossal mucous glands and colonic goblet cells of rabbit	
(b) Sulfate esters not on vic-glycols	Guinea pig colon; exorbital lacrimal gland of mouse	
(2) Positive to oxidation with periodic acid (a) Metachromatic with 0.02% azure A at or above pH 2	Glossal mucous glands and rectosigmoid colonic goblet cells of mouse and rat	
(b) Weak or negative metachromasia with 0.02% azure A at or above pH 4.5	Some duodenal goblets and pyloric glands and some laryngotracheal glands in mouse and rat	

*Zugibe, F. T.: Diagnostic histochemistry, St. Louis, 1970, The C. V. Mosby Co.

Table 9-1. Carbohydrate classification—cont'd

Substance and chemical characterization	Location	Staining reactions
2. Nonsulfated mucosubstances		Positive staining with AlBl
a. Sialic acid–rich (sialoglycoproteins; these contain sialic acid; reactive groups are carboxyl groups and vic-glycols)		at pH 2.5; negative at pH 0.5; metachromatic
(1) Connective tissue mucosubstances, Connective tissue sialomucins	Cartilage (?)	with azure A and toluidine blue at pH 3 and above; negative at pH 2
(2) Epithelial mucosubstances (epithelial sialomucins, acid glycoproteins)		and below; variable PAS reaction depending on subtype
(a) Very susceptible to *Vibrio cholerae* sialidase; PAS-positive; metachromatic with azure A	Sublingual glands of mouse, Syrian hamster, and guinea pig	
(b) Slowly digested by *V. cholerae* sialidase		
[1] PAS-positive	Vaginal epithelium of pregnant mouse	
[2] PAS-negative	Rectosigmoid mucous cells of mouse	
(c) Not digested by *V. cholerae* sialidase		
[1] Rendered metachromatic and susceptible to enzyme by prior saponification	Sublingual gland of rat	
[2] Resistant to sialidase even after saponification		
[a] PAS-positive	Human and monkey sublingual glands	
[b] PAS-negative	Mammary gland secretion of lactating mouse	
b. Hexuronic acid–rich (contain hyaluronic acid and reactive groups are carboxyl groups)		As above except PAS-negative
(1) Hyaluronic acid, chondroitin	Uterine cervical stroma of estrogen-treated mouse; cock's comb; ganglion cysts of synovial membranes and vitreous humor in man	
D. *Mucoproteins* Composed of polysaccharide and protein; carbohydrate content is greater than 4%	Basement membranes, mucoid cells of pituitary	PAS-positive
E. *Glycoproteins* Composed of polysaccharide and protein; carbohydrate component is less than 4%	Collagen, reticular fibers, serum albumin	PAS-positive
F. *Mucolipids (glycolipids)* Carbohydrate and lipid compounds containing fatty acid, sphingosine, and hexose	Cerebrosides, gangliosides	PAS-positive; lipid methods positive on frozen sections

Table 9-2. Carbohydrate demonstration methods

Method	Demonstrates
Periodic acid–Schiff (PAS)	Simple polysaccharides, neutral mucosubstances, some acid mucosubstances, basement membranes, certain pigments, mucolipids, certain amyloid deposits, fungus, mucoid cells of pituitary
Periodic acid–phenylhydrazine–Schiff (PAPS)	Distinguish neutral polysaccharides and glycoproteins from sialic acid–containing mucosubstances
Periodic acid–borohydride–KOH–PAS method	Differentiate lower gastrointestinal tract mucins from other mucins in primary or metastatic tumors
Periodic acid–methenamine silver (PAM)	Basement membranes, fungi, mucin, glycogen
Best's carmine	Glycogen
Bauer-Feulgen	Glycogen, fungus
Metachromatic staining methods (such as toluidine blue)	Acid mucosubstances, mucins
Metachromatic methods with controlled pH levels	Strongly acidic from weakly acidic mucosubstances
Alcian blue-Kernechtrot	Acid mucosubstances
Alcian blue with controlled pH levels	Carboxylated from sulfated mucosubstances
Alcian blue–PAS	Neutral and acid mucosubstances and mixtures of neutral and acid mucosubstances
Alcian blue–aldehyde fuchsin	Acid mucosubstances, sulfated mucosubstances, and mixtures of both types
Aldehyde fuchsin	Sulfated mucosubstances
Colloidal iron	Acid mucosubstances
High iron diamine	Sulfate esters
Low iron diamine	Sulfated and nonsulfated mucins
Mixed diamine	Periodic unreactive acid mucosubstances from periodic-reactive neutral and acidic mucosubstances
Critical electrolyte concentration methods (CEC)	Carboxylated acid mucosubstances from sulfated mucosubstances
Mucicarmine	Epithelial mucins

DEMONSTRATION METHODS

Some commonly used demonstration methods and their purpose are listed in Table 9-2.

DIAGNOSTIC APPLICATIONS OF CARBOHYDRATE DEMONSTRATION TECHNICS
Periodic acid–Schiff (PAS) reaction

Some of the many uses of the PAS reaction include the following:
1. Demonstration of PAS-positive reticulum fibers and basement membranes
2. Indication of presence of PAS-positive glycolipids (cerebrosides and gangliosides) in certain disease states
3. Distinguishing a secreting adenocarcinoma (PAS-positive) from undifferentiated squamous cell carcinoma (PAS-negative)
4. Demonstration of fungus in tissue secretions
5. Demonstration of certain types of PAS-positive mucosubstances secreted by epithelia of various organs, such as those in the digestive tract, lungs, and cervix.

Glycogen demonstrations

Glycogen is normally present in varying amounts in many cells, notably skin, liver, parathyroid glands, and skeletal and cardiac muscle. Amounts of glycogen are increased in certain congenital pathologic conditions, such as in von Gierke's disease, a defect of glycogen mobilization affecting the liver and kidneys primarily, and Pompe's disease, affecting the heart. Glycogen may also be increased in areas of inflammatory reaction around necrotic tissues. Cytoplasmic liver glycogen is decreased in wasting diseases and diabetes mellitus. However, liver cell nuclei in diabetes mellitus show an increased glycogen content. Nodules of myocardial fibers distended with glycogen are observed in cases of rhabdomyosarcoma. The benign clear cell tumor of the lung ("sugar" tumor) contains large amounts of cytoplasmic glycogen.

Technics for glycogen demonstration include the PAS reaction with diastase digestion, Best's carmine, and Bauer-Feulgen. The first of these methods is considered to have histochemical specificity. The dimedone-PAS method is useful for demonstrating glycogen in areas where its visualization is difficult because of the proximity of diastase-resistant PAS-positive substances.

Mucin stains

"Mucin" is a term given to a secretion produced by a variety of epithelial and connective tissue cells. Excess mucin is secreted by epithelial cells in certain inflammations. Amounts secreted are also increased in certain intestinal carcinomas. A mucinous material formed by connective tissue cells may be found in subcutaneous tissue in cases of thyroid deficiency (myxedema) and in myxomas.

Mucins are not single compounds but are composed of a number of chemical substances. Although mucins differ chemically depending on the cells from which they are derived, they nonetheless have similar reactions to certain staining technics. Mucins are usually PAS-positive, metachromatic, and basophilic. Certain mucins with acid groups also stain with alcian blue and colloidal iron methods. If derived from epithelial sources, they will frequently color when treated with a mucicarmine solution.

The mucicarmine technic may be useful in the determination of the site of a primary tumor. For example, finding mucin-positive tumor cells in an area of the body that normally lacks mucin-positive cells would indicate that the tumor cells did not arise from that area. The location of the primary lesion would be in an area that normally secretes mucin. The technic is also useful in distinguishing undifferentiated mucin-negative squamous cell carcinoma from mucin-positive adenocarcinoma.

Acid mucosubstances

The mucopolysaccharidoses are a group of genetic disorders of acid mucosubstance metabolism, but the exact nature of the basic mucosubstance defect is not yet fully understood. Six subtypes have been classified according to clinical, genetic, and biochemical criteria. The mucosubstances in the six subtypes are found principally in phagocytic cells of the spleen, liver, lymph nodes, and marrow; in hepatocytes; in endocrine epithelial cells; in neurons; and in "gargoyle cells" of connective tissue.

Excessive amounts of hexuronic acid–rich, nonsulfated acidic mucosubstances are seen in mesotheliomas. Amounts of various kinds of acid mucosubstances are increased in the collagen diseases.

Certain acid mucosubstances (hyaluronic acid, chondroitin sulfates A and C, dermatan sulfate, and heparan sulfate) occur normally in blood vessel walls. Their amounts are increased in early lesions of spontaneous and experimentally induced atherosclerosis.

With advancing age, the amounts of acid mucosubstances present tends to decline. Histochemically, the mucosubstances may be demonstrated with metachromatic stains or by the alcian blue methods. The use of various hyaluronidases can also assist in identification.

FIXATIVES FOR CARBOHYDRATE DEMONSTRATION

The advantages and disadvantages of various fixative solutions for carbohydrate preservation has been a subject of investigation by numerous authors. Since many carbohydrates are themselves water soluble, it was once believed that only nonaqueous fixatives should be employed for carbohydrate preservation. In tissue, however, most carbohydrates are covalently bonded to protein. Either aqueous or alcoholic solutions can function to preserve the protein and thereby preserve the carbohydrate bound to the protein. Even non–protein bound glycogen can be preserved if the tissue proteins surrounding it are satisfactorily fixed.

Glycogen fixatives. Lillie[3] considers alcoholic formalin or acetic alcoholic formalin the best preservatives for glycogen. Formalin and glutaraldehyde solutions may also be used. However, because of the presence of free aldehyde groups in glutaraldehyde-fixed material, nonspecific PAS-positive staining will occur. These free aldehydes must first be neutralized after fixation in a dialdehyde solution,[4] as follows:

1. Deparaffinize and bring sections to 95% ethanol.
2. Treat slides with aniline oil solution for 1 hour. Prepare this solution by mixing 88 ml of aniline oils with 12 ml of glacial acetic acid. Discard after use.
3. Rinse slides quickly in 2 changes of 95% alcohol.
4. Wash slides in running tap water for 10 minutes.
5. Rinse slides in distilled water and proceed with the PAS technic.

Murgatroyd[5] evaluated glycogen preservation after various routine histologic fixatives and concluded that formol-alcohol and Rossman's fluids used at 4° C preserved the most glycogen. Neutral 10% formalin gave good preservation at 4° C but not at 18° C. Mercuric chloride–

containing fixatives (Susa's, Zenker's, Helly's) produce an uneven glycogen staining pattern with noticeable streaming regardless of the temperature at which the fixative was allowed to act. Cold formol alcohol was the only fixative that preserved threshold values of glycogen and the silver methenamine method (p. 187) is recommended for the demonstration of these small amounts since the silver grains are deposited around the individual glycogen granules and render them more visible.

Other carbohydrates. Lillie recommends fixatives containing acid or alcohol, or both, for mucin preservation. Solutions that have been employed include neutral buffered formalin, alcoholic formalin mixtures, Carnoy's, Newcomer's, and formol-calcium. Cetylpyridinium chloride in 10% formalin and cetyltrimethylammonium bromide–formalin have been employed as fixatives for acid mucosubstances, but their overall value for fixation of these substances has been questioned. Acid mucosubstances fixed in glutaraldehyde show a lessened staining intensity with alcian blue and colloidal iron methods.[4]

STAINING REACTIONS FOR CARBOHYDRATES
Iodine[3]

The oldest staining reactions for polysaccharides involve color formations on exposure to iodine solutions. Plant starch and its partial decomposition products, amylose and amylopectin, give a blue color; glycogen and amyloid give a red-brown reaction.

Method
Tissues should be fixed in acetic alcohol formalin, alcohol formalin, or Carnoy's fluid. Tissues are routinely processed and embedded in paraffin. Hydrate sections, and expose to Gram's iodine for 5 to 10 minutes. Dehydrate sections with 2 changes of 2% iodine in absolute alcohol; clear and mount in oil of origanum.

Periodic acid–Schiff reaction[6]
Staining mechanisms and technical comments

Principle. Tissue sections are first oxidized by periodic acid (Fig. 9-1). The oxidative process results in the formation of aldehyde groupings through carbon-to-carbon bond cleavage (Fig. 9-2). Free hydroxyl groups should be present for oxidation to take place, and if these groups are involved in ester or glycosidic linkages, the reaction will not take place. Periodic acid will not oxidize newly formed aldehyde groups to further

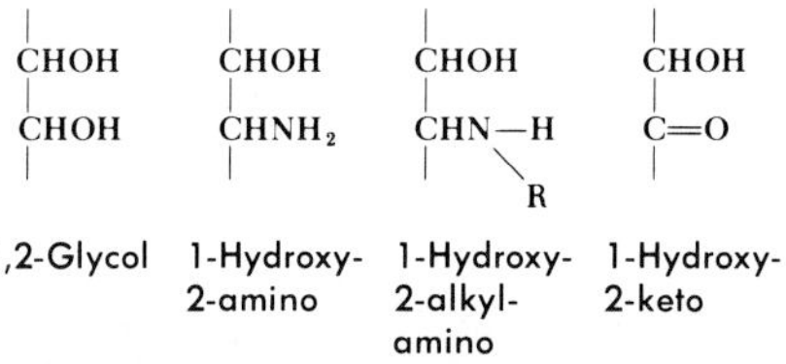

Fig. 9-1. Chemical groupings oxidized by periodic acid.

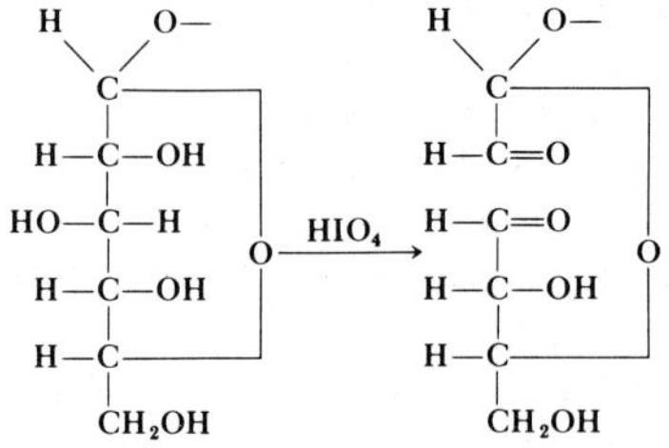

Fig. 9-2. Aldehyde end product resulting from the oxidative action of the periodic acid.

breakdown products (which would decrease staining intensity); oxidation is completed when it reaches the aldehyde stage.

The presence of the newly formed aldehyde groups is detected by the Schiff reagent (or leucofuchsin). The first-stage reaction involves the formation of a colorless, unstable dialdehyde addition compound that is then transformed to the colored final product by restoration of the quinoid chromophoric grouping (Fig. 9-3).

Sulfurous rinses usually follow the Schiff reagent treatment and serve to remove excess reagent and prevent false pigmentation of the tissue section because of air oxidation of the adsorbed Schiff reagent. This false pigmentation would usually occur after the section has been coverslipped. After the sulfurous rinses, the sections are washed in running tap water to intensify the color and then are suitably counterstained.

Depending on the specific technic, there will be some variability in the concentration of periodic acid (HIO_4 or H_5IO_6) required. In addition, different procedures will state varying treatment times with both periodic acid and Schiff reagent. Generally, an oxidation time of 5 minutes using 0.5% aqueous periodic acid is sufficient. Depending on the strength of the Schiff reagent and the temperature at which it is used, the exposure time to this solution will range from 10 to 30 minutes. Thinner sections (1 to 3 μm) require longer times in both the oxidizing agent

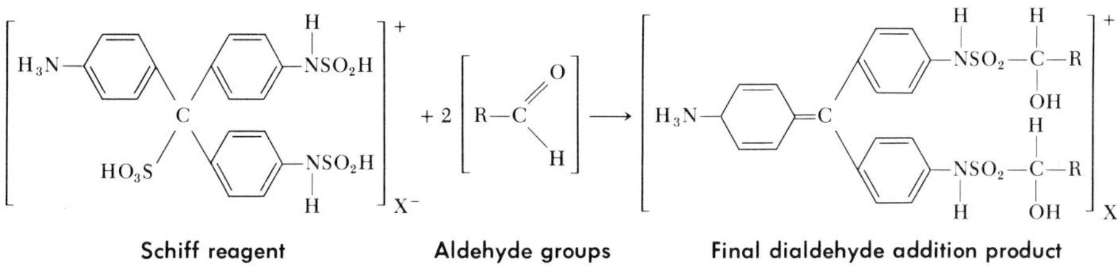

Fig. 9-3. Reaction of aldehydes with Schiff reagent results in formation of a colored end product.

and the Schiff reagent. The periodic acid should be *freshly* prepared in such cases; the Schiff reagent should be changed weekly.

Some technics refer to a Schiff reagent and others to a leucofuchsin reagent. Studies with leucofuchsin have shown that two different types of leuco compounds may be formed with a reduction reaction. Leucofuchsin is formed through a simple reduction process; Schiff reagent is prepared through a reduction with sulfurous acid or a sulfite. It was originally believed that Schiff reagent was the same as leucofuchsin, but the color formed on subsequent reoxidation because of the aldehyde groups was a distinct purple-red, not a simple red as it would be on a simple reoxidation basis. This would indicate a chemical change taking place in the dye, in addition to its simple reduction to a leuco compound. Schiff reagent is formed in two steps in the presence of excess SO_2. The first step introduces a sulfite ester at the central carbon atom of the pararosanilin (basic fuchsin) molecule. The result is pararosanilin–leucosulfonic acid and is colorless because of the reduction of the quinoid grouping of the basic fuchsin molecule. In the second step, amino groupings add sulfur dioxide to form the sulfinic acid derivative of pararosanilin–leucosulfonic acid, which is the actual Schiff reagent.

The intensity of PAS staining will vary with different structures depending on the fixative employed, and the reason for this is not known. Aldehyde groups derived from different compounds will produce different color shades on combination with the Schiff reagent, and this may indicate that different structural complexes are being formed as addition products with the Schiff reagent.

Lillie's "cold Schiff" solutions[3]

1. Weigh 1 gm of basic fuchsin and 1.9 gm of sodium metabisulfite ($Na_2S_2O_5$). Dissolve these in 100 ml of 0.15 N hydrochloric acid. (For 2 gm of basic fuchsin, Lillie recommends the use of 0.25 N hydrochloric acid and 3.4 gm of sodium metabisulfite.)
2. Shake the above at intervals until the solution is clear and a yellow to tan color (mechanical shaker for 2 hours). If the solution is not the proper color, allow it to stand overnight in a dark place.
3. Add approximately 500 mg/dl of *fresh activated* charcoal and shake well for 1 to 2 minutes. It is important that the charcoal be activated.
4. Using a double layer of Whatman no. 1 filter paper, filter the solution into a bottle. The filtrate itself should be clear as water.
5. Restore to original volume with some distilled water and store in refrigerator.

Schiff reagent of Barger and DeLamater[7]

1. Dissolve 1 gm of basic fuchsin in 400 ml of distilled water, using heat if necessary.
2. Add 1 ml of thionyl chloride ($SOCl_2$), stopper the flask, shake well, and allow to stand for 12 hours in the dark at room temperature.
3. Add 2 gm of *activated* charcoal to the solution. Shake well and filter. Store in a well-stoppered brown bottle at 4° C. Solution should remain stable for several months.

Tests for Schiff reagent

Chemical (AFIP).[8] Pour 10 ml of 37% to 40% formalin into a watch glass. To this add a few drops of the Schiff reagent to be tested. A good Schiff reagent will rapidly turn a red-purple color. A deteriorating Schiff reagent will give a delayed reaction and the color produced will be a deep blue-purple.

Histologic (Lillie).[3] Stain a cross section of human appendix. If the Schiff reagent is good, a fine red meshwork of sarcolemma between individual smooth muscle cells should be visible.

• • •

Prolonging the time of exposure to Schiff reagent can compensate for a weaker solution;

however new Schiff reagent should be prepared.

Schiff reagent, once prepared, should be stored at 4° C and discarded when it develops a pink tinge. Shelf life of Schiff reagent varies, depending on use. Luna[9] states 3 months.

McManus' periodic acid–Schiff reaction[6]

Fixation. See p. 163.

Embedding. Cut paraffin sections at 5 μm.

Solutions

0.5% aqueous periodic acid
Schiff reagent (p. 165)
1 N hydrochloric acid

Distilled water	916.5 ml
Concentrated hydrochloric acid (specific gravity 1.19)	83.5 ml

Always add the concentrated acid to the water!
10% aqueous sodium metabisulfite
Sulfurous rinse (prepare fresh when needed)

Distilled water	300 ml
1 N hydrochloric acid	15 ml
10% sodium metabisulfite	18 ml

Harris's hematoxylin counterstain (p. 142)

Method

1. Hydrate slides.
2. Immerse in periodic acid for 5 minutes. Discard solution.
3. Rinse in several changes of distilled water.
4. Immerse in Schiff reagent for 15 minutes. Filter back.
5. Rinse slides in sulfurous rinse, 3 changes of 2 minutes each change. Discard each change.
6. Wash in running tap water for 10 minutes.
7. Counterstain in Harris's hematoxylin for 1 minute. Filter back.
8. Wash in running tap water for 10 minutes.
9. Dehydrate and coverslip using a synthetic mounting medium.

Additional counterstains for PAS reaction

Other alum hematoxylin solutions may be substituted for Harris's formula. A working solution of light green may be used instead of hematoxylin.

A counterstain of Weigert's hematoxylin followed by a picro-indigo-carmine solution may be employed after step 6 of the PAS reaction as follows:

1. Use working Weigert's iron hematoxylin (p. 190), 3 minutes.
2. Wash in tap water for 10 minutes.
3. 15 dips in 1% aqueous hydrochloric acid.
4. Rinse in tap water.
5. 15 dips in 5% aqueous sodium bicarbonate.
6. Rinse in tap water; rinse in distilled water.
7. 10 dips in picro-indigo-carmine solution:

Saturated aqueous picric acid	100 ml
Indigo carmine	0.25 gm

8. Dehydrate rapidly, clear, and coverslip using a synthetic mounting medium.

Results

PAS reactions (see PAS results, below)
Collagen—blue
Muscle and cell cytoplasm—yellow

PAS results (Plate 2, *K*). Reaction intensities will vary; however, the following substances will show a PAS-positive reaction: glycogen, neutral mucosubstances, certain epithelial sulfomucins, certain epithelial sialomucins, certain hyalin substances, colloid material of thyroid and pars intermedia of pituitary, beta cell granules of pancreatic islets and adenohypophysis, basement membranes, reticular fibers, collagen fibers, juxtaglomerular granules, fungal cell walls.

Glycolipids, phospholipids, and some pigments of a lipid nature, such as ceroid, are PAS-positive. Unsaturated lipids also may stain with the reaction, though the mechanism is believed to be that of an oxidation of double bonds through the addition of hydroxyl groupings. These are, in turn, oxidized to the aldehyde groups that are demonstrated with the Schiff reagent.

The pale background reaction seen in the PAS reaction is believed to be caused by the presence of proteins. However, it may be small amounts of carbohydrates instead.

Glycogen demonstration methods

Stains for glycogen include the iodine reaction (p. 164), PAS with diastase digestion, Best's carmine, and the Bauer-Feulgen methods. The PAS with diastase or α-amylase digestion has histochemical specificity. Histochemical demonstration of glycogen may also be achieved with a dimedone blockade after periodic acid oxidation. The periodic acid–methenamine silver method (p. 187) may also be used; however, other substances will react besides glycogen.

Bauer-Feulgen reaction[10]

Principle. Chromic acid is the oxidizing agent used in this technic and functions similarly to the periodic acid already discussed. Chromic acid does have the tendency to further oxidize the newly formed aldehyde groups to carboxylic acids and other breakdown products, which will then not combine with the Schiff reagent.

Weaker reactions, such as those of collagen and reticulin, are suppressed because of this further oxidizing process, leaving only glycogen and certain strongly PAS positive mucins to be demonstrated. The reaction of the aldehyde groups with the Schiff reagent and the purpose of the sulfurous rinses are discussed in the PAS section.

Fixation. See p. 163.

Embedding. Cut paraffin sections at 5 μm.

Solutions

    4% of aqueous chromium trioxide (chromic acid)
    Schiff reagent (p. 165)
    0.05 M aqueous sodium bisulfite
    Harris's hematoxylin (p. 142)

Method

1. Hydrate slides to distilled water.
2. Chromic acid solution for 1 hour. Discard after use.
3. Running tap water for 5 minutes.
4. Schiff reagent for 15 minutes. Filter back.
5. Rinse in 0.05 sodium bisulfite for 3 changes, 90 seconds each change. Discard after use.
6. Wash in running tap water for 10 minutes. Positive reactions are pink at this stage.
7. Counterstain lightly for 10 to 15 seconds in Harris's hematoxylin. Filter back.
8. Wash in running tap water for 10 minutes.
9. Dehydrate, clear, and coverslip using a synthetic mounting medium.

Results

Glycogen, fungus, and certain mucins—red-purple

Nuclei—blue

Best's carmine technic[11]

Principle. Best's carmine is an empirical stain that will produce a brilliant red staining of glycogen under certain conditions. This technic appears to demonstrate less glycogen than does the PAS method, and where glycogen is being studied histochemically, the PAS reaction, with diastase digestion, should be done. Hydrogen bonding is believed to play a role in the staining of glycogen using Best's carmine solution.[12] The pH of the staining solution ranges between 9 and 11, and at this pH the phenolic groups of the dye ionize to the anion $-O^-$, which, in turn, can bind to the glycol groups of the glycogen by hydrogen bonding.

Fixation. Tissue must be fixed in absolute alcohol or Carnoy's fluid.

Embedding. Cut paraffin sections at 5 μm.

Solutions

    Carmine stock solution
        Carmine   2 gm

Potassium carbonate	1 gm
Potassium chloride	5 gm
Distilled water	60 ml

Boil gently and cautiously for several minutes. When it is cool, add 20 ml of 28% ammonium hydroxide. Store in refrigerator.

    Working solution of carmine

Stock carmine solution	10 ml
28% ammonium hydroxide	15 ml
Methanol	15 ml

    Differentiating solution

Absolute alcohol	20 ml
Methanol	10 ml
Distilled water	25 ml

    Harris's hematoxylin (p. 142)

Method

1. Hydrate sections.
2. Stain nuclei with Harris's hematoxylin for 5 minutes. Filter back.
3. Wash in running tap water for 15 minutes.
4. Stain in working carmine solution for 30 minutes. Discard after use.
5. Differentiate in differentiating solution for a few seconds. Do *not* rinse in distilled water between steps 4 and 5.
6. Rinse quickly in 80% ethanol.
7. Dehydrate and clear as usual. Coverslip, using a synthetic mounting medium.

Results

Glycogen—pink to red

Nuclei—blue

Diastase and amylase digestions

Diastase and α-amylase act on glycogen to depolymerize it, and the resultant breakdown products of smaller sugar units are washed away in the water wash after diastase treatment. Parallel sections are hydrated to water. One slide (the "extracted" section) is treated with a solution of diastase in buffer. The parallel slide (the "unextracted" section) is treated with buffer only. Incubation times in the two solutions are the same. After incubation with either the diastase in the buffer solution or the buffer only, sections are washed in water and the PAS method is performed. (Alternatively, Best's carmine technic could be performed.)

Slides are examined with the light microscope. Areas of PAS-positive staining on the unextracted section that appear PAS-negative in the diastase-extracted section are assumed to be glycogen.

Fixation of tissue may influence the digestion process. Glycogen fixed in a picric acid–containing fixative, for example, may be slightly more resistant to the digestion process. Do not celloidinize sections prior to diastase treatment, since the celloidin film will inhibit the digestion reaction.

Solutions

Buffer solution

Freshly boiled distilled water	1	liter
Anhydrous disodium phosphate (dibasic)	0.28	gm
Sodium phosphate (monobasic)	1.97	gm
Sodium chloride	8	gm

Dissolve the solid ingredients in the distilled water. When it is cool, add a few drops of thymol as a preservative. Store in the refrigerator at 5° C.

Extraction solution

Malt diastase	0.1 gm
Buffer solution	100 ml

Alternatively the 0.1% malt diastase may be prepared with distilled water being used as the solvent. The extraction solution using α-amylase is 0.5% in distilled water. The pH of this solution should be adjusted to about 5.5 to 6.0 with the use of 4 mM acetates.[3]

Method

1. Preheat needed amounts of buffer solution and extraction solution in separate labeled staining dishes (or Coplin jars) for 1 hour at 37° C.
2. Appropriately label the parallel test slides as to their future treatment with either the extraction solution or the buffer only. Hydrate these slides. Known positive controls should also be appropriately labeled and included in the digestion and staining processes.
3. Incubate the slides in their respective preheated solutions for 1 hour at 37° C.
4. When incubation is completed, discard the solutions, wash the slides for 5 to 10 minutes in running tap water, rinse in 2 changes of distilled water, and proceed with the PAS technic.

Note: Human saliva has been used as a glycogen digestant by some workers.

Dimedone blockade[13]

The dimedone (5,5-dimethylcyclohexane-1,3-dione) method is considered useful for demonstration of glycogen in areas that also contain large amounts of nonglycogen PAS-positive materials. In such cases, judging the amount of glycogen that could be extracted by diastase treatment is more difficult. Dimedone blocks the PAS reaction of many materials but, with the incubation times employed, the PAS-positive reaction of glycogen remains intact.

Time of exposure to the dimedone may vary depending on the nature of the other PAS-positive materials in the vicinity. Nonglycogen materials that resist dimedone actions are few and of limited distribution.

Method

1. Deparaffinize sections, rinse in several changes of absolute alcohol, and celloidinize (p. 131).
2. Oxidize for 10 minutes in 0.5% aqueous periodic acid. Discard after use.
3. Wash sections in several changes of distilled water.
4. Incubate in a 5% dimedone solution in absolute alcohol for 3 hours at 60° C.
5. Wash sections well in several changes of distilled water.
6. Treat with Schiff reagent (p. 165) for 10 minutes. Filter back.
7. Three changes of sulfurous rinses (p. 166) for 2 minutes each change. Discard solutions after use.
8. Wash in running tap water for 10 minutes.
9. Dehydrate, clear, and coverslip, using a synthetic mounting medium.

Mucin and acid mucosubstance demonstration methods

Mucin is defined on p. 163; the classification of the various kinds of acid mucosubstances is detailed in Table 9-1. Diagnostic applications and a list of the major staining methods are described on pp. 162 and 163.

Mucicarmine technics[11]

Principle. This stain is largely empirical, and the carmine, with the aluminum mordant, stains the mucin a deep rose to red. It is a valuable technic to demonstrate mucin derived from epithelial sources. Connective tissue mucin stains poorly. The aluminum is believed to form a chelation complex, binding the acid groups of the mucin and attaching the red color to the complex in a dye-lake formation. Iron hematoxylin is used to stain the nuclei, and the metanil yellow is the counterstain.

Fixation. Any well-fixed tissue will stain with this method.

Embedding. Cut paraffin sections at 5 μm.

Solutions

Working solutions of Weigert's iron hematoxylin (p. 190)

Mucicarmine solutions. Either Mayer's or Southgate's may be used.

Mayer's stock mucicarmine solution

Carmine (alum lake)	1 gm
Anhydrous aluminum chloride	0.5 gm
Distilled water	2 ml
50% ethanol	100 ml

Combine the dry reagents in a Pyrex beaker, and add the 2 ml of distilled water. Heat over a small flame for approximately 2 minutes. The liquid should turn dark purple and become syrupy. Agitate the solution with a glass rod during the heating process. Do not allow the solution to dry out or burn. When the end point has been reached, pour 100 ml of 50% ethanol into the beaker. Allow this solution to remain at room temperature for 24 hours. (If dye has adhered to the glass rod, allow it to remain immersed in the solution during the room temperature incubation time.) Filter and store at 4° C. Solution is stable for 4 to 6 months.

Southgate's stock mucicarmine solution

Carmine (alum lake)	1 gm
Aluminum hydroxide	1 gm
50% ethanol	100 ml

Add these reagents to a Pyrex flask. Shake well and to the mixture add 0.5 gm of anhydrous aluminum chloride. Place the flask in a boiling water bath, bring the solution to a boil rapidly, and allow it to boil for 2½ to 3 minutes. Agitate flask during the heating process. When complete, cool the solution (flask may be held under tap water for this). Make up to original volume with 50% ethanol, filter, and store at 4° C.

Working solutions. Traditionally, the working solutions are 1:4 dilutions of the stock and the diluent is tap water. Stronger or weaker dilutions may be needed, depending on the strength of the stock solution.

Metanil yellow solution (p. 247)

Method
1. Hydrate sections.
2. Stain in working solution of Weigert's hematoxylin for 10 minutes.
3. Wash in running tap water for 10 minutes.
4. Stain in diluted mucicarmine for 30 minutes or longer. This step may take several hours. Check control slide under microscope. *Note:* Staining time is decreased by incubation at either 37° C or 56° C.
5. When staining is complete, discard the mucicarmine solution and rinse slides in 2 or 3 changes of distilled water.
6. Stain with metanil yellow for 15 seconds to 1 minute.
7. Rinse quickly in distilled water.
8. Dehydrate, clear, and coverslip, using a synthetic mounting medium.

Results (Plate 2, *I*)
Mucin—deep rose to red
Capsule of *Cryptococcus*—deep rose to red
Nuclei—black
Other tissue elements—yellow
Note: The rose color attributable to carmine staining will be obscured if sections are overcounterstained with metanil yellow. Freshly prepared metanil yellow solutions stain rapidly, about 15 sec-

onds; longer times, up to 1 to 2 minutes, may be needed for an older solution. Metanil yellow is stable for about 2 months.[9]

Rapid mucin stain[32]

Fixation. Formalin-fixed tissue is preferred.

Solutions
Weigert's iron hematoxylin solution (p. 190)
1% acetic acid solution
Fast green stain (1:5000)

Fast green FCF	0.2 gm
Distilled water	1 liter

Basic fuchsin stain

Basic fuchsin	0.1 gm
Distilled water	100 ml
Glacial acetic acid	1 ml

Method
1. Hydrate slides.
2. Place in working Weigert's iron hematoxylin for 1 minute.
3. Wash in running tap water to develop blue color.
4. Place in 1:5000 aqueous fast green FCF for 3 minutes.
5. Wash in 1% acetic acid.
6. Stain 4 minutes in the basic fuchsin solution.
7. Dehydrate with 95% alcohol and 2 changes of absolute alcohol.
8. Clear through 3 changes of xylene, and coverslip, using a synthetic mounting medium.

Results
Nuclei—black
Cytoplasm—gray-green
Mucin, cartilage, mast cell granules—red

Metachromatic methods

Metachromatic dyes such as thionin and toluidine blue may be used to demonstrate certain mucins and acid mucosubstances. Because of the presence of large amounts of oriented ionized groupings, these two substances are among the most active naturally occurring materials that will stain metachromatically. The actual reaction involves a single dye selectively coloring a tissue structure or component a color different from that of the dilute dye solution, and with most metachromatic staining, the color shift is from blue hues to red-purple. The mechanism of metachromatic staining and precautions to be followed are discussed on p. 126.

TOLUIDINE BLUE STAIN FOR MUCIN (pH 4.5)[14]

Fixation. 10% neutral buffered formalin, alcoholic formalin mixtures, formol-calcium.

Embedding. Cut paraffin sections at 5 μm.

Solutions

Veronal acetate–HCl buffer, pH 4.5

Veronal acetate solution	5 ml
0.1 M hydrochloric acid	11 ml
Distilled water	9 ml

The Veronal acetate solution is prepared when 1.943 gm of sodium acetate and 2.943 gm of sodium barbiturate are added and diluted to a volume of 100 ml.

Staining solution

0.25 gm of toluidine blue (C.I. 52040) dissolved in 100 ml of the above buffer

Method

1. Hydrate sections.
2. Stain in buffered toluidine blue for 10 seconds.
3. Rinse in distilled water.
4. Blot sections with filter paper and allow to dry. When dry, dip slide in xylene and coverslip using a synthetic mounting medium.

Results

Mucins and certain acid mucosubstances (such as sialic acid–rich nonsulfated mucosubstances) are metachromatic and appear red to red purple. Background color is blue.

Note: Other basic dyes have been employed in similar metachromatic technics, notably azure A (C.I. 52005), azure C (C.I. 52002), new methylene blue (C.I. 52015), and thionin (C.I. 52000).

Metachromasia at a controlled pH.[15] A range of buffered metachromatic dyes (such as those listed above) may be used to distinguish strongly acidic from weakly acidic mucosubstances. For most purposes, staining at pH 3.0 and at pH 1.5 is sufficient. Strongly acidic mucosubstances show metachromasia at both pH levels; weakly acidic mucosubstances show metachromasia at the higher pH value only.

Periodic acid–phenylhydrazine– PAS method[16]

Principle. This technic may be used to distinguish neutral polysaccharides and glycoproteins from certain PAS-positive epithelial sulfomucins and epithelial sialomucins. Phenylhydrazine blocks the periodic acid–induced aldehydes of the neutral polysaccharides and glycoproteins from reacting with the Schiff reagent; the other carbohydrate substances mentioned are apparently unaffected by the blocking process and appear magenta colored.

Technic

1. The use of parallel slides for comparison purposes is suggested. Hydrate slides to distilled water.
2. Oxidize in freshly prepared 1% aqueous periodic acid. Discard solution after use.

3. Wash in running tap water for 5 minutes; rinse in several changes of distilled water.
4. Treat one of the test slides with 0.5% aqueous phenylhydrazine hydrochloride for 30 minutes. Discard solution after use. Allow the alternate slide to remain in distilled water for 30 minutes.
5. Wash slides well in several changes of distilled water.
6. Place both slides in Schiff reagent (p. 165) for 10 to 15 minutes. Filter back.
7. Give slides 3 changes of sulfurous rinse (p. 166) for 2 minutes each change. Discard rinses after use.
8. Wash in running tap water for 10 minutes.
9. Counterstain, if desired, in Harris's hematoxylin for 1 minute. Wash in tap water for 10 minutes.
10. Dehydrate, clear, and coverslip, using a synthetic mounting medium.

Results

PAS staining from neutral polysaccharides and glycoproteins should be abolished in the phenylhydrazine-treated section but should be present in the nonblocked section. PAS reactivity from certain epithelial sulfomucins and sialomucins will appear in both sections.

Periodic acid–borohydride–KOH– PAS technic[17]

Principle. Epithelial mucins of human normal terminal ileum, cecum, colon, and rectum will stain with this technic. Periodic acid functions to release aldehyde groups as previously described. Released aldehydes are reduced and rendered unreactive with the sodium borohydride treatment and, if sections were treated with Schiff reagent after this step, there would be no color produced. However, this method requires that sections be treated with potassium hydroxide (KOH) after the borohydride reduction. The KOH is believed to deacylate the side chains of O-acylated sialic acid, and these groups, once revealed, are reactive with Schiff reagent.

Mucin containing these O-acylated sialic acids is produced by the epithelial cells mentioned above. Mucin-producing metastases from adenocarcinomas of the lower gastrointestinal tract can be identified as such when positive staining occurs with this method. Such identification can assist in the determination of the primary tumor site, if not known. Approximately 70% of lower gastrointestinal metastases will give a positive reaction.

Fixation. 10% neutral buffered formalin or formol-calcium

Embedding. Cut paraffin sections at 5 μm.

Technic

1. Hydrate appropriately labeled parallel sections to distilled water.
2. Oxidize in freshly prepared 1% aqueous periodic acid for 30 minutes. Discard after use.
3. Wash sections in running tap water for 10 minutes.
4. Treat with 0.1% sodium borohydride in 1% disodium hydrogen phosphate for 30 minutes. Discard after use.
5. Wash well in several changes of distilled water. Allow one of the parallel slides to remain in distilled water.
6. Treat the alternate slide with 0.5% KOH in 70% ethanol for 5 to 30 minutes. Rinse in 70% ethanol. Wash in slowly running tap water for 10 minutes. Rinse in several changes of distilled.
7. Perform the PAS technic (p. 166) on both slides.

Results

Compare sections for increased PAS positivity in the section treated with the KOH. Substances responsible for the increased staining in the KOH section may be epithelial mucins from terminal ileum, cecum, colon, and rectum. (Culling notes that myelin sheaths also show increased PAS staining after KOH treatment.)

Müller-Mowry colloidal iron technic[18]

Principle. The first step in the procedure employs an acidified colloidal solution of ferric hydroxide. Acid mucosubstances and certain acidic mucins are the principal substances in a tissue section that absorb the colloidal ferric ions. The exact basis of the affinity of colloidal ferric hydroxide to attach to the acid carbohydrates, and occasionally to nuclei, is not known. It is believed that the initial linkage is an ionic bond of the ferric ion with the free carboxyl group of the protein (Fig. 9-4). Iron bound to tissue substances is then demonstrated by the Prussian blue reaction. On treatment with potassium ferrocyanide, the ferric ion forms ferric ferrocyanide, or Prussian blue. Positive staining is therefore indicated by a blue color (Fig. 9-5).

Nonspecific staining is reduced by acidified colloidal solutions and acidified washings. The intensity of the final blue color varies with the amount and degree of polymerization of the acid mucosubstances; however, the color is usually a deeper shade than that produced by alcian blue methods. The colloidal iron method does not have the histochemical specificity of some of the alcian blue technics.

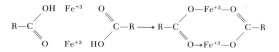

Fig. 9-4. Electrostatic bond of ferric ion with carboxyl groups of tissue protein.

$$4Fe^{+3} \quad + \quad 3Fe(CN)_6^{-4} \longrightarrow Fe_4[Fe(CN)_6]_3$$

Ferric iron   Ferrocyanide   Prussian
bound to tissue   ion   blue

Fig. 9-5. Formation of Prussian blue end product used to indicate sites of acid mucosubstance distribution.

Fixation. 10% neutral buffered formalin. Carnoy's or alcoholic formalin preferred. Chromate fixatives should not be used.

Embedding. Cut paraffin sections at 5 μm.

Solutions

Stock colloidal iron solution

Bring 250 ml of distilled water to a boil. While the water is boiling, pour 4.4 ml of 29% ferric chloride solution (USP XI) into it. Stir while adding the ferric chloride, and keep boiling until the solution becomes a dark red color. Remove from heat and allow to cool.

Free acid and ionizable iron salt may be removed by dialysis. Transfer 25 ml portions of the dark red solution to 41 mm dialysis tubes containing a glass marble weight at the lower end of the tube. Suspend each tube in individual 250 ml cylinders and add distilled water to fill the cylinder and surround each dialysis tube. Change the water twice during the 24-hour dialysis period. When the dialysis period is complete, remove the dialysis tubes and filter the contents through a *very fine* filter paper to remove particulate iron oxide. Store the filtrate in a brown bottle labeled as stock colloidal iron. It is stable for many months when stored at room temperature.

Working solution of colloidal iron (prepare fresh)

Stock colloidal iron	10 ml
Distilled water	18 ml
Glacial acetic acid	12 ml

12% aqueous acetic acid

Ferrocyanide–hydrochloric acid solution (prepare fresh)

2% potassium ferrocyanide	30 ml
1% hydrochloric acid	60 ml

Nuclear fast red *(Kernechtrot)* counterstain (p. 183).

If PAS reaction is to serve as the counterstain, periodic acid–Schiff reagent and sulfurous rinses will be needed. See pp. 165 and 166.

Technic
1. Hydrate slides.
2. 12% acetic acid for 30 seconds. Discard after use.
3. Working colloidal iron solution for 10 to 60 minutes. Discard after use.
4. Rinse sections in 12% acetic acid, 3 changes at 3 minutes each change. Discard after use.
5. Immerse in ferrocyanide–hydrochloric acid solution for 10 minutes. Discard after use.
6. Rinse thoroughly using several changes of distilled water.
7. Counterstain with either a. or b.:
   a. *Kernechtrot* for 3 to 5 minutes followed by 2 or 3 rinses in distilled water. Dehydrate, clear, and coverslip, using a synthetic mounting medium.
   b. The PAS reaction, up to and including the 10-minute water wash following the sulfurous rinses (that is, omit Harris's hematoxylin). Dehydrate, clear, and coverslip, using a synthetic mounting medium.

Results (Plate 2, *G*)
Acid mucosubstances and certain acidic mucins appear bright blue. With the *Kernechtrot* counterstain, nuclei are colored pink-red and cytoplasm a pale pink. With the PAS counterstain, PAS-positive materials are colored magenta. Mixtures of both neutral and acidic mucosubstances are stained a purple color because of reactions with both colloidal iron and PAS procedures.

Technics using alcian blue

Alcian blues are a group of polyvalent basic dyes that are water soluble and colored blue because of the presence of copper in the molecule. In aqueous solutions, alcian blues react to compounds containing anionic groups, for example, acid mucosubstances, acidic mucins, and DNA. Salt linkages have been postulated as the binding forces, though there is not complete agreement on this mechanism.

There are numerous technics available that employ alcian blue:
1. A "general" method that uses an alcian blue solution of pH 2.5. Use of this solution will color many acidic mucins and acid mucosubstances. Counterstaining is optional but is usually done with either *Kernechtrot* or the PAS reaction.
2. Alcian blue solutions at different pH levels. Generally pH values of 2.5 and 1.0 are used. With the higher pH value (that is, pH 2.5) both carboxylated and sulfated acidic mucosubstances and mucins are colored blue. With the lower pH value (that is, pH 1.0) only sulfated acidic mucosubstances are stained blue. Counterstaining is optional, but is usually done with either *Kernechtrot* or the PAS reaction.
3. Alcian blue solutions containing varying electrolyte concentrations. Different molar concentrations of magnesium chloride are added and, depending on the staining pattern, acidic mucins and acid mucosubstances may be distinguished as being carboxylated and sulfated, weakly and strongly sulfated, strongly sulfated, very strongly sulfated, or keratan sulfate.
4. Alcian blue may be used as a counterstain after aldehyde fuchsin staining. The procedure stains acidic nonsulfated mucosubstances a blue to blue-green color; weakly sulfated mucosubstances, purple; and strongly sulfated mucosubstances, a deep purple. (Aldehyde fuchsin has also been employed by itself at varying pH levels to distinguish strongly from weakly sulfated mucosubstances.)
5. Staining with alcian blue may be preceded by various digestion procedures such as testicular hyaluronidase to increase specificity for the various acid mucosubstances.

ALCIAN BLUE METHOD (pH 2.5[19])

Fixation. 10% neutral buffered formalin or Bouin's solution.

Embedding. Cut paraffin sections at 5 μm.

Solutions

    3% glacial acetic acid
    Alcian blue staining solution

3% glacial acetic acid	100 ml
Alcian blue 8GX	1 gm

        Add a crystal of thymol to prevent mold growth. Solution may be filtered back and reused. pH should be 2.5. Solution is stable for about 2 months.
    Nuclear fast red (*Kernechtrot*) counterstain (p. 183) or the PAS reaction (p. 166) may be used.

Technic
1. Hydrate slides to distilled water.
2. Stain in the alcian blue solution for 30 minutes. Filter back.
3. Wash in running tap water for 2 minutes; rinse in distilled water.
4. Counterstain, if desired, with *Kernechtrot* for 3 to 5 minutes, followed by several changes of distilled water. Dehydrate, clear, and coverslip. Alternatively, the PAS reaction may be performed (p. 166) up to and including the 10-minute water wash after the sulfurous rinses. Dehydrate, clear, and coverslip, using a synthetic mounting medium.

Results

Carboxylated and sulfated acid mucosubstances and acidic mucins (with the exception of the strongly sulfated variety) are stained blue. With the *Kernechtrot* counterstain, nuclei are colored pink-red and the cytoplasm is a pale pink. With the PAS counterstain, PAS-positive materials are colored magenta. Mixtures of both neutral and acidic mucosubstances are stained a purple color because of positive reactions with both the alcian blue stain and the PAS reaction.

ALCIAN BLUE STAIN (pH 1.0) FOR SULFATED MUCOSUBSTANCES[19]

1. Hydrate sections.
2. Stain in 1% alcian blue 8GX in 0.1 N hydrochloric acid for 30 minutes. Filter back.
3. Rinse sections briefly in 0.1 N HCl.
4. Blot sections dry with fine filter paper. Do not wash in water, since this can change the pH and cause nonspecific staining to occur.
5. Counterstain, if desired. See preceding method, step 4. Otherwise, dehydrate, clear, and coverslip, using a synthetic mounting medium.

Results

Sulfated mucosubstances—blue
For counterstain interpretation, see preceding sections.

ALCIAN BLUE WITH VARYING ELECTROLYTE CONCENTRATIONS[20]

Fixation. 10% neutral buffered formalin or 95% ethanol at 4° C.

Embedding. Cut paraffin sections at 5 μm. Mount on albuminized slides.

Solutions

Alcian blue 8GX (C.I. 74240) in 0.025 M acetate buffer, pH 5.8
To separate 100 ml portions of alcian blue solution, add the following amounts of magnesium chloride to achieve the required molar concentration:

Grams of MgCl$_2$	Molar concentration
1.20	0.06
6.10	0.3
10.15	0.5
14.20	0.7
18.30	0.9

Note:
1. The pH of 5.8 is used because background protein staining and glycoprotein staining is just faintly positive. A lower pH solution will mask the critical electrolyte concentration effect.
2. The alcian blue employed should be 8GX and not other varieites such as GS, 5GX, or

7GX. It should be fresh, be soluble in water to 5%, and not precipitate for at least 24 hours when mixed in 2 M MgCl$_2$ buffered to pH 5.7 with 0.025 M acetate buffer.

Method

1. Hydrate slides.
2. Stain for 18 hours at 25° C in each of the solutions listed above.
3. Rinse in a stream of distilled water, dehydrate, clear, and coverslip, using a synthetic mounting medium.

Results

With increasing concentrations of MgCl$_2$, alcian blue stains with increasing selectivity. With the various molar concentrations, blue staining will be shown by the following substances:

Molar concentration	Substance stained
0.06	Carboxylated and sulfated mucosubstances and mucins
0.3	Weakly and strongly sulfated mucosubstances and mucins
0.5	Strongly sulfated mucosubstances and mucins
0.7	Highly sulfated connective tissue mucosubstances
0.9	Keratan sulfate

ALDEHYDE FUCHSIN–ALCIAN BLUE METHOD[21]

Principle. An aldehyde fuchsin solution may be used to demonstrate sulfated mucosubstances. Nonsulfated mucosubstances do not react with the aldehyde fuchsin, but will color with the alcian blue (pH 2.5) solution.

Solutions

Aldehyde fuchsin (p. 197)
Substitute 60% ethanol solvent for the traditional Gomori 70% ethanol solvent. The pH of this solution is about 1.7.
Alcian blue solution, pH 2.5 (p. 172)

Technic

1. Hydrate sections to 70% ethanol.
2. Stain in aldehyde fuchsin for 10 to 20 minutes. (Fresh aldehyde fuchsin will generally stain more specifically and in a shorter time period.) Filter back.
3. Rinse sections in 70% ethanol.
4. Wash in running tap water.
5. Stain in alcian blue solution (pH 2.5) for 5 minutes. Filter back.
6. Wash in running tap water.
7. Dehydrate, clear, coverslip, using a synthetic mounting medium.

Results

Strongly sulfated acidic mucosubstances—deep purple

Weakly sulfated acidic mucosubstances—purple
Nonsulfated acidic mucosubstances—blue

ALDEHYDE FUCHSIN STAINING OF SULFATED MUCOSUBSTANCES[22]

The first four steps of the preceding procedure may be used to show the reaction of sulfated mucosubstances only. Highly sulfated mucosubstances may be shown by staining in an aldehyde fuchsin solution whose pH has been lowered to a value of 1.0 by the addition of concentrated hydrochloric acid. A working solution of light green is an optional counterstain.

Hyaluronidase digestions[2]

Various kinds of hyaluronidases have been used to identify various kinds of acid mucosubstances, as follows:

Enzyme	Acid mucosubstance depolymerized
Streptococcal hyaluronidase	Hyaluronic acid
Testicular hyaluronidase	Hyaluronic acid
	Chondroitin 4-sulfate (chondroitin sulfate A)
	Chondroitin 6-sulfate (chondroitin sulfate C)
Flavobacterium heparinum extract adapted to chondroitin sulfate A	Hyaluronic acid
	Chondroitin 4-sulfate (C.S. A)
	Chondroitin 6-sulfate (C.S. C)
	Dermatan sulfate (C.S. B)
Flavobacterium heparinum extract adapted to heparitin sulfate	Hyaluronic acid
	Chondroitin 4-sulfate (C.S. A)
	Chondroitin 6-sulfate (C.S. C)
	Heparitin sulfate, heparin

General procedure. Parallel test sections are hydrated to water. One slide (the "extracted section") is treated with a solution of the specific enzyme in buffer. The alternate slide (the "unextracted section") is treated with buffer only for the same time and at the same temperature as the extracted section. After incubation, both sections are washed and stained with alcian blue (pH 2.5 or pH 1.0). Extracted and unextracted sections are examined for positive staining. Positive staining in an area of the unextracted section that does not stain in the extracted section is assumed to be composed of the component or components depolymerized by the enzyme. Appropriate control slides should be included for each run.

Information about the *Flavobacterium* digestions may be found in references 2 and 23. Specific details on the streptococcal and testicular hyaluronidase procedures follow.

DIGESTION WITH STREPTOCOCCAL HYALURONIDASE

1. Hydrate sections to water.
2. Rinse in acetic acid–acetate buffer, pH 5.0 (p. 389).
3. Place appropriately labeled sections in preheated solutions of either
   a. acetic acid–acetate buffer pH 5.0 or
   b. acetic acid–acetate buffer containing streptococcal hyaluronidase (1500 TRU/dl) 0.1 M NaCl and 0.05% gelatin.
4. Incubate for 24 hours at 37° C. Discard solution.
5. Rinse in several changes of distilled water.
6. Stain with alcian blue, pH 2.5.

Results
Staining from hyaluronic acid will be blue in the unextracted slide and unstained in the extracted slide.

TESTICULAR HYALURONIDASE DIGESTION METHOD

1. Hydrate sections.
2. Place appropriate labeled sections in preheated solutions of either
   a. acetic acid–acetate buffer, pH 6.0 (p. 389) or
   b. acetic acid–acetate buffer, pH 6.0, containing 0.05% testicular hyaluronidase
3. Incubate 2 hours at 37° C. Discard solution.
4. Rinse sections in several changes of distilled water.
5. Counterstain with alcian blue, pH 2.5 or pH 1.0.

Results
Staining from hyaluronic acid, with or without chondroitin 4-sulfate and with or without chondroitin 6-sulfate, will be blue in the unextracted sections and unstained in the extracted sections.
Note: If the PAS reaction is used as the counterstain (after the alcian blue stain), the reaction may be increased in terms of color intensity in the extracted section. This is believed to be caused by an increased number of terminal groups released because of the enzyme depolymerization process. These terminal groups provide additional sites for the periodic acid to attack; hence more aldehyde groups are released, and the increased PAS positivity is noted.

SIALIDASE DIGESTION[24]

Staining of many, but not all, sialic acid–containing mucosubstances may be abolished by pretreatment with sialidase (neuraminidase).

Method

1. Hydrate sections.
2. Place appropriately labeled slides in preheated solutions containing either
   a. 0.05 M acetate buffer, pH 5.5 (p. 389) containing 0.1% calcium chloride or
   b. the buffer listed in (a) to which has been added 100 units of sialidase (neuraminidase) per milliliter.
3. Incubate sections for 24 hours at 37° C.
4. Rinse in several changes of distilled water.
5. Stain with alcian blue, pH 2.5.

Results

Staining from sialic acid–containing mucosubstances and mucins will appear blue in the unextracted section and unstained in the extracted section, provided that the substance was not a sialic acid–containing compound that is resistant to the sialidase treatment. Such compounds cannot be histochemically identified.

Iron diamine methods[16,25]

The mechanism of staining with diamine solutions is by salt formation between the cationic stain and the anionic groups present in the tissues.

High iron diamine method

1. Hydrate sections to distilled water.
2. Stain for 24 hours in the following solution:
   N,N-dimethyl-m-phenylenediamine   120 mg
      dihydrochloride
   N,N-dimethyl-p-phenylenediamine   20 mg
      hydrochloride
   Dissolve the above reagents in 50 ml of distilled water. Add 1.4 ml of 40% aqueous ferric chloride; pH should be 1.5 to 1.6. Prepare this solution fresh and use immediately.
3. After incubation, discard the solution, rinse rapidly in distilled water, dehydrate, clear, and coverslip, using a synthetic mounting medium.

Results

Sulfated mucins—gray-purple-black
Nonsulfated mucins—unstained
Note: After the water rinse at step 3, sections may be stained with 1% alcian blue (pH 2.5). If this counterstaining is performed, nonsulfated mucins present would be colored blue in the final result.

Low iron diamine method

1. Hydrate sections.
2. Stain for 24 hours in the following solution:
   N,N-dimethyl-m-phenylenediamine   30 mg
      dihydrochloride
   N,N-dimethyl-p-phenylenediamine   5 mg
      hydrochloride
   Dissolve the above reagents in 50 ml of distilled water. Add 0.5 ml of 40% ferric chloride. Prepare fresh and use immediately.
3. After incubation, rinse very quickly in distilled water.
4. Stain in alcian blue 8GX, pH 2.5, for 30 minutes.
5. Rinse very quickly in distilled water, dehydrate, clear, and coverslip, using a synthetic mounting medium.

Results

Sulfated and many acid nonsulfated mucins stain black; some acid nonsulfated mucins will color blue with the alcian blue.

Mixed diamine method

1. Preheat 1 N HCl for 30 to 45 minutes at 60° C.
2. Hydrate parallel sections.
3. Hydrolyze both sections in the preheated 1 N HCl for 10 minutes. This will remove background nuclear staining. Discard solution and wash sections for 5 minutes in running tap water; rinse in several changes of distilled water.
4. Oxidize one of the sections in 1% aqueous periodic acid for 10 minutes. Discard solution and wash in running tap water for 5 minutes. Rinse in several changes of distilled water.
5. Stain both sections for 24 hours in the following solution:
   N,N-dimethyl-m-phenylenediamine   30 mg
      dihydrochloride
   N,N-dimethyl-p-phenylenediamine   5 mg
      hydrochloride
   Dissolve the above reagents in 50 ml of distilled water. Adjust the pH of this solution to a range of 3.4 to 4.0 using 0.2 M sodium phosphate dibasic (Na_2HPO_4). This will require about 0.15 to 0.65 ml of the phosphate. Prepare this solution fresh.
6. At the conclusion of incubation, rinse sections in distilled water; dehydrate, clear, and coverslip, using a synthetic mounting medium.

Results

In the section that was *oxidized* with periodic acid: periodic acid–unreactive acidic mucosubstances stain purple; periodic acid–reactive neutral and acidic mucosubstances color gray to gray-brown.
In the *unoxidized* section, both types of acid mucosubstances color purple.

AMYLOID

Amyloid is primarily a protein material that is deposited in tissues in various pathologic conditions. Carbohydrate components may or may not be present. With the light microscope, amyloid deposits are observed to be homogeneous and eosinophilic. Transmission electron microscopy has revealed that amyloid consists of protein fibrils with certain constant physical characteristics. Amyloid deposits are intercellular and may become sufficiently large to cause significant damage to the surrounding tissues. The exact origins of amyloid are unknown, but they are believed to represent a tissue localization of a circulating abnormal protein complex arising from an immune reaction.

Studies on amyloid from different animal species and humans have indicated that it is not a uniform substance either physically, chemically, or ultrastructurally; various kinds of amyloids have certain similarities and certain differences.

Amyloid may be classified either according to types or according to patterns of localization. The types are as follows:

1. Primary (not associated with a predisposing disease)
2. Secondary (occurs as a sequel to certain chronic inflammatory conditions, for example, rheumatoid arthritis)
3. Associated with multiple myeloma
4. Hereditary (this type may occur, for example, in patients with familial mediterranean fever)
5. Associated with diabetes mellitus

There are four major patterns of amyloid distribution:

1. Deposits may be found in the tongue, heart, gastrointestinal tract, skeletal and smooth muscles, nerves, skin, and carpal ligaments. Types 1 and 3 tend to have this localization pattern.
2. Deposits may involve the liver, spleen, kidneys, and adrenals. Types 2 and 4 tend to have this pattern.
3. Mixed distribution involving areas of the above two patterns.
4. Localized distribution involving a single tissue or organ.

Demonstration technics for amyloid include staining with Congo red followed by examination with the light and polarizing microscopes, fluorescent staining with thioflavine T, and metachromatic methods using crystal violet or methyl violet. None of these technics produces consistent staining results, and the age of the amyloid deposit and the disease type it is associated with are variables affecting the reactions produced.

A useful reaction for distinguishing the homogeneous deposits of amyloid from other homogeneous deposits in gross tissue employs an iodine solution. Amyloid will stain a dark brown color that may be changed to blue-violet by the addition of sulfuric acid after the iodine solution. Mallory states that "sometimes, instead of turning a blue-violet, the color may merely turn a deeper brown."

Iodine reaction of amyloid[3,11]

Fixation. Absolute alcohol or 10% formalin.

Method

1. If paraffin sections are used, hydrate to water. If frozen sections are employed, they may be stained directly.
2. Stain sections in Lugol's iodine (p. 131) for 2 to 3 minutes.
3. Wash in water; mount in either water or glycerol.

Result

Amyloid—dark brown

With decomposed tissue, this reaction will not take place because of the alkalinity of the tissue. Treat with dilute acetic acid before performing the above technic and the amyloid will react.

Metachromatic stains for amyloid
Crystal violet stain for amyloid[26]

Principle. The usual mechanism for metachromasia depends on the fact that tissue with electronegative radicals and periodic negative surface charges will bind a dye in such a way that interaction between the dye molecules can occur. When polymerized in this way, dye molecules will show a new metachromatic absorption maximum and a color shift is observed. Dye-binding experiments with amyloid have revealed that amyloid possesses only a few strong anionic binding sites; so metachromasia seen with amyloid may depend on a different type of dye binding than that seen with ordinary metachromasia. Acid may be added to the crystal violet solution to prevent heavy orthochromatic staining of the cytoplasm. Acid rinses may follow the staining also with a similar function.

Fixation. 10% neutral buffered formalin, alcohol, Bouin's solution.

Embedding. Cut paraffin sections at 10 μm.

Solutions

Stock staining solution

Crystal violet (C.I. 42555)	1 gm
Methyl violet (C.I. 42535)	0.5 gm

The methyl violet gives a redder color to the solution.

Absolute alcohol	10 ml
Distilled water	90 ml

Working solution

Stock crystal violet–methyl violet staining solution	10 ml
Distilled water	90 ml

1% aqueous acetic acid

Method

1. Hydrate sections to distilled water. Include a control slide.
2. Stain in working solution for 7 minutes.
3. Wash slides in 1% aqueous acetic acid.
4. Wash in tap water for 10 to 20 minutes (a minimum of 10 minutes).
5. Lay slides out on filter paper and dry thoroughly. Dip section in xylene and coverslip, using a synthetic mounting medium.[27]

Lieb's crystal violet stain for amyloid[28]

Fixation. 10% neutral buffered formalin, alcohol, Bouin's fluid.

Embedding. Cut paraffin sections at 10 μm.

Solutions

Stock crystal violet solution

95% alcohol	100 ml
Crystal violet (C.I. 42555)	14 gm

This is a saturated solution, since it is soluble in alcohol to 13.87%.

Working solution of crystal violet

Stock solution	10 ml
Distilled water	300 ml
Hydrochloric acid	1 ml

Method

1. Hydrate slides to distilled water. Include a control slide.
2. Stain in working solution of crystal violet for 5 minutes to 24 hours. Luna[8] recommends 5 hours as a routine time. *Check with microscope.*
3. Wash well in tap water and mount from water in Highman's modification of Apathy's gum syrup or allow slide to air-dry thoroughly, and then dip in xylene and coverslip, using a synthetic mounting medium.

Results

Amyloid—purplish violet
Other tissue elements—blue

Highman's methyl violet method[29]

Fixation. 10% neutral buffered formalin, alcohol, Bouin's fluid.

Embedding. Cut paraffin sections at 10μm.

Solutions

Methyl violet	0.1 gm
Distilled water	2.5 ml
Glacial acetic acid	97.5 ml

Method

1. Hydrate sections to distilled water. Include a control slide.
2. Stain in staining solution for 10 to 30 minutes. *Check with microscope.*
3. Wash in running water and mount in Apathy's gum syrup *or* allow slide to air-dry thoroughly, dip in xylene, and coverslip, using a synthetic mounting medium.

Results (Plate 2, *N*)
Amyloid—red-purple

Nuclei may be stained prior to the amyloid staining with Weigert's iron hematoxylin. This does, however, give a denser stain.

Congo red technics for demonstration of amyloid

Principle. Much of the staining of amyloid by Congo red appears to depend on dye configuration. The Congo red dye is a linear molecule, and this configuration permits hydrogen bonding of the azo and amine groups of the dye to similarly spaced hydroxyl radicals of the amyloid. Some technics employ a section pretreatment with alkali that aids in releasing native internal hydrogen bonding between adjacent protein chains, and these technics release, as a result, more potential sites available for dye binding. A hematoxylin counterstain is usually performed and will color the nuclei blue. Amyloid is also birefringent after staining with Congo red.

Sections stained with Congo red are permanent, in contrast to the crystal violet or methyl violet stains, which have a tendency to fade.

Puchtler's modification of Bennhold's Congo red[30]

Fixation. Best result with Carnoy's fluid or absolute alcohol; 10% neutral buffered formalin and Bouin's fluid may be used.

Embedding. Cut paraffin sections at 10 μm (small amounts of amyloid are more easily demonstrated at this thickness).

Solutions

Mayer's hematoxylin (p. 142)
1% aqueous sodium hydroxide
Stock saturated solution of sodium chloride in 80% ethanol
Stock Congo red solution
100 ml of this solution may be prepared by the addition of 0.2 gm of Congo red to 100 ml of the saturated solution of sodium chloride in 80% ethanol.

Method

1. Hydrate sections to distilled water. Include a control slide.
2. Stain in Mayer's acid hemalum for 10 minutes. Filter back.
3. Wash in 3 changes of distilled water.
4. Transfer slides to alkaline sodium chloride solution for 20 minutes (to 100 ml of saturated sodium chloride solution in 80% alcohol, add 1 ml of 1% sodium hydroxide just before using).

5. Stain 50 minutes in freshly alkalinized solution of Congo red (to 100 ml of the stable stock solution of Congo red, add 1 ml of 1% sodium hydroxide). *Filter and use within 15 minutes.*
6. Dehydrate *quickly* in 3 changes of absolute alcohol. Clear in xylene and mount in synthetic resin in xylene.

Results with light microscopy (Plate 2, *H*)
Amyloid—red to pink-red
Nuclei—blue
Elastic fibers—lighter red
Other tissue elements—unstained
When examined with the polarizing microscope, amyloid deposits show a green birefringence, provided that sections have been cut between 5 and 10 μm. Sections not in this thickness range will not show the birefringence. Tissue fixed in solutions other than formalin may display false positive birefringence.

Thioflavine T fluorescent stain[31]

Fixation. 10% neutral buffered formalin.
Embedding. Cut paraffin sections at 5 to 10 μm. Frozen sections may also be used.

Solutions
Mayer's hematoxylin (p. 142).
1% aqueous thioflavine T (Roboz Surgical Instrument Co., Washington, D.C.)
1% aqueous acetic acid
Apathy's mounting medium (p. 278)

Method
1. Hydrate sections to distilled water.
2. Stain in Mayer's hematoxylin for 2 to 5 minutes. This will quench nuclear fluorescence. Do not differentiate or blue the stain. Filter the hematoxylin back.
3. Wash in running tap water for 1 to 2 minutes.
4. Stain in thioflavine T for 3 minutes. Discard solution.
5. Rinse in several changes of distilled water.
6. Differentiate in the acetic acid solution for 10 to 20 minutes.
7. Wash in running tap water for 2 minutes.
8. Mount in Apathy's medium (p. 278).

Results
Examine with the fluorescent microscope. Use of BG12 exciter filter with an OG4 or OG5 barrier filter will show yellow amyloid deposits on a black background. Use of a UG1 or UG2 exciter filter with a colorless ultraviolet barrier filter will demonstrate amyloid brighter yellow against a blue background. Culling recommends the latter filter sequence for demonstrating the finest amyloid deposits.

REFERENCES
1. Spicer, S. S., Leppi, T. J., and Stoward, P. J.: Suggestions for a histochemical terminology of carbohydrate-rich tissue components, J. Histochem. Cytochem. **13**:599, 1965, The Histochemical Society, The Williams & Wilkins Co. (agent).
2. Zugibe, F. T.: Diagnostic histochemistry, St. Louis, 1970, The C. V. Mosby Co.
3. Lillie, R. D., and Fullmer, H. M.: Histopathologic technic and practical histochemistry, ed. 4, New York, 1976, McGraw-Hill Book Co.
4. Yanoff, M., Zimmerman, L. E., and Fine, B. E.: Glutaraldehyde fixation of whole eyes, Am. J. Clin. Pathol. **44**:167-171, 1965.
5. Murgatroyd, L. B.: Chemical and spectrometric evaluation of glycogen after routine histological fixatives, Stain Technol. **46**:111-119, 1971, The Williams & Wilkins Co.
6. McManus, J. F. A.: The histological and histochemical uses of periodic acid, Stain Technol. **23**:99-108, 1948, The Williams & Wilkins Co.
7. Barger, J. D., and DeLamater, E. D.: The use of thionyl chloride in the preparation of Schiff's reagent, Science **108**:121-122, 1948.
8. Luna, L. G., editor: Manual of histologic staining methods of the Armed Forces Institute of Pathology, ed. 3, New York, 1968, McGraw-Hill Book Co.
9. Luna, L. G., editor: Stability of more commonly used special staining solutions, Histo-Logic **5**(3):2, July 1975.
10. Lillie, R. D., and Fullmer, H. M.: Histopathologic technic and practical histochemistry, ed. 4, New York, 1976, McGraw-Hill Book Co. Original reference: Bauer, H.: Mikroskopisch-chemischer Nachweis von Glykogen und einigen anderen Polysacchariden, Z. Mikrosk. Anat. Forsch. **33**:143-159, 1933.
11. Mallory, F. B.: Pathological technique, New York, 1961, Hafner Publishing Co.
12. Horobin, R. S., and Murgatroyd, L. B.: The staining of glycogen with Best's carmine and similar hydrogen bonding dyes: a mechanistic study, Histochem. J. **3**:1-9, 1971.
13. Bulmer, D.: Dimedone as an aldehyde blocking reagent to facilitate the histochemical demonstration of glycogen, Stain Technol. **34**:95-98, 1959, The Williams & Wilkins Co.
14. Vassar, P. S., and Culling, C. F. A.: Fibrosis of breast, Arch. Pathol. **67**:128, 1959.
15. Highman, B.: Staining of mucus with buffered solutions of toluidine blue O, thionin and new methylene blue N, Stain Technol. **20**:85-87, 1945, The Williams & Wilkins Co.
16. Leppi, T. J., and Spicer, S. S.: The histochemistry of mucins on certain primate salivary glands, Am. J. Anat. **118**:833-860, 1967.
17. Culling, C. F. A., Reid, P. E., Burton, J. D., and Dunn, W. L.: A histochemical method of differentiating lower gastrointestinal tract mucin from other mucins in primary or metastatic tumors, J. Clin. Pathol. **28**:656-658, 1975.
18. Mowry, R. W.: Improved procedure for the staining of acidic polysaccharides by Müller's colloidal

(hydrous) ferric oxide and its combination with the Feulgen and the periodic acid Schiff reactions, Lab. Invest. **7:**566-576, 1958.

19. Lev, R., and Spicer, S. S.: Specific staining of sulphate groups with alcian blue at low pH, J. Histochem. Cytochem. **12:**309, 1964, The Histochemical Society, The Williams & Wilkins Co. (agent).

20. Scott, J. E., and Dorling, J.: Differential staining of acid glycosaminoglycans (mucopolysaccharides) by alcian blue in salt solutions, Histochemie **5:**221, 1965.

21. Spicer, S. S., and Meyer, D. B.: Histochemical differentiation of acid mucopolysaccharides by means of combined aldehyde fuchsin–alcian blue staining, Am. J. Clin. Pathol. **33:**453-460, 1960, and in Tech. Bull. Regist. Med. Technol. **30:**53-60, 1960, Williams & Wilkins Co.

22. Halmi, N. S., and Davies, J.: Comparison of aldehyde fuchsin staining, metachromasia and periodic acid–Schiff reactivity of various tissues, J. Histochem. Cytochem. **1:**447-459, 1953, The Histochemical Society, The Williams & Wilkins Co. (agent).

23. Zugibe, F. T.: The demonstration of the individual acid mucopolysaccharides in human aortas, coronary arteries and cerebral arteries. I. The methods, J. Histochem. Cytochem. **10:**441, 1962, The Histochemical Society, The Williams & Wilkins Co. (agent).

24. Quintarelli, G., Tsuiki, S., Hasimoto, Y., and Pigman, W.: Studies of sialic acid–containing mucins in bovine submaxillary and rat sublingual glands, J. Histochem. Cytochem. **9:**176, 1961, The Histochemical Society, The Williams & Wilkins Co. (agent).

25. Spicer, S. S.: Diamine methods for differentiating mucosubstances histochemically, J. Histochem. Cytochem. **13:**211-234, 1965, The Histochemical Society, The Williams & Wilkins Co. (agent).

26. Modification used in Laboratory of Surgical Pathology at Hospital of the University of Pennsylvania, Philadelphia, Pennsylvania.

27. Personal communication, Helen N. Futch, M. D. Anderson Hospital, Houston, Texas.

28. Lieb, E.: Permanent stain for amyloid, Am. J. Clin. Pathol. **17:**413-414, 1947.

29. Highman, B.: Improved methods for demonstrating amyloid in paraffin sections, Arch. Pathol. **41:**559-562, 1946.

30. Puchtler, H., Sweat, F., and Levine, M.: On the binding of Congo red by amyloid, J. Histochem. Cytochem. **10:**355-363, 1962, The Histochemical Society, The Williams & Wilkins Co. (agent).

31. Vassar, P. S., and Culling, C. F. A.: Fluorescent stains, with special reference to amyloid and connective tissues, Arch. Pathol. **68:**487-498, 1959.

32. Carson, F. L., Matthews, J. L., and Pickett, J. P.: Preparation of tissue for laboratory examination. In Race, G. J., editor: Laboratory medicine, New York, 1977, Harper & Row, Publishers, vol. 3, chapter 22, p. 36.

Connective tissue and muscle fiber stains

Connective tissue is the most diverse of the four primary tissues and is the most widespread in the body.[1] Generally, connective tissue is considered to be composed of comparatively few cells and a large amount of intercellular substance. The cell types seen will vary depending on the exact type of connective tissue and may include fibroblasts, mast cells, histiocytes, adipose cells, reticular cells, osteoblasts and osteocytes, chondroblasts and chondrocytes, blood cells and blood-forming cells. The intercellular substance is usually composed of both amorphous (for example, nonsulfated and sulfated mucopolysaccharides) and formed elements (for example, collagen, reticular fibers, and elastic fibers).

Connective tissues are derived embryologically from mesoderm through an intermediate stage called mesenchyme. Mesenchyme consists of pale-staining cells with extended processes lying in a gelatin-like matrix; later in development the mesenchymal cells and matrix differentiate into the various types of connective tissues. In the adult, connective tissues may be subdivided into five main groups:

1. Connective tissue proper (including loose [areolar], dense irregular, dense regular, reticular, adipose)
2. Cartilage (including hyaline, elastic cartilage, and fibrocartilage)
3. Bone (including spongy [cancellous], and dense [cortical])
4. Blood
5. Blood-forming (hemopoietic)

Each of the five major groups are in turn subdivided and some of the subdivisions are indicated above. As indicated previously, each subdivision has characteristic cells and intercellular substances.

Some of the functions of the various types of connective tissues include support, restraint, binding, and separating of other tissues; transport of metabolites; storage of water, salts, and fats; protection against trauma and pathogens; and repair of damaged tissue by the process of fibrosis.

Additional details on the formed fibers (reticulum, collagen, and elastic) as well as muscle tissue are given prior to each section for their demonstration.

DEMONSTRATION METHODS FOR RETICULAR FIBERS AND BASEMENT MEMBRANES

Electron microscopic studies have shown that reticular fibers are young collagen or perhaps a small bundle of collagen. These fibers are not visible with the H & E stain but do possess a carbohydrate component that allows coloration in many situations by the periodic acid–Schiff reaction. It may be the same carbohydrate compound responsible for the affinity for silver that is one of the main characteristics of reticular fibers. Both ammoniacal and methenamine silver solutions have been employed, with the former type being more widely used.

Basement membranes, a modified connective tissue membrane upon which epithelial cells rest, may also be demonstrated, depending on the technic. Usually the PAS reaction and the Jones methenamine silver method are employed for basement membrane demonstration.

Diagnostic applications

In certain tumors, reticulum is located in a characteristic position in relation to the actual tumor cells. Reticulum stains can therefore be an important diagnostic tool for the differential diagnosis of certain types of tumor. For example, in most carcinomas, reticulum surrounds nests of tumor cells and provides support on the outer surface. In sarcomas, the reticulum pattern is more meshlike, with each cell surrounded by some reticulum. Lymphosarcoma is a tumor that arises in lymph nodes and here the pattern of reticular fibers is between individual cells.

Reticular fibers have a support function. They are normally found throughout the body but are most abundant in liver, spleen, and kidney. A normal liver, for example, will show well-defined strands of reticular fibers but a necrotic or cirrhotic liver will show a discontinuous pattern. Reticulum stains, especially modifications such as the Jones method, are also valuable for the study of glomerular basement membranes and the changes they undergo in renal diseases.

Ammoniacal silver methods

Most of the ammoniacal silver methods are similar in mechanism. Prior to beginning the technics, removal of mercury deposits, if necessary, should be performed (pp. 46 and 131). Because of the alkalinity of the silver solution, paraffin sections will sometimes float free of the slide. Tissues may be coated with celloidin (p. 131) to help prevent section loss.

Following are the major steps in the ammoniacal silver methods:

Oxidation
Sensitization
Exposure to the silver solution
Reduction
Toning
Removal of unreacted silver
Appropriate counterstaining

Oxidation of the tissues serves to enhance subsequent staining of the reticular fibers. Oxidants used vary with the procedure. In Wilder's technic, the oxidizing agent is phosphomolybdic acid, and in this case the hexavalent molybdenum of the molybdic acid is reduced easily to a lower valence. In the Foot and the Laidlaw methods, potassium permanganate is the oxidizing agent, followed by an oxalic acid treatment to remove excess permanganate from tissue. Gridley's method uses periodic acid. The washing step done after the oxidation is completed serves to remove excess reagent.

A sensitizing step may be employed next, and, as a rule, it is an impregnation procedure using a metal salt. It is believed that the metal forms metal-organic compounds with the tissue, and the sensitizing metal is subsequently replaced by silver from the silver compound. Sensitizers that may be used include uranyl nitrate (Wilder's technic) and a dilute solution of silver nitrate (Foot and Gridley).

After sensitization, tissues are treated with the ammoniacal silver solution. In the preparation of ammoniacal silver solutions, concentrated ammonium hydroxide (NH_4OH; strongly basic) is added to an aqueous solution of silver nitrate ($AgNO_3$; pH approximately 5). The addition of the ammonium hydroxide raises the pH of the silver nitrate solution almost immediately to 9.5

and a brown-black precipitate of silver hydroxide (AgOH) or silver oxide (AgO) is formed.[2]

$$AgNO_3 + NH_4OH \rightarrow NH_4NO_3 + AgOH \downarrow$$

Continued addition of ammonium hydroxide results in a gradual clearing of the precipitate by the formation of a silver diamine complex, $Ag(NH_3)_2^+$. A point is reached when practically all of the silver hydroxide precipitate has disappeared, and at this stage, the addition of a small amount of ammonium hydroxide will raise the pH to a range of 11 to 12, and the silver solution is then ready for use. At this pH, the concentration of silver diamine complex is high and the concentration of silver ions is low.

In the Laidlaw method, lithium carbonate is added to the silver nitrate producing an immediate precipitate of yellow-white silver carbonate. As ammonium hydroxide is added, however, brown-black silver oxide precipitate is formed, and the addition of more ammonium hydroxide results in the formation of a silver diamine complex as described previously. Similar considerations apply when sodium hydroxide is added in the silver solution preparation as is the case with Wilder's method.

Times for exposure to the silver solution vary with the procedure. Usually no gross color change in the tissue is evident until sections are reduced. This reduction process is sometimes called developing, and diamine silver technics require the use of varying concentrations of formalin (formaldehyde, HCHO) as the reducing agent. The formaldehyde itself becomes oxidized to formic acid (HCOOH) during the reduction process, and the silver diamine complex is reduced to visible metallic silver on those tissue structures that have been selectively impregnated with the silver diamine complex:

$$2Ag(NH_3)_2OH + HCHO \rightarrow$$
$$2Ag \downarrow + HCOOH + H_2O + 4NH_3$$

The metallic silver visible as a result of the reduction process may appear brown or black depending on the amount present and the particle size. These brown-black deposits may be transformed or "toned" into purple-black deposits of metallic gold by treatment with yellow or brown gold chloride ($AuCl_3$ or $HAuCl_4$). The metallic silver is oxidized to silver ions, and the gold chloride is reduced to metallic gold:

$$3Ag^0 \downarrow + AuCl_3 \rightarrow Au^0 \downarrow + 3AgCl$$

The metallic gold is more stable than the metallic silver, and toned sections show better contrast and clarity than do untoned sections.

The final treatment prior to counterstain is immersion in a sodium thiosulfate solution (hypo, $Na_2S_2O_3$). Thiosulfate ions form soluble silver complexes with any unreacted ionic silver present in the section:

$$Ag^+ + 2Na_2S_2O_3 \rightarrow Na^+ + Na_3Ag(S_2O_3)_2$$

The removal of the unreacted silver will prevent a later nonspecific reduction to metallic silver by light. The sodium thiosulfate will also remove any excess gold chloride that may be present.

Counterstains follow according to what other components are to be demonstrated.

Some common ammoniacal silver procedures are included in the following section. For all, acid-cleaned glassware should be used for solution preparation and staining. Nonmetallic forceps should also be used for slide transferral until after the sodium thiosulfate reaction is completed. This will prevent silver precipitate from forming on slides.

Wilder's reticulum technic[3]

Fixation. 10% neutral buffered formalin; Zenker's, Helly's, or Orth's.

Embedding. Paraffin, celloidin, or frozen sections may be used. Cut paraffin sections at 5 μm.

Solutions
10% aqueous phosphomolybdic acid
1% aqueous uranium nitrate
Ammoniacal silver hydroxide solution
   To 5 ml of a 10.2% aqueous solution of silver nitrate, add 28% (concentrated) ammonium hydroxide drop by drop until the precipitate that forms is *almost* dissolved. Add 5 ml of a 3.1% aqueous solution of sodium hydroxide and barely dissolve the resulting precipitate with a few drops of the 28% ammonium hydroxide. Make the solution up to 50 ml with distilled water. Use at once. *Note:* Use fresh ammonium hydroxide for best results. Overdissolving the precipitates can result in uneven staining.
Reducing solution
   Make fresh just prior to beginning the staining procedure.

Distilled water	100 ml
37% to 40% formalin	1 ml
1% aqueous uranium nitrate	3 ml

0.2% gold chloride solution

1% stock aqueous gold chloride	10 ml
Distilled water	40 ml

Note: The gold chloride may be filtered back and reused for approximately 100 slides.

5% aqueous sodium thiosulfate

Nuclear fast red *(Kernechtrot)* counterstain

Use a Pyrex beaker to prepare this solution. Dissolve 0.1 gm of nuclear fast red in a 5% aqueous solution of aluminum sulfate with the aid of heat. Cool, filter, and add a grain of thymol as a preservative.

Other counterstains, for example, working light green or alum hematoxylin may also be used.

Technic

1. Hydrate slides to distilled water.
2. De-Zenkerize if necessary. See p. 131.
3. Wash well in distilled water.
4. Phosphomolybdic acid solution for 1 minute. Discard solution. Wash sections well in running tap water until yellow color is removed.
5. Rinse in several changes of distilled water.
6. Treat with 1% uranium nitrate for 1 minute. Discard solution after use.
7. Wash in distilled water for 10 seconds.
8. Place in ammoniacal silver solution (freshly prepared) for 1 minute. Give sections 2 changes of this solution for best results. Discard solution after use.
9. Dip *very quickly* in 95% ethanol and immediately proceed with step 10.
10. Place in reducing solution for 1 minute. Give slides 2 changes in this solution during the 1-minute time period. Discard solution after use. Agitate slides gently during the reduction process.
11. Rinse well in distilled water.
12. Tone sections in gold chloride solution for approximately 1 minute until sections lose their yellow color and turn gray-lavender. Prolonged toning produces undesirable red tones. Control toning by rinsing in distilled water and microscopically checking for lavender-gray background with black reticular fibers.
13. Rinse sections in several changes of distilled water.
14. Treat with 5% sodium thiosulfate for 1 minute.
15. Wash sections well in tap water for approximately 1 minute.
16. Counterstain, if desired, with nuclear fast red solution for 3 to 5 minutes. Solution may be filtered back and reused. Rinse well in several changes of distilled water after this counterstain.
17. Dehydrate, clear, and coverslip, using a synthetic mounting medium.

Results

Reticulum fibers—black

Nuclei—pink-red if *Kernechtrot* is used

Background—pale pink if *Kernechtrot* is used

Foot's modification of Bielschowsky's method for reticulum [4]

Fixation. May be used on any well-fixed tissue.

Embedding. Cut paraffin sections at 5 µm.

Solutions

0.25% aqueous solution of potassium permanganate

5% aqueous solution of oxalic acid

2% aqueous silver nitrate

Ammoniacal silver nitrate solution

To 20 ml of a 10% solution of silver nitrate, add 20 drops of 40% solution of sodium hydroxide. The resulting brownish precipitate is dissolved with 28% ammonium hydroxide, which is added slowly, with continual shaking. About 2 ml will be needed, so it is well to add ammonium hydroxide drop by drop as this point is neared until the precipitate is almost dissolved. It is better to filter out a few undissolved granules than to run the risk of adding too much ammonium hydroxide. The resulting solution is made up to 80 ml with distilled water and filtered before use. This solution must be made fresh.

5% aqueous neutral formalin solution (Add excess calcium carbonate to 37% to 40% formalin to prepare neutral formalin.)

Gold chloride solution

1% gold chloride solution	1 ml
Distilled water	100 ml

5% aqueous sodium thiosulfate

Technic

1. Hydrate sections.
2. De-Zenkerize if necessary (p. 131).
3. Rinse in distilled water.
4. Potassium permanganate solution for 5 minutes. Discard solution after use.
5. Wash well in distilled water.
6. Oxalic acid solution for 15 minutes. Discard solution after use.
7. Wash thoroughly in tap water and rinse in distilled water.
8. Place sections in 2% silver nitrate solution for 48 hours in subdued light. Discard solution after use.
9. Rinse in distilled water.
10. Place in ammoniacal silver solution for 30 minutes. Discard after use.
11. Rinse very quickly in distilled water.
12. Reduce in 5% neutral formalin solution for 30 minutes. Two changes of 15 minutes each is preferred.
13. Rinse in tap water.
14. Tone in aqueous gold chloride solution for 1 hour. See gold chloride comments under Wilder's technic (p. 182).
15. Rinse in distilled water.

16. Place in sodium thiosulfate solution for 2 minutes.
17. Wash thoroughly in running tap water.
18. Counterstain if desired.
19. Dehydrate, clear, and coverslip, using synthetic mounting medium.

Results
Reticulum—dark violet to black
Background—depends on counterstain

Gridley modification of the silver impregnation method of staining reticular fibers [5]

Fixation. Formalin-fixed tissue is preferred. Zenker's, Bouin's, alcohol, or Carnoy's may be used.
Embedding. Cut paraffin sections at 5 μm.

Solutions
0.5% aqueous solution of periodic acid
2% silver nitrate solution (aqueous)
Ammoniacal silver nitrate solution
  Using a graduated cylinder with a ground glass stopper, add 20 drops of 10% sodium hydroxide to 20 ml of 5% silver nitrate. Add concentrated strong ammonium hydroxide solution drop by drop until there is a layer of granules left on the bottom of the cylinder. Add distilled water to make 60 ml. The ammonium hydroxide should be fresh and only a minimum amount used. Prepare immediately before use.
30% formalin solution

Formalin (40%), commercial	30 ml
Distilled water	70 ml

Gold chloride solution

1% gold chloride solution	10 ml
Distilled water	40 ml

5% aqueous solution of sodium thiosulfate

Technic
1. Hydrate section to distilled water.
2. Place in periodic acid solution for 15 minutes. Discard solution after use.
3. Rinse in distilled water.
4. 2% silver nitrate solution for 30 minutes. Discard solution after use.
5. Rinse in distilled water.
6. Place in ammoniacal silver nitrate solution for 15 minutes. Discard solution after use.
7. Rinse as quickly as possible in distilled water and go immediately into step 8.
8. 30% formalin solution for 3 minutes. Discard solution after use.
9. Wash in several changes of distilled water.
10. Tone in gold chloride solution for 5 minutes or until sections have lost all yellow color. See gold chloride comments under Wilder's technic (p. 182).
11. Wash in distilled water.

12. Fix in 5% sodium thiosulfate solution for 3 to 5 minutes.
13. Wash well in running tap water.
14. Counterstain if desired.
15. Dehydrate, clear in xylene, and coverslip, using a synthetic mounting medium.

Results
Fine reticulum fibers are stained black. Background is colored taupe if no counterstain is used; otherwise it is colored according to the counterstain.

Reticulum-staining procedure of Nassar and Shanklin [6]

Fixation. 10% neutral buffered formalin.
Embedding. Cut paraffin sections at 5 μm.

Solutions
Equal-parts mixture of 0.5% aqueous potassium permanganate and 0.5% aqueous sulfuric acid
2% aqueous oxalic acid
Freshly prepared 2% aqueous silver nitrate
  Add 3 drops of pyridine for every 10 ml of silver solution.
Silver diamine hydroxide solution (approximately 50 ml volume)
  Place 1 ml of 28% ammonium hydroxide in a flask. To this add 7 ml of 10% silver nitrate rapidly. Solution should appear clear right away. Add more 10% silver nitrate drop by drop. Shake between each additional drop. At about 22 ml volume a slight turbidity will remain. Dilute this with an equal amount of distilled water. For every 10 ml of diamine silver solution, add 3 drops of pyridine.
Reducing solution
  Equal-parts mixture of 2% neutral formalin and absolute alcohol. Prepare 2% formalin by diluting 5 ml of 10% neutral formalin to a final volume of 25 ml with distilled water.
0.2% or 0.1% aqueous gold chloride
5% aqueous sodium thiosulfate
Harris's hematoxylin (counterstain)

Technic
1. Hydrate sections to distilled water.
2. Oxidize in equal parts of 0.5% potassium permanganate and 0.5% sulfuric acid for 1 to 2 minutes, until sections turn a brownish color. The solution should be changed frequently.
3. Rinse in distilled water and decolorize in 2% oxalic acid for 2 minutes. Wash under tap water for 5 minutes and dehydrate up to 95% alcohol.
4. Place in the 2% silver nitrate solution for 1 hour at 50° C.
5. Rinse quickly in 95% alcohol and impregnate in silver–diamine hydroxide solution.
6. Rinse quickly in 95% alcohol and reduce in the reducing solution for 2 minutes.

7. Wash in distilled water and tone in 0.2% or 0.1% aqueous gold chloride until sections turn grayish, about 1 minute.
8. Treat with 5% sodium thiosulfate for 2 minutes.
9. Wash in tap water and counterstain in Harris's hematoxylin for 1 minute.
10. Decolorize in acid alcohol if necessary and wash in tap water for 5 minutes. Dehydrate, clear, and coverslip, using a synthetic mounting medium.

Results
Reticular fibers—black
Nuclei—blue

Laidlaw's silver stain for reticulum [7]

Fixation. Bouin's preferred. May be done on formalin-fixed tissues.
Embedding. Cut paraffin sections at 5 μm.

Solutions
1% iodine in 95% ethanol
5% sodium thiosulfate
0.25% potassium permanganate
  Prepare fresh before use.
5% oxalic acid
Modified lithium-silver solution of Hortega
  In a 250 ml glass-stoppered graduate dissolve 12 gm of silver nitrate in 20 ml of distilled water. Add 230 ml of a saturated solution of lithium carbonate in distilled water (about 1.33%); shake well; let settle to about 70 ml of precipitate. Pour off supernatant fluid. Add distilled water to 250 ml and let precipitate settle to 70 ml four times. Pour off supernatant fluid after last wash and settling of precipitate to 70 ml. Add ammonium hydroxide (26% to 28%), shaking constantly until the fluid is *almost* clear. Add distilled water to a total of 120 ml; shake and filter into a brown bottle.
1% formalin
0.2% aqueous gold chloride

Technic
1. Hydrate sections to distilled water.
2. Wash Bouin's fixed sections in running tap water for 20 minutes—formalin-fixed sections in running tap water for 5 minutes.
3. Place sections in a 1% alcoholic solution of iodine for 3 minutes.
4. Treat with 5% sodium thiosulfate for 3 minutes.
5. Tap water for 5 minutes.
6. Place in 0.25% freshly prepared potassium permanganate for 3 minutes.
7. Rinse in distilled water.
8. Place in 5% oxalic acid for 3 minutes.
9. Wash in running tap water for 10 minutes.
10. Wash in 3 changes of distilled water over a 10-minute period.

11. Stain in the lithium silver solution. Heat the stock solution in a 60° C oven and stain in oven for 5 minutes. The used solution can be filtered and reused a dozen times or more.
12. Rinse slides by carefully pouring distilled water over them several times.
13. Treat section with 1% formalin for 3 minutes, changing the solution 4 or 5 times.
14. Rinse slides well with distilled water.
15. Immerse slides in the gold chloride solution at room temperature for 10 minutes. (See gold chloride comments under Wilder's technic, p. 182.)
16. Rinse in distilled water.
17. Pour 5% sodium thiosulfate over slides, changing the solution as often as it becomes turbid for 10 minutes.
18. Wash well in running tap water.
19. Counterstain if desired.
20. Dehydrate, clear in xylene, and coverslip, using a synthetic mounting medium.

Results
Reticular fibers—black
Background—depending on counterstain

Snook's reticulum stain [8]

Fixation. 10% formalin
Embedding. Paraffin, celloidin, or frozen sections. Cut 5 μm sections.

Solutions
0.25% aqueous potassium permanganate
5% aqueous oxalic acid
1% aqueous uranium nitrate
1% aqueous formalin
5% aqueous sodium thiosulfate (hypo)
5% aqueous silver nitrate solution
10% aqueous sodium hydroxide
Ammoniacal silver solution
  To 20 ml of 5% silver nitrate solution in an acid-clean graduated glass cylinder, add 20 drops of 10% sodium hydroxide solution. Then add ammonium hydroxide, drop by drop, until only a few granules of the resulting precipitate remain on the bottom of the cylinder. Add distilled water to make 60 ml and use at once. The ammonium hydroxide must be fresh.

Technic
1. Hydrate sections.
2. Oxidize with potassium permanganate solution for 5 minutes.
3. Rinse in tap water and distilled water.
4. 5% oxalic acid until sections are clear.
5. Rinse in tap water, place in distilled water. Use acid-clean Coplin jars and nonmetallic forceps for steps 6 through 15. Replace solutions after 10 or 12 slides have been processed, one slide at a time.
6. 1% uranium nitrate for 5 seconds (sensitizer).

7. Rinse in distilled water, 2 changes.
8. Place in ammoniacal silver solution for 1 minute.
9. Dip once in distilled water.
10. Place in 1% formalin solution for 1 minute. Section should turn yellowish brown.
11. Rinse in distilled water, 2 changes.
12. 1% gold chloride solution for 1 minute. Section should turn gray-black.
13. Rinse in distilled water, 2 changes.
14. 5% sodium thiosulfate for 30 seconds to 1 minute.
15. Rinse in distilled water, two changes.
16. Counterstain (if desired) in nuclear fast red (*Kernechtrot*) stain for 3 to 5 minutes. Rinse well in distilled water.
17. Dehydrate, clear, and coverslip, using a synthetic mounting medium.

Results (Plate 1, *U*)
Reticulum fibers—lavender gray to black
Background—pink to rose

Methenamine silver methods

The Jones and Gomori methenamine silver methods rely on the production of aldehyde groups from the carbohydrate components of the reticular fibers and basement membranes after exposure to a periodic acid solution. The released aldehydes then reduce the silver of the methenamine silver complex to visible metallic silver. The gold chloride solution functions to tone the tissue section, and sodium thiosulfate functions to remove excess unreacted silver and gold.

Jones' method for reticulum and basement membranes [9]

Fixation. 10% neutral buffered formalin, Bouin's, or Zenker's.

Embedding. Cut paraffin sections at 1 to 4 μm; 5 μm sections do not stain so well.

Solutions
0.5% aqueous periodic acid freshly prepared
3% aqueous methenamine (hexamethylenetetramine)
5% aqueous silver nitrate
Borate buffer, pH 8.2

0.2 M boric acid	6.5 ml
0.25 M sodium borate	3.5 ml

Working methenamine silver solution. Prepare fresh just before use.

3% methenamine	42.5 ml
5% silver nitrate	2.5 ml
Mix and add:	
Borate buffer, pH 8.2	12 ml

Mix again and filter into a chemically clean Coplin jar. When used at 70° C, the working silver solution is stable for about 60 to 75 minutes; solution stability may be prolonged somewhat by staining at 65° C. Solution instability is indicated by the deposition of a black precipitate on the slides.

Gold chloride solution, 0.2%

1% gold chloride stock solution	10 ml
Distilled water	40 ml

The working solution may be filtered back and reused for approximately 100 slides.

3% aqueous sodium thiosulfate
Counterstain: nuclear fast red (*Kernechtrot*) or Harris's hematoxylin

Notes:
1. The second to fifth solutions mentioned above should be prepared in acid-cleaned glassware (p. 134).
2. Glassware for the technic itself should also be acid-cleaned and rinsed well in distilled, deionized water.
3. Additional suggestions [10]
   a. The Coplin jars that are to be used for the actual silver impregnation should be rinsed in distilled water, upended on gauze pads, and allowed to drain dry in the paraffin oven. This preheating assists in preventing cracking of the jar when it is placed in the 70° C water bath.
   b. Prevent condensation and silver dilution by removing the water-bath lid during the silver incubation period. Use ground-glass lids to cover the Coplin jars during the incubation period.
   c. Prepare an extra quantity of working silver solution and use half for the regular incubation at 70° C. The other half can be placed in the paraffin oven (56° to 58° C). If the regular silver solution begins to precipitate but the reaction is not yet fully completed, the slides may be transferred to the prepared 56° C preheated solution and the incubation then continued at 70° C with the fresh silver solution.
   d. Although the method traditionally calls for silver incubation to take place at 70° C, the use of a 65° C water bath can work just as well with a somewhat lessened possibility of precipitate production. Staining time in the silver may take a little longer, however, to compensate for the decreased temperature.
   e. The technic seems to work better on slides that have been alcohol cleaned.

Technic
1. Hydrate sections to distilled water.
2. Oxidize in periodic acid solution for 11 minutes. Discard solution after use.
3. Rinse thoroughly in distilled, deionized water.
4. Place slides in the Coplin jar containing the freshly prepared and filtered working methe-

namine silver solution. Place this Coplin jar in a 70° C water bath. Place another Coplin jar containing distilled, deionized water in the 70° C water bath. This water will be used for later rinses. Check slides *macro*scopically at 20 minutes for any precipitate formation. The total staining time is approximately 60 to 75 minutes when sections are incubated at 70° C. Generally, tissue fixed in formalin or paraformaldehyde will require slightly longer incubation times than does Bouin's fluid–fixed material. Tissue that has been allowed to remain in any fixative for more than a few days will tend to take longer to stain.

5. *Microscopic check:* Numerous microscopic checks tend to favor precipitate formation and should not be necessary once experience has determined proper time guidelines.

When sections show a medium brown color stain, remove from the silver solution, rinse in the 70° C distilled deionized water, and check microscopically for a dark yellow-brown background and black reticular fibers and basement membranes. Renal tubular basement membranes will blacken prior to the glomerular capillary basement membranes, but for a satisfactory stain, the latter basement membranes should also appear brown-black.

An understained section should be rinsed in the 70° C distilled, deionized water, returned to the 70° C silver solution, and checked every 5 to 10 minutes until proper intensity is reached. An overstained section may be "destained" by 1 or 2 dips in a very dilute potassium ferricyanide solution.

Do not allow slides to cool significantly during the microscopic check; otherwise uneven staining will occur.

6. Rinse sections well in distilled water.
7. Tone in gold chloride solution for 1 minute. Sections should turn gray-black. Overtoning produces red tones. If overtoned, treat sections with 3% sodium metabisulfite for 1 to 3 minutes.
8. Rinse in several changes of distilled water.
9. Treat with sodium thiosulfate for 1 to 2 minutes. Discard solution.
10. Wash in running tap water for 10 minutes.
11. Rinse in distilled water.
12. Counterstain as desired. Nuclear fast red for 3 to 5 minutes (filter back), followed by several changes in distilled water may be used. Or sections may be counterstained with Harris's hematoxylin for 1 to 3 minutes (filter back) followed by a brief rinse in tap water, differentiation in acid alcohol, a rinse in tap water, bluing in ammonia water, and several washes of tap water.
13. Dehydrate, clear in xylene, and coverslip, using a synthetic mounting medium.

Results

Reticular fibers and basement membranes—black
Other tissue elements—colored according to counterstain employed

Gomori's periodic acid–methenamine silver method[11]

Fixation. 10% formalin, Carnoy's, Bouin's.
Embedding. Cut paraffin sections at 5 μm.

Solutions

0.5% aqueous periodic acid
Stock methenamine silver solution

3% methenamine	100 ml
5% silver nitrate	5 ml

Use chemically clean glassware for preparation and storage. Add the silver nitrate solution in small amounts to the methenamine solution, mixing after each addition. There will form a white precipitate that redissolves on shaking. Stock solution should be clear for use. Filter the stock solution into a brown bottle. Solution is stable for several months if stored at 4° C.

Working methenamine silver solution

Stock methenamine silver solution	50 ml
5% sodium borate (borax) solution	5 ml

Mix well. Filter into a chemically clean Coplin jar and *allow to preheat* for approximately 20 to 30 minutes at 45° to 60° C prior to actual use. Allow another Coplin jar containing distilled water to preheat also.

0.2% gold chloride (p. 182).
3% sodium thiosulfate
Stock solution of light green counterstain

Light green SF yellowish	1 gm
Distilled water	500 ml
Glacial acetic acid	1 ml

Mix well and filter. Stock solution is stable for 2 to 3 months.

Working solution of light green

Stock light green solution	10 ml
Distilled water	50 ml

Mix. Working solution may be discarded after use.

Technic

1. Hydrate sections to distilled water.
2. Oxidize in periodic acid solution for 15 minutes at room temperature.
3. Rinse slides well in distilled water.
4. Using nonmetallic forceps, transfer the slides into the *preheated* methenamine silver solution. Check slides at half-hour intervals and note development of a yellow-brown color. At this point, rinse slides in the hot distilled water, and check microscopically for blackened reticulum fibers and basement membranes against a yellow-brown background. Staining times will vary depending on preheat time and incubation temperature.

5. When sections have reached the proper intensity, wash in distilled water.
6. Tone in gold chloride solution (see comments under Wilder's technic, p. 182).
7. Rinse in distilled water.
8. Treat with sodium thiosulfate solution for 2 minutes.
9. Wash in running tap water for 10 minutes.
10. Counterstain in working light green solution for 1 to 2 minutes. Discard solution after use. Other counterstains may also be used instead of light green (for example, nuclear fast red or H & E).
11. Dehydrate, clear in xylene, and coverslip, using a synthetic mounting medium.

Results (Plate 1, *E*)
Basement membranes, reticular fibers—black
Background—green, if light green counterstain is used

COLLAGEN AND MUSCLE DEMONSTRATION METHODS
HISTOLOGIC CONSIDERATIONS

Collagen is the commonest protein in the body and, when viewed with the light microscope, appears as slender, threadlike structures woven in varying degrees of density and commonly referred to as collagen fibers.

Four genetically distinct types of collagen have been identified in mammalian tissues: type 1 collagen is found in tendon, bone, adult skin, and human aorta; type 2 is found in cartilage and intervertebral discs; type 3 has been described in newborn human skin, human aorta, and many other organs—this type may be identical with reticular fibers, type 4 is found in basement membranes.

The collagen fibers are themselves composed of still finer, threadlike structures, visible with the electron microscope called "microfibrils." These microfibrils exhibit "axial periodicity" along their length because of the distinctive spatial arrangement of the molecules that comprise the microfibrils. These molecules are called "tropocollagen" and are secreted, in most cases, by fibroblast cells. Once the tropocollagen is secreted out of the cell body, the molecules polymerize into the collagen microfibrillary units.

In the fresh state, collagen appears white; with the hematoxylin and eosin technic it is eosinophilic. Collagen appears as different colors in various selective staining methods.

Muscle tissue, another of the four primary tissues, is composed of (1) muscle cells (usually called muscle fibers because of their fiberlike appearance) and (2) the connective tissues that serve to bind the muscle fibers together. There are three major types of muscle fibers, and the distinctions are made primarily on a morphologic and functional basis:

Smooth muscle (nonstriated muscle)—involuntary; usually associated with viscera; lacks the cross-striations seen in the other two muscle types; cells elongated; tapered at the ends; cells possess a single centrally located nucleus.

Striated muscle (skeletal muscle)—voluntary; has distinctive banding patterns (striations); large cylindric fibers; multinucleated; nuclei located on periphery of fiber.

Cardiac muscle—involuntary; striated; centrally located nucleus; composed of branching and anastomosing fibers connected by junctions called "intercalated discs."

DIAGNOSTIC APPLICATIONS

The use of trichrome and other staining methods that distinguish collagen from muscle are useful in the histopathology laboratory for indicating fibrotic change (that is, an increased amount of collagen). Fibrotic change can occur, for example, in cirrhosis of the liver and in various renal diseases such as pyelonephritis. A Gomori trichrome variant is considered useful for distinguishing histologic changes that occur in neuromuscular diseases. Trichrome methods are also helpful in distinguishing tumors that have arisen from muscle cells, from tumors that have arisen from fibroblasts. Phosphotungstic acid–hematoxylin (PTAH) is another collagen-and-muscle demonstration method that is also a routine method in neuropathologic work because of its simplicity and ability to distinguish abnormal fibrous astrocytes. The PTAH technique is also considered particularly suitable for striated muscle. In certain muscle diseases, individual muscle cells can degenerate and lose their striations. The PTAH technic can help in diagnosis of such dystrophic change in muscle tissue.

Collagen and muscle may be demonstrated by
1. Acid aniline dye mixtures with picric acid
2. Trichrome procedures employing phosphomolybdic and phosphotungstic acids
3. Phosphotungstic acid hematoxylin variants
4. Periodic acid–oxidation methods

DEMONSTRATION METHODS
Acid aniline dye mixtures with picric acid

The exact mechanism for collagen staining by use of acid aniline dyes is unknown, but demonstration depends on the selectivity of the collagen fiber for acid dyes from strongly acid solutions.[12] The most commonly used dyes in these technics include indigocarmine, aniline blue, methyl blue, and acid fuchsin. These are used in solution with picric acid, which provides the acidic pH necessary for selective staining and also acts as a dye itself in counterstaining muscle and cell cytoplasm. It is important to maintain a low pH of the staining solution, as selective staining of the collagen fiber will not occur at higher pH levels. Another important factor is the saturation of the picric acid solution. Should it not be saturated, the collagen would appear pale pink to pale orange; muscle and cytoplasm might stain the same color as the connective tissue, or may appear unstained.

Van Gieson's picric acid–fuchsin stain [13]

Fixation. Any well-fixed tissue can be used.
Embedding. Cut paraffin sections at 5 μm.

Solutions

1% aqueous acid fuchsin solution
Saturated aqueous solution of picric acid
Weigert's iron hematoxylin (p. 190)
Van Gieson's stain

1% aqueous acid fuchsin	5 ml
Saturated aqueous picric acid	100 ml

This solution may be employed in many technics (for example, reticulum demonstration methods) as a counterstain. Lillie[14] states that the addition of 0.25 ml of concentrated hydrochloride acid can sharpen the distinction between the mucle and collagen color shades. A variant sometimes used for counterstaining nervous tissues may be prepared as follows:

1% aqueous acid fuchsin	15 ml
Saturated aqueous picric acid	50 ml
Distilled water	50 ml

Technic

1. Hydrate sections to distilled water.
2. Stain sections rather deeply with Weigert's iron hematoxylin 10 to 20 minutes. The nuclear stain must be deep because the picric acid extracts it to some extent.
3. Wash in tap water for 10 minutes.
4. Stain in Van Gieson's stain for 5 minutes. Discard solution after use.
5. Transfer directly to 95% alcohol and dehydrate as usual; clear in xylene, and coverslip, using a synthetic mounting medium.

Results

Collagen—brilliant red
Smooth and striated muscle—yellow
Cornified epithelium and cell cytoplasm—yellow
Neuroglia fibrils—yellow
Nuclei—blue-black

Trichrome procedures employing phosphomolybdic and phosphotungstic acids

These technics are sequence procedures employing a plasma stain, followed by a phosphotungstic or phosphomolybdic acid mixture, followed by a collagen-fiber stain. Staining is done at an acid pH to increase selectivity for the collagen fiber. Although the exact mechanism of how the stain works is unknown, some theories are available.

Acid dyes are used to stain the acidophilic cytoplasm and muscle fibers; Biebrich scarlet is a common example. Collagen fibers are also acidophilic but, on the final result, color differently from the muscle and cell cytoplasm because of the action of the phosphomolybdic (or phosphotungstic) acid. One theory of why this is so suggests that the acid (phosphomolybdic or phosphotungstic) is taken up by the connective tissue and then replaced by aniline blue or similar dyes (light green, fast green, and so on). Aniline blue is more of a group of related dyes rather than a single dye, but the group is considered to act as an acid dye. According to this theory, the mechanism would act as a substitution reaction of one acid for another.

Further work has shown that the dyes used in the trichrome methods for staining after the phosphomolybdic or phosphotungstic acid treatment are not strictly acid dyes, but rather amphoteric and as such can act as either acid dyes or basic dyes depending on the staining situation. Studies have shown that the polymeric and pentavalent phosphomolybdic and phosphotungstic acids actually become located in the fibers that are stained selectively by the trichrome methods.[15] These structures are rich in basic groups. On a comparative basis, the phosphomolybdic and phosphotungstic acids have more acidic groups than the substrate tissue has basic groups. As a result numerous acidic groups are left free to bind dyes that are rich in basic groups. Dyes falling in this category include the basic dyes, and the amphoteric dyes with strong basic groups of which aniline blue is an example. The phosphomolybdic or phosphotungstic acid thus acts as a link connecting basic groups of the connective tissue fiber to the basic groups of the dye. The phosphomolybdic or phosphotungstic acid treatment has the ultimate effect of making an amphoteric dye that would ordinarily act as an acid dye to change and act as a basic dye.

Another factor to be considered concerns the differential permeabilities of collagen versus the other acidophilic constituents in the tissue. Collagen is readily entered by almost any dye, as it is of comparatively loose texture. Cytoplasm has lesser permeability and is more selective to a dye. In Masson's trichrome, for example, the acid plasma stain (Biebrich scarlet–acid fuchsin solution) enters all the acidophilic tissue constituents including the collagen. Because of the lesser permeability of the cytoplasm, it will remain there even when the sections are exposed to the action of the phosphomolybdic and phosphotungstic acid. Acid causes the Biebrich scarlet to diffuse out of the collagen, and one purely physical reason may be that the loose texture of the collagen aids in dye diffusion. pH factors may also play a role, as the pH may not be sufficiently acidic to give selective collagen staining with the first treatment of Biebrich scarlet. Since there is no chemical combination with the Biebrich scarlet, the dye will easily diffuse out on subsequent treatments, enabling it to be differentially stained with the aniline blue on the chemical basis mentioned above.

Masson's trichrome stain[16]

Fixation. Bouin-fixed tissue is preferable; 10% neutral buffered formalin may be used.

Embedding. Cut paraffin sections at 5 μm.

Solutions

Bouin's fluid (p. 47)

Weigert's iron hematoxylin

Stock solution A

Hematoxylin	1 gm
95% alcohol	100 ml

Stock solution B

29% aqueous ferric chloride	4 ml
Distilled water	95 ml
Hydrochloric acid	1 ml

For *working solution* of Weigert's iron hematoxylin, use equal parts of solution A and solution B.

Working solution of Biebrich scarlet–acid fuchsin

1% aqueous stock Biebrich scarlet	90 ml
1% aqueous stock acid fuchsin	10 ml
Glacial acetic acid	1 ml

Mix. Filtering prior to use can assist in prevention of deposition of red-staining artifact.

Phosphomolybdic-phosphotungstic acid solution

Phosphomolybdic acid	5 gm
Phosphotungstic acid	5 gm
Distilled water	200 ml

Aniline blue solution

Aniline blue	2.5 gm
Acetic acid	2 ml
Distilled water	100 ml

Acetic water

Glacial acetic acid	1 ml
Distilled water	100 ml

Technic

1. Hydrate slides to distilled water.
2. Place in Bouin's fixative for 1 hour at 56° C or overnight at room temperature. Make sure dish or jar is covered. Cool for 5 to 10 minutes if slides are postfixed with heat, before proceeding with step 3.
3. Wash in running water until sections are colorless.
4. Rinse in distilled water.
5. Weigert's iron hematoxylin solution for 10 minutes. Wash in running tap water for 10 minutes.
6. Rinse in distilled water.
7. Biebrich scarlet–acid fuchsin solution for 15 minutes.
8. Rinse in distilled water.
9. Phosphomolybdic-phosphotungstic acid solution for 10 to 15 minutes. Discard solution.
10. Transfer directly to the aniline blue solution for 10 to 20 minutes. Solution may be filtered back and reused.
11. Rinse in distilled water.
12. 1% acetic water for 3 to 5 minutes. Discard solution.
13. Dehydrate, clear in xylene, and coverslip, using a synthetic mounting medium.

Results (Plates 1, S, and 2, X)

Nuclei—black

Cytoplasm, keratin, muscle fibers—red

Collagen, mucin—blue

Note: When 2 to 4 μm paraffin sections of renal biopsy specimens are being stained, staining times may be shortened as follows:

Biebrich scarlet–acid fuchsin solution	5 min
Phosphomolybdic-phosphotungstic acid solution	10 to 12 min
Aniline blue solution	3 min

Mallory's aniline blue collagen stain[17]

Fixation. Tissue must be Zenker-fixed.

Embedding. Cut paraffin sections at 5 μm.

Solutions

Acid fuchsin solution

Acid fuchsin	0.5 gm
Distilled water	100 ml

Aniline blue-orange G solution

Aniline blue, water soluble	0.5 gm
Orange G	2 gm
Phosphotungstic acid	1 gm
Distilled water	100 ml

Technic

1. Hydrate sections.
2. Remove mercury deposits (pp. 46 and 131).
3. Wash well in running water.
4. Stain sections in acid fuchsin solution for 1 to 5 minutes. (This step may be omitted so that the collagenous fibers may be brought out more sharply.)
5. Transfer directly to aniline blue solution for 30 minutes to 1 hour or longer.
6. Dehydrate, clear in xylene, and coverslip, using a synthetic mounting medium.

Results

Nuclei—red

Collagenous fibrils—blue

Ground substance, cartilage, mucin, amyloid—varying shades of blue

Erythrocytes, myelin—yellow

Elastic fibrils—pale pink, pale yellow, or unstained

Heidenhain's aniline blue stain[13] or azan technic

Fixation. Zenker's, Helly's, Bouin's, or Carnoy's fluids.

Embedding. Cut paraffin sections at 5 μm.

Solutions

Azocarmine B solution

Azocarmine B	1 gm
Distilled water	200 ml
Glacial acetic acid	1 ml

Bring azocarmine and distilled water to a boil. Filter at 56° C. Cool and add glacial acetic acid. This solution contains fine needlelike crystals that will go into solution at 56° C. Store at 4° C. Refilter before use.

Aniline alcohol solution

Aniline oil	0.1 ml
95% alcohol	100 ml

Acetic alcohol

Glacial acetic acid	1 ml
95% alcohol	100 ml

Phosphotungstic acid solution

Phosphotungstic acid	5 gm
Distilled water	100 ml

Aniline blue solution

Aniline blue	0.5 gm
Orange G	2 gm
Acetic acid	8 ml
Distilled water	300 ml

Technic

1. Hydrate sections to distilled water.
2. Remove mercury precipitate if necessary (pp. 46 and 131).

3. Stain in filtered preheated azocarmine solution for 15 minutes at 56° C.
4. Rinse in distilled water.
5. Differentiate in aniline oil solution until cytoplasm and connective tissue are pale pink and nuclei stand out sharply.
6. Control differentiation by rinsing in 1% acetic alcohol.
7. Mordant in 5% phosphotungstic acid for 10 to 15 minutes.
8. Rinse in distilled water.
9. Counterstain with aniline blue solution until the finest connective tissue fibers are sharply stained. About 15 minutes.
10. Rinse in distilled water.
11. Dehydrate, clear in xylene, and coverslip, using a synthetic mounting medium.

Results (Plate 2, X)

Chromatin, osteocytes, neuroglia—red

Cytoplasm—pink to blue

Collagen and reticulum—blue

Muscle—red to yellow

Gomori's one-step trichrome stain[18]

Principle. Gomori's one-step trichrome is a staining procedure that combines the plasma stain (chromotrope 2R) and connective fiber stain (either light green or fast green FCF) in a phosphotungstic acid solution to which glacial acetic acid has been added. Pretreatment of sections with hot Bouin's solution intensifies the staining colors. Phosphotungstic acid favors the red shades of muscle and cytoplasm. The collagen fibers specifically take up the tungstate ion and the fast green is subsequently bound to this complex, coloring the collagen green. The acetic acid rinse makes the color shades more transparent, but does not alter the color balance.

Fixation. Any well-fixed tissue.

Embedding. Cut paraffin sections at 5 μm.

Solutions

Bouin's fluid (p. 47)

Weigert's iron hematoxylin (p. 190)

Trichrome stain

Chromotrope 2R	0.6 gm
Light green SF yellowish or fast green FCF	0.3 gm
Acetic acid	1 ml
Phosphotungstic acid	0.8 gm
Distilled water	100 ml

Keep stain in refrigerator. Aniline blue may substitute as the fiber dye.

0.5% acetic acid

Technic

1. Hydrate sections.
2. Place in Bouin's fixative for 1 hour at 56° C or overnight at room temperature. Make sure dish

or jar is covered. Cool for 5 to 10 minutes if slides are postfixed with heat, before proceeding with step 3.

3. Wash well in running water to remove all yellow color.
4. Stain nuclei with Weigert's iron hematoxylin for 10 minutes.
5. Wash in tap water for 10 minutes.
6. Trichrome stain for 15 to 20 minutes. Solution may be filtered back and reused.
7. Rinse in 0.5% acetic water for 2 minutes. If the stain is too dark, decolorize in 1% acetic water plus 0.7% phosphotungstic acid solution.
8. Dehydrate, clear in xylene, and coverslip, using a synthetic mounting medium.

Results

Cell cytoplasm, muscle fibers—red
Collagen—green (a blue if aniline blue was used in the trichrome solution)
Nuclei—blue to black

Trichrome method for muscle biopsies[19]

Solutions

Harris's hematoxylin (p. 142)
Gomori's trichrome stain

Chromotrope 2R	0.6 gm
Fast green FCF	0.3 gm
Phosphotungstic acid	0.6 gm
Glacial acetic acid	1 ml
Distilled water	to make 100 ml

Adjust the pH of the above mixture to 3.4 using 1 N NaOH. Solution should be freshly prepared each week.
0.2% acetic acid

Technic

1. Freeze the unfixed muscle using chilled isopentane (p. 294).
2. Pick up 2 to 10 μm frozen sections using cool coverslip. Allow sections to dry for 2 to 20 minutes at room temperature.
3. Stain sections in Harris's hematoxylin for 5 minutes.
4. Rinse briefly in 3 changes of distilled water.
5. Stain for 10 minutes in the Gomori's trichrome solution, pH 3.4.
6. Differentiate using 0.2% acetic acid. A few dips should be sufficient.
7. Dehydrate, clear in xylene, and coverslip, using a synthetic mounting medium.

Results

Nuclei—red-purple
Normal muscle myofibrils—green with distinct A and I bands.
Intermyofibrillar muscle—red
Interstitial collagen—green

Phosphotungstic acid–hematoxylin methods

Hematoxylin solutions employing a tungsten mordant in the form of phosphotungstic acid may be used to demonstrate collagen and muscle fibers. (Additional uses are described under the heading Diagnostic Applications, p. 188.)

There are numerous modifications of the PTAH procedure. Most call for fixation or postmordanting in Zenker's fluid. Although it is true that the mercuric chloride component of the Zenker's could increase affinity for the dye, the requirement for the Zenker's is probably not totally necessary. Potassium permanganate is the second major solution in many PTAH modifications and is believed to function as a dye-trapping agent. What factors determine which cells retain the permanganate and which cells lose it after the oxalic acid treatment are unknown, but cell-membrane permeabilities are believed to be involved, rather than some chemical reaction with a specific chemical component of the cell.[20] Fixation would, of course, have some effect on permeabilities.

The results seen after staining with PTAH are interesting because the single solution gives two major colors, blue and reddish brown. In the staining solution, the ratio of phosphotungstic acid is far in excess of hematein (20:1). One theory states that all the available hematein is bound by the tungsten to give a blue-colored lake, and this lake provides the blue color to selected tissue components. The components demonstrated red-brown are believed to be stained by the phosphotungstic acid, which is reddish colored and present in excess. Tissue components colored by the phosphotungstic acid lose their red color with water or prolonged alcohol washes, hence the necessity for rapid dehydration after staining.

PTAH solutions are stable for prolonged periods, especially if, after ripening, they are kept in a brown bottle and stored in the dark at room temperature.[10]

Appropriate control tissues that may be used to check the strength of the PTAH solution include (1) striated muscle and (2) brain. Striated muscle should color deep blue with well-defined striations. Brain sections should show the following colors:

Axons, dendrites, neuronal nuclei—blue to blue-purple
Neuronal cytoplasm and collagen—red-brown

An overoxidized PTAH solution will fail to show proper density of blue tones and should be replaced.

Mallory's phosphotungstic acid–hematoxylin stain [13]

Fixation. Zenker's fluid; 10% neutral buffered formalin.

Embedding. Paraffin. Cut sections at 5 μm.

Solutions

Zenker's fluid (p. 46)

Phosphotungstic acid–hematoxylin

Hematoxylin	1 gm
Phosphotungstic acid	20 gm
Distilled water	1 liter

Dissolve the solid ingredients in separate portions of the water. Use gentle heat to dissolve the hematoxylin. Combine the two when cool. The solutions ripen in several weeks and this naturally ripened solution works best. If the stain is needed for immediate use however, Mallory recommends adding 0.177 gm of potassium permanganate to the solution. Solution artificially ripened is reddish brown when ready for use.

0.25% potassium permanganate

Potassium permanganate	0.25 gm
Distilled water	100 ml

5% oxalic acid

Oxalic acid	5 gm
Distilled water	100 ml

Technic

1. Hydrate slides. Mordant, if tissues are not Zenker-fixed, for 3 hours in Zenker's fixative at 56° C.
2. Rinse in distilled water. De-Zenkerize tissues to remove mercury precipitate (p. 131).
   Note: If tissue from the central nervous system is being stained, do *not* use sodium thiosulfate to decolorize excess iodine during the mercury precipitate removal process; otherwise, subsequent staining will be impaired. Instead, decolorize in 95% ethanol for 1 hour or longer.[22]
3. Place in 0.25% potassium permanganate solution for 10 minutes.
4. Wash in water.
5. Place in 5% oxalic acid solution for 10 minutes.
6. Wash thoroughly in several changes of tap water. Rinse in distilled water.
7. Stain in PTAH solution 12 to 24 hours at room temperature or for 2 hours at 56° C. Stain may be filtered back and reused.
8. Transfer slides from stain directly to 95% ethanol; follow this with several changes of absolute alcohol. Dehydration should be carried out QUICKLY as alcohol treatment may extract the red shades from the tissue.
9. Clear in xylene and coverslip, using a synthetic mounting medium.

Results (Plate 1, *R*)

Nuclei—blue
Cytoplasm—blue

Collagen—brown-pink
Fibrin—blue
Coarse elastic fibers—purplish
Mitotic figures—blue
Mitochondria and astrocytes—blue
Striated muscle fibers—blue
Neuronal and glial cell processes—blue-purple

Rapid PTAH method [23]

Solutions

Langeron's iodine (p. 131)
5% sodium thiosulfate
PTAH solution (see preceding technic)

Technic

1. Hydrate sections.
2. Langeron's iodine for 10 minutes. Discard solution after use.
3. 5% sodium thiosulfate for 5 minutes. Discard solution.
   Note: Even tissues fixed in a non–mercury containing fixative must go through steps 2 and 3.
4. Wash in running tap water for 5 minutes.
5. Stain in PTAH solution for approximately 1 hour at 60° C.
6. Rapidly dehydrate in 2 changes of 95% ethanol and 2 changes of absolute ethanol, clear in xylene, and coverslip, using a synthetic mounting medium.

Results

Nuclei, muscle, cytoplasm, fibrin, keratin—various shades of blue
Collagen, reticulum, basement membranes, cartilage—various shades of red to red-brown

Long PTAH method [14,24]

Solutions

Zenker's fluid (p. 46)
Weigert's iodine (p. 131)
5% sodium thiosulfate
0.5% potassium permanganate—prepare fresh
5% oxalic acid
4% ferric alum
PTAH solution (See column on left.)

Technic

1. Hydrate sections.
2. Treat with Zenker's fixative for 24 hours at room temperature. Discard after use. Rinse slides in distilled water.
3. Weigert's iodine for 5 minutes. Discard after use.
4. 5% sodium thiosulfate for 5 minutes. Discard after use.
5. Rinse in running tap water for 5 minutes.
6. 0.5% potassium permanganate for 5 minutes. Discard after use.
7. Wash in tap water for 3 minutes. Rinse in distilled water.
8. Decolorize with 5% oxalic acid for 4 minutes. Discard solution after use.

9. Wash in tap water. Rinse in distilled water.
10. Mordant 1 hour in 4% ferric alum at room temperature. Discard solution after use.
11. Rinse in tap and distilled water.
12. Stain in PTAH solution for 18 to 24 hours at room temperature in the dark. Refilter solution for reuse.
13. Rapidly dehydrate in 95% to 100% ethanol, clear in xylene, and coverslip, using a synthetic mounting medium.

Results

See preceding method.

Periodic acid oxidation methods

There are two methods, using periodic acid as oxidant, that may be used to demonstrate collagen, reticular fibers, and basement membranes. The first technique is the periodic acid–Schiff technic, and fibers stain red–purplish red (see PAS discussion). In collagen the positive reaction is given largely by the nonglucosamine polysaccharide complex that is conjugated with the collagen.[25]

Lillie's allochrome procedure is the second method in this classification and differentiates between collagen, reticular fibers, and basement membranes. The sequence procedure employs, first, the periodic acid–Schiff technic, followed by a nuclear stain using Weigert's iron hematoxylin, followed by a selective collagen stain as a counterstain to the PAS reaction. This selective collagen stain is a mixture of picric acid with methyl blue and exhibits a strong selectivity for collagen. The collagen fiber shows a color change from red to blue during the staining process. Glomerular and renal tubule basement membranes are usually red, whereas fine reticular fibrils and more delicate basement membranes are intermediate in their reaction and vary in color from red to violet-black to blue.

Lillie's allochrome procedure[26]

Fixation. Any well-fixed tissue may be used.
Embedding. Paraffin. Sections cut at 5 μm.

Solutions

1% aqueous periodic acid
Schiff reagent (p. 165)
0.5% sodium metabisulfite
Weigert's iron hematoxylin (p. 190)
Collagen stain: 40 mg of methyl blue (C.I. 42780) dissolved in 100 ml of saturated aqueous picric acid.

Method

1. Hydrate slides.
2. Oxidize 10 minutes in 1% aqueous periodic acid.

3. Wash 5 minutes in running water to remove excess traces of the acid.
4. Place in Schiff's reagent for 10 to 15 minutes.
5. Immerse in three separate changes of 0.5% sodium metabisulfite, 2 minutes each change. Wash 10 minutes in running water.
6. Stain 2 minutes in Weigert's iron hematoxylin.
7. Wash 10 minutes in running tap water.
8. Stain 6 minutes in collagen stain.
9. Dehydrate and differentiate in 2 changes each of 95% and absolute alcohol, clear in xylene, and coverslip, using a synthetic mounting medium.

Results (Plate 1, V)

Nuclei—black, gray, or brown
Cytoplasm and muscle cells—gray-green to greenish yellow
Collagen—blue
Reticular connective tissue—usually blue
Glomerular basement membranes—red-purple

ELASTIC FIBERS

Elastic fibers constitute the third type of connective tissue fiber and are highly refractive, elastic, and usually thinner than collagen fibers. Ultrastructural studies have shown that elastic fibers contain at least two distinct components, a central amorphous constituent called elastin and a microfibrillar component.[27-29] Elastic fibers stain with acid dyes and also may be colored deeply by certain specific dyes such as orcein, resorcin-fuchsin, orcinol–new fuchsin, aldehyde fuchsin, and Verhoeff's stain.

Diagnostic applications of elastic fiber methods

Elastic fiber demonstration methods are useful in demonstrating atrophy of elastic tissue, as may be seen, for example, in cases of emphysema. The technics can show thinning and loss of elastic fibers that can occur as a result of arteriosclerosis. Breaks, splitting, and reduplication of elastic lamellae that occur in various other vascular diseases can also be demonstrated.

Elastic fiber technics that incorporate a nuclear stain are valuable for determining if a particular cancer has progressed so far that it has invaded blood vessels. Evidence of tumor metastasis, of course, may change treatment plans and affect overall prognosis.

Elastic fiber–staining procedures
Weigert's resorcin-fuchsin[30]

The first step in the staining procedure is the nuclear staining with Weigert's iron hematoxylin. The iron hematoxylin is used rather than an alum hematoxylin because the high acidity and alcohol content of the resorcin-fuchsin, which follows in the sequence procedure, would over-differentiate an alum hematoxylin. An iron hematoxylin is not affected this way. The resorcin-fuchsin solution is actually a complex formed from an iron resorcin lake of the basic fuchsin, and it is this complex that attaches to the elastic fibers and renders them blue-black. The mode of attachment is not known but may be through formation of hydrogen bonds of some part of the elastic tissue with the phenol groups of the resorcin. A Van Gieson counterstain follows the elastic fiber stain and renders collagen red and other tissue elements yellow. This counterstain takes advantage of the fact that picric acid solutions combine with many dyes to form a complex that has a particular affinity for collagen. Here the collagen is bright red because fuchsin is the dye used with the picric acid. A further note on staining with resorcin-fuchsin is that the counterstain should always follow the actual resorcin-fuchsin stain. Silver impregnations, if performed, should precede the resorcin-fuchsin staining.

Fixation. Alcohol or 10% formalin is preferable, but other fixing reagents give excellent results.

Embedding. Cut paraffin sections at 5 μm.

Solutions
Weigert's hematoxylin (p. 190)
Resorcin-fuchsin solution

Basic fuchsin	2 gm
Resorcinol	4 gm

(It should be fresh and crystalline.)

Distilled water   200 ml

Bring the solution to boil in an enamel dish, and when it is briskly boiling, add 25 ml of a 29% aqueous solution of ferric chloride. Stir and boil for 2 to 5 minutes more. Cool and filter. The filtrate is discarded. Leave the precipitate on the filter paper until it is thoroughly dry. Then return filter paper and precipitate to the enamel dish, which should be dry but still contain whatever part of the precipitate remains adherent to it. Add 200 ml of 95% alcohol and heat carefully. Stir constantly and discard the filter paper when the precipitate on it has dissolved. Cool, filter, and add 95% alcohol to make up the 200 ml. Add 4 ml of hydrochloric acid. The solution keeps well for months.

Van Gieson solution (p. 189)

Technic
1. Hydrate slides.
2. Weigert's hematoxylin solution for 10 minutes.
3. Wash in tap water for 10 minutes.
4. Stain in resorcin-fuchsin solution for 30 to 60 minutes. Check with microscope and stain until elastic fibers are black.
5. Wash off excess stain in 95% alcohol.
6. Wash in tap water.
7. Counterstain in Van Gieson's solution for 1 minute.
8. Dehydrate, clear in xylene, and coverslip, using a synthetic mounting medium.

Results
Elastic fibers—blue-black to black
Nuclei—blue to black
Collagen—pink-red
Other tissue elements—yellow

Alternately, one may stain sections overnight in the following resorcin-fuchsin mixture:

Hart's resorcin-fuchsin solution[13,22]

Stock resorcin-fuchsin	10 ml
70% ethanol	100 ml
Concentrated hydrochloric acid	2 ml

After staining, sections may be rinsed briefly in acid alcohol and the procedure outlined above continued at step 9.

Orcinol–new fuchsin[31]

The orcinol–new fuchsin technic stains elastic tissue only, and this is an advantage over other elastic tissue methods, which, in addition to coloring elastic tissue, also stain nuclei, collagen, and certain other cells and granules to some degree. The orcinol–new fuchsin reagent is prepared much like Weigert's resorcin-fuchsin, but no hydrochloric acid is added. Elimination of this acid was found to increase the selectivity of the reagent for the elastic fiber. Exact mechanism of the reaction is unknown.

Fixation. Any well-fixed tissue.

Embedding. Cut paraffin sections at 5 μm.

Solutions
Orcinol–new fuchsin
Staining solution

Two grams of new fuchsin and 4 gm of orcinol (highest purity) are added to 200 ml of distilled water, and the solution is boiled for 5 minutes; 25 ml of 10% aqueous ferric chloride solution is added and the solution is boiled for 5 minutes longer. After cooling, the precipitate is collected on a filter (washing and drying are unnecessary) and dissolved in 100 ml of 95% ethanol. The solution is ready for immediate use.

Technic
1. Deparaffinize sections in xylene and take them to absolute alcohol.
2. Stain for 15 minutes at 37° C with orcinol–new fuchsin staining solution.

3. Differentiate in 70% alcohol for 15 minutes (3 changes of 5 minutes each).
4. Dehydrate through absolute alcohol, clear in xylene, and coverslip, using a synthetic mounting medium.

Results

Elastic fibers—deep violet with a brownish tinge
Collagen—unstained

Verhoeff–Van Gieson technic[13]

The first step in the procedure is an overstaining of the tissue section with a soluble lake of hematoxylin–ferric chloride–iodine. Ferric chloride and iodine both serve mordant functions primarily and oxidizing functions secondarily. The latter characteristic will assist in the conversion of hematoxylin dye to hematein. In addition, the iodine may serve as a dye-trapping agent,[20] thereby retarding dye loss from selected components during the subsequent differentiation process.

Elastic-fiber staining shows properties that indicate a nonelectrostatic type of bond, and the proposed dye-binding mechanism is hydrogen bonding.[32] The identity of the chemical groups that form the hydrogen bonds with the hematoxylin has not been determined. As noted previously, ultrastructural studies show elastic fibers to be composed of a central amorphous substance called "elastin" surrounded by microfibrils. The elastin portion stains more densely with the Verhoeff mixture than does the microfibrillar component. The only residues present in the elastin, but lacking in the microfibrils, are desmosine, isodesmosine and n(5-amino,5-carboxypentyl) lysine, hence the selective staining by hydrogen bonding is believed to occur at these sites.

Other tissue constituents have been described as staining with Verhoeff's iron hematoxylin at an ultrastructural level, including ribosomes, heterochromatin, and secretory granules.[27] Evidence indicates that the staining of these structures is not by hydrogen bonds but is electrostatic in nature. This, in turn, suggests that the Verhoeff solution is amphoteric, or perhaps more than one staining moiety is present in the Verhoeff mixture.[27]

Differentiation, a necessary step in any overstaining process, is accomplished by use of excess mordant (a dilute solution of ferric chloride) to break the tissue-mordant-dye complex. The dye distributes itself partly as a soluble lake with the free mordant, and partly as a component of the insoluble complex. Since the amount of mordant in the complex is small in comparison with the amount in the differentiating fluid, nearly all the dye will eventually associate itself with the differentiator. Since this is soluble, it will be removed in the next washings. The elastic tissues, having the strongest affinity for the insoluble complex, retain it the longest and so are colored black in the final result.

Sodium thiosulfate (hypo) is used to remove the excess iodine from the solution, and tap water removes both from the tissue section. The Van Gieson solution of acid fuchsin and picric acid is used as the counterstain and colors the collagen bright red and other tissue elements yellow.

The period of counterstaining with the Van Gieson solution must not be prolonged, since the picric acid will then act to further differentiate the stain.

Fixation. Any well-fixed tissue. 10% neutral buffered formalin or Zenker's preferred. It is not necessary to remove mercury deposits if tissues have been fixed in a mercury-containing fixative, since they will be removed by the staining solution.

Embedding. Cut paraffin sections at 5 μm.

Solutions

5% hematoxylin solution in absolute ethanol
Dissolve the hematoxylin in the absolute ethanol with the aid of gentle heat. Filter. A small amount of this solution may be prepared as needed for immediate use in the staining solution. Alternatively, a larger amount may be prepared and stored for later use. Solution is stable for several months.

10% aqueous ferric chloride (prepare fresh)

Weigert's iodine solution (p. 131)
This solution may be prepared fresh as needed or made in larger quantities and stored in a brown bottle in the dark at room temperature.

Verhoeff's staining solution
The working staining solution should be made up *fresh* for best results. It will not stain satisfactorily if it is kept more than one working day.

Prepare the working solution by adding *in order* the following reagents:

5% alcoholic hematoxylin	20 ml
10% freshly prepared ferric chloride	8 ml
Weigert's iodine solution	8 ml

Mix the above amounts (or needed proportions thereof) well. Solution should be jet black. Use immediately.

2% aqueous ferric chloride (prepare fresh)
5% aqueous sodium thiosulfate
Van Gieson's counterstain (p. 189)

Technic

1. Hydrate slides to distilled water.
2. Stain in Verhoeff's solution for 1 hour. Tissue should be completely black. At the conclusion of the staining time, pour the Verhoeff mixture into a container and save it until after the differentiation process has been properly completed. If it should prove necessary to restain, this saved solution may be used.
3. Rinse in tap water with 2 or 3 changes.
4. Differentiate in 2% ferric chloride. Agitate slides gently during this process. Stop differentiation with *several* changes of tap water and check microscopically for black elastic fiber staining and gray background. Repeat 2% ferric chloride treatment and tap water rinses as necessary for adequate demonstration. Kidney and myometrium are good controls. If the elastic fiber staining is too pale, restain in the saved Verhoeff's solution for 30 minutes and then proceed with the differentiation process.
   It is better to *slightly* underdifferentiate the tissue, since the subsequent Van Gieson's counterstain can extract the elastic stain somewhat.
5. Wash slides in tap water.
6. Treat with 5% sodium thiosulfate for 1 minute. Discard solution.
7. Wash in running tap water for 5 minutes.
8. Counterstain in Van Gieson's solution for 3 to 5 minutes.
9. Dehydrate, clear in xylene, and coverslip, using a synthetic mounting medium.

Results (Plate 1, *W*)

Elastic fibers—blue-black to black (fine elastic fibrils may not be stained by this method)
Nuclei—blue to black
Collagen—red
Other tissue elements—yellow

Gomori's aldehyde fuchsin[33]

This technic may be employed for staining elastic fibers in tissue sections but has other uses as a special stain for demonstrating beta cells of pancreatic islets and hypophyseal granules. The staining solution is prepared by the addition of hydrochloric acid and paraldehyde to basic fuchsin in an alcohol solution. Paraldehyde, a trimer of acetaldehyde, increases the depth of the stain by linking with the basic fuchsin and forming aldehyde fuchsin. The aldehyde and fuchsin form Schiff bases, which have an unexplained affinity for elastic fibers and color them a deep purple. Beta cells, mentioned above, are also basophilic and are colored purple. Other tissue elements are stained according to the counterstain employed.

Fixation. Avoid chromate fixation. Formalin and Bouin's fluid give colorless backgrounds, and mercury fixatives give a pale lilac. Formalin preferred.

Embedding. Cut paraffin sections at 5 μm.

Solutions

Working light green counterstain (p. 187)
Aldehyde fuchsin solution

Basic fuchsin	1 gm
70% alcohol	200 ml
Hydrochloric acid	2 ml
Fresh paraldehyde	2 ml

Let stand at room temperature for 2 to 3 days or until stain is deep purple in color. Filter and store in refrigerator. *Note:* A 60% ethanol solution may be used instead of the traditional 70% concentration with good results.[34]

Solution and technic variables

1. *Fresh* paraldehyde should be used in the solution preparation. Do not use bottles or vials that have been previously opened.
2. Allow the solution to ripen sufficiently at room temperature prior to use.
3. Solutions that contain basic fuchsin that is mainly rosanilin (C.I. 42510) will not stain properly fixed substances that are reported to stain with aldehyde fuchsin. The aldehyde fuchsin solution should be made from basic fuchsin that is mainly pararosanilin (C.I. 42500).[36] Consult reference 36 for further details.
4. Inadequate tissue fixation and insufficient staining time will produce poor results even when a good solution of the dye is used.
5. Aldehyde fuchsin is stable for approximately 2 to 3 months when stored at 4° C; deteriorating solutions show poorly stained elastic fibers. It is suggested that 50 ml of ripened aldehyde fuchsin stock solution be kept in a separate Coplin jar, used for a 1-week period, and then discarded. Although the actual tissue staining takes place at room temperature, the aldehyde fuchsin solution should be returned to 4° C as soon as possible. Newly ripened aldehyde fuchsin is required for proper demonstration of beta cells and sulfated mucopolysaccharides.
6. An aldehyde fuchsin crystalline artifact can occur if sections are not quickly rinsed in 95% ethanol after completion of the stain.[35]

Technic

1. Hydrate sections to 70% ethanol.
2. Stain in aldehyde fuchsin. Freshly ripened solution will stain elastic fibers in 10 minutes, but beta cells of pancreatic islets in 30 minutes to 2 hours.
3. Rinse excess stain with a quick rinse in 95% ethanol, followed by 2 or 3 changes of distilled water, and check microscopically for proper staining. If further staining is necessary, rinse in 70% ethanol and return to aldehyde fuchsin. If further differentiation is necessary, it may be accomplished with additional rinse in 70%

ethanol. Control differentiation with distilled water rinses. Refilter aldehyde fuchsin after use.
4. Rinse slides in distilled water.
5. Counterstain with a working solution of light green for 1 to 2 minutes. Discard solution.
6. Dehydrate, clear in xylene, and coverslip, using a synthetic mounting medium.

Results (Plate 1, *T*)

Elastic fibers, mast cell granules, gastric chief cells, beta cells of pancreatic islets, and certain of the hypophyseal granules—violet to purple
Other tissue elements—green

Orcein methods

Paraffin sections of formalin-fixed tissues may be hydrated to 70% ethanol and stained for 30 minutes in the following solution[37]:

Acid orcein solution

Synthetic orcein (Harleco Co.)	0.2 gm
70% alcohol	100 ml
Concentrated hydrochloric acid	0.6 ml

Solution is ready for staining immediately and improves on standing. It is stable for many months. A wash in running tap water for 15 minutes follows the orcein solution. Elastic fibers should be stained a dark brown.

Tissues may be counterstained overnight in a dilute Giemsa solution (2 drops of Giemsa stock to 40 ml distilled water adjusted to pH 7 with phosphate buffer). Alternatively, the following counterstains may be employed: Unna's polychrome methylene blue (p. 150) for 1 minute; alum hematoxylin (p. 142) for 3 to 6 minutes; picroindigocarmine (p. 166) for 6 minutes. Dehydrate, clear, and coverslip in a synthetic resin. Tissue elements other than elastic fibers will color according to the counterstain used.

MISCELLANEOUS CONNECTIVE TISSUE AND MUSCLE DEMONSTRATION METHODS
Movat's pentachrome [38]

Principle. An alcian blue solution is used to color the acid mucopolysaccharide component of ground substance blue to blue-green. (See mechanism under alcian blue staining.) The alkaline alcohol solution next employed functions to convert the alcian blue staining into insoluble monastral fast blue. This conversion is necessary because of the length of time needed to complete the procedure and because the high acid and alcohol content of the resorcin-fuchsin solution used would decolorize the alcian blue stain. Resorcin-fuchsin demonstrates the elastic tissue and the suggested mechanism for this procedure has been discussed previously. The diluted resorcin-fuchsin is used instead of Weigert's stock resorcin-fuchsin because the latter

does not give good results with tissues fixed in mercury-containing solutions, the preferred fixative fluids for this method. Weigert's iron hematoxylin functions as a nuclear stain. Woodstain scarlet–acid fuchsin (both components being acid dyes) stain muscle, cell cytoplasm, collagen, and reticular fibers and overlies the monastral fast blue stain of the ground substance. Differentiation with phosphotungstic acid functions to remove the woodstain scarlet–acid fuchsin stain from the extracellular connective tissue fibers (collagen and reticulum) and ground substance. When the woodstain scarlet–acid fuchsin solution is removed from the ground substance, the staining with the insoluble monastral fast blue is again shown. The phosphotungstic acid solution is removed with an acetic water wash, and alcoholic saffron, functioning as an acid dye, is then used to demonstrate collagen and reticular fibers.

Fixation. Movat recommends that the tissue specimens be fixed for 12 to 18 hours in acetic formalin sublimate (mercuric chloride, 4 gm; 37% to 40% formaldehyde, 20 ml; distilled water, 80 ml; glacial acetic acid, 5 ml). Specimens fixed in neutral buffered formalin or Bouin's fluid may also be used.

Embedding. Cut paraffin sections at 5 μm.

Solutions

Alcian blue
Alcian blue 8GS	1 gm
Distilled water	100 ml
Glacial acetic acid	1 ml

Mix and filter before use.
Alkaline alcohol
95% ethanol	100 ml
28% ammonium hydroxide	in drops

Add ammonium hydroxide to the alcohol, drop by drop, until a pH of 8 or higher is reached.
Hart's resorcin-fuchsin solution (p. 195)
Weigert's iron hematoxylin (p. 190)
Woodstain scarlet stock solution
Woodstain scarlet NS	0.1 gm
(E. I. Du Pont de Nemours & Co., Inc., Wilmington, DE 19898)	
Glacial acetic acid	0.5 ml
Distilled water	to make 100 ml

Mix and filter.
Acid fuchsin stock solution
Acid fuchsin	0.1 gm
Glacial acetic acid	0.5 ml
Distilled water	to make 100 ml

Mix and filter.
Working woodstain scarlet–acid fuchsin solution
Stock woodstain scarlet	80 ml
Stock acid fuchsin	20 ml

0.5% aqueous acetic acid
5% aqueous phosphotungstic acid

Alcoholic saffron

> Saffron (Safran du Gâtinais) (Roboz Surgical Instrument Co., Washington, DC 20006)   6 gm
>
> Absolute ethanol   to make 100 ml
>
> Place the saffron in the alcohol in an airtight container at 56° to 58° C for 48 hours. Keep in an airtight brown bottle.

Technic

1. Hydrate sections to distilled water. Remove mercury precipitates if necessary (p. 131) and follow this removal with several rinses in distilled water.
2. Alcian blue solution for 20 to 30 minutes.
3. Running tap water for 3 minutes.
4. Alkaline alcohol solution for 2 hours.
5. Running tap water for 10 minutes.
6. Rinse in 70% ethanol.
7. Resorcin-fuchsin for 16 hours.
8. Running tap water for 10 minutes.
9. Rinse in distilled water.
10. Weigert's iron hematoxylin for 10 minutes.
11. Running tap water for 10 minutes.
12. Rinse in distilled water.
13. Working solution of woodstain scarlet–acid fuchsin for 5 minutes.
14. Rinse in 0.5% acetic acid.
15. 5% phosphotungstic acid for 10 to 20 minutes. Check microscopically. Continue differentiation until collagen is pale pink in color and the ground substance, initially colored red, becomes bluish in color.
16. Rinse in 0.5% acetic acid.
17. Wash thoroughly in 3 changes of *absolute* ethanol.
18. Alcoholic saffron for 15 minutes. Use a screw-capped Coplin jar for this step, and keep the jar sealed during the staining procedure. If collagen is not sufficiently yellow, stain for a longer period.
19. Dehydrate in 3 changes of absolute alcohol, clear in xylene, and coverslip, using a synthetic mounting medium.

Results

Nuclei—black
Cell cytoplasm, muscle—red
Fibrinoid—intense red
Ground substance—blue to blue-green
Elastic fibers—dark purple to black
Collagen, reticular fibers—yellow

Hematoxylin–basic fuchsin–picric acid method for myocardial ischemia [39]

Principle. The H & E method does not reveal unequivocal morphologic changes in cases of myocardial infarction until 15 to 20 hours have elapsed after the onset of the injury. The HBFP technic detects early changes of myocardial infraction by coloring affected fibers red.

Normal and frankly ischemic myocardium colors yellow. The differential staining results are believed to be caused by an unstable protein complex present in the early phases of myocardial ischemia.

Fixation. 10% neutral buffered formalin.

Embedding. Cut paraffin sections at 5 μm.

Solutions

Alum hematoxylin (solution A)

Ammonium aluminum sulfate	6 gm
Hematoxylin	0.5 gm
Yellow mercuric oxide	0.25 gm

Mix these 3 ingredients in 70 ml of distilled water. Boil 10 minutes. Cool and add 30 ml of glycerol and 4 ml of glacial acetic acid. Filter before use.

0.1% basic fuchsin in distilled water (solution B)
0.1% picric acid in absolute acetone (solution C)

Technic

1. Deparaffinize and hydrate to distilled water.
2. Stain in solution A for 5 minutes. Filter back.
3. Wash in running tap water for 5 minutes.
4. Stain in solution B for 3 minutes. Discard solution.
5. Rinse briefly (5 to 10 seconds) in distilled water.
6. Rinse briefly (5 to 10 seconds) in absolute acetone.
7. Differentiate in solution C until the red color ceases to run off the section—usually about 20 seconds for human tissue; 15 seconds for animal tissue. Too much or too little decolorization produces false positives and false negatives, respectively. Solution should be changed for every 3 to 5 slides.
8. Rinse briefly (5 to 10 seconds) in absolute acetone.
9. Clear in xylene and coverslip, using a synthetic mounting medium.

Results

Acutely ischemic myocardium—crimson red
Normal myocardium—light brown
Nuclei—blue-purple
Red blood cells, fibrin, plasma, proteins, elastic fibers, collagen—red
Note: The irregular fuchsin staining of myocardial cells along the edge of the section is considered an artifact.

Pamihall connective tissue stain [40]

Fixation. 10% buffered neutral formalin.

Embedding. Cut paraffin sections at 5 μm.

Solutions

1.5% alcian blue solution

Alcian blue, 8GS (C.I. 74240)	1.5 gm
Distilled water	100 ml
Glacial acetic acid	1 ml

Iodine solution

Iodine	2 gm

Potassium iodide	4 gm
Distilled water	100 ml

Hematoxylin solution

15% hematoxylin (C.I. 75290) in absolute ethanol	25 ml
Absolute ethanol	25 ml
15% aqueous ferric chloride	25 ml
Iodine solution	25 ml

5% aqueous sodium thiosulfate

2% aqueous ferric chloride

Crocein scarlet–acid fuchsin solution

Stock solution A

Crocein scarlet 7B (C.I. 27165)	0.125 gm
Distilled water	100 ml
Glacial acetic acid	0.5 ml

Stock solution B

Acid fuchsin (C.I. 42685)	0.125 gm
Distilled water	100 ml
Glacial acetic acid	0.5 ml

Working solution

Mix 10 parts of solution A with 2 parts of solution B.

Note: Biebrich scarlet may be substituted for crocein; however, it lacks the staining brilliance of crocein.

0.5% aqueous acetic acid

5% aqueous phosphotungstic acid

Collagen stains

for blue fibers:

Aniline blue solution

Aniline blue (C.I. 42755)	1 gm
Distilled water	100 ml
Glacial acetic acid	0.5 ml

for green fibers:

Light green solution

Light green SF yellowish (C.I. 42095)	0.2 gm
Distilled water	100 ml
Glacial acetic acid	1 ml

for taupe fibers:

Metanil yellow–basic fuchsin solution

0.5% aqueous metanil yellow stock (C.I. 13065)	40 ml
0.1% aqueous basic fuchsin stock (C.I. 42510)	10 ml

Note: Alcian blue, crocein scarlet, and metanil yellow may be purchased from Roboz Surgical Instrument Co., Inc. (810-18th Street, N.W., Washington, DC 20006).

Technic

1. Hydrate sections to distilled water.
2. Stain in alcian blue for 15 minutes.
3. Wash in running water.
4. Rinse in distilled water.
5. Stain in hematoxylin for 10 minutes (stain will stay stable approximately 3 weeks).
6. Rinse in water.
7. Differentiate in 2% ferric chloride.
8. Rinse in water. Check slide under microscope for nuclear detail (mucopolysaccharides should appear green).
9. Place in sodium thiosulfate for 1 minute.
10. Wash in running water (mucopolysaccharides should appear light sea blue).
11. Stain in crocein scarlet fuchsin for 5 minutes.
12. Rinse in 0.5% acetic acid water, 2 changes.
13. Place slides in 5% phosphotungstic acid for 1 minute.
14. Rinse in 0.5% acetic acid water.

For taupe fibrous tissue:

15. Stain in metanil yellow-basic fuchsin solution for 5 minutes.
16. Rinse very quickly in 95% alcohol.
17. Rinse in absolute alcohol, 2 changes very quickly.
18. Clear in xylene, and coverslip, using a synthetic mounting medium.

For green fibrous tissue:

15. Stain in light green for 5 minutes.
16. Rinse in 95% alcohol, 2 changes quickly.
17. Rinse in absolute alcohol, 2 changes.
18. Clear in xylene, and coverslip, using a synthetic mounting medium.

For blue fibrous tissue:

15. Stain in aniline blue for 2 minutes.
16. Rinse in 0.5% acetic acid water, 2 changes.
17. Rinse in absolute alcohol, 2 changes.
18. Clear in xylene, and coverslip, using a synthetic mounting medium.

Results

Nuclei and elastic fibers—black

Sulfated acid mucopolysaccharides—black cytoplasmic granules

Ground substance, mucin—light sea blue

Skeletal muscle—deep red

Smooth muscle—light red

Erythrocytes, fibrinoid, fibrin—crimson

Fibrous tissue

Royal blue, if aniline blue solution was used

Green, if light green solution was used

Taupe, if metanil yellow–basic fuchsin solution was used

REFERENCES

1. Ham, A. W.: Histology, ed. 7, Philadelphia, 1974, J. B. Lippincott Co.
2. Feigin, I., and Naoumenko, J.: Some chemical principles applicable to some silver and gold staining methods for neuropathological studies, J. Neuropathol. & Exp. Neurol. **35:**495-507, 1976.
3. Wilder, H. C.: An improved technic for silver impregnation of reticulum fibers, Am. J. Pathol. **11:** 815-819, 1935.
4. Foot, N. C.: A technic for demonstrating reticulum fibers in Zenker-fixed paraffin sections, J. Lab. Clin. Med. **9:**777-781, 1924.
5. Gridley, M. F.: A modification of the silver impregnation method of staining reticular fibers, Am. J. Clin. Pathol. **21:**897-899, 1951.
6. Nassar, T. K., and Shanklin, W. M.: Simplified procedure for staining reticulum, Arch. Pathol. **71:**611-614, 1961.

7. Laidlaw, G. F.: Silver staining of the skin and its tumors, Am. J. Pathol. **5:**239-248, 1929.

8. Snook, T.: The guinea-pig spleen; studies on the structure and connections of the venous sinuses, Anat. Rec. **89:**413-427, 1944.

9. Jones, D. B.: Inflammation and repair of the glomerulus, Am. J. Pathol. **27:**991-1009, 1951 (modification).

10. Personal communication, Polly Stanton, Ohio State University Hospitals, Columbus, Ohio, 1978.

11. Gomori, G.: A new histochemical test for glycogen and mucin, Am. J. Clin. Pathol. **16:**177-179, 1946 (modification).

12. Lillie, R. D.: Studies on selective staining of collagen with acid anilin dyes, J. Tech. Meth. **25:**1-43, 1945.

13. Mallory, F. B.: Pathological technique, New York, 1961, Hafner Publishing Co.

14. Lillie, R. D., and Fullmer, H. M.: Histopathologic technic and practical histochemistry, ed. 4, New York, 1976, McGraw-Hill Book Co.

15. Puchtler, H., and Isler, H.: The effect of phosphomolybdic acid on the stainability of connective tissue by various dyes, J. Histochem. Cytochem. **6:**265-270, 1958. The Histochemical Society, Baltimore, The Williams & Wilkins Co. (agent).

16. Masson, P.: Trichrome stainings and their preliminary technique, J. Tech. Meth. **12:**75-90, 1929.

17. Mallory, F. B.: The anilin blue collagen stain, Stain Technol. **11:**101-102, 1936, The Williams & Wilkins Co.

18. Gomori, G.: A rapid one-step trichrome stain, Am. J. Clin. Pathol. **20:**661-664, 1950.

19. Engel, W. K., and Cunningham, G. G.: Rapid examination of muscle tissue: an improved trichrome method for fresh frozen biopsy sections, Neurology **13:**919, 1963, Harcourt, Brace & Jovanovich, Inc.

20. Thompson, S. W.: Selected histochemical and histopathological methods, Springfield, Ill., 1966, Charles C Thomas, Publisher.

21. Luna, L. G., editor: Stability of more commonly used special staining solutions, Histologic 5(3):2, July 1975.

22. Luna, L. G., editor: Manual of histologic staining methods of the Armed Forces Institute of Pathology, ed. 3, New York, 1968, McGraw-Hill Book Co.

23. Puchtler, H., Sweat, F., and Doss, N.: A one-hour phosphotungstic acid hematoxylin stain, Tech. Bull. Reg. Med. Technol. **33:**144-147, 1963.

24. Lieb, E.: Modified phosphotungstic acid–hematoxylin stain, Arch. Pathol. **45:**559-560, 1948.

25. Bangle, R., Jr., and Alford, W. C.: The chemical basis of the periodic acid Schiff reaction of collagen fibers with reference to periodate consumption of collagen and insulin, J. Histochem. Cytochem. **2:**62-76, 1954.

26. Lillie, R. D.: The allochrome method: a differential method segregating the connective tissues, collagen, reticulum and basement membranes into two groups, Am. J. Clin. Pathol. **21:**484-488, 1951.

27. Brissie, R. M., Spicer, S. S., Hall, B. J., and Thompson, N. T.: Ultrastructural staining of thin sections with iron hematoxylin, J. Histochem. Cytochem. **22**(9):895-907, 1974, The Histochemical Society, Baltimore, The Williams & Wilkins Co. (agent).

28. Brissie, R. M., Spicer, S. S., and Thompson, N. T.: Variable fine structure of elastin visualized with Verhoeff's iron hematoxylin, Anat. Rec. **181:**83-94, 1975.

29. Ross, R.: The elastic fiber: a review, J. Histochem. Cytochem. **21**(3):199-208, 1973, The Histochemical Society, Baltimore, The Williams & Wilkins Co. (agent).

30. Mallory, F. B.: Pathological technique, New York, 1961, Hafner Publishing Co.; original reference: Weigert, C.: Ueber eine Methode zur Färbung elastischer Fasern, Zentralbl. Allg. Pathol. **9:**289-292, 1898.

31. Fullmer, H. M., and Lillie, R. D.: A selective stain for elastic tissue, Stain Technol. **31:**27-29, 1956, The Williams & Wilkins Co.

32. Goldstein, D. J.: Ionic and nonionic bonds in staining, with special reference to the action of urea and sodium chloride on the staining of elastic fibres and glycogen, Q. J. Micro. Sci. **103:**477-489, 1962.

33. Gomori, G.: Aldehyde fuchsin—a new stain for elastic tissue, Am. J. Clin. Pathol. **20:**665-666, 1950.

34. Lambert, C., and Futch, H. N.: An evaluation of elastic tissue staining, Am. J. Med. Technol. **42:** 305-309, 1976.

35. Thompson, S. W., and Luna, L. G.: An atlas of artifacts, Springfield, Ill., 1978, Charles C Thomas, Publisher.

36. Mowry, R. W.: Aldehyde fuchsin staining, direct or after oxidation: problems and remedies, with special reference to human pancreatic β cells, pituitaries, and elastic fibers, Stain Technol. **53:** 141-154, 1978, Baltimore, The Williams & Wilkins Co.

37. Pinkus, H.: Acid orcein–giemsa stain (modification of Unna-Taenzer method): useful routine stain for dermatologic sections, Arch. Dermatol. Syph. **49:**355-356, 1944.

38. Movat, H. Z.: Demonstration of all connective tissue elements in a single section, Arch. Pathol. **60:**289-295, 1955.

39. Lie, J. T., Holley, K. E., Kampa, W. R., and Titus, J. L.: New histochemical method for morphological diagnosis of early stages of myocardial ischemia, Mayo Clin. Proc. **46:**319-327, 1971.

40. Personal communication, G. F., Pawlick, O. B. Mitchell, and M. C. Hall, The Permanente Medical Group, San Francisco, California, 1978.

CHAPTER 11

Lipids

CLASSIFICATION

Lipids are a structurally heterogeneous group of substances with the common characteristic of solubility in organic solvents. Classically they may be classified into simple lipids, compound lipids, or derived lipids.[1] *Simple lipids* are esters of fatty acids with alcohols and include fats, oils, and waxes. Fats are neutral esters of glycerol with saturated or unsaturated fatty acids; oils are similar substances but liquid instead of solid at room temperature. Waxes are esters of higher alcohols with long-chain fatty acids (generally C_{34} to C_{36}). Simple fats or triglycerides usually occur in the body as energy stores in adipose tissue. Waxes, though components of some plant and animal species, are not involved in the metabolism of higher species. *Compound lipids* consist of a fatty acid, an alcohol (usually glycerol), and one or more additional groups such as phosphorus or nitrogen. These compound lipids may be subdivided into phospholipids (lecithin, cephalins, and sphingomyelins), glycolipids (cerebrosides and gangliosides), and sulfolipids. These are found primarily in the brain and other nervous tissue. *Derived lipids* refer to the various fatty acids that can be derived from the simple and compound lipids by hydrolysis. Sterols and their esters are usually placed in this class, and specific examples include cholesterol, bile acids, and sex and adrenocortical hormones.

More recently,[2] lipids have been classified as follows:

Triglycerides (including fats and oils)
Glycerophosphatides (including phosphatidic acids, phosphatidyl esters, lysophosphatides, inositol, and acetal phosphatides)
Sphingolipids (including sphingomyelins, cerebrosides, and gangliosides)
Waxes (including true waxes, steryl esters, and vitamin A and D_3 esters)

Lipids may occur in cells either in the form of microscopic droplets or in the form of bound or "masked" lipids that are attached to other tissue components. Free lipid droplets, with little or no binding to the other tissue components, are readily demonstrated by convenient methods, but it is important not to expose such tissue to any fat solvents such as alcohol, acetone, chloroform, xylene, and paraffin. Since these substances are routinely used in the preparation of ordinary histologic sections, simple fats are not preserved in these sections. To be able to demonstrate simple fats, use frozen sections for staining. The lipids that show a moderate to strong binding capacity to other tissue components may resist routine paraffin embedding after fixation and be demonstrated by Sudan dyes or chemical methods using oxidation or mordanting procedures. Examples of such bound lipids include phospholipids, some lipofuscins, and granules of leukocytes. For fat fixation neutral buffered formalin is preferred. A formol-calcium fixative is good for phospholipid preservation.

Demonstration technics for lipids include physical methods without dyes (polarized light, primary fluorescence), physical methods with dyes (lipid soluble dyes such as the Sudans that may or may not be accompanied by various extraction procedures), and chemical methods for various complex lipids.

DEMONSTRATION METHODS WITHOUT DYES
Polarized light[2-5]

So far polarization microscopy has not been used clinically since similar optical patterns may be seen with oriented molecular arrangements of chemically different substances, and thus no conclusions as to the chemical nature of the lipids seen may be drawn.

Results with polarization are variable depending on the state of the lipid at the time of examination. Generally, any lipid in a crystalline state may be anisotropic or birefringent. Cholesterol and its esters may be seen as birefringent, rhomboid needles, or as Maltese-cross patterns. Neutral fats and fatty acids are usually isotropic (monorefringent). The fatty nature of any birefringence seen should be confirmed by examination of a control slide that has been extracted for 10 minutes in a 2:1 chloroform-methanol solution.

Primary fluorescence[2,3,5]

Although some lipids and their oxidized derivatives will exhibit distinct fluorescence, primary fluorescence is still not used as a positive clinical tool for lipid identification. Lipofuscins, certain corticosteroids, and estrogens are some of the better known fluorescent lipids.

METHODS WITH SUDAN AND RELATED DYES

The following methods using the Sudan dyes and oil red O are among the oldest and simplest technics for lipid demonstration.

Staining mechanism

These technics involve primarily physical processes in contrast to most staining procedures, which involve chemical mechanisms. The dye is dissolved in a lipid solvent, and sections are treated with the dye-solvent solution. Since the dye is comparatively more soluble in the lipid in the tissue section than in the original solvent, the dye will move out of the solvent and color the tissue lipid. Substances stainable by such methods are referred to as sudanophilic. Boundary-surface adsorption plays a prominent role in the process. Since the staining is of such a physical nature, chemically different lipids cannot be distinguished by any of the following methods because they will exhibit similar staining characteristics.

The temperature at which a lipid melts will determine to a large extent whether the lipid will stain by the oil-soluble dyes. Usually only liquid lipids take up these stains, but if the staining is carried out at 60° C, a lipid that is solid at room temperature is more likely to melt and admit the dye and consequently be stained. The lipid staining effect of a given method depends both on the dye and its solvent. Fat-staining ability increases with the molecular weight of the dye, and this factor parallels the solubility of the dye itself. Dyes used should be strongly colored, soluble in fat but not soluble in water, not attach to any tissue constituents except by solution, and be more soluble in fat than in the solvents in which they are dissolved.

Lipid extraction[5,6]

A lipid extraction process involves examining an unextracted control tissue and a piece of tissue that has been extracted by any of a number of different methods. Different lipids are removed by the different extraction processes. Cold acetone, for example, removes glycerides; hot acetone removes cerebrosides; hot ether removes lecithins and cephalins; a mixture of hot chloroform and methanol will remove all lipids. After extraction, the tissue is fixed in formalin and washed, and frozen sections are prepared and usually stained. Sections are compared with the nonextracted control tissue that has been fixed in formol-calcium during the period of extraction. Comparison of the extracted and nonextracted tissue will indicate the general distribution of lipid material.

Diagnostic applications of simple fat stains

Simple fat stains such as oil red O and sudan black B are useful for the following:
1. One can demonstrate fat in an abnormal place, such as in the kidneys or in the brain. Bone fractures or crushing injuries to areas of the body containing fat may sometimes cause the fat to be released into the circulation and may ultimately cause a

fat embolism. Fat stains would verify a fat embolism as being the cause of the loss of function or a cause of death.

2. When cells undergo degenerative change, membrane lipid becomes disoriented and stainable with the simple fat stains. In other disease states there is a disturbance of fat metabolism within the cell and the fat can coalesce into droplets. Provided that the tissue is specially processed, the oil red O technic could distinguish between these fine lipid droplets and fine droplets of glycogen.

3. Fat stains may be used in distinguishing a tumor of bizarre morphology. Sometimes it is difficult to determine if a tumor is arising from fat cells or other cell types (such as liposarcoma from rhabdomyosarcoma). Diagnosis would then affect treatment and prognosis.

General comments on procedure when staining with simple fat stains

Fixative considerations. The best fixatives are neutral buffered formalin or formol-calcium. Alcoholic fixatives, or those solutions containing organic solvents, should not be used because of their lipid solubility. Fixation of tissue in mercuric chloride solution tends to produce hardening, and this can cause difficulty with section production. Tissues fixed in a picric acid–containing fixative, such as Bouin's, tend to be difficult to freeze, making frozen-section production a problem.

Processing and sectioning. Simple lipid stains that are supposed to demonstrate the presence or absence of simple lipids are performed on *frozen* sections. The sections may be cut by either a clinical freezing microtome or a cryostat. Generally, free-floating sections stain more rapidly than those mounted on slides. (Simple fat stains may also be done on paraffin sections to demonstrate, for example, lipofuscin or ceroid. Of course, simple lipids themselves will not be shown in such a section because of the solvent action of the reagents used in the preparation.)

Staining. A number of solvents for the simple lipid dyes have been described including 70% ethanol, acetone-ethanol mixtures, isopropanol, and propylene glycol. It is important that the dye solvent not dissolve out any of the tissue lipid. There is minimal removal of tissue lipids with an isopropanol solvent, but no removal with a propylene glycol solvent.

The actual staining process should be carried out in a *closed* container; otherwise, some of the dye solvent can evaporate and the dye itself can precipitate on the tissue.

Coverslipping. Aqueous mounting media, such as glycerol gelatin (glycerin jelly), are used to mount the finished slide. If a synthetic resin is used, the organic solvents present in the medium would dissolve the dye-lipid complex.

If air bubbles are present after coverslipping, they should *not* be pressed out, since this process will displace stained lipid. Instead, reimmerse the slide in warm water until the cover slip falls off; re-wipe excess water from the slide and re-coverslip.

Glycerol gelatin (glycerin jelly) mounting medium is solid at room temperature and has to be warmed prior to use. The solution should not be allowed to get too hot for coverslipping but should be warm enough to be spread easily on the slide.

The formula for Kaiser's glycerin jelly is as follows:

Gelatin	10 gm
Distilled water	52.5 ml
Glycerol	62.5 ml
Phenol crystals	1.25 ml

After mixing, store aliquots of the solution in small brown bottles. Melt as needed for use. Glycerol gelatin (glycerin jelly) is also available commercially.

Demonstration technics
Sudan black B in propylene glycol[7]

Fixation. Formalin or Bouin's.
Embedding. Cut frozen sections at 10 μm.

Solutions
Sudan black B solution
Dissolve 0.7 gm of Sudan black B in 100 ml of propylene glycol. Add a small amount at a time with stirring. Heat to 100° C (not over 110°) for a few minutes, stirring constantly. *Do not exceed 110° C.* Filter through Whatman no. 2 filter paper. Cool to room temperature and filter through fritted glass filter of medium porosity with suction. Store in the oven at 60° C, and the stain will keep almost indefinitely. If precipitate forms in Sudan black B, remove it by skimming the top with a piece of thin paper.
Nuclear fast red (*Kernechtrot*) stain (p. 183)
85% propylene glycol
Kaiser's glycerin jelly (above)
Warm glycerol gelatin prior to use.

Technic

1. Dehydrate for 10 to 15 minutes in absolute propylene glycol.
2. Stain for 10 minutes in Sudan black B.
3. Differentiate in 85% propylene glycol.
4. Wash in distilled water.
5. Counterstain for 1 minute in nuclear fast red.
6. Wash well through several changes of distilled water.
7. Mount in glycerol gelatin.

Results (Plate 2, *P*)

Fat—blue-black
Background—red

Oil red O in propylene glycol[8]

Fixation. Formalin or Bouin's.

Embedding. Cut frozen sections at 10 μm.

Solutions

Oil red O solution
    Dissolve 0.7 gm of oil red O in 100 ml of propylene glycol. Add a small amount at a time with stirring. Heat to 100° C (not over 110°) for a few minutes, stirring constantly. *Do not exceed 110° C.* Filter through Whatman no. 2 filter paper. Cool to room temperature and filter through fritted glass filter of medium porosity with suction. Store in the oven at 60° C and stain will keep almost indefinitely. If precipitate forms in the oil red O, remove it by skimming the top with a piece of thin paper.

Harris's hematoxylin (p. 142)

Ammonia water (p. 143)

Technic

1. Cut frozen sections at 10 μm and place in distilled water. A drop or two of ammonia may be added to aid in straightening out the sections. If ammonia is used, rinse in fresh distilled water.
2. Drain water off section and place in 100% propylene glycol for 5 minutes. Agitate with a glass rod to be *sure of complete dehydration. Do not carry any water over into the oil red O.*
3. Place in the oven in oil red O (which has been kept in the oven at 60° C) for 7 minutes. Agitate occasionally.
4. Place in 85% propylene glycol 3 minutes, stirring section gently with a glass rod.
5. Place in a small dish of distilled water to prevent tearing of the section.
6. Transfer to a large dish of distilled water.
7. Counterstain in Harris's hematoxylin (diluted two parts of distilled water to one part hematoxylin). (If differentiation is necessary, use 1% aqueous acetic acid.)
8. Blue in tap water to which is added several drops of ammonia water.
9. Place sections in distilled water. Coverslip, using an aqueous mounting medium.

Results (Plate 2, *O*)

Fat—red
Nuclei—blue

Oil red O—isopropanol method[9]

Solutions

Stock solution
    Saturated solution of oil red O (300 mg/dl) in 99% isopropanol

Working solution
    Mix 6 parts of stock oil red O with 4 parts of distilled water. Allow to stand for 10 minutes. Filter this solution using Whatman no. 42 filter paper. Working solution is stable for 1 to 2 hours.

Ehrlich's or Harris's hematoxylin

0.05% aqueous lithium carbonate

Technic

1. Rinse sections in distilled water.
2. Stain in working solution of oil red O for 6 to 15 minutes.
3. Clear background if necessary, using 60% isopropanol.
4. Wash well in distilled water.
5. Counterstain nuclei, using Ehrlich's hematoxylin for 2 minutes or Harris's hematoxylin for 30 seconds to 1 minute.
6. Rinse in tap water.
7. Blue sections in 0.05% lithium carbonate.
8. Rinse well in several changes of tap water or distilled water.
9. Coverslip, using an aqueous mounting medium.

Results

Lipids—red
Nuclei—blue

Variant method

A variant of the preceding method has been described.[27] Attached cryostat sections are rinsed in distilled water and then in 60% isopropanol and stained for 15 minutes in a working solution of:

    60 ml of stock saturated oil red O in 99% isopropanol

    40 ml of 1% aqueous dextrin

This working solution is mixed, allowed to stand 10 minutes, and then filtered, using a Büchner funnel with vacuum. The addition of the dextrin is reported to decrease the presence of nonspecific precipitate and prolong the shelf life of the working solution to 1 to 2 weeks. After being stained, the sections are rinsed in 60% isopropanol and then distilled water, counterstained with alum hematoxylin, blued, washed, and coverslipped with use of an aqueous mounting medium.

Results

Fats—red
Nuclei—blue

Method for gross staining of arteries[10]

Gross staining of arterial vessels facilitates the detection of atherosclerotic lesions for observation and grading. Selection of tissue samples for further processing is also aided.

After fixation in 10% neutral buffered formalin, individual samples of intact arteries are placed in separate Erlenmeyer flasks and stained for 16 hours in a supersaturated Sudan IV solution in 38% isopropanol. The optical density of this solution should read 0.22 ± 0.01 at 520 nm. Approximately 125 ml of staining solution is used per flask, and the stain should not be reused more than twice. It is helpful to circulate the stain during the staining process (such as with a mechanical shaker). After staining is done, the arteries are washed in running tap water for 1 hour. After being washed, the specimen may be examined grossly. Fatty atherosclerotic plaques color red; fibrous plaques remain unstained but appear more distinct than they do in the fresh state; mixed fatty-fibrous plaques color a paler red.

Secondary fluorescent methods

Solutions containing phosphine 3R or 3,4-benzpyrene may be used for fluorescent detection of lipids in formalin-fixed frozen sections. The phosphine method is more permanent; the benzpyrene method more sensitive. Sections may be examined using an ultraviolet (UG1 or UG2) or blue (BG12) exciter filter and a colorless ultraviolet barrier filter.

PHOSPHINE 3R TECHNIC[11]

1. Wash frozen sections in distilled water.
2. Stain in 0.1% aqueous phosphine 3R for 3 minutes.
3. Rinse quickly in water.
4. Coverslip, using 90% glycerol and examine.

Results

Most lipids fluoresce silver-white; fatty acids, soaps, and cholesterol show no fluorescence with this method.

3,4-BENZPYRENE TECHNIC[12]

Staining solution

Make a saturated aqueous solution of caffeine (approximately 1.5%). Allow it to stand overnight at room temperature. Filter. To each 100 ml of caffeine filtrate, add 0.002 gm of 3,4-benzpyrene. Allow this solution to incubate for 2 days at 37° C. Filter this solution and add an equal volume of distilled water. *Note:* Benzpyrene is carcinogenic and should be handled with appropriate care.

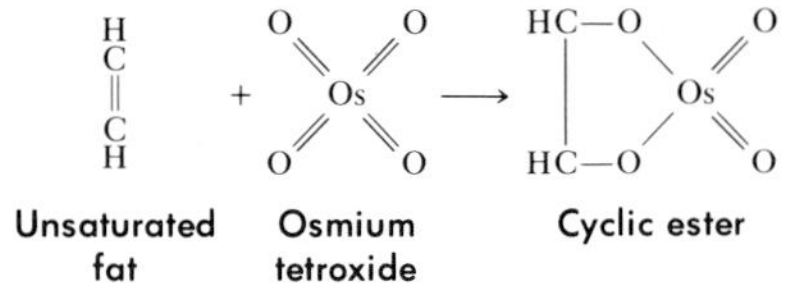

Fig. 11-1. Osmium reduction compound formation.

Technic

1. Rinse frozen sections in distilled water.
2. Filter the staining solution onto the sections. Allow it to stain for 20 minutes.
3. Rinse in distilled water.
4. Coverslip, using distilled water, and examine immediately.

Results

Lipids fluoresce a brilliant blue-white. The reaction fades rapidly, hence the necessity for immediate examination. This method will demonstrate even very minute lipid droplets.

CHEMICAL METHODS FOR LIPID DEMONSTRATION
Osmium tetroxide technic for unsaturated lipids[13]

Principle. Osmium tetroxide (osmic acid) is one of the oldest fat stains, and unsaturated fatty acids, such as oleic acid, have been traditionally considered to be responsible for the reduction reaction. There is also the possibility that certain protein and carbohydrate groups contribute to the reaction. Osmium tetroxide is soluble in fats and forms a black reduction compound with them by the addition to the double carbon-to-carbon bonds in the proportion of one molecule of osmium tetroxide to one double bond (Fig. 11-1). The ester may in turn attach to other double bonds forming double coordinate linkages. Complexes formed are no longer soluble in the usual fat solvents, but when mounted in synthetic resins, the osmium will oxidize and be decolorized because of the oxidation; hence sections are not permanent.

Fixation. Formalin-fixed tissue.

Cutting. Cut frozen sections at 10 to 15 μm.

Solutions
Osmium tetroxide solution

Osmium tetroxide	1 gm
Distilled water	100 ml

Score a 1 gm ampule of osmium tetroxide with a file and drop into closed cylinder containing the distilled water. Vigorous shaking will break the ampule safely.

Technic

1. Place frozen sections in distilled water.

2. Allow the sections to remain in osmium tetroxide solution for 24 hours.
3. Wash in several changes of water for 6 to 12 hours.
4. Place in absolute alcohol for several hours.
5. Wash well in distilled water.
6. Coverslip using glycerol gelatin, or dehydrate, clear, and coverslip, using a synthetic mounting medium.

Results
Fat—black
Background—yellow to brown

Precaution. Vapor is harmful and osmium compounds can cause damage to eyes. Use only under a fume hood.

Schiff reactions for unsaturated lipids[5]

The neuraminic acid or galactose residues of glycolipids (cerebrosides and gangliosides) are believed to be responsible for a positive periodic acid–Schiff (PAS) reaction. A control using dimedone (5,5-dimethyl-1,3-cyclohexanedione) may be employed to block aldehyde groups. Additional controls can be employed with use of extraction procedures since glycolipids are resistant to cold acetone treatment and are extracted with hot acetone.

A performic or peracetic acid–Schiff reaction may also be used to demonstrate unsaturated lipids in paraffin or frozen sections of formol-saline or Zenker's fixed tissue.

Solutions
Performic acid (p. 221)
Peracetic acid (p. 221) (also available commercially)
Schiff reagent (p. 165)

Technic
1. Hydrate sections to water and remove mercury precipitate if necessary. Blot sections.
2. Oxidize with performic or peracetic acid for 2 to 5 minutes (Culling). Lillie prefers 2 hours in the peracetic acid and 90 minutes in the performic acid.
3. Treat with Schiff reagent for 30 minutes.
4. Wash in warm running water for 10 minutes.
5. Coverslip, using an aqueous mounting medium such as glycerol gelatin.

Results
Unsaturated lipids—magenta

Nile blue sulfate technic for neutral and acidic lipids[14]

Principle. This technic demonstrates neutral and acidic lipids in tissue sections. Staining tissue sections with a Nile blue sulfate solution involves both chemical and physical mechanisms, since some of the components of the staining solution dye lipids in a physical adsorption type of staining, and other components react chemically with lipid derivatives contained in tissue.

The three principle components of the Nile blue solution are (1) the dark blue, water-soluble, oxazine salt of the Nile blue; (2) the free base of the oxazine, insoluble in water, soluble in lipids, and red in color; and (3) the Nile red oxazone derivative, insoluble in water and soluble in lipids. Generally these latter two components are present in low amounts in a Nile blue solution; their amount may be increased by boiling the Nile blue solution with dilute sulfuric acid. The following reactions are believed to occur when a tissue is treated with the Nile blue solution: neutral lipids will stain red with the Nile red solution component. Acidic lipids, being lipid in nature, have a tendency to also color red. However, these acidic lipids also have the capacity to form salts with the free base present in the staining solution, and the salt formed is lipid soluble and dark blue in color. This dark blue may mask the red color with which the acidic lipids may also stain. Most fatty acids are stained blue with the Nile blue sulfate component.

Solutions
Formol-calcium solution for fixation of tissue
1% acetic acid
1% Nile blue sulfate

Test the 1% Nile blue sulfate for the presence of the Nile red oxazone component by adding some xylene and shaking the mixture well. If there is a good Nile red component, the xylene should turn red in 20 to 30 seconds. If the xylene does not turn red, increase the Nile red component by boiling the 1% Nile blue sulfate in 5% sulfuric acid for 1 to 2 hours in a reflux condenser.[3]

Method
1. Fix tissue pieces for 48 to 72 hours in formol-calcium. After fixation, rinse tissues well with tap water.
2. Cut frozen sections (6 to 8 μm).
3. Stain with 1% Nile blue sulfate at 60° C for 5 minutes.
4. Rinse with 60° C distilled water.
5. Rinse for 30 seconds with 1% acetic water to remove dye bound to nonlipid structures.
6. Rinse in distilled water and mount in glycerol gelatin.

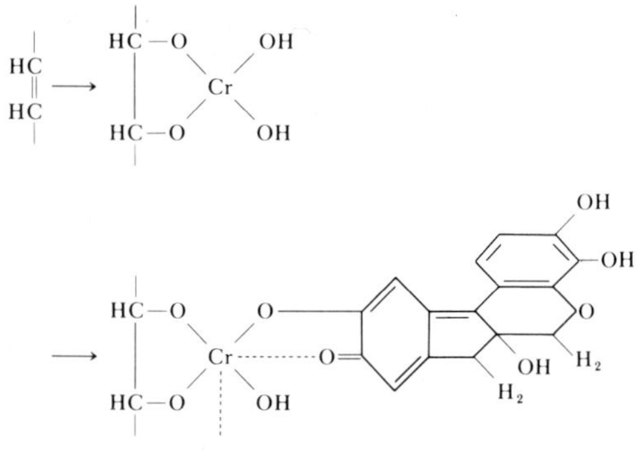

Fig. 11-2. Proposed structure of chromium-lipid complex and its attachment to acid hematein. (From Lillie, R. D.: Histochemie **20**:338, 1969.)

Results

Neutral lipids (triglycerides, cholesterol esters, steroids)—red to pink
Acidic lipids (fatty acids, phospholipids)—blue
Nuclei—blue
Cytoplasm—pale blue

Baker's acid hematein method for phospholipids[15]

Principle. Tissues are fixed in calcium-formol to prevent dissolution of the phospholipids. Tissues are then chromated, and phospholipids and certain other nonlipid acidic substances form chelate complexes.

The mechanism of how the chromate ion is taken up by the tissue has been investigated by a number of authors.[15-17] The most likely occurrence is that the dichromate functions to render the phospholipids insoluble through a polymerization process with the end product being a complex lipid polymer containing chelated chromium.[16,17] Several structures have been postulated; the one shown in Fig. 11-2 is considered the most likely, since it provides the necessary hydroxyls for the formation of the chelate ring with the acid hematein. After the dichromate mordanting process, sections are stained with acid hematein, resulting in the formation of dye lakes of blue to brown colors with the bound chromium. Differentiation with the borax ferricyanide solution removes most of the dye bound to nonphospholipid substances, but very dark blue staining components containing phosphoric acid are almost completely resistant to the decolorization process.

Two conditions are important for the reaction: (1) The time of chromate mordanting should not be lengthened because, in the amount of time allowed for the chromation, phospholipids will absorb relatively more of the chromate ion than will other substances. If chromated too long, other substances will nonspecifically pick up the chromate ion. (2) The differentiation step should not be shortened for similar reasons. The mordant-phospholipid complex is relatively more resistant to the differentiation than are the other substances, which may have formed a complex with the ion. A long differentiation will permit these substances to be decolorized while leaving the phospholipids demonstrated. The lipid character of the stained substance is confirmed by a pyridine extraction process. Phospholipids are soluble in a pyridine solution, and staining is not seen in extracted sections. Unextracted slides, run simultaneously, show the blue-black color indicating their presence.

Stain specificity for phospholipids has been questioned. If acid hematein technics are used on brain tissue, there is a difference seen in gray-matter versus white-matter staining, yet chemical analysis of both shows that there is little difference in the amount of phospholipid and unsaturated lipid between the gray and white matter. Some studies indicate that the phospholipid component per se is not so important as the actual structure of the lipids.[18] Myelin, present in large amounts in white matter, is a multilamellar structure, and it is believed that this configuration can hold the chromium ions in a stable, three-dimensional structure that is resistant to the differentiation step. Erythrocytes also stain with the acid hematein methods, and it was formerly assumed that this staining was attributable to the phospholipid content of the erythrocyte. The fact that erythrocyte staining was present even after lipid-extraction procedures had been performed prior to staining was interpreted to mean that the phospholipid present was very firmly bound to tissue protein. Biochemical analysis of the erythrocyte has revealed that less than 1% of the dry weight is phospholipid, and further work has shown that the hemoglobin present is the component responsible for the positive staining with the acid hematein methods.[19] This, of course, indicates that tests such as Baker's acid hematein are neither sensitive nor specific for phospholipids. There is one way of distinguishing lipid versus nonlipid acid hematein–positive substances by use of a sulfosalicylic acid–Sudan III counterstain after the acid hematein staining.[20] If the substance staining with the acid hematein is phospholipid in nature, it will color with the Sudan III counterstain. If the staining is attributable to components other than phospholipids, for example, hemoglobin, the blue-black color will be retained even after the counterstain has been applied.

Solutions
Fixative solution—formol-calcium

37% to 40% formalin	10 ml
10% anhydrous calcium chloride	10 ml
Distilled water	80 ml

5% potassium dichromate containing 1% calcium chloride

Potassium dichromate	5 gm
Calcium chloride	1 gm
Distilled water	100 ml

This solution is stable.

Acid hematein

Hematoxylin	0.05 gm
1% sodium iodate	1 ml
Glacial acetic acid	1 ml
Distilled water	48 ml

Place hematoxylin and sodium iodate in a flask; add the distilled water; heat to boiling; cool; add acetic acid. Use on day of preparation. Solution is not stable.

Differentiating solution

Borax	0.25 gm
Potassium ferricyanide	0.25 gm
Distilled water	100 ml

Solution is stable, but should be stored in the dark.

Method
1. Fix small tissue pieces in formol-calcium for 6 hours. This time may be prolonged.
2. Transfer into dichromate and calcium chloride solution for 18 hours at room temperature.
3. Transfer blocks into fresh dichromate solution for 24 hours at 60° C.
4. Wash in tap water for 6 hours.

5. Cut 10 μm frozen sections.
6. Place sections in the dichromate–calcium chloride solution for 1 hour at 60° C.
7. Wash 5 minutes in running tap water; rinse in distilled water.
8. Treat for 5 hours at 37° C with the acid hematein solution.
9. Rinse in distilled water; differentiate in differentiating solution for 18 hours at 37° C.
10. Wash in tap water for 10 minutes; rinse in distilled water.
11. Mount in glycerol gelatin.

Results
Phospholipids—dark blue or blue-black
Nucleoproteins—dark blue or blue-black
Cytoplasm—pale yellow

Pyridine extraction for Baker's acid hematein technic

Solutions
Dilute Bouin's solution

Saturated aqueous picric acid	50 ml
37% to 40% formalin	10 ml
Glacial acetic acid	5 ml
Distilled water	35 ml

70% ethanol; 50% ethanol
Pyridine

Method
1. Fix tissue pieces in dilute Bouin's solution overnight. Bouin's fixation is supposed to aid in complete removal of the phospholipids by the pyridine.
2. Immerse pieces in 70% ethanol for 1 hour.
3. Wash in 50% ethanol for 30 minutes.
4. Extract with pyridine for 1 hour at room temperature. Change solution at the end of the hour and treat for another hour at room temperature.
5. Treat with pyridine solution for 24 hours at 60° C.
6. Wash in tap water for 2 hours.
7. Place in dichromate–calcium chloride solution and proceed as in step 2 of the Baker's technic.

Osmium tetroxide–α-naphthylamine (OTAN) method for hydrophobic and hydrophilic lipids[21]

The OTAN procedure distinguishes hydrophilic phospholipids (including cephalins, lecithins, cerebrosides, and sphingomyelins) from hydrophobic lipids (such as triglyceride and cholesterol esters, and fatty acids). Osmium tetroxide reacts with the nonpolar ethylene bonds of the hydrophobic lipids and becomes reduced to a black reduction compound. Unsaturated hydrophilic lipids color orange-red to orange-brown because of chelation with the α-naphthylamine. Intermediate color shades result from mixtures of hydrophilic and hydrophobic lipids. The reduction reaction that colors the hydrophobic lipids may be prevented by an extraction treatment with cold acetone (4° C) for a 2-hour period prior to the staining procedure.

Fixation and processing. Use formol-calcium–fixed tissue. Cut free-floating frozen sections at 10 to 15 μm.

Solutions
Osmium tetroxide–potassium chlorate solution (solution A)

1% OsO_4	1 part
1% $KClO_3$	3 parts

Saturated α-naphthylamine (solution B)
Prepare a saturated solution by adding an excess amount of α-naphthylamine to distilled water. Heat this solution to 40° C. Filter.
2% alcian blue in 3% acetic acid (optional counterstain)

Precautions. Both solutions A and B should be prepared under a fume hood. Osmium tetroxide vapor is harmful and can cause eye damage. The α-naphthylamine may contain the volatile carcinogen β-naphthylamine. Disposable gloves should be used. All staining containers should be tightly sealed to prevent evaporation and should be opened under the fume hood.

Technic
1. Immerse free-floating sections in the OsO_4-$KClO_3$ solution for 18 hours. Fill the container and seal it tightly.
2. When incubation is completed, open the container under a fume hood and transfer the sections to distilled water. Wash sections well in distilled water and mount on slides.
3. Treat the sections with the saturated α-naphthylamine solution for 10 to 20 minutes at 37° C. The shorter period of time is suggested for the thicker sections, since colors will appear darker in these sections. Exposure of thinner sections for longer than 20 minutes will also produce darker colors. Too short a staining time can produce an orange-brown color in lipids that should stain black.
4. Open the α-naphthylamine staining container under the fume hood and transfer sections to distilled water. Wash in distilled water for 5 minutes.
5. Optional: Counterstain in alcian blue solution for 15 seconds to 1 minute. Rinse in distilled water after the counterstain.
6. Coverslip, using an aqueous mounting medium.

Results
Hydrophilic lipids (unsaturated phospholipids and normal myelin)—orange-red or orange-brown
Hydrophobic lipids (cholesterol esters, triglyceride esters, unsaturated fatty acids, degenerating myelin)—black

Color density should not be a factor in quantitative estimation of the amount of lipid present.

Sodium hydroxide–OTAN technic for sphingomyelin[22]
Solutions
2 N sodium hydroxide (NaOH)
1% acetic acid
Solutions as listed under OTAN method

Technic
1. Preheat sections with 2 N NaOH at 37° C for 1 hour.
2. Wash sections gently in distilled water.
3. Treat with 1% acetic acid for 1 minute.
4. Rinse in distilled water and transfer to osmium tetroxide solution. Proceed with OTAN technic step 1.

Results
Alkali-resistant lipids—orange-red
The most important alkali-resistant lipid is sphingomyelin, and this method may be useful in demonstrating the sphingomyelin content in Niemann-Pick cells.
Alkali-labile lipids are hydrolyzed and do not stain. Cholesterol and triglyceride esters are only partly hydrolyzed; however, a preliminary acetone extraction (see OTAN technic) may be employed to remove these and other hydrophobic lipids.

Fischler's technic for fatty acids[23]
Principle. Fatty acids usually do not occur in sufficient quantity in tissue to allow for their demonstration. An exception to this would be found in certain cases of fat necrosis. The Fischler technic for fatty acids depends on the affinity of fatty acids and their calcium soaps for heavy metals such as copper. Tissues are first mordanted in an aqueous solution of copper acetate. After the mordant treatment, sections are immersed in a lithium-hematoxylin solution. The result is the formation of black lakes that are resistant to decolorization with a borax-ferricyanide differentiating solution.

Solutions
Weigert's lithium-hematoxylin
Solution A
10% hematoxylin in absolute alcohol
Solution B
Lithium carbonate solution: 10 ml saturated aqueous lithium carbonate diluted to 100 ml volume with distilled water
Working solution
Mix equal parts of solutions A and B.
Saturated aqueous cupric acetate
Borax-ferricyanide differentiating solution

Potassium ferricyanide	25 gm
Sodium borate (borax)	20 gm
Distilled water	make to 1 liter

Method

1. Fix tissues in 10% formalin and cut frozen sections 10 μm.
2. Mordant sections at 37° C for 24 hours in saturated aqueous cupric acetate.
3. Wash in distilled water and stain 20 minutes in the above hematoxylin solution.
4. Differentiate in borax-ferricyanide until the red cells are nearly colorless.
5. Wash in distilled water and mount in glycerol gelatin.

Results

Fatty acids and their calcium soaps appear dark black. To distinguish the calcium soaps from the fatty acids, some of the tissue sections may be exposed for 24 hours to an absolute alcohol–ether (equal-parts) mixture. Only calcium soaps will remain in the extracted sections, and the fatty acids are soluble in the alcohol-ether solution. When stained by the above method, the calcium soaps will be colored black, and the fatty acids will not stain because of their being dissolved.

Cholesterol and its esters

Cholesterol and its esters occur in varying amounts in animal tissue. Pathologic deposits of these substances are seen in certain types of atherosclerotic lesions. Patients with Hand-Schüller-Christian syndrome may develop cholesterol deposits in some bones, notably the flat bones of the skull. Cholesterol will usually exhibit birefringence when viewed with polarized light and the birefringence seen in discrete chronic lesions is frequently attributable to the presence of cholesterol. However, positive birefringence does not preclude the presence of other birefringent lipids, certain proteins, amyloid, or even formalin artifact.

Cholesterol and its esters may be demonstrated by the perchloric acid–naphthoquinone (PAN) technic and by the Schultz method. Nonesterified cholesterol may be shown by the digitonin procedure. These methods are described in the next section.

More recently, a histochemical procedure employing cholesterol hydrolase and cholesterol oxidase to demonstrate free and esterified cholesterol in free-floating tissue sections has been described.[24] This method depends on the production of hydrogen peroxide from free cholesterol by the action of cholesterol oxidase; cholesterol esters may be demonstrated as cholesterol after hydrolysis with cholesterol ester hydrolase. Sites of hydrogen peroxide production are demonstrated by the formation of a benzidine-brown reaction product after a peroxidase-catalyzed reaction between the newly formed peroxide and diaminobenzidine.

Perchloric acid–naphthoquinone (PAN) method for cholesterol[25]

Principle. Perchloric acid acts on cholesterol, and cholesta-3,5-diene is formed. This latter substance then reacts with naphthoquinone to produce a dark blue color marking the site of sterol presence. This coloration only lasts a few hours. The PAN method is considered to be more sensitive than the Schultz method for sterol detection.

Fixation and processing. Cut frozen sections. Immerse sections in formol-calcium fixative for a minimum of 1 week to ensure adequate oxidation of cholesterol. Mount sections on slides and proceed with technic.

Solutions

PAN reagent

0.1% 1,2-naphthoquinone-4 sulfonic acid in ethanol	4 ml
60% perchloric acid	2 ml
40% formalin	0.2 ml
Distilled water	1.8 ml

60% perchloric acid

Technic

1. Cover sections with a minimum amount of PAN reagent.
2. Heat slides at 60° to 70° C for 5 to 10 minutes. Use a hot plate for this step. Discontinue heating when the original red color changes to blue.
3. Place a drop of 60% perchloric acid on the section and then apply a coverslip over this. No mounting medium as such is used. Examine immediately.

Results

Cholesterol and its esters—dark blue

Schultz's method for cholesterol and its esters[26]

Principle. This technic is a modification of the Liebermann-Burchard reaction, and the reaction depends on the oxidation of cholesterol to oxycholesterol. This oxidation may be accomplished through ultraviolet light or, more commonly, with ferric ammonium sulfate. The exact mechanism of the color reaction of the cholesterol with the concentrated sulfuric–glacial acetic acid is not fully understood, but it is believed that 7-hydroxycholesterol is mainly responsible for the blue-green characteristic color. The test is not specific for cholesterol and its esters, since carotene will produce a similar color in the tissue if present.

Fixation. Fix tissues in formalin.

Sectioning. Cut frozen sections.

Solutions

Iron alum solution

Iron alum	2.5 gm
Distilled water	100 ml

Concentrated sulfuric–glacial acetic acid mixture
Add the sulfuric acid slowly to an equal volume of glacial acetic acid, stirring and cooling all the while. (Only the purest acids are suitable and the sulfuric acid must contain at least 98% sulfuric acid. The reagent is hygroscopic and must be protected from atmospheric moisture.)

Technic

1. Place formalin-fixed frozen sections in the iron alum solution for 3 days at 37° C.
2. Rinse in distilled water.
3. Mount on slides and blot with fine filter paper.
4. Add a few drops of the acid mixture and cover with a cover glass.

Results

A positive test for cholesterol, or its esters, is indicated by the appearance of a blue-green color, which reaches its maximum intensity within a few minutes. Within 30 minutes the sections acquire a brown discoloration. The appearance of large numbers of bubbles results from using impure acids. Adrenal cortex can be used as a control.

Digitonin reaction[2]

Principle. This reaction will demonstrate nonesterified cholesterol in sections. Digitonin, a naturally occurring glucoside, is a precipitating agent and forms crystalline complexes with nonesterified cholesterol.

Fixation. Formalin-fixed tissue or fresh tissue may be used.

Sectioning. Cut frozen sections.

Solutions

0.5% solution of digitonin in 50% alcohol

Technic

1. Cut frozen sections.
2. Immerse sections in a 0.5% solution of digitonin in 50% alcohol in a small covered dish for several hours.
3. Rinse in 50% alcohol.
4. Counterstain part of the sections only, using the Sudan IV or oil red O technic.
5. Mount all sections in Apathy's gum syrup or a glycerol gelatin.

Results

Examine the uncounterstained sections under polarized light. Needles or rosettes of complex cholesteryl digitonides are formed. Because of the coarseness of the needles and rosettes, localization is not precise. In the counterstained preparations the cholesterol compound remains doubly refractile and does not stain, but the cholesteryl ester compound colors with the oil-soluble dye and loses its birefringence.

Note: The crystals are insoluble in cold 95% alcohol, acetone, ether, or water; slightly soluble in hot ethanol and in methanol; readily soluble in glacial acetic acid; and very soluble in pyridine and in chloral hydrate.

REFERENCES

1. Bloor, W. R.: Biochemistry of fats, Chem. Rev. **2:**243-300, 1925.
2. Lillie, R. D.: Histopathologic technic and practical histochemistry, ed. 4, New York, 1976, McGraw-Hill Book Co.
3. Culling, C. F. A.: Handbook of histopathological and histochemical techniques, ed. 3, London, Eng., 1974, Butterworth & Co. (Pubs.) Ltd.
4. Zugibe, F. T.: Diagnostic histochemistry, St. Louis, 1970, The C. V. Mosby Co.
5. Pearse, A. G. E.: Histochemistry, theoretical and applied, ed. 3, vol. 1, London, 1968, J. & A. Churchill, Ltd.
6. Keilig, I.: Über Spezifitätsbreite und Grundlagen der Markscheidenfärbungen; nach Untersuchungen an fraktioniert extrahierten Gehirnen, Virchows Arch. Pathol. Anat. **312:**405, 1944.
7. Chiffelle, T. L., and Putt, F. A.: Propylene and ethylene glycol as solvents for Sudan IV and Sudan black B, Stain Technol. **26:**51-56, 1951, Baltimore, copyright The Williams & Wilkins Co.
8. Luna, L. G., editor: Manual of histologic staining methods of the Armed Forces Institute of Pathology, ed. 3, New York, 1968, McGraw-Hill Book Co.
9. Lillie, R. D., and Ashburn, L. L.: Super-saturated solutions of fat stains in dilute isopropanol for demonstration of acute fatty degenerations not shown by Herxheimer technique, Arch. Pathol. **36:**432, 1943.
10. Guzman, M. A., McMahan, L. A., McGill, H. C., Strong, J. C., et al.: Selected methodologic aspects of the International Atherosclerosis Project, Lab. Invest. **18:**479-497, 1968, U.S.-Canadian Division of the International Academy of Pathology, Baltimore, The Williams & Wilkins Co. (agent).
11. Popper, H.: Distribution of vitamin A in tissue as visualized by fluorescence microscopy, Physiol. Rev. **24:**205-224, 1944.
12. Berg, N. O.: A histological study of masked lipids: stainability, distribution and functional variations, Acta Pathol. Microbiol. Scand. (Supp. **90**) p. 1, 1951.
13. Mallory, F. B.: Pathological technique, New York, 1961, Hafner Publishing Co.
14. Cain, A. J.: The use of Nile blue in the examination of lipoids, Q. J. Micro. Sci. **88:**383, 1947.
15. Baker, J. R.: The histochemical recognition of lipine, Q. J. Micro. Sci. **87:**409, 1946.
16. Baker, J. R.: Principles of biological microtechnique, New York, 1958, John Wiley & Sons, Inc.

17. Lillie, R. D.: Mechanisms of chromation hematoxylin stains, Histochemie 20:338, 1969.

18. Roozemond, R. C.: The staining and chromium binding of rat brain tissue and of lipids in model systems subjected to Baker's acid hematein technique, J. Histochem. Cytochem. 19:244-251, 1971.

19. Elleder, M., and Lojda, A.: Studies in lipid histochemistry. II. The nature of the material stained with the acid hematein test with the OTAN reaction in red blood cells, Histochemie 24:21-28, 1970.

20. Jordanov, J., and Zapnianova, E.: A technique combining Baker's acid hematein and Hadjioloff's hydrotropic Sudan III stains for identification of choline-containing phospholipids within the same tissue section, Acta Histochem. 42:360-366, 1972.

21. Adams, C. W. M.: A histochemical method for the simultaneous demonstration of normal and degenerating myelin, J. Pathol. Bacteriol. 77:648, 1959.

22. Adams, C. W. M., and Bayliss, O. B.: Histochemical observations on the localization and origin of sphingomyelin, cerebroside and cholesterol in the normal and atherosclerotic human artery, J. Pathol. Bacteriol. 86:113, 1963.

23. Fischler, C.: Ueber die Unterscheidung von Neutral Fetten, Fettsäuren und Seiten im Gewebe, Zentralbl. Allg. Pathol. 15:913, 1904.

24. Emeis, J. J., VanGent, C. M., and Van Sabben, C. M.: An enzymatic method for the histochemical localization of free and esterified cholesterol separately, Histochem. J. 9:197-204, 1977.

25. Adams, C. W. M.: A perchloric acid–naphthoquinone method for the histochemical location of cholesterol, Nature 192:331, 1961.

26. Weber, A. F., Phillips, M. G., and Bell, J. T.: An improved method for the Schultz cholesterol test, J. Histochem. Cytochem. 4:308-309, 1956, Baltimore, copyright The Williams & Wilkins Co.

27. Catalano, R. A., and Lillie, R. D.: Elimination of precipitates in oil red O fat stain by adding dextrin, Stain Technol. 50:297-299, 1975, Baltimore, copyright The Williams & Wilkins Co.

Pigments and minerals

Pigments that may be encountered in normal and pathologic conditions may be classified into two general groups—those that are "artifact" and those that are actually present within the cells. The distinction between the two groups is that artifact pigment will lie on top of the cells or in the interstitial tissue, but not within the cell. Artifact pigment is also present in a section because of processing technics; this is not the case with nonartifact pigment. Pigments found within tissues and cells may be classified as endogenous or exogenous. Endogenous pigments may be subdivided into hematogenous (including hemoglobin, hemosiderin, porphyrins, and bile pigments) and nonhematogenous (melanin, chromaffin, lipofuscin, and ceroid). Exogenous pigments are present because of an outside agent such as carbon inhalation or therapeutic agents.

The most common examples of artifact pigment are formalin pigment, mercury pigment, and chrome deposits. Chrome deposits are formed when chromate fixatives such as Zenker's or Helly's are used. They appear as black granules and are prevented from forming by washing the tissue in running tap water prior to dehydration and the completion of processing.

Formaldehyde pigment, a dark brown crystalline birefringent substance, is formed when acid aqueous solutions of formaldehyde act on blood-rich tissues. It will resist extraction by concentrated sulfuric, hydrochloric, phosphoric, and acetic acids, as well as by water, alcohol, acetone, fat solvents, etc. It can be bleached within an hour by concentrated nitric acid, or partially by 90% formic acid, and in 30 minutes by 3% hydrogen peroxide. It can be extracted by treatment with weak alcoholic, water-acetone solutions of the hydroxides (sodium, potassium, or ammonium hydroxide). The most convenient method to remove the pigment immediately from a tissue section is by use of a saturated alcoholic solution of picric acid. It is this method that is most commonly used in the laboratory (see p. 130 for details). Lillie states that the pigment itself will not be formed in tissues that have been fixed in neutral phosphate buffered formalin (pH 7). Formalin mixtures at pH levels from 3.0 to 5.0 will form large quantities of the pigment and will form in formalin below pH 5.6.

Mercury pigment is the third example of an artifact pigment and is formed in tissue sections as the result of fixation in mercuric chloride fixatives. It appears as a fine brown granular deposit, more abundant at the center of a section rather than at the periphery, because of the solubility of the pigment in the alcohols used to dehydrate the tissue. It is removed by treatment of the sections with a solution of iodine followed by treatment with sodium thiosulfate. In the iodine treatment, the mercury is oxidized to mercuric iodide or some mercuric iodide complex. Free brown iodine left is removed by the sodium thiosulfate (hypo) and changes into the colorless iodide ion. A water wash follows this treatment to ensure removal of all excess reagent from the section. (See p. 131 for details.)

ENDOGENOUS PIGMENTS OF HEMATOGENOUS ORIGIN[1-3]

Hemoglobin is a basic protein containing closely bound iron, which is usually nonreactive for iron-ion tests. Tests that may be used for the recognition of hemoglobin include staining characteristics, enzyme reactions, and near-specific coloring reactions.

Staining characteristics include coloring with acid dyes, appearing as pink to red with eosin, bright red with phloxine combinations, and red-orange in Mallory variants. Certain basic aniline dyes, such as toluidine blue O and thionin, when used in 1:1000 neutral aqueous solution will stain the red cells that contain the hemoglobin a brilliant green or yellow green. For these and other hemoglobin demonstration methods that follow, one should note that hemoglobin outside the red blood cells is much less easily demonstrated, since none of the available tests possess a true specificity for the hemoglobin molecule.

"Histochemical" technics for hemoglobin include Lison's zinc leuco dye stain and benzidine methods. These technics depend on the presence of peroxidases within the red cell. Authorities believe that freshly broken-down hemoglobin colors with both of these histochemical methods but loses its ability to react with the zinc leuco dye method after a few days outside the red cell.

Semispecific coloring reactions for hemoglobin include Sudan black B, Baker's phospholipid technic, Fischler's fatty acid stain, and Luxol fast blue. Staining may be caused partly by phospholipid coating of the red cell. Hemoglobin may also be stained by alizarin dye as in Okajima's method.

HEMOGLOBIN
Dunn-Thompson hemoglobin stain[4]

Principle. The purpose of this coloring reaction is to demonstrate hemoglobin in tissue sections. The exact mechanism is unknown, but the empiric basis is that alum hematoxylin colors red cells, presumably because of the hemoglobin content, a deep green. A picrofuchsin counterstain is used to distinguish cytoplasm (yellow) from collagen (red). Nuclei are stained with the hematoxylin also and are the usual purple-gray.

Solutions
Aqueous alum hematoxylin

Hematoxylin	2.5 gm
Ammonium alum	50 gm

Dilute with 1000 ml of distilled water.
Allow to ripen 10 days at room temperature (immediate ripening may be achieved by addition of 0.44 gm of potassium permanganate). Add 2.5 gm of thymol to solution as a preservative.
It remains stable 2 to 3 months.
4% iron alum
Picrofuchsin solution

1% aqueous acid fuchsin	13 ml
Saturated aqueous picric acid	87 ml

Method
1. Hydrate sections.
2. Stain 15 minutes in the above hematoxylin solution. (Lillie states that almost any unacidified hematoxylin will do.)
3. Wash in tap water to remove excess hematoxylin from slides.
4. Mordant 1 minute in 4% iron alum.
5. Rinse in tap water.
6. Stain 15 minutes in the above picrofuchsin solution.
7. Dehydrate and differentiate 3 minutes in 1 change (or more) of 95% alcohol. Completely dehydrate with absolute alcohol, 2 changes; clear in xylene and coverslip, using a synthetic mounting medium.

Results
Cytoplasm—brown to yellow
Hemoglobin casts, phagocytosed particles, and red cells—emerald green
Collagen—red
Nuclei—brown, purple, gray-black

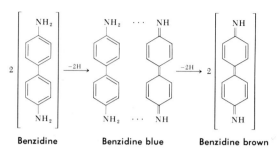

Fig. 12-1. Oxidation of benzidine to benzidine blue.

Benzidine methods

Principle. Ralph's method for hemoglobin and Lepehne's method for hemoglobin work on the same principle. The staining solution consists of benzidine and hydrogen peroxide. Hemoglobin and its derivatives (oxyhemoglobin, reduced hemoglobin, methemoglobin, carboxyhemoglobin, and acid hematin) possess peroxidases that decompose the hydrogen peroxide to water and nascent oxygen. The oxygen released from this action oxidizes benzidine, a colorless crystalline compound, to benzidine blue, a quinoid oxidation product. This benzidine blue possesses a blue-green color that turns a stable brown on standing (Fig. 12-1).

Ralph method for hemoglobin[5]

Fixation. Absolute alcohol, Carnoy's fluid, or formalin-fixed tissue.

Embedding. Cut paraffin sections at 5 μm.

Solutions
Benzidine solution

Benzidine	1 gm
Methanol, absolute	99 ml

Important! Precautions and disposal for benzidine solutions are described on p. 322.
Peroxide reagent
25% superoxol in 70% alcohol
Nuclear fast red stain (*Kernechtrot*) counterstain (p. 183)

Technic
1. Hydrate sections to distilled water.
2. Flood slide with benzidine reagent for 1 minute.
3. Drain off and flood with the peroxide reagent for 1½ minutes.
4. Wash in distilled water for 15 seconds.
5. Counterstain for a few seconds in nuclear fast red.
6. Rinse in distilled water, 2 changes.
7. Dehydrate, clear in xylene, and coverslip, using a synthetic resin.

Results
Hemoglobin—dark brown

Lepehne method for hemoglobin[6]

Fixation. 10% formalin-fixed tissue. Results may be impaired if left too long in formalin solution.

Embedding. Cut frozen sections.

Solutions
Benzidine peroxide solution
A small knife tip of benzidine is dissolved in 2 ml of 95% alcohol in a test tube, and a freshly prepared mixture of 0.5 ml of strong hydrogen peroxide plus 4.5 ml of 70% alcohol is added. *Important!* Precautions and disposal for benzidine solutions are described on p. 322.
Nuclear fast red solution (p. 183)

Technic
1. Place sections in distilled water for a few seconds.
2. Stain sections in freshly prepared benzidine-peroxide solution in a watch glass for 1 to 3 minutes. Care must be taken that sections do not fold or swim on the surface of the solution.
3. Transfer into 50% alcohol.
4. Wash in distilled water.
5. Stain for a few seconds in nuclear fast red.
6. Wash in several changes of distilled water.
7. Dehydrate, clear in xylene, and coverslip, using a synthetic mounting medium.

Results
Erythrocytes and hemoglobin—dark brown
NOTE: To avoid errors in doubtful cases with hemosiderin, proceed after step 3 for ½ to 1 hour in equal parts of 2% potassium ferrocyanide and 1% hydrochloric acid. Color results are then:
Hemoglobin—brown
Hemosiderin—blue

Okajima's stain for hemoglobin[7]

Principle. The positive reaction in tissue sections is caused by the affinity of hemoglobin for alizarin red S, an acid dye. Phosphomolybdic acid is used to enhance the results obtained with the acid dye. Red cells are stained red-orange, as are renal tubular casts in hemoglobinuria.

Solutions
10% phosphomolybdic acid
Staining solution

10% phosphomolybdic acid	10 ml
7.7% aqueous alizarin red S	30 ml

Harris's hematoxylin (see hematoxylin formulas)

Method
1. Hydrate sections.
2. Place sections in phosphomolybdic acid solution for 1 minute.
3. Wash in distilled water.
4. Stain 1 to 2 hours in staining solution.
5. Wash in distilled water; then tap water.

6. Counterstain in Harris's hematoxylin for 1 minute.
7. Wash in running tap water for 5 minutes.
8. Dehydrate, clear in xylene, and coverslip, using a synthetic mounting medium.

Results
Hemoglobin—orange to orange-red
Nuclei—blue
Background—reddish brown

HEMOSIDERIN

Hemosiderin, which occurs as yellow to brown intercellular granules, is a crystalline aggregate of ferritin. Hemosiderin is insoluble in alkalis but soluble in strong acid solutions. After formalin fixation, it is slowly soluble in dilute acids. The iron contained in hemosiderin pigment is easily unmasked and exhibits one or more of the reactions of ionic iron.

Diagnostic applications

Small amounts of ferric iron are found normally in the spleen and bone marrow. Excessive amounts are present in hemochromatosis and hemosiderosis.

The cause of hemochromatosis is unknown. The iron deposits are found mainly in the liver and pancreas, and there is significant damage to the tissue because of this deposition.

The abnormally excessive iron deposits seen in hemosiderosis may result from a variety of causes including (1) increased destruction of red cells because of transfusion reactions, hemolytic diseases, or pernicious anemia; (2) excessive iron intake or absorption; and (3) local hemorrhages and chronic congestive conditions. In these cases, the stainable iron is found principally in the liver, spleen, and lymph nodes.

Hemosiderin may also be demonstrated in macrophages of the efferent lymphatics and alveolar spaces of the lung. These macrophages have been called "heart failure cells" because they are associated with cardiac decompensation conditions. In certain cases, the yellow-brown granules themselves color blue with the Prussian-blue reaction; in other cases, only blue halos around the unstained granules are observed.

Two of the classic methods for the demonstration of iron are the Prussian blue reaction and Turnbull's blue reaction. Prussian blue reaction involves the treatment of sections with acid solutions of ferrocyanides. Any ferric ion (+3) present in the tissue combines with the ferrocyanide and results in the formation of a bright blue pigment called Prussian blue, or ferric ferrocyanide. This is one of the most sensitive histochemical tests and will demonstrate even single granules of iron in blood cells. It is a stable pigment and numerous other stains, such as the PAS reaction, may follow it.

Turnbull's blue reaction involves the treatment of sections with potassium ferricyanide. The ferricyanide will combine with any ferrous (+2) ion present in the tissue and will result in the formation of a stable, bright blue pigment called Turnbull's blue or ferrous ferricyanide. The ferrous ion may be found in some foreign pigment and in some disease situations, but is not so common as the ferric form.

It is important to use iron-free reagents for these technics. Masked iron, such as that present in hemoglobin, may be rendered positive for reaction in the iron technics when sections are first exposed to an unmasking treatment with hydrogen peroxide (see p. 228 for details). It is assumed that this treatment will destroy the organic part of the iron complex; however, it is not known whether all the masked iron is released by this treatment.

With easily demonstrated, loosely bound ions, hydrochloric acid treatment is sufficient to release the ferric or ferrous form from its combination with the tissue, hence the necessity for including acid in the reaction solution. Some technics, such as modified Gomori, include a preliminary exposure to ferrocyanide before the use of mixed ferrocyanide and hydrochloric acid, since the ferrocyanide molecules are believed to diffuse more slowly through the tissue.

Technics for demonstration
Gomori's iron reaction [8]

Fixation. Any well-fixed tissue will give good results.

Embedding. Cut paraffin sections at 5 μm.

Solutions
20% aqueous solution of hydrochloric acid
10% aqueous solution of potassium ferrocyanide
Nuclear fast red solution (p. 183)

Technic
1. Hydrate sections to distilled water.
2. Mix equal parts of hydrochloric acid and potassium ferrocyanide prepared immediately before use. Use chemically clean glassware. Reaction may take 20 minutes.
3. Wash thoroughly in distilled water.
4. Counterstain with nuclear fast red for 2 minutes.
5. Rinse twice in distilled water.
6. Dehydrate, clear in xylene, and coverslip, using a synthetic mounting medium.

Results

Iron (ferric form)—bright blue
Nuclei—red
Cytoplasm—pink

Gomori's modified iron stain (Prussian blue)[8]

Solutions

    10% potassium ferrocyanide
    20% hydrochloric acid
    Counterstain (*Kernechtrot*, eosin, etc.)

Method

1. Hydrate slides.
2. Immerse in 10% potassium ferrocyanide for 5 minutes.
3. Immerse in equal parts of potassium ferrocyanide and 20% hydrochloric acid for 30 minutes. Do not mix these two solutions together until just before use.
4. Wash thoroughly in distilled water.
5. Counterstain as desired (*Kernechtrot* for 5 minutes *or* 3% eosin for 30 seconds *or* 0.25% aqueous acid fuchsin for 20 seconds).
6. Rinse twice in distilled water.
7. Dehydrate, clear, and coverslip, using a synthetic mounting medium.

Results (Plate 1, X)

Iron (ferric form)—bright blue
Background—depends on counterstain used

Siderocyte demonstration in smears[9]

Siderocytes are red cells that contain nonhemoglobin iron-containing granules. They are demonstrated with the Prussian blue reaction.

Smear preparation. Blood or bone marrow smears are air-dried and fixed in absolute methanol for 15 minutes at room temperature. The smears are allowed to dry free of alcohol.

Solutions

    2% potassium ferrocyanide
    0.2 N hydrochloric acid
    0.1% aqueous eosin

Technic

1. Mix equal volumes of the 2% potassium ferrocyanide and 0.2 N hydrochloric acid.
2. Place the dried fixed smears in a Coplin jar containing the staining solution. Stain for 10 minutes at 56° C.
3. Wash slides in running tap water for 20 to 30 minutes.
4. Counterstain for 5 to 10 seconds in 0.1% aqueous eosin. Rinse away excess eosin with distilled water.
5. Air-dry slides and examine *or* dehydrate, clear in xylene, and coverslip, using a synthetic mounting medium.

Results

Siderocyte granules—blue
Normal blood contains 0.4% to 0.6% siderocytes.
The findings in some diseases are as follows:

Microcytic hypochromic anemia	1% to 3%
Infections	6% to 10%
Severe burns	3% to 10%
Pernicious anemia	8% to 14%
Lead poisoning	10% to 30%

Lillie's technic for Turnbull's blue reaction[1]

Solutions

    0.06 N hydrochloric acid
    Potassium ferricyanide   400 mg
        Dissolve the 400 mg potassium ferricyanide in 40 ml of 0.06 N hydrochloric acid.
    1% acetic acid or 0.01 N hydrochloric acid
    0.5% basic fuchsin in 1% acetic acid

Method

1. Hydrate slides.
2. Immerse slides in a fresh solution of potassium ferricyanide in 0.06 N hydrochloric acid for 1 hour.
3. Wash slides in 1% acetic acid or 0.01 N HCl.
4. Stain 5 to 10 minutes in 0.5% basic fuchsin in 1% acetic acid.
5. Wash in distilled water.
6. Dehydrate, clear in xylene, and coverslip, using a synthetic mounting medium.

Results

Iron (ferrous form)—bright blue
Background—pink-red

APOSIDERIN

Aposiderin is believed to be formed from hemosiderin by the action of acid fixatives. It is a brown granular pigment and negative to the usual tests for iron such as Prussian blue and Turnbull's blue. Schmorl's reaction is also negative for aposiderin and for the hemosiderin from which it is probably formed. Authorities believe that the action of the acid fixatives on the tissue either removes the iron or renders it inactive to these tests. Aposiderin is very resistant to extraction processes; however, its formation may be prevented by the use of neutral buffered formalin. Clinically it is important to distinguish aposiderin from the lipofuscin pigment, which may also be present in tissue and present a similar appearance.

PORPHYRINS

Porphyrins are cyclic tetrapyrroles and are precursors of the heme part of hemoglobin. They accumulate in tissues in certain forms of porphyria. They are insoluble in dilute acids and alkalis and are normally not present in sufficient amounts in tissue to be recognized microscopically. If present, they will give a positive Gmelin test and will fluoresce orange to red with ultraviolet light (365 nm).

BILE PIGMENTS

Bile pigments are the straight-chain tetrapyrrole derivatives of heme. Bilirubin is the principal bile pigment and is a normal product of red cell degradation. Excessive amounts of bile pigment in the liver may be found in cases of intrahepatic or extrahepatic biliary obstruction. Hematoidin, a pigment similar to bilirubin, is formed locally in tissues as a result of reduced oxygen tension and hemorrhage.

Bile pigments will not give primary fluorescence. Tests for their identification include positive staining with the Gmelin test, Stein's method, and Hall's technic using Fouchet's reagent.

Stein's bile pigment stain[10]

Principle. Stein's iodine test depends on the oxidation of the bile pigment to green biliverdin upon exposure to the iodine solution. The reaction will not be reversed by removal of excess iodine by sodium thiosulfate—a further indication of the oxidative process.

Fixation. Fix for a short period of time in alcohol or 10% formalin.

Embedding. Cut paraffin sections at 5 μm.

Solutions

Tincture of iodine

Iodine	7.5 gm
Potassium iodide	5 gm
Distilled water	5 ml
95% alcohol	sufficient to make 100 ml

Lugol's solution

Iodine	1 gm
Potassium iodide	2 gm
Distilled water	100 ml

Stein's iodine reagent

Tincture of iodine	1 volume
Lugol's solution	3 volumes

Sodium thiosulfate solution
5% aqueous solution of sodium thiosulfate
Counterstain (nuclear fast red [*Kernechtrot*] may be used; see p. 183)

Technic

1. Hydrate sections to distilled water.
2. Iodine reagent for 6 to 12 hours.
3. Wash in distilled water.
4. Decolorize with 5% sodium thiosulfate for 15 to 30 seconds.
5. Wash in distilled water.
6. Counterstain with nuclear fast red for 5 minutes.

7. Wash twice in distilled water.
8. Dehydrate quickly in acetone.
9. Clear in xylene, and coverslip, using a synthetic mounting medium.

Results

Bile pigments—emerald green
Localizations cannot be considered reliable because of the diffusibility of the reactants and the final color.

Gmelin's test[10]

Gmelin's test involves a rapid microscopic examination. After the tissue is deparaffinized and hydrated to water, a coverslip is placed over the section and a nitric-nitrous acid mixture allowed to diffuse beneath it. The tissue is destroyed in the process from the action of the acid, and a positive test consists in observation of color changes from violet to blue to green in the presence of bile pigments. Tests should be done on two or three slides before being diagnosed as negative. A nitric-nitrous acid mixture may be prepared by the addition of a crystal or two of sodium nitrite to nitric acid, which will make the desired 1% to 2% nitrous acid component in the concentrated acid.

Hall's technic for bilirubin[11]

Principle. The oxidizing action of Fouchet's reagent converts the bile pigment to green biliverdin. Colors that may be observed range from olive green to emerald green depending on the concentration of bile pigment present.

Fixation. 10% neutral buffered formalin.

Embedding. Cut paraffin sections at 5 μm.

Solutions

Fouchet's reagent

Trichloroacetic acid	25 gm
Distilled water	100 ml

Mix the above. When the acid has dissolved, add 10 ml of 10% ferric chloride. Prepare fresh before use.

Van Gieson's solution (p. 189)

Technic

1. Hydrate sections.
2. Immerse in Fouchet's reagent for 5 minutes.
3. Rinse in several changes of tap water, followed by distilled water.
4. Counterstain in Van Gieson's solution for 5 minutes.
5. Dehydrate, clear, and coverslip, using a synthetic mounting medium.

Results

Bile pigments—various shades of green
Muscle and cell cytoplasm—yellow
Collagen—red

HEMATINS

Hematins usually occur in tissues as granular black crystalline deposits and are of three general types. The first is formalin pigment (already discussed), malarial pigment, and acid hematin. Malarial pigment occurs in the plasmodium parasites and in the reticuloendothelial cells. Its appearance and properties are similar to formalin pigment. It is soluble in 5% alcoholic solutions of sulfuric, nitric, and hydrochloric acid at 40° to 50° C in 1 day or less. Lillie has described an acid hematin found in material fixed in neutral buffered formalin. The microcrystalline brown pigment occurs in autolyzed spleens in the surface next to the stomach and is seen in fresh material fixed in neutral formalin in focal hemorrhages of gastric mucosa. It gives no iron reaction and is dissolved by alcoholic picric acid solutions and by alkalis. It is resistant to strong organic, and dilute mineral, acids. It will also resist extraction by concentrated sulfuric acid.

ENDOGENOUS PIGMENTS OF NONHEMATOGENOUS ORIGIN

These pigments are found within tissue cells and may be normally present (melanins), formed as the result of "wear and tear" (lipofuscins), or formed as the result of disease process (ceroid).

MELANIN

Melanins comprise a group of naturally occurring compounds that are complex polymeric substances closely bound to proteins. They are characteristically brown-black and derive from tyrosine or tyrosine-containing compounds. They are present in the cells as granules.

Diagnostic applications

Melanin pigment is normally present in the melanocytes and melanophores of skin, hair and hair follicles, retina, iris, and certain parts of the nervous system. When present in large concentrations, it is easy to recognize. In some cases, the amount of the pigment may obscure nuclear detail and mitotic figures, and a bleaching reaction may be necessary. When melanin is present in lesser concentrations, it appears brown and may be confused with hemosiderin. In such cases, the Prussian blue reaction for hemosiderin and the various melanin identification technics are requested. These same technics are useful for the detection of small concentrations of melanin pigment.

Melanin pigmentation is increased in Addison's disease (adrenal insufficiency) and decreased in hyperadrenal function. In cases of hemochromatosis, there is increased melanin and increased iron deposits seen. Melanin identification methods as well as the Prussian blue reaction are used in such cases to distinguish the two pigments.

Melanin demonstrations are most important when a diagnosis of malignant melanoma is to be established. Classically, the tumor cells have a characteristic appearance, and contain melanin pigment that can be identified as such in the lab when bleaching reactions, argentaffin reactions, the ferrous-ion uptake procedure, and Schmorl's reduction reaction are used. Occasionally the cells of a melanocarcinoma will lack melanin pigment, and this is referred to as a "nonpigmented melanoma." Cells at either the primary or metastatic site or sites may exhibit this nonpigmented phenomenon. Although these cells lack the melanin granules, they do possess the capacity to produce the melanin, and the dopa oxidase reaction is used to indicate this melanin-producing potential.

Identification of melanin pigment

Identification of melanin may be made on the basis of general characteristics of the substance and certain tests. Melanin is insoluble in organic solvents and weak acids and bases; however, it dissolves in strong alkali. Melanin is *bleached* by oxidizing agents. Agents used in the oxidizing process include hydrogen peroxide, acidified potassium permanganate, and performic and peracetic acids. Melanin is *argentophilic:* that is, it reduces silver nitrate to metallic silver. It possesses this capacity in acid, neutral, and alkaline solutions of the silver nitrate. This is a sensitive, but not strictly specific reaction. With dilute Nile blue solution in 1% sulfuric acid, melanins are stained dark green. Melanin is *strongly basophilic* and is stained by acidified solutions of basic dyes. It *forms complexes with ferrous ion,* which can then be demonstrated by the Turnbull's blue reaction. It will also give a *positive Schmorl's reaction*. It will give a negative iron reaction for intrinsic iron content, a negative periodic acid–Schiff reaction, and a negative acid-fast reaction, and it will not stain with lipid dyes.

Bleaching reactions for melanin[1]
POTASSIUM PERMANGANATE BLEACHING

Bleaching with acidified potassium permanganate is the most convenient way to bleach melanin. Use albuminized slides, since sections tend to fall off during the treatment process. Run duplicate sections of the same case—one bleached and one not bleached to serve as a control. Additional known controls treated in the same manner are also suggested.

Solutions

Bleaching solution

Prepare 0.3% sulfuric acid by adding 0.3 ml of concentrated sulfuric acid to approximately 95 ml of distilled water. Mix. Dilute to a final volume of 100 ml. To this add 0.3 gm of potassium permanganate.

1% oxalic acid

Nuclear fast red counterstain (optional) (p. 183)

Technic

1. Hydrate slides.
2. Treat with the bleaching solution for 10 minutes to several hours. Skin melanin is usually bleached by permanganate treatment in 20 minutes; neuromelanin, in 1 to 5 minutes; ocular melanin in 2 to 4 hours.
3. Rinse in several changes of distilled water.
4. Remove excess brown-colored permanganate with 1% oxalic acid for 1 to 2 minutes. Sections should turn white.
5. Wash in gently running tap water for 20 to 30 minutes.
6. Counterstain, if desired, with nuclear fast red for 3 to 5 minutes. Rinse in several changes of distilled water.
7. Dehydrate, clear in xylene, and coverslip, using a synthetic mounting medium.

Results

Melanin is bleached in 4 hours or less with the permanganate solution. A second test slide that has not been exposed to the bleaching solution should be reserved for comparison purposes. Nuclei are red and cytoplasm pink if the nuclear fast red counterstain is used.

HYDROGEN PEROXIDE BLEACHING

Solution

10% hydrogen peroxide

Method

Treat sections with the above solution for 1 to 2 days.

Result

Melanin should be bleached after a 2-day treatment.

PERFORMIC OR PERACETIC ACID BLEACHING

Solutions

Performic acid may be prepared by the addition of 31 ml of 30% hydrogen peroxide and 0.22 ml of concentrated sulfuric acid to 8 ml of 90% formic acid. This gives a 4.7% concentration of performic acid in 2 hours. The acid is unstable and decomposes in several hours.

Peracetic acid may be prepared by the addition of 259 ml of 30% hydrogen peroxide and 2.2 ml of concentrated sulfuric acid in 95.6 ml of glacial acetic acid. Stir at 22° to 23° C. Maximum concentration (8.6%) is reached in 80 to 90 hours. Sodium pyrophosphate may be added to the solution for stability, and the solution is stable for months if stored in the refrigerator.

Method

Treat sections to either of the above acid solutions for several hours.

Result

Melanin should be bleached within 24 hours with the above solutions.

Argentaffin reaction for melanin

Principle. Melanins are argentaffin; that is, they possess the capacity to bind silver from a silver solution and reduce it directly to visible metallic silver in the section without the aid of a separate reducing agent. Acid, neutral, or alkaline solutions may be used, and the different melanins differ in their capacity to react with the different pH strengths of the solutions. Neuromelanin, for example, reduces acid silver nitrate very slowly.

Ammoniacal silver solution and methenamine silver solution are not specific for melanin as other pigments may reduce the alkaline silver complexes. Methenamine silver solution is considered less sensitive, and greater time is required for blackening. The first step in the procedure, after hydration of the slides to water, is the treatment of the sections with an iodine solution. This iodine is a mild oxidizing agent and will oxidize some of the other reducing agents present in tissue so that they will not subsequently reduce the silver nitrate. The iodine also has a mild oxidizing effect on the melanin itself and oxidizes it to the quinone form (Fig. 12-2). Not all the melanin is thus oxidized, however. Lillie states that the melanin in tissues is probably an intermediate form between a reduced o-diphenol and an oxidized quinone, and this intermediate form, called a quinhydrone, is most likely responsible for the reducing capacity of melanogenic sites. The oxidation of melanin completely to the quinone would render the section nonargentaffin, but as it is, the exposure to the mild action of the iodine is not sufficient to render all the reducing sites to the quinone state, and there are left sufficient quinhydrone groupings to reduce the silver nitrate to metallic silver. The thiosulfate is used to remove the ex-

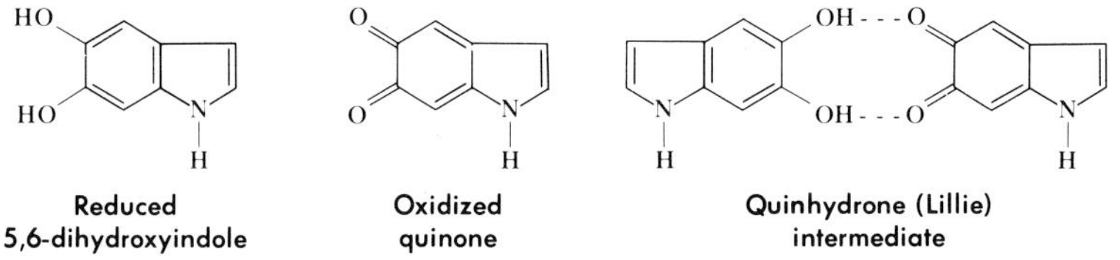

Fig. 12-2. Final-stage products of the Raper cycle. (From Lillie, R. D., and Fullmer, H. M.: Histopathologic technic and practical histochemistry, ed. 4, copyright 1976, with permission of McGraw-Hill Book Co.)

cess iodine from the tissue section after the iodine treatment. After the silver solution has acted, sections are again treated with the sodium thiosulfate solution to "fix" the reaction in the tissue and remove unreacted silver.

GOMORI'S METHENAMINE SILVER ARGENTAFFIN REACTION FOR MELANIN[12]

Solutions

Gram's or Weigert's iodine (p. 131)
5% sodium thiosulfate
Methenamine silver
  Stock solution (p. 187)
  Working solution
  Mix equal volumes of stock solution and distilled water. Add 3 ml of borate buffer, pH 8.2. Filter.
0.2 M borate buffer, pH 8.2
  0.2 M boric acid   65 ml
  0.05 M sodium borate   35 ml
0.2% safranin in 0.2 M acetic acid *or Kernechtrot* (p. 183)

Method

1. Hydrate sections.
2. Treat 10 minutes with either Gram's or Weigert's iodine.
3. Rinse in distilled water.
4. Rinse in 5% sodium thiosulfate; rinse in distilled water.
5. Place sections in the working methenamine silver solution and keep in the dark for 18 to 24 hours.
6. Rinse in distilled water.
7. Wash 2 minutes in 5% sodium thiosulfate. Rinse in distilled water.
8. Counterstain for 2 minutes in safranin or 5 minutes in *Kernechtrot*. Rinse in distilled water.
9. Dehydrate in 2 changes each of 95% and absolute alcohol; clear in xylene; mount in a synthetic mounting medium.

Results (Plate 2, *D*)

Melanin granules—black
Nuclei—red
Background—pink
The positive reaction, as mentioned previously, is not diagnostic for melanin.

Precautions. Glassware for this technic should be chemically clean. Use nonmetallic forceps for handling slides.

FONTANA-MASSON ARGENTAFFIN REACTION

See p. 277.

ACID SILVER NITRATE ARGENTAFFIN REACTION[1]

Solutions

0.1 M (1.7%) silver nitrate in 0.1 M acetate buffer, pH 4
0.1 M acetate buffer, pH 4
  0.1 M acetic acid   164 ml
  0.1 M sodium acetate   36 ml
5% sodium thiosulfate
Nuclear fast red (*Kernechtrot*) (p. 183)

Technic

1. Hydrate sections. Rinse well in distilled water.
2. Immerse sections in silver nitrate solution for 1 hour in the dark at 25° C.
3. Wash in distilled water for 1 to 2 minutes.
4. 5% sodium thiosulfate for 1 minute.
5. Wash in running tap water for 10 minutes.
6. Counterstain, if desired, with nuclear fast red for 3 to 5 minutes. Rinse well in distilled water.
7. Dehydrate, clear, and coverslip, using a synthetic mounting medium.

Results

Lillie states the preceding metal reduction procedure is the crucial histochemical test for cutaneous, ocular, and pial melanin. These pigments should blacken within the time allotted for immersion in the silver solution. Human neuromelanin requires 3 days for reduction of the silver to occur at 25° C in the dark.

Ferrous-ion uptake for melanin[1]

Principle. Lillie states that this is a specific reaction for melanin. Sections are exposed to a solution of ferrous sulfate, and the melanin forms complexes with the ferrous ion (most likely chelate complexes of the ion with the *o*-quinhydrone form of melanin). The ferrous ion taken up is then demonstrated by means of Turnbull's blue reaction. Sections are treated with potassium ferricyanide, and this combines with the ferrous iron to form ferrous ferricyanide, a blue end product to indicate melanin sites.

Solutions
2.5% ferrous sulfate

1% potassium ferricyanide in 1% acetic acid

Counterstain (optional) (*Kernechtrot;* Van Gieson's solution, or others)

1% acetic acid

Method
1. Hydrate sections.
2. Place sections in the 2.5% ferrous sulfate solution for 1 hour.
3. Wash in four changes of distilled water for 5 minutes each change.
4. Treat sections with the 1% potassium ferricyanide solution in 1% acetic acid for 30 minutes.
5. Wash in 1% acetic acid.
6. Counterstain as desired.
7. Dehydrate in 2 changes each of 95% alcohol and absolute alcohol; clear in xylene; mount in synthetic medium.

Results
Melanin—dark blue to dark green

Background—colored according to counterstain used

Note: The trace ferrous iron content present in hemosiderin may also react with the ferricyanide solution and produce a positive reaction. Specificity for melanin is controlled by the Prussian blue reaction.

Schmorl's ferric ferricyanide reduction test[1]

Principle. The purpose of this test is to indicate sites of reducing activity in tissue sections. A positive reaction is presumptive evidence of the presence of melanin, though other reducing substances react, including ascorbic, oxalic, and uric acids, phenols, indoles, aryl amines, thiols, and others. These reducing substances reduce the ferric ions present in the staining solution to the ferrous form, and the ferrous form, in turn, combines with the ferricyanide, also present in the staining solution, to form Turnbull's blue (ferrous ferricyanide) as the end product.

Solutions
Ferricyanide solution

  3 parts of 1% ferric chloride

  1 part freshly prepared 1% potassium ferricyanide

  Mix fresh just before use.

1% neutral red or *Kernechtrot* counterstain

Method
1. Hydrate slides.
2. Immerse sections in ferricyanide solution for 5 minutes.
3. Wash several minutes in running tap water.
4. Counterstain in 1% neutral red for 3 minutes or *Kernechtrot* for 5 minutes. Rinse well in distilled water.
5. Dehydrate in 2 changes each of 95% and absolute alcohol; clear in xylene; mount in synthetic medium.

Results (Plate 2, *E*)
Reducing substances—blue

Nuclei—red

Dopa oxidase[13]

Tyrosinase is an enzyme that catalyzes the oxidation of tyrosine to dopa (3,4-dihydroxyphenylalanine) and the oxidation of dopa to melanin through various intermediate steps. It has been found that a melanin or melanin-like pigment is deposited in cells called melanocytes when fresh frozen tissue sections are exposed to a buffered solution of dopa. This is most evident with skin sections. This melanin formation is attributed to an enzyme called dopa oxidase. The exact relation of this dopa oxidase to tyrosinase is not yet fully known, but there is a considerable degree of similarity in their enzyme activity. Some authors believe that the two enzymes should be considered to form a complex enzyme system with the common name of tyrosinase.

The histochemical reaction is performed by incubation of the sections with dopa, and activity caused by dopa oxidase is indicated by deposition of black to brown melanin granules. Evaluation of enzyme activity may be difficult where there is already present in the tissue section large amounts of preformed melanin pigment. The deposition of the newly formed pigment is useful in determining microscopic sites of melanogenesis; however, using dopa as a substrate does not imply specificity, since other active oxidizing systems, such as the cytochromes and the peroxidases, may cause nonspecific staining reactions.

Solutions
0.1% L-dopa in 0.1 M phosphate buffer, pH 7.4 (DL-dopa may also be used.)

0.1 M phosphate buffer, pH 7.4

0.1 M KH_2PO_4 or $NaH_2PO_4 \cdot H_2O$	8 ml
0.1 M Na_2HPO_4	42 ml

Controls
To check on the presence of preformed pigment, incubate some tissue sections in buffer only. Skin serves as a known positive control.

Method 1

1. Fix tissues in formalin for 1 to 2 hours at room temperature or overnight at 4° C.
2. Cut thin slices from fixed tissue blocks (surface layers preferred) and wash in water for 3 minutes.
3. Incubate tissue slices for 1 hour at 37° C in the dopa solution. Change solution at the end of the hour and continue incubation for 10 to 12 hours at 37°.
4. Wash tissue in running tap water.
5. Fix in Bouin's fixative or formalin for 24 hours.
6. Dehydrate in alcohols. Clear with benzene or toluene. Embed in paraffin.
7. Cut sections at 5 μm. Hydrate slides and counterstain as desired.
8. Dehydrate, clear, and coverslip, using a synthetic mounting medium.

Method 2

For fresh frozen postfixed sections or formalin-fixed frozen sections:

1. Rinse sections in distilled water.
2. Immerse sections in the staining solution at 37° C for 45 minutes.
3. Transfer sections to fresh staining solution at 37° C for 2 to 3 hours. Check results at half-hour intervals.
4. Rinse sections in gently running tap water for 5 minutes.
5. Optional: counterstain in nuclear fast red for 3 to 5 minutes. Rinse well in distilled water after counterstaining.
6. Dehydrate, clear in xylene, and coverslip, using a synthetic mounting medium.

Results

Positive reaction from dopa oxidase (or phenolase complexes, or others) is indicated by the deposit of black-brown melanin granules.

LIPID PIGMENTS

Lipid pigments found in tissue sections are an ill-defined group of nonhemoglobin pigments that possess the common properties of yellow brown coloration and a presumed lipid precursor. Many names have been applied to this general class of pigments: "wear and tear" pigment, lipochromes, ceroid, yellow pigment, lipofuscins, and others, and these various subdivisions are characterized essentially by indeterminate differences in reactivity to a number of special staining and histochemical tests.

Lipofuscins

Lipofuscin pigment is frequently seen in human tissue, but its differentiation from other similar-appearing pigments may be difficult. The amount of lipofuscin present within a cell generally increases with age. Certain cells, for example, neurons, are more prone to accumulate this pigment. Lipofuscin granules are believed to be derived from secondary lysosomes and represent remnants of undigested substances. The chemical composition of the lipofuscins is variable and complex.

The pigments are yellow brown and iron-negative and give a brownish fluorescence in ultraviolet light. The granules are also basophilic and positive with the periodic acid–Schiff reaction and performic and peracetic acid–Schiff reactions. They resist alcoholic dehydration and paraffin embedding. They may be demonstrated with lipid stains such as Nile blue sulfate and Sudan black B after paraffin treatment. Lipofuscins may be decolorized by a brief (20 seconds to 5 minutes) treatment in acetone, examined from water or glycerol, washed, and then restained by the original fat stain used. The destain-restain procedure may be repeated several times with no apparent lessening of reactivity. Certain lipofuscins (especially ceroid) will also show acid-fast characteristics after prolonged treatment with a carbol fuchsin solution. (See p. 237 for details.) Lipofuscins will also give a weakly positive Schmorl reaction and will reduce silver salts.

Staining characteristics of this substance are variable and differences in staining are observed, depending on the pigment's location in the body. Pearse suggested that these pigments are derived from the oxidation of unsaturated lipid substances and undergo characteristic changes as the oxidation process continues. The changes that the molecules undergo as they are oxidized are reflected in the final result of the staining reactions. He states that pigmentation, fluorescence, basophilia, and reducing capacity increase with progressive oxidation, whereas solubility in lipid solvents and staining with the oil-soluble dyes diminish with progressive oxidation. Varying degrees of acid fastness and positive reactions with periodic, peracetic, and performic acid–Schiff reactions are found only at certain stages in the development of the pigment, hence the variable staining reactions to these and the above technics. See Lillie, R. D., and Fullmer, H. M., loc. cit., pp. 513-517, for expected staining reactions of lipofuscins in various histologic locations.

Hemofuscin

Hemofuscin, now classified as a lipofuscin, was first described in 1889. It is found associated with hemosiderin in the liver and in other tissues in cases of hemochromatosis. Hemofuscin is a brown, iron-free pigment that is non–acid fast and stains with oil-soluble dyes in frozen sections, but not after paraffin embedding. Mallory recommends a fuchsin stain for demonstration because hemofuscin has an affinity for fuchsin dyes and relatively good resistance to decolorization with alcohol after the staining. This technic may be combined with the Prussian blue reaction to give a complete pigment picture in hemochromatosis. In this case, the fuchsin stain should follow the iron stain.

Mallory's hemofuscin method[6]

Solutions
Nuclear stain—any alum hematoxylin
0.5% basic fuchsin
Dissolve 0.5 gm of basic fuchsin in 100 ml of equal parts distilled water and 95% alcohol.

Method
1. Hydrate sections.
2. Stain 5 to 10 minutes in alum hematoxylin.
3. Wash well in water.
4. Stain 5 to 20 minutes in basic fuchsin solution.
5. Wash in water; differentiate in 95% alcohol.
6. Dehydrate in absolute alcohol; clear in xylene, and coverslip, using a synthetic mounting medium.

Results
Nuclei—blue
Hemofuscin—bright red (ceroid may also be stained)
Melanin and hemosiderin—unstained

Ceroid

Ceroid was originally described in 1941 as a brown acid-fast pigment occurring in rat livers with experimental cirrhosis. In gross preparations it is a yellow-brown substance and occurs in liver cells, large phagocytes, and surrounding fat globules. The exact origin and chemical composition of the pigment is not known, but the pigment most likely derives from fat substances through the oxidation of long-chain fatty acids. Pearse believes that it is a mixture of substances and a typical lipofuscin in an early stage of oxidation. The ceroid pigment is insoluble in alcohols, acetone, ether, dilute acids and alkalis, chloroform, carbon tetrachloride, and pyridine. It gives a variable Prussian blue reaction, usually negative, and stains by Mallory's hemofuscin method. The periodic acid–Schiff reaction is also variable but usually most of the pigment will color magenta. Clear small unstained globules may be seen within the positive

PAS–staining mass. They will also stain with acid-fast and lipid stains. Fluorescence with frozen sections shows a green-yellow that fades to pale yellow. In paraffin sections a golden brown fluorescence is seen, and it is these fluorescent characteristics plus the acid-fast stain that are the chief tests for identification of the ceroid pigment. (It should be noted, however, that other lipofuscins may give similar reactions with these two tests.)

ENDOGENOUS DEPOSITS
Uric acid and sodium urate crystals

Persons suffering from gout, a disorder of uric acid metabolism, may accumulate urate crystals around joints and occasionally in soft tissues. In other disease conditions (such as leukemia), excessive cellular destruction may occur, followed by a breakdown of the nucleoprotein contained in the cells. Ultimately, urate deposits may appear in the renal tubules.

Urate crystals are soluble in the usual aqueous fixatives; hence alcoholic fixatives must be used for their subsequent demonstration. Their presence may be conveniently shown by use of Gomori's methenamine silver technic.

Fixation and processing
1. Place specimens immediately in absolute alcohol for 24 hours. Change several times.
2. Place in 3 changes of acetone, 1½ hours each change.
3. Place in equal-parts mixture of acetone and benzene for 1 hour, changing tissue into a fresh mixture three times during the course of the hour.
4. Place in 2 changes of benzene, 30 minutes each change.
5. Give tissue 2 changes of paraffin, 1 hour each change.
6. Embed in paraffin.

Gomori's methenamine silver technic for urate crystal demonstration[14]

Solutions
Methenamine silver working solution
Stock methenamine silver (p. 187)   25 ml
Distilled water   25 ml
5% sodium borate   3 ml
0.1% gold chloride
3% sodium thiosulfate
Light green working solution (p. 187)

Technic
1. Deparaffinize with xylene and rinse with 3 changes of absolute alcohol.
2. Transfer slides into the preheated working solution of methenamine silver.

3. Incubate for 30 minutes at 60° C. Urate crystals should be black.
4. Rinse sections in distilled water.
5. Tone with gold chloride for 5 minutes.
6. Give sections 4 or 5 rinses of distilled water.
7. 3% sodium thiosulfate for 5 minutes.
8. Wash in tap water for 5 minutes.
9. Rinse in distilled water.
10. Counterstain in light green working solution for 2 minutes.
11. Dehydrate in 2 changes of 95% alcohol and 2 changes of absolute alcohol, clear in xylene, and coverslip, using a synthetic mounting medium.

Results (Plate 2, *B*)
Urate crystals—black
Background—green

EXOGENOUS PIGMENTS IN TISSUES

The most common exogenous pigment found in tissues is the anthracosis pigment caused by accumulation of coal dust and carbon particles in the lungs and lymphatic tissue. Its distribution may be focal or may affect the entire organ. It has been occasionally found in liver and spleen. Under intense light, it appears as yellow-brown granules when finely divided and black when clumped. It resists all the usual chemical reactions for pigment identification, is insoluble to all types of solvents, and will not bleach. Individuals with anthracosis may also show a pigment that is related more to oil and tar inhalation rather than carbon. This will appear as a browning of the cytoplasm, barely colors with Sudan IV, and is negative to other methods for pigment demonstration.

INORGANIC ELEMENTS

The components of tissues and cells are for the most part of an organic nature, yet metals contribute significantly to cell organization also. *Microincineration* is the process employed to study mineral content in tissues and gives information on the amount and distribution of the minerals without the organic elements interfering. Calcium, magnesium, silicon, and iron are among those substances that can be identified in an incinerated section.

Preparation of the tissue for this process should not add extrinsic mineral elements; therefore fixatives with chromate and mercuric salts should be avoided. Processing should not remove any elements already present. Although freeze-dried material and cryostat sections have been used, the usual procedure is done on paraffin sections. Fixation may be accomplished with 10% neutral buffered formalin, or in a mixture of 9 volumes of absolute alcohol to 1 volume of neutral commercial formalin. This latter fixative is preferred. Dehydration, clearing, and embedding proceed as usual. Sections are cut at 4 μm in a series that allows for alternate sections to be used for the actual microincineration process and the rest for routine staining technics (H & E) or special stains. Sections for the microincineration are mounted on slides made of quartz or hard glass that will not melt during the heating process. The usual albumin fixative is not used. Contact with water should be avoided.

Incineration is done in a suitable furnace with a flat floor or one in which flat copper strips can be placed horizontally to hold the slides. Incineration usually starts at 70° C and the temperature is gradually elevated by 70° C each 5 minutes until a final temperature of 650° C is reached. Generally 45 to 50 minutes are required for actual incineration time, but this can vary. Sections containing a great deal of collagen, for example, will take longer, as the first 70° C rise should be slow and sections should stay at 70° C for 1 hour before proceeding with the temperature elevation. Incomplete incineration is indicated by the presence of a brown-black carbonized structure of the remaining, incompletely burned off, organic matter. The end point is empirically determined, the oven is turned off, and the slides are allowed to slowly cool inside the oven. After cooling, sections are removed, coverslipped with a glycerol mounting medium, and examined.

Examination may be done with transmitted light, polarized light, or dark-field illumination. Examination with dark-field light is most suitable. Calcium and magnesium appear as a similar white amorphous ash. Iron is present as red to yellow ferric oxide. Silicon appears as a white birefringent crystalline substance. It is recommended that further chemical tests and stains be done on the nonincinerated sections to definitely identify the inorganic material.

IDENTIFICATION OF METALS IN TISSUE SECTIONS

Calcium, iron, zinc, copper, and lead are the common metals that may be identified in tissue sections.

Calcium

Calcium salts are normally present in bones and teeth. Abnormal deposits may be found in

$$Ca^{++}CO_3^- + 2[Ag^+NO_3^-] \longrightarrow Ag_2CO_3 + Ca^{++} + 2NO_3^-$$

$$2H^+ + Ag_2CO_3 \xrightarrow[\text{strong light}]{\text{reduction by}} 2Ag\downarrow + H_2O + CO_2$$

Metallic
silver

Fig. 12-3. Chemical reactions in the Von Kossa test for calcium.

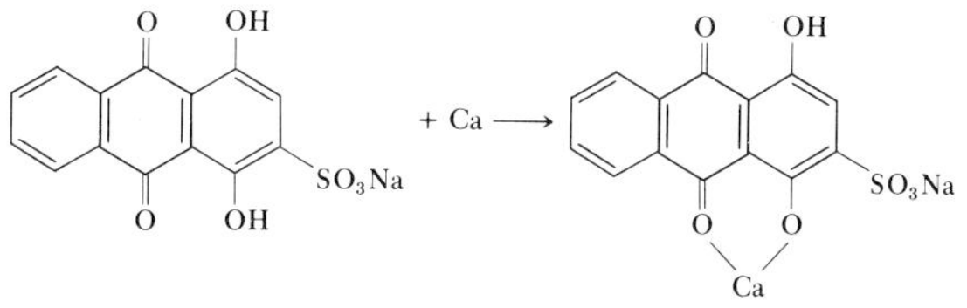

Alizarin red S   Alizarin red S–calcium complex

Fig. 12-4. Chelation of calcium with alizarin red S.

any area including arterial elastic lamellae, foci of infection with *Mycobacterium tuberculosis* or *Histoplasma capsulatum,* hyaline cartilage, lymph nodes, fibroids, and so forth.

With an H & E stain, most calcium salts are colored a deep blue-purple. Special stains for its identification include the Von Kossa technic, the alizarin red S stain, and the chloranilic acid method.

Von Kossa silver test for calcium[10]

Principle. This is a metal substitution technic for demonstration of calcium and depends on the anionic part of the calcium salt and hence is not specific for the calcium ion itself. Phosphate and carbonate are the most common anions in calcium deposits, and treatment with a metal results in the transformation of the calcium salt into the corresponding metal salt, which is then visualized in different ways. The transformation depends in part on the relative solubilities of the calcium and metal salts, and quantitative transformation occurs only if the metal salt is considerably less soluble than the original salt. In this technic, sections are treated with a silver nitrate solution and the silver is deposited, presumably by replacing the calcium, reduced by the action of strong light, and thereby visualized as metallic silver (Fig. 12-3).

Fixation. Alcohol preferred; formalin may be used. Avoid calcium in the fixative solution.

Embedding. Frozen or paraffin sections.

Solution

5% aqueous silver nitrate solution
5% sodium thiosulfate
Nuclear fast red (p. 183)

Technic

1. Hydrate sections to distilled water.
2. Immerse slides in (or flood slides with) the 5% silver nitrate solution.
3. Expose the immersed (or flooded) slide to bright sunlight or ultraviolet light for 10 to 20 minutes or to a 60-watt electric bulb at a range of 4 to 5 inches for 60 minutes. Stop exposure when calcium salts are black-brown.
4. Wash slides in several changes of distilled water.

5. Remove unreacted silver with 5% sodium thiosulfate for 2 minutes.
6. Counterstain for 3 to 5 minutes with nuclear fast red. Filter back.
7. Rinse slides well in several changes of distilled water.
8. Dehydrate, clear in xylene, and coverslip, using a synthetic mounting medium.

Results

Calcium salts—black to brown-black
Nuclei—red
Cytoplasm—pink
Note: Oxalate salts are usually believed to give a negative Von Kossa reaction.

Alizarin red S[15]

Principle. Alizarin red S, an anthraquinone derivative, may be used to demonstrate calcium in tissue sections. The reaction is not strictly specific for calcium, since magnesium, manganese, barium, strontium, and iron may interfere, but these elements usually do not occur in sufficient concentration to interfere with the staining. Demonstration depends on a chelation process with the dye, and the end product is believed to have the structural formula shown in Fig. 12-4.

Fixation. Neutral buffered formalin or alcoholic formalin. Avoid calcium in the fixative solution.

Embedding. Cut paraffin sections at 5 μm.

Solution

Staining solution

Alizarin red S (C.I. 58005)	2 gm
Distilled water	100 ml

Mix. Adjust the pH of this solution to a range of 4.1 to 4.3 with dilute ammonium hydroxide.

Technic

1. Hydrate slides to 50% alcohol.
2. Rinse rapidly in distilled water.
3. Cover the section with the alizarin red S solution.
4. Observe the reaction under a microscope and remove when a red-orange lake forms (30 seconds to 5 minutes). The lake should be heavy but not too diffuse.

5. Shake off excess dye and blot carefully.
6. Dehydrate in acetone for 10 to 20 seconds and in acetone-xylene (50:50) for 10 to 20 seconds.
7. Clear in xylene and mount in a synthetic mounting medium.

Results

Calcium deposits (except oxalate)—orange-red
This precipitate is birefringent.

Carr's chloranilic acid technic for calcium [16]

Principle. Chloranilic acid (2,5-dichloro-3,6-dihydroxy-*p*-quinone) is a strong dibasic organic acid that forms a number of salts with cations including calcium, copper, manganese, barium, strontium, zinc, and silver. Cations that do not form salts with this reagent include sodium, potassium, ammonium, iron, and magnesium. The contours of the stained calcium deposits are irregular, and numerous thin sharp crystals of calcium chloranilate project from their borders.

Fixation. 10% neutral buffered formalin.

Embedding. Cut paraffin sections at 5 μm.

Solutions

Chloranilic acid solution

Distilled water	100 ml
Sodium hydroxide	0.4 gm
Chloranilic acid	1 gm

Shake solution until all the chloranilic acid is dissolved. Some crystallization may occur; however, staining ability is not impaired. Filter through fine filter paper prior to use.
Working solution of light green (p. 187)

Technic

1. Hydrate sections to distilled water.
2. Stain in chloranilic acid solution for 30 minutes. Discard after use.
3. Wash in running distilled water for 15 minutes or dip 50 times in a dish of distilled water.
4. Counterstain in light green working solution for 2 to 3 minutes. Discard after use.
5. Rinse in distilled water.
6. Dehydrate, clear, and coverslip, using a synthetic mounting medium.

Results

Background—green
Calcium—red brown
Under polarized light, calcium deposits are brilliantly birefringent.

Pizzolato's method for calcium oxalate [17]

Familial primary oxalosis has an autosomal recessive mode of inheritance, and oxalate deposits may be found in the heart, renal parenchyma, bone, testes, and medial layer of vessels.

Calcium oxalate will not color with hematoxylin or alizarin red. Oxalate salts are considered to give usually a negative von Kossa reaction, but there is disagreement concerning this characteristic.

Principle. Hydrogen peroxide converts oxalate present in tissue to carbonate. See the Von Kossa method (p. 227) for the theory of staining carbonate salts.

Fixation. Neutral buffered formalin.

Embedding. Cut several paraffin sections at 5 to 7 μm. Avoid excessive albumin adhesive.

Solutions

30% hydrogen peroxide
5% silver nitrate
0.1% safranin in 1% acetic acid

Technic

1. Hydrate slides.
2. Mix equal volumes of the hydrogen peroxide and silver nitrate solutions. Prepare enough to allow 2 ml of the mixture for each slide. Flood slides with the mixture.
3. Expose flooded sections to a 60-watt tungsten-filament electric lamp (or a 25-watt fluorescent bulb). The light should be approximately 15 cm above the sections. Exposure time varies from 15 to 30 minutes. If excessive bubbling is noted, replace the reagent mixture with a fresh one.
4. Rinse thoroughly in distilled water.
5. Counterstain, if desired, for 2 to 3 minutes with safranin. Rinse in distilled water.
6. Dehydrate, clear, and coverslip, using a synthetic mounting medium.

Results

Calcium oxalate—black
Nuclei—red (if counterstained)
Note: Calcium fluoride and calcium and barium sulfates do not react by this method.

Iron

Iron-containing complexes may be divided into two general categories—complexes in which the iron is loosely bound to proteins (as in hemosiderin) and complexes where the iron is strongly bound (as in hemoglobin). Loosely bound iron complexes release the ion (ferric usually) by mild acid treatment. The strongly bound iron, sometimes known as "masked iron," is released with stronger treatment employing hydrogen peroxide. A few drops of 30% hydrogen peroxide that has been alkalinized by the addition of a small amount of dilute ammonium hydroxide or sodium carbonate, is placed on the hydrated tissue section and allowed to remain for 30 minutes. After this incubation, the tissue sections are washed in tap water before one proceeds with staining reac-

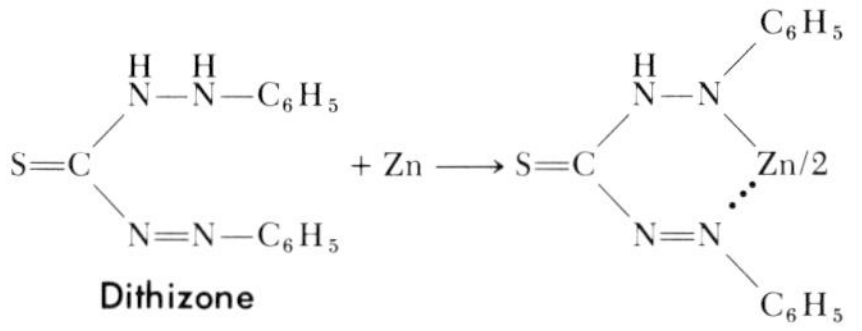

Fig. 12-5. Formation of zinc-dithizone complex. (From Mager, M., McNary, W. F., Lionetti, F.: Histochemical detection of zinc, J. Histochem. Cytochem. **1**:493, 504, 1953, The Histochemical Society, Baltimore, The Williams & Wilkins Co. [agent].)

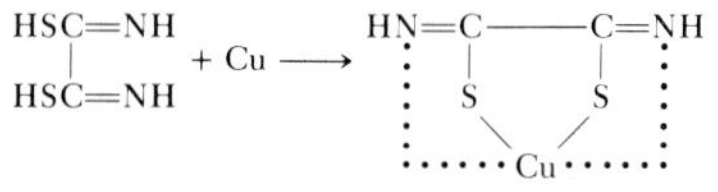

Fig. 12-6. Reaction of copper with rubeanic acid. (From Barka, T., and Anderson, P.: Histochemistry, New York, 1965, Harper & Row, Publishers.)

tions. The two main reactions—Prussian blue (for ferric ion) and Turnbull's blue (for ferrous ion)—have already been discussed.

Zinc[18]

Zinc has been reported to occur in pancreatic islet cells, parietal cells of the stomach, and prostatic epithelial cells. The dithizone reaction may be used for demonstration.

Principle. Diphenylthiocarbazone (dithizone) will form insoluble colored complex salts with a number of heavy metals, including zinc. The reaction will proceed in acid, neutral, or aqueous solutions and the complex formed with zinc is red-purple (Fig. 12-5).

The specificity of the dithizone reaction is increased by the use of complex-forming buffer solutions. Most heavy metals that might interfere with the reaction are not present in sufficient amounts to cause much interference.

Solutions

Complexing buffer

Dissolve 55 gm of sodium thiosulfate, 9 gm of sodium acetate, and 1 gm of potassium cyanide in 100 ml of distilled water. Shake in a separatory funnel with several successive portions of dithizone in carbon tetrachloride until the carbon tetrachloride layer is clear green. (This removes traces of zinc.)

Stock dithizone

Dissolve 10 mg of dithizone in 100 ml of anhydrous acetone (reagent grade). Store in brown glass bottle in the refrigerator.

1 N acetic acid

20% aqueous solution of sodium potassium tartrate (Rochelle salt)

Working solution

Mix 24 ml of stock dithizone solution with 18 ml of distilled water. Adjust with 1 N acetic acid to pH 3.7. Add 5.8 ml of the complexing buffer solution and 0.2 ml of the Rochelle salt solution. Solution should be used immediately.

Technic

1. Use freeze-dried or cryostat sections for this technic. If cryostat sections are used, postfix for 1 hour in absolute ethanol or methanol.
2. Stain with the working solution for 10 minutes.
3. Flood slides with chloroform to remove excess stain.
4. Rinse quickly in distilled water and mount in an aqueous mounting medium such as glycerol gelatin.

Results

Zinc—red-purple granules or diffuse red

Copper

Copper is usually not present in sufficient amounts in tissue sections to allow for demonstration. When present in excessive pathologic amounts, such as in Wilson's disease and some forms of cirrhosis, it may be demonstrated by the rubeanic acid method. The technic is sensitive and specific, but staining is variable at times, probably attributable to protein binding of the copper ion. Copper may also be demonstrated by use of p-dimethylaminobenzalrhodanine.

Rubeanic acid method[19]

Principle. Sections are treated with an alcoholic solution of rubeanic acid, which reacts with copper to form a dark green-black precipitate of copper rubeanate. Nickel and cobalt react in a similar manner, but are soluble in the presence of acetate, hence the inclusion of sodium acetate in the staining solution. The complex is a salt of the diimido form of rubeanic acid with the copper ion (Fig. 12-6).

Solutions

0.1% rubeanic acid in absolute ethanol

10% aqueous sodium acetate

70% and absolute ethanol

Method

1. Fix tissue in formalin.
2. Process as usual and embed in paraffin. Cut 5 μm sections. Hydrate sections.
3. Immerse sections for 12 to 24 hours at 37° C in

the following solution: 5 ml of stock rubeanic acid and 100 ml of 10% sodium acetate.
4. Wash in 2 changes of 70% alcohol for 30 minutes each change.
5. Wash overnight in several changes of absolute alcohol.
6. Clear in xylene and mount in synthetic medium.

Results
Copper—green-black precipitate of copper rubeanate

Note: Reagents should not be contaminated with copper. If it is desired to release the protein-bound copper, place hydrated sections downward over a beaker containing concentrated hydrochloric acid for 15 minutes.

Rhodanine* method for copper[20]

Fixation. 10% buffered neutral formalin.
Embedding. Cut paraffin sections at 6 to 10 μm. (Thicker sections may stain better.)

Solutions
Distilled water, preferably deionized, should be used in all solutions and rinses.
Rhodanine saturated solution *(stock solution)*

p-Dimethylaminobenzalrhodanine*	0.2 gm
Absolute ethanol	100 ml

(Make sure jar has crystals on bottom.)
Rhodanine solution *(working solution)*

Rhodanine saturated solution	6 ml
Distilled water	94 ml

Note: Shake stock solution before measuring and mixing solutions and shake working solution when pouring it on slides.
Diluted Mayer's hematoxylin

Mayer's hematoxylin	50 ml
Distilled water	50 ml

0.5% aqueous sodium borate (borax)

Technic
1. Hydrate slides to distilled water.
2. Incubate in rhodanine working solution at 37° C for 18 hours.
3. Wash well in several changes of distilled water.
4. Stain in diluted Mayer's hematoxylin for 10 minutes.
5. Rinse with distilled water.
6. Quickly rinse in 0.5% sodium borate.
7. Rinse well with distilled water.
8. Dehydrate through 95% alcohol to absolute alcohol, clear in xylene, 2 changes each, and coverslip, using a synthetic mounting medium.

---

*Rhodanine is p-dimethylaminobenzalrhodanine, or 5-[p-(dimethylamino)benzylidene]rhodanine; Catalog no. 2748, Eastman Organic Chemicals Distillation Products Industries, Rochester, N.Y.

Results
Copper—bright red to red yellow
Nuclei—light blue

Note: With low copper concentrations in tissue, slight fading may occur after coverslipping and the golden precipitate may be difficult to distinguish from lipofuscin.

Mallory's stain for iron and copper[21]

Principle. This technic uses fresh, unoxidized hematoxylin without mordant salts. A metal chelate reaction takes place between the hematoxylin and the ferric or cupric ions, or both, present in the tissue, giving a black color with the iron salts and a dark blue with the copper salts.
Fixation. Fix tissues in alcohol. Formalin fixation will result in yellow-brown colors with the iron salts. Embed in paraffin. Cut sections at 5 μm.

Solutions
Hematoxylin solution
Dissolve 5 to 10 mg of hematoxylin in 0.5 to 1 ml of absolute alcohol. Add 10 ml of carbon dioxide–free distilled water (boil distilled water 5 minutes to drive off CO_2).

Method
1. Hydrate sections.
2. Stain sections 1 hour or more in the above hematoxylin solution.
3. Wash in several changes of tap water.
4. Dehydrate in alcohols, clear in xylene, and coverslip, using a synthetic mounting medium.

Results
Nuclei—bluish-gray
Hemosiderin—black
Copper—dark blue

Lead
Mallory-Parker stain for lead and copper[21]

Principle. Lead may also be present in tissue sections and can be demonstrated by this method. The mechanism is a metal chelate reaction, with the lead ion forming a dark gray-blue color on combination with the fresh hematoxylin.
Fixation. Fix tissue in 95% or absolute alcohol; formalin may be used for copper.
Embedding. Cut paraffin or celloidin sections at 5 to 6 μm.

Solutions
Hematoxylin reagent
Dissolve 5 to 10 mg of hematoxylin in a few drops of 95% alcohol and add 10 ml of freshly filtered 2% dibasic potassium phosphate.

Technic

1. Hydrate sections to distilled water.
2. Stain sections in hematoxylin solution for 2 to 3 hours at 54° C.
3. Wash in tap water for 10 to 60 minutes.
4. Dehydrate, clear in xylene, and coverslip, using a synthetic mounting medium.

Results

Lead—light to dark grayish blue
Nuclei—deep blue
Copper or hemofuscin pigment—intense blue
(Alcohol fixation) inorganic iron or hemosiderin—black
(Formalin fixation) inorganic iron or hemosiderin—dark brown

Note: Even slightly aged hematoxylin will give a brown color and is useless. Nonreducing resins should be used as mounting media, otherwise the stain colors will turn brown.

Gold[22]

Administration of colloidal gold as a therapeutic agent for rheumatoid arthritis may lead to its accumulation in tissue. A hydrogen peroxide method may be used for demonstration of the metal; with this technic, gold is reduced to the metallic state and other tissue pigments are bleached.

Hydrogen peroxide method

Fixation. Formalin.

Solution

3% hydrogen peroxide

Method

1. Hydrate paraffin sections.
2. Incubate sections for 1 to 3 days in 3% hydrogen peroxide at 37° C.
3. Wash well in distilled water; dehydrate, clear, and coverslip, using a synthetic mounting medium.

Counterstaining is not recommended, since slides are better evaluated without it. If necessary, hematoxylin may be used since it won't interfere too much with interpretation.

Results

Gold—rose-colored with some purple, blue, and black

Asbestos

Asbestos may occur in tissues either as long, thin, crystalline needles or as asbestos bodies that appear as beaded rods with large, rounded ends. They are golden-yellow in the unstained state and will usually give a positive Prussian blue reaction.

Aluminum

Aluminum is not usually present in sufficient amounts in tissue to allow for its demonstration. Increased amounts have been reported to occur in Alzheimer's disease. Aluminum forms a salt with morin (C.I. 75660) in acetic acid or neutral conditions, and when examined with ultraviolet light, this salt compound fluoresces an intense green.[23] Hydrated frozen or paraffin sections are pretreated in 1% aqueous hydrochloric acid for 10 minutes, rinsed in distilled water, and then rinsed in 85% ethanol. Sections are then stained for 10 minutes in 0.2% morin (3,5,7,2',4'-pentahydroxyflavone) in 85% ethanol containing 0.5% acetic acid. After staining, rinse sections in distilled water, dehydrate, clear, and coverslip, using a low-fluorescent mounting medium (such as DPX or HSR).[24] Exciter filters are BG38 and BG12; barrier filters are 50 and 65.

REFERENCES

1. Lillie, R. D., and Fullmer, H. M.: Histopathologic technic and practical histochemistry, ed. 4, New York, 1976, McGraw-Hill Book Co.
2. Barka, T., and Anderson, P.: Histochemistry, New York, 1965, Harper & Row, Publishers.
3. Zugibe, F. T.: Diagnostic histochemistry, St. Louis, 1970, The C. V. Mosby Co.
4. Dunn, R. C., and Thompson, E. C.: A new hemoglobin stain for histologic use, Arch. Pathol. **39:**49-50, 1945, copyright, Chicago, The American Medical Association.
5. Ralph, P. H.: The histochemical demonstration of hemoglobin in blood cells and tissue smears, Stain Technol. **16:**105-106, 1941, Baltimore, The Williams & Wilkins Co.
6. Mallory, F. B.: Pathological technique, New York, 1961, Hafner Publishing Co.
7. Okajima, K.: On the selective staining of the erythrocyte, Anat. Rec. **11:**295-296, 1916.
8. Gomori, G.: Microtechnical demonstration of iron, Am. J. Pathol. **12:**655-663, 1936.
9. Modification used at Ohio State University Hospitals, Columbus, Ohio.
10. McManus, J. F. A., and Mowry, R. W.: Staining methods: histologic and histochemical, New York, 1960, Harper & Row, Publishers.
11. Hall, M. J.: A staining reaction for bilirubin in sections of tissue, Am. J. Clin. Pathol. **34:**313-316, 1960.
12. Burtner, H. J., and Lillie, R. D.: A five-hour variant of Gomori's methenamine silver method for argentaffin cells, Stain Technol. **24:**225-227, 1949, Baltimore, The Williams & Wilkins Co.
13. Laidlaw, G. F., and Blackberg, S. N.: Melanoma studies. II. A simple technique for the dopa reaction, Am. J. Pathol. **8:**491-498, 1932.
14. Pearse, A. G. E.: Histochemistry, theoretical-ap-

plied, ed. 3, vol. 1, London, 1968, Churchill Livingstone.

15. McGee-Russell, S. M.: Histochemical methods for calcium, J. Histochem. Cytochem. **6:**22-42, 1958, The Histochemical Society, Baltimore, The Williams & Wilkins Co. (agent).

16. Carr, L. B., Rambo, O. N., Feichtmeir, T. V.: A method of demonstrating calcium in tissue sections using chloranilic acid, J. Histochem. Cytochem. **9:**415-417, 1961, The Histochemical Society, Baltimore, The Williams & Wilkins Co. (agent).

17. Pizzolato, P.: Histochemical recognition of calcium oxalate, J. Histochem. Cytochem. **12:**333-336, 1964, The Histochemical Society, Baltimore, The Williams & Wilkins Co. (agent).

18. Mager, M., McNary, W. F., and Lionetti, F.: Histochemical detection of zinc, J. Histochem. Cytochem. **1:**493-504, 1953, The Histochemical Society, Baltimore, The Williams & Wilkins Co. (agent).

19. Uzman, L. L.: Histochemical localization of copper with rubeanic acid, Lab. Invest. **5:**299-305, 1958.

20. Lindquist, R. R.: Studies on the pathogenesis of hepatolenticular degeneration, Arch. Pathol. **87:**370-379, 1969, copyright, Chicago, The American Medical Association.

21. Mallory, F. B., and Parker, F., Jr.: Fixing and staining methods for lead and copper in tissues, Am. J. Pathol. **15:**517-522, 1939.

22. Elftman, H., and Elftman, A. G.: Histologic methods for the demonstration of gold in tissues, Stain Technol. **20:**59-62, 1945, Baltimore, The Williams & Wilkins Co.

23. Feigl, F.: Spot tests in inorganic analysis, ed. 5, Amsterdam, 1958, Elsevier North Holland Biomedical Press.

24. DeBoni, U., Scott, J. W., and Crapper, D. R.: Intracellular aluminum binding: a histochemical study, Histochemie **40:**31-37, 1974.

Microorganisms

Microorganisms are life forms so small that their detection requires microscopic observation. Microorganisms of medical importance are subdivided into the following groups:

Bacteria
Fungi
Viruses
Protozoa

Control tissues containing the appropriate organisms should be used when one does microorganism demonstrations. Smears made from commercially available material have been employed as known positive controls for bacterial and fungal staining.[1,30]

BACTERIA

Bacteria are microscopic unicellular organisms widely distributed in soil, air, food products, various parts of the body, etc. Their size varies from 0.2 to 5 μm, with the average being approximately 1.5 μm. They may be classified into three groups on the basis of shape: spheric, rod shaped, or spiral. Like plants, they possess a cell wall, but unlike true plants they lack chloro-

phyll and are colorless. To study their morphology, therefore, one needs to use dyes. Classification of bacteria does not rest solely on morphology and staining characteristics, however, since bacteria may be similar in these respects yet differ widely in others, including pathogenicity. The most commonly used staining methods in the histopathology lab for demonstrating bacteria include the Giemsa methods (p. 155), Gram stains, acid-fast technics, and certain silver procedures.

TECHNICS FOR DIFFERENTIAL DEMONSTRATION
Gram reaction
Diagnostic applications

The most informative routine stain for demonstrating bacteria in tissue sections is the Gram stain, and this technic differentiates the bacteria into the gram-positive and the gram-negative categories. Variants of the Gram stain are useful in the determination of whether an abscess or necrosis is bacterial in origin. Gram-positive fungal filaments of *Nocardia* and *Actinomyces* may also be shown.

Principle. Basically, the procedure involves the application of a crystal violet solution, followed by an iodine mordant to form a dye lake. Both gram-positive and gram-negative cells are colored blue-black after these two steps. (In any modification of the Gram stain, the mordant must be applied after the actual dye application. If sections are exposed to the mordant first, followed by the dye, decolorization will be similar in action with both the positive and negative organisms.) Decolorization is the third major step, and its purpose is to render the gram-negative cells colorless while leaving the blue-black dye lake in the gram-positive cells. The decolorizer penetrates the entire cell, and the step is a relative rather than an absolute one. If sections are exposed too long to the action of the decolorizing agent, even gram-positive cells will lose the dye lake and become colorless. The final major step is counterstaining; usually safranin or basic fuchsin is employed for this purpose, and the gram-negative cells are dyed pink-red.

There are numerous theories that attempt to explain the gram reaction. Although the dye lake is most likely distributed throughout the entire cell, the cell wall of the bacteria is believed to play a role in keeping the dye lake within the gram-positive cell. Studies have shown that gram-positive cells have walls three or four layers thick and measure 15 to 25 nm in thickness; gram-negative cells consist of only two layers about 8 to 12.5 nm thick. This would explain differential decolorization on a somewhat physical basis because the gram-negative cell wall would not be thick enough to resist decolorization relative to the gram-positive cell wall. Another factor is that gram-positive cell walls have a greater proportion of lipoprotein and polysaccharide components within them; hence they are relatively more impermeable cell walls compared to the gram-negative cell walls. This lesser permeability would aid in dye-lake retention once the lake had entered the gram-positive cell. A chemical factor may also be involved in Gram staining as experiments have shown that gram-positive cells contain an acidic substance within the wall. This particular substance, known as magnesium ribonucleate, is known to form insoluble complexes with crystal violet and iodine, and these complexes do not decolorize with conventional decolorizing agents. Gram-negative cells lack this substance.

Taylor's Brown-Brenn modified Gram stain[2]

Fixation. Bouin's, 10% formalin, Zenker's, Helly's.

Embedding. Embed in paraffin and cut 5 μm sections.

Solutions

Harris's hematoxylin (p. 142)

Hucker's ammonium oxalate crystal violet

Crystal violet, 10% alcoholic solution	2 ml
Distilled water	18 ml
Ammonium oxalate, 1% aqueous solution	80 ml

Mix and filter before use. Solution is stable for 3 to 6 months.

Gram's iodine (p. 131)

1% hydrochloric acid in 70% ethanol

Filtered saturated aqueous lithium carbonate

Ether-acetone solution

Equal-parts mixture of ether and acetone

Note: Ethyl ether is extremely flammable and volatile. Extinguish all open flames and cigarettes when using this reagent. Store in an explosion-proof refrigerator.

Alcoholic basic fuchsin

Stock solution

0.1% basic fuchsin diluted with 95% ethanol

Working solution

5 ml of stock solution diluted to 60 ml with distilled water

Picric acetone solution

Anhydrous picric acid	0.1 gm
Acetone	100 ml

The picric acid component should be nearly anhydrous and possess no greenish tint. If greenish, it is unsuitable for use. Dehydrate by spreading over calcium chloride in a dessicator jar until it is nearly whitish. *Note:* Anhydrous picric acid has explosive tendencies.

Technic

1. Hydrate slides.
2. Stain in freshly filtered Harris's hematoxylin for 5 to 10 minutes. Refilter solution.
3. Wash in running tap water to remove excess hematoxylin from slides.
4. Wash in 1% acid alcohol. One brief rinse is sufficient to obtain the desired brick-red color.
5. Wash in tap water for 3 minutes.
6. Wash in saturated lithium carbonate to intensify the blue color.
7. Wash in tap water 1 to 5 minutes. Proceed with the technic carrying one slide through at a time in a Coplin jar sequence.
8. Stain 2 minutes in Hucker's solution.
9. Wash quickly with water.
10. Mordant in iodine solution for 1 minute. Sections should turn black. Discard after use.
11. Wash with water; blot with water-moistened filter paper.
12. Decolorize with ether acetone until blue no longer comes off the section.
13. Stain for 3 minutes in working solution of alcoholic basic fuchsin. Discard after use.

14. Wash with water; blot sections.
15. Dip in acetone until sections begin to decolorize (10 to 15 seconds).
16. Pass quickly to picric acetone to decolorize background tissue until it becomes brownish red-yellow (15 to 30 seconds).
17. Pass quickly through acetone-xylene mixture I (1:2), acetone-xylene mixture II (1:3), and xylene 2 changes. Coverslip, using a synthetic mounting medium.

Results (Plate 1, *J* and *K*)
Gram-positive cells—blue-black
Gram-negative cells—pink-red
Cytoplasm—brownish yellow
Red blood cells—red to greenish yellow
Connective tissue—red
White blood cells—red
Necrotic tissue—yellow-green

Special precautions. Sections should not be allowed to dry at any time during the staining process, as drying will tend to favor the formation of insoluble compounds that will not be decolorized when the ether-acetone is used.

Brown-Hopps modified Gram stain[3]

Fixation. 10% neutral buffered formalin; 2.5% buffered glutaraldehyde; or Helly's. Bouin's fixed tissues do not stain satisfactorily.
Embedding. Cut paraffin sections at 5 μm.

Solutions
1% aqueous crystal violet
   Filter before use.
Gram's iodine (p. 131)
Cellosolve (ethylene glycol monoethyl ether)
0.5% aqueous basic fuchsin
Gallego's differentiating solution

Distilled water	50 ml
37% to 40% formalin	1 ml
Glacial acetic acid	0.5 ml

1.5% aqueous tartrazine

Technic
1. Hydrate sections to distilled water.
2. Place slides in staining rack and stain with crystal violet for 2 minutes.
3. Drain off the crystal violet and rinse with distilled water.
4. Mordant in Gram's iodine for 5 minutes.
5. Rinse in distilled water.
6. Differentiate in a Coplin jar of Cellosolve until blue color ceases to stream away from the section. This will take about 5 to 10 seconds. Timing is critical.
7. *Quickly* rinse in distilled water.
8. Stain in basic fuchsin solution for 5 minutes.
9. Rinse in distilled water.
10. Differentiate and fix the basic fuchsin stain with Gallego's solution for 5 minutes.
11. Rinse thoroughly in distilled water. Blot slides lightly to remove excess water but do not allow tissue to dry.
12. Tartrazine solution for 3 seconds. Timing is critical. Immediately blot away excess but not to dryness.
13. 3 changes of Cellosolve—6 *quick dips in each change*.
14. 3 changes of xylene—10 dips in each change. Coverslip, using a synthetic mounting medium.

Results
Gram-positive organisms—blue to blue-violet
Gram-negative organisms—red
Background—yellow

Gram stain for smears[4]
1. Heat-fix air-dried smears.
2. Place on a staining rack and cover with a solution of crystal violet (1% aqueous, or Hucker's solution, p. 234).
3. Drain off crystal violet and rinse with distilled water.
4. Cover slides with Gram's iodine (p. 131) and mordant for 30 seconds to 1 minute.
5. Drain off iodine and decolorize for 30 to 60 seconds with 95% ethanol, or for 5 to 10 seconds with acetone.
6. Wash with distilled water.
7. Counterstain 30 to 60 seconds in a 0.1% to 0.5% aqueous solution of safranin O.
8. Wash in distilled water, air-dry, and examine with oil immersion.

Results
Gram-positive organisms—blue to blue-black
Gram-negative organisms—red

Acid-fast technics
Applications of acid-fast technics

Acid-fast methods are most frequently used to demonstrate the presence of acid-fast bacteria in tissue sections. Acid-fast bacteria belong to the genus *Mycobacterium,* of which several species are pathogenic for man, including *Mycobacterium tuberculosis* (causative agent for tuberculosis), *Mycobacterium leprae* (causative agent for leprosy), and various other species that cause atypical mycobacteriosis. *Mycobacterium leprae* is best shown with Wade's modification of Fite's new fuchsin formaldehyde technic.

Certain fungal species also exhibit acid-fast characteristics (*Nocardia* species), and a modification of Fite's stain may be used for demonstration of this organism (p. 237).

Certain lipofuscins (ceroid) and intranuclear inclusion bodies will show positive acid-fast characteristics after a prolonged staining time with Ziehl-Neelsen carbol fuchsin (p. 237).

Human sperm are acid-fast positive and may be stained with Berg's stain (p. 281). Russell bodies (variable-shaped bodies that occur in plasma cell cytoplasm and are frequently seen in cancer cells) are also positive with acid-fast technics.

Principle. Most acid-fast stains involve the application of a phenylmethane dye (such as pararosaniline, rosaniline, or new fuchsin) in a phenol solution. Phenol enhances the staining and appears to combine with the fuchsin dye within the acid-fast bacilli. It also functions to dissolve the fuchsin dye. Alcohol is usually added to the carbol-fuchsin solution both to enhance the staining and dissolve the dye. When the carbol-fuchsin is applied, all cells, including the normally hard-to-stain acid-fast varieties, are colored red.

The next step in the procedure involves the application of the acid alcohol decolorizer. More uniform decolorization is obtained with use of an alcoholic, rather than aqueous, solution. At the decolorization stage, all tissue elements except the acid-fast ones, are rendered colorless. This is the classic acid-fast phenomenon; that is, acid-fast elements (in this case, acid-fast bacilli) retain a carbol-fuchsin stain and resist decolorization with acid treatment.

There are several opinions as to why the acid-fast bacteria stain and resist decolorization as they do. One concept states that acid-fastness is determined by selective permeability of the cell wall, and should the cell be mechanically disrupted, the acid-fast property will be lost. There also seems to be a correlation between the lipid content of the acid-fast bacteria and the ability to stain. Experiments have shown that a particular lipid fraction (mycolic acid) exists within the cell wall of *Mycobacterium*. This fraction, in combination with cellular polysaccharides, demonstrates the acid-fast phenomenon. The only problem in accepting this fraction as the sole cause of acid-fastness is the fact that in vitro demonstration of acid-fastness of mycolic acid requires many times the amount of the substance ordinarily contained in an acid-fast bacterium. The presence of the mycolic acid fraction therefore is more likely a contributing factor in the mechanism.

Other bacterial types may be demonstrated by the counterstain employed, usually methylene blue (malachite green, light green, or fast green FCF may also be used). The final result shows the acid-fast bacteria a bright red, and other tissue elements are colored according to the counterstain used.

The property of acid-fastness is one of degree because there are differences in the resistance to decolorization depending on the amount of acid used in the decolorizing agent. Acid-fast cells may also appear beaded rather than homogeneously colored, and this beading is believed to be a staining artifact. It may be avoided by use of pure dyes and the chloride (rather than the acetate) salt of the basic fuchsin in the staining solution. Drying of a section after the carbol-fuchsin staining produces a compound that is resistant to decolorization. Attempts to remove this compound with repeated exposure to the acid alcohol will render the acid-fast organisms completely unstained.

Kinyoun's acid-fast stain[4]

Fixation. Formalin preferred. Other fixatives may be used.

Embedding. Embed in paraffin and cut 5 μm sections.

Solutions

Kinyoun's carbol-fuchsin

Basic fuchsin	4 gm
Phenol crystals, melted	8 gm
95% ethanol	20 ml
Distilled water	100 ml

Filter before use. Discard if precipitate adheres to the sides of the storage bottle. Stable for 1 to 2 months.

Acid alcohol

95% ethanol	99 ml
Concentrated hydrochloric acid	1 ml

Methylene blue

Stock solution

Methylene blue	0.7 gm
95% ethanol	50 ml

Filter into a stock bottle. Stable about 3 months.

Working solution

Stock solution	5 ml
Tap water	45 ml

Technic

1. Hydrate slides to distilled water.
2. Stain in Kinyoun's carbol-fuchsin for 1 hour at room temperature.
3. Wash well in tap water.
4. Decolorize in two changes of acid alcohol; tissue should be pale pink.
5. Wash in tap water.
6. Counterstain in working solution of methylene blue for a few seconds. For better control of the stain intensity, individual slides may be carried through a Coplin-jar sequence of counterstain, alcohols, and xylene.
7. 95% alcohol, 2 changes.

8. Absolute alcohol, 2 changes.
9. Xylene, 2 changes. Coverslip, using a synthetic mounting medium.

Results (Plate 1, *A*)
Acid-fast bacilli—bright red
Background—blue

Ziehl-Neelsen stain[6]

Fixation. Any well-fixed tissue may be used.
Embedding. Embed in paraffin and cut 5 μm sections.

Solutions
Carbol fuchsin solution

Basic fuchsin	0.5 gm
Distilled water	50 ml
Absolute ethanol	5 ml
Melted phenol crystals	2.5 ml

Filter solution before use.
Decolorizing solution
1% hydrochloric acid in 70% ethanol
or
1% aqueous sulfuric acid solution
Working methylene blue counterstain (p. 236)

Technic
1. Hydrate sections to distilled water.
2. Carbol fuchsin solution, 1 hour at room temperature.
3. Decolorize sections until tissue appears pale pink using either of the decolorizing solutions listed above.
4. Wash for 5 to 10 minutes in running tap water.
5. Continue with steps 6 to 9 described in the preceding Kinyoun's method.

Results
Acid-fast bacilli—bright red
Red blood cells—yellow orange
Other tissue elements—blue

The use of heat and prolonged staining times with the Ziehl-Neelsen carbol-fuchsin may be used to demonstrate the acid-fast characteristics of certain lipofuscins (ceroid) as well as intranuclear inclusion bodies that may occur in cases of chronic lead or bismuth poisoning. Hydrated sections are stained with the carbol-fuchsin solution for 3 hours at 60° C, decolorized with acid alcohol until red blood cells are faint pink, and directly counterstained with an unacidified aqueous alum hematoxylin. After counterstaining, sections are washed in running tap water for 5 minutes, rinsed in distilled water, dehydrated, cleared, and coverslipped as usual.

Fite's stain[9]

Fixation. 10% Formalin. Zenker's also gives good results.

Embedding. Embed in paraffin and cut 5 μm sections.

Solutions
Xylene petrolatum mixture

Liquid petrolatum (paraffin oil)	1 part
Xylene	2 parts

Ziehl-Neelsen carbol-fuchsin (see Ziehl-Neelsen stain, left column)
Working methylene blue solution (p. 236)
Acid alcohol

70% alcohol	99 ml
Concentrated hydrochloric acid	1 ml

Technic
1. Remove paraffin with xylene-petrolatum mixture. Allow two changes of 12 minutes each.
2. Drain slides, wipe off excess oil, and blot to opacity. It is important to blot well; otherwise, residual oil will produce a staining artifact.[8] Rinse in water until slide is clear.
3. Stain for 30 minutes at room temperature in the carbol-fuchsin solution.
4. Wash in tap water.
5. Decolorize with acid alcohol. Tissue should be pale pink. One to 2 minutes may be required.
6. Wash in tap water.
7. Counterstain with working solution of methylene blue for 30 seconds.
8. Wash in tap water.
9. Blot, allow tissue to dry out well, and mount directly in a synthetic mounting medium.

Results
Acid-fast bacilli—red
Background—blue

Nocardia demonstration. For demonstration of *Nocardia species*,[9] stain 10 minutes (timing is critical) in the carbol-fuchsin solution. Decolorize in 1% aqueous sulfuric acid for 5 to 10 minutes. Agitate slides frequently to remove background staining. Counterstain lightly in methylene blue; rinse in tap water to remove excess methylene blue. Blot dry and allow tissue to air-dry. Coverslip directly, using a synthetic mounting medium.

Results
Nocardia—red
Background—light blue

Fite's new fuchsin formaldehyde technic[10]

Principle. Sections are treated with a phenol solution of new fuchsin. (New fuchsin is believed to give better staining results than those obtained with solutions of rosaniline or pararosaniline.) After being stained, sections are treated with a concentrated formalin solution, which is considered an aldehyde-mordanting procedure that results in cells highly resistant to decolorization. The formaldehyde also changes the color of the fuchsin-stained cells from red to violet. Acid alcohol is employed as the decolorizing agent, and at this step all cells, except the acid-fast variety, are decolorized. Sections are again immersed in the formalin solution to reintensify the stain in the acid-fast bacilli. Counterstaining is done with hematoxylin to color nuclei and Van Gieson's solution to color collagen, muscle, and cell cytoplasm.

Fixation. 10% neutral buffered formalin or Zenker's.

Embedding. Cut paraffin sections at 5 μm.

Solutions
New fuchsin staining solution

Phenol	5 gm (melted)
Ethanol or methanol	10 ml
New fuchsin	1 gm
Distilled water	to make 100 ml

Concentrated (40%) formalin
2% hydrochloric acid in 95% ethanol
Harris's hematoxylin (p. 142)
Van Gieson's solution (p. 189)

Technic
1. Hydrate sections.
2. Stain in new fuchsin solution for 60 minutes. Rinse well in tap water.
3. Immerse in concentrated formalin for 5 minutes.
4. Decolorize with acid alcohol. Rinse well in tap water.
5. Immerse in formalin again for a few seconds. Rinse well in tap water.
6. Counterstain with Harris's hematoxylin for 2 minutes.
7. Wash in water.
8. Stain 3 minutes with Van Gieson's solution.
9. Dehydrate, clear, and coverslip, using a synthetic mounting medium.

Results
Acid-fast bacilli—violet
Muscle and cytoplasm—yellow
Collagen—red
Nuclei—bluish

Wade's modification of Fite's new fuchsin formaldehyde[11]

Principle. Not all acid-fast bacilli are young and readily stained, and Wade's technic is used primarily when older, less easily stained forms are present in the tissue sections. It may also be used to demonstrate the lepra bacillus, which is more difficult to color than are the more conventional acid-fast forms. Not only may the bacilli themselves be inherently difficult to stain by the conventional technics already discussed, but the tissue-processing technics may also cause difficulty in their demonstration. Numerous steps are involved in the preparation of a tissue for paraffin embedding, and the reagents used in the dehydrating and clearing may affect the waxy components of the bacillus capsule in such a way that when slides are deparaffinized, acid-fast components are extracted. If this is the case, the cells will be decolorized when exposed to the action of the acid alcohol. One may overcome this difficulty to a certain extent by not exposing the slides to the action of xylene in the deparaffinization process. Instead, paraffin is removed by a "protective" mixture of turpentine and paraffin oil. This mixture will not extract acid-fast components, and there is a minimum of section shrinkage. A longer staining time in the fuchsin solution is done so that all acid-fast cells, even the deteriorated ones, will be stained. Formalin treatment functions as it does in the Fite's new fuchsin formaldehyde technic. Sulfuric acid solution is used as the decolorizing agent. Potassium permanganate is an oxidizer and removes excess fuchsin from the tissue; oxalic acid is used to bleach the excess permanganate from the section. Van Gieson's counterstain functions to color the muscle, cytoplasm, and collagen.

Solutions
Deparaffinizing solution

Rectified turpentine	2 parts
Paraffin oil (liquid petrolatum)	1 part

Fite's new fuchsin solution (see preceding technic)
40% formalin
5% sulfuric acid
1% potassium permanganate
2% oxalic acid
Van Gieson's solution (p. 189)

Technic
1. Deparaffinize with two 5-minute changes of the deparaffinizing solution.
2. Drain slide; wipe back and edges of slides; blot with filter paper until section appears opaque. Blot well or the residual oil may produce a staining artifact. Clear slide in water.
3. Stain overnight (18 to 24 hours) in new fuchsin solution.
4. Wash in water for 2 minutes and immerse in 40% formalin. Acid-fast bacilli should turn blue, and sections may also turn blue or remain reddish.
5. Immerse in 5% sulfuric acid for 1 minute. Wash in water for 5 minutes.
6. Treat sections with 1% potassium permanganate for 3 minutes. Rinse in water.
7. Bleach with 2% oxalic acid. Timing should not

exceed 1 minute. Rinse in several changes of running tap water.

8. Stain 3 minutes in Van Gieson's solution.
9. Dehydrate rapidly in 95% ethanol, change absolute ethanol twice, clear in xylene, and coverslip, using a synthetic mounting medium.

Results
Acid-fast bacilli—dark blue
Collagen—red
Muscle and cytoplasm—yellow

Note: Wade recommends a carbowax embedding procedure rather than paraffin for the purpose of demonstrating leprosy bacilli. Acid-fast staining may be increased in these bacilli when they are treated with the paraffin oil and turpentine mixture for 6 to 10 hours, as this aids in "refatting" the deteriorated bacilli, hence making them more readily stained.

Auramine-rhodamine fluorescent technic[12]

Tissue suspected of containing *Mycobacterium tuberculosis* or other acid-fast bacilli may be rapidly examined under low magnification with this technic. Auramine O and rhodamine B are both basic dyes and fluoresce in the ultraviolet range; the use of both dyes in the staining solution gives better results than using either separately. The exact mechanism of their staining of the acid-fast bacilli is not known.

Fixation. Neutral buffered formalin.

Embedding. Embed in paraffin and cut 5 μm.

Solutions
Auramine-rhodamine solution

Auramine O (C.I. 41000)	10.5 gm
Rhodamine B (C.I. 45170)	5.25 gm
Glycerol	525 ml
Phenol	70 ml
Sterile distilled water	350 ml

Rinse all glassware in sterile distilled water before using it to make up this solution. Place the solution in the oven (60° C) overnight and filter it the next day into brown bottles. Store the solution at room temperature.

0.5% acid alcohol

70% ethanol	995 ml
Concentrated hydrochloric acid	5 ml

In making 70% ethanol from 95% or absolute ethanol, use sterile distilled water as the diluent. Rinse all glassware in sterile distilled water before use.

0.5% potassium permanganate

Dissolve 5 gm of potassium permanganate in distilled water and dilute up to 1 liter.

Use a positive and a negative control in each Coplin jar or staining dish. It is not necessary to include a control for each case stained. The negative control is normal lung.

Technic
1. Deparaffinize sections and hydrate to sterile distilled water. Avoid regular distilled water.
2. Stain slides in the auramine-rhodamine solution by placing the slides in a 60° C to 70° C oven for 1 hour *or* by placing the slides in a water bath at 45° to 50° C for 5 minutes and transferring slides to a 60° C to 70° C oven for 20 minutes.
3. Discard auramine-rhodamine solution. Differentiate in acid alcohol until the sections are colorless. While differentiating, quickly pour acid alcohol on and off the slides while agitating the slides. Use fresh acid alcohol as needed. Differentiate as quickly as possible.
4. Rinse slides in distilled water *or* wash in running tap water for 5 minutes followed by a few rinses in distilled water.
5. Counterstain in potassium permanganate for 2 minutes. Discard solution.
6. Rinse slides in distilled water, dehydrate, clear in xylene, and coverslip, using HSR, Permount, or Fluormount.
7. Examine using a high-dry objective with a UG1 or UG2 exciter filter and a colorless ultraviolet barrier filter.

Results (Plate 1, *C*)
Acid-fast bacilli fluoresce reddish yellow.
Background is green-black.
Note: Deparaffinization by the Fite mixture (p. 237) increases the fluorescence of the acid-fast bacilli.

Spirochetes

Spirochetes are spiral-shaped bacteria, and several varieties are pathogenic for man, including the following:

Treponema. This type is difficult to demonstrate by routine methods and requires silver impregnation procedures to be visualized in tissue sections. These silver methods will be described shortly. *Treponema pallidum* causes syphilis; *Treponema pertenue* causes yaws, a tropical disease similar, but not identical to, syphilis; *Treponema carateum* causes pinta, primarily a skin disease.

Borrelia. Organisms of this genus may be demonstrated with the Wright or Giemsa technics and color pink-red with the Gram stain. *Borrelia recurrentis* causes relapsing fever, and *Borrelia vincentii* contributes to trench-mouth infection.

Leptospira. Organisms in this genus require silver impregnation procedures for best demonstration. Weil's disease (spirochetal jaundice) is caused by *Leptospira icterohaemorrhagiae;* other similar but rare diseases caused by *Leptospira* have also been reported.

Levaditi's classic method for staining tissue blocks that are suspected of containing spirochetes has been abandoned in favor of silver procedures that may be done on tissue sections. The Warthin-Starry and Dieterle methods are most commonly used. The Dieterle method has also proved useful for the demonstration of the causative agent of Legionnaires' disease (*Legionella pneumophilia*). Recently[31] it was reported that the Steiner and Steiner method can also be used to stain *Legionella pneumophilia* as well as spirochetes.

Warthin-Starry technic[13,14]

Principle. Spirochetes are argyrophilic; that is, they will adsorb silver from a silver solution but need a separate solution of a reducing agent to reduce the adsorbed silver to the visible metallic state. The effective reducing agent in the Warthin-Starry technic is hydroquinone, a phenolic compound that becomes oxidized to a quinone as the silver is reduced to the metallic state.

Fixation. Formalin.

Embedding. Embed in paraffin and cut 5 μm.

Special precautions. Add a positive control slide to each batch of slides run. All glassware should be cleaned in acid-dichromate solution, washed well in tap water, and rinsed several times in triply distilled water. (Any water is acceptable if a silver nitrate solution is mixed with it and remains clear for several hours.) Metal instruments should not be used to transfer slides. Use Teflon instruments or coat metal forceps with paraffin.

Solutions

Acidulated water
  Acidulate 1 liter of triply distilled water with a weak solution of citric acid (1% or less solution of the citric acid) to a pH of 3.8 to 4.4. pH of 4.0 is ideal for spirochete demonstration. Donovan bodies of granuloma inguinale may be demonstrated if the pH is 3.6. Phosphate buffer may be used instead of the acidulated water.

2% silver nitrate solution (for developer)
Silver nitrate C.P. crystals	2 gm
Acidulated water	100 ml

1% silver nitrate solution (for impregnation)
Silver nitrate C.P. crystals	1 gm
Acidulated water	100 ml

0.15% hydroquinone solution
Hydroquinone (photographic quality crystals)	0.15 gm
Acidulated water	100 ml

5% gelatin solution
Sheet gelatin (or granulated gelatin of high degree of purity)	10 gm
Acidulated water (heat before adding gelatin)	200 ml

Technic

1. Hydrate slides to triply distilled water. Rinse twice in the triply distilled water.
2. Place in 1% silver nitrate solution for 30 minutes at 43° C. A water bath may be used for warming.
3. Have the following solutions in separate acid-cleaned flasks warmed to 54° to 56° C in a water bath: 2% silver nitrate; 5% gelatin; 0.15% hydroquinone.
4. About 5 minutes before step 2 is completed, prepare the developer solution. The components of the developer should be added in the order given and the flask rotated after each addition:
   Developer solution
2% silver nitrate in acidulated water	1.5 ml
5% gelatin in acidulated water	3.75 ml
0.15% hydroquinone	2 ml
   Acid-cleaned pipettes should be used to measure the above amounts.
5. When step 2 is completed, place slides horizontally on a slide rack and cover with developer. Allow sections to develop until they are light golden brown or yellow. Time of development may vary from 3 to 12 minutes, but under standardized procedures the time is constant.
6. Rinse quickly and thoroughly in hot tap water (about 56° C).
7. Rinse in distilled water.
8. Dehydrate in 95% ethanol and absolute ethanol, clear in xylene, and mount in a synthetic mounting medium.

Results (Plate 1, *D*)
Spirochetes—black (if well developed)
Background—pale yellow to light brown.

The spirochetes appear yellow in underdeveloped sections. Check the known positive control to see that all the spirochetes are black and background is pale enough to allow good contrast. If all spirochetes are not black, either develop other slides to the desired intensity or rehydrate the slide to distilled water, add freshly mixed developer, and develop to the desired intensity.

Note: Melanin, nuclei, and certain pigments have a greater affinity for the silver solution than do the spirochetes. Spirochetes are not sharply demonstrated if they are near these elements, but prolonged development and a lower pH may aid in revealing their presence. Other areas of the section may overstain, however, if this method is followed.

Modification of Dieterle's spirochete stain[15,16]

Materials and methods. Tissue is formalin

fixed, embedded in paraffin, cut at 4 to 6 μm and affixed to glass slides with either egg albumin or by the use of gelatin in the flotation bath. Glass or plastic staining racks may be used to stain 10 to 25 slides at a time, eliminating hand dipping.

A known positive spirochete control is used in *each* staining rack. Care is taken that racks and glassware are clean and that no metal comes into contact with the staining solutions.

Solutions

5% alcoholic uranyl nitrate
  50 gm of uranyl nitrate in 1 liter of 70% ethanol
  Store at 4° C.
10% alcoholic gum mastic
  100 gm of gum mastic in 1 liter of absolute ethanol
  Allow 2 to 3 days to dissolve, and then filter and store in well-stoppered bottle in the refrigerator.
1% silver nitrate
  10 gm of silver nitrate in 1 liter of distilled water
  Store in the refrigerator and discard if solution becomes dark. Preheat the silver solution at 55° to 58° C for approximately 30 minutes prior to use.
Developer (mix in order)

Hydroquinone	15 gm
Sodium sulfite	2.5 gm
Distilled water	600 ml
Acetone	100 ml
Formalin (37% to 40%)	100 ml
Pyridine	100 ml
10% alcoholic gum mastic	100 ml

Swirl gently as each reagent is added. Solution becomes milky yellow as gum mastic solution is added and medium brown on standing in a well-lighted area. *Developer should be made when the procedure is begun* because aging of the developer is required for proper development—about 6 hours. Developer may be used for 2 to 3 days or until the color becomes dark brown.

Gum mastic from O. G. Innes Corp., 10 East 40th Street, New York, N.Y. 10016.

Control tissue available from Center for Disease Control, Attention: Mrs. Pat Greer, Control Tissue Repository, Pathology Division, Building 1-2330, Atlanta, GA 30333.

Staining procedure

1. Preheat the 5% alcoholic uranyl nitrate solution in a 55° to 58° C oven for at least 30 minutes. (Do not exceed temperature of 60° C because silver solutions will precipitate.)
2. Deparaffinize and hydrate sections to distilled water.
3. Place sections in preheated 5% alcohol uranyl nitrate in 55° to 58° C oven for 30 minutes.
4. Distilled water, 1 dip.
5. 95% alcohol, 1 dip.
6. 10% alcoholic gum mastic, 3 minutes.
7. 95% alcohol, 1 quick dip.
8. Distilled water, 1 minute, and then allow slides to drain for 15 to 20 minutes until almost dry.
9. Place sections in preheated 1% silver nitrate solution in 55° to 58° C oven in the dark for 4 hours.
10. Distilled water, 2 dips.
11. Developer—dip until sections are pale yellow to light tan.
12. Distilled water, 2 dips.
13. 95% ethanol, 2 dips.
14. Acetone, 2 dips.
15. Xylene I, 2 dips.
16. Xylene II, 2 dips.
17. Coverslip, using a synthetic mounting medium.

Results

Legionella pneumophilia, spirochetes, and other bacteria including *Calymmatobacterium granulomatis*—black to dark brown
Background—pale yellow to tan
Other structures that stain are melanin granules, chromatin, formalin pigment, and some foreign material in macrophages.

Steiner and Steiner method[32]

Fixation. Neutral buffered formalin.
Embedding. Cut paraffin sections at 5 μm.

Solutions

1% uranyl nitrate
1% silver nitrate
Reducing solution component A
  2.5% gum mastic in absolute ethanol
  The gum mastic will need 24 hours to dissolve in the ethanol. Age this dissolved solution for 1 week prior to use. Filter until clear prior to use.
Reducing solution component B
  Silver nitrate–sodium potassium tartrate solution

Silver nitrate	2 gm
Boiling distilled water	1000 ml

  Dissolve the silver nitrate in the boiling distilled water. To this solution carefully add:

Sodium potassium tartrate powder	1.65 gm

  When cool, filter this solution into a chemically clean brown glass bottle. Solution will appear whitish after filtering.
Reducing solution component C
  1.8% hydroquinone (prepare fresh as needed)
Reducing solution
  Measure 20 ml of component A and put in chemically clean cylinder. Into this 20 ml, pour 20 ml of component B. Immediately prior to use, add 60 ml of component C. Do *not* reverse the order of these components. The final solution will have a milky appearance.

Note: Prepare sufficient fresh reducing solution so that each Coplin jar of slides will have a fresh change. Discard the reducing solution after use.

Technic
1. Hydrate sections to distilled water.
2. Treat with uranyl nitrate for 3 minutes.
3. Rinse well in several changes of distilled water.
4. Treat slides with the 1% silver nitrate at 56° C for 2 hours.
5. Wash well in distilled water.
6. Rinse in 2 changes of 95% ethanol; followed by 2 changes of absolute ethanol.
7. Treat with 2.5% gum mastic solution for 5 minutes.
8. Treat with reducing solution for 5 to 15 minutes. Sections should be a light brown when this step is complete.
9. Rinse well in distilled water.
10. Dehydrate, clear, and coverslip, using a synthetic mounting medium.

Results
Bacteria (including spirochetes and *Legionella pneumophilia*), Donovan bodies, and fungi—black
Background—yellow to brown

Rickettsias and chlamydias

Rickettsias are now classified with the bacteria; however they are obligate intracellular parasites and, with the exception of *Rickettsia quintana,* require living cells to multiply. Like bacteria, rickettsias reproduce by binary fission, contain both DNA and RNA, and can be detected with light microscopic observation, appearing intracellularly as small pleomorphic coccobacilli. The ratio of cytoplasm to chromatinic body (nucleus) is responsible for the pleomorphism and, because of this, variations in tinctorial properties of the stained rickettsial preparation are not uncommon.

Some of the diseases caused by rickettsial subgroups include typhus (epidemic and murine), spotted fever (Rocky Mountain spotted fever, boutonneuse fever, rickettsial pox), tsutsugamushi disease (scrub typhus), Q fever, and trench fever.

Giemsa technic

The Giemsa technic is good for demonstrating rickettsias, especially when sections are differentiated in an alcoholic colophonium (rosin) solution (p. 156). A modification of Wright's stain and the Pinkerton method may also be used. Descriptions of these last two procedures follow.

Wright's stain for rickettsias[26]
Fixation. 10% neutral buffered formalin.

Embedding. Cut paraffin sections at 3 to 5 μm.

Technic
1. Hydrate sections to distilled water.
2. Stain section with Wright's stock stain on staining rack for 6 minutes.
3. Differentiate with Wright's stock buffer for 6 minutes.
4. Dehydrate quickly and coverslip, using a synthetic mounting medium.

Results
Rickettsial cytoplasm—reddish pink
Nucleus—blue

Pinkerton's method for rickettsias[27]
Fixation. 10% neutral buffered formalin (NBF), Regaud's, Zenker's.
Embedding. Embed in paraffin and cut 5 μm sections.

Solutions
1% aqueous methylene blue
0.25% aqueous basic fuchsin
0.5% aqueous citric acid solution

Technic
1. Hydrate sections to distilled water.
2. Remove mercury crystals if necessary (p. 131).
3. Stain in methylene blue solution overnight.
4. Rinse in 95% ethanol for 5 seconds.
5. Rinse quickly in distilled water for 2 to 3 seconds.
6. Stain in basic fuchsin solution for 30 minutes.
7. Decolorize rapidly in citric acid solution for 1 to 2 seconds, never more than 3 seconds.
8. Continue differentiation in absolute ethanol until nuclei stand out blue and rickettsias are red.
9. Clear in 2 changes of xylene and coverslip, using a synthetic mounting medium.

Results
Rickettsias—bright red
Red blood cells—red
Nuclei—blue
Other structures—light blue

Chlamydias

Organisms that belong to the genus *Chlamydia* include causative agents of psittacosis, lymphogranuloma venereum, trachoma, and inclusion conjunctivitis. Cat-scratch fever may also be caused by a member of this genus. Chlamydias are now classified with the bacteria. They are obligate intracellular parasites but possess both DNA and RNA. Chlamydias reproduce by binary fission and resemble the rickettsias in size and staining characteristics.

FUNGI

Fungi are primitive plants that possess no roots, stems, leaves, or chlorophyll. The study of fungi is called mycology, and the diseases produced by fungi are called mycoses. Fungi are a large and varied group and their identification depends primarily on culture appearance and microscopic morphology. Fungi of medical importance are divided into four groups:

Filamentous fungi
Yeasts
Yeastlike fungi
Dimorphic fungi

The filamentous fungi, also called molds, have as a basic structure a filament known as a "hypha." As the fungus grows, it produces more and more hyphae and this collection of hyphae is called a "mycelium." Mycelia may be classified as vegetative or reproductive, and it is the latter variety that produces the spores that are characteristic for each fungal type.

Yeasts are single, round or oval cells that reproduce by forming small buds that enlarge and develop into new yeast cells.

Yeastlike fungi also reproduce by budding, but in this class the buds produced tend to elongate into filamentous structures called "pseudohyphae." The pseudohyphae link together in chains that somewhat resemble the mycelia of the filamentous fungi. Unlike their filamentous counterparts, the pseudohyphae production of the yeastlike fungi does not result in spore formation, nor does true branching occur with the pseudohyphae.

Dimorphic fungi possess two morphologies depending on temperature. The dimorphic fungi (1) have a yeast morphology when growing either in the body or when cultured on artificial media at 37° C and (2) have a filamentous appearance when growing either in the soil or when cultured on artificial media at room temperature (25° C).

Pathogenic fungi can be divided into three groups:

1. Those fungi that affect the superficial keratinized layers of skin. These are called superficial fungi or dermatophytes. Ringworm and athlete's foot are caused by superficial fungi.
2. Those fungi that affect the deeper tissues or organs. These are called the deep or systemic fungi and are usually dimorphic. Examples of this type include *Blastomyces dermatitidis, Coccidioides immitis, Histoplasma capsulatum,* and *Sporotrichum*

schenckii. One systemic fungus highly pathogenic for man is *Cryptococcus neoformans,* which exists in a single yeastlike phase only.
3. Fungi that are capable of producing either deep or systemic disease. The major representative of this group is *Candida albicans.*

Certain hardy fungal species can grow in many of the reagent solutions used in the lab. During staining, these fungi may be deposited on the sections. Their presence is, naturally, not associated with an inflammatory response. Reagents displaying evidence of fungal growth should be discarded and the storage bottles thoroughly washed. The inclusion of thymol crystals in certain solutions can serve to inhibit mold growth; ethanol in hematoxylin solutions has a similar function.

There are a number of staining technics that may be used to demonstrate fungus in tissue sections, and these include hematoxylin and eosin, Giemsa, acid-fast technics, Brown-Brenn gram stain, Hotchkiss-McManus and Bauer procedures, and Grocott and Gridley technics. The H & E stain, though not primarily a fungus stain, does suggest the organism's presence in sections and makes further studies necessary. The Giemsa technic usually does not provide a sharp color contrast between tissue cells and fungal forms. Acid-fast technics are useful when the organism possesses acid-fastness as a chemical characteristic; if this is not the case, the methylene blue counterstain usually employed in acid-fast stains will nonspecifically demonstrate the fungal form. The Brown-Brenn modified Gram stain, discussed previously, is a gram technic followed by a picric acetone decolorization of the host tissue. For this to be a successful fungus demonstration technic, the organism must have a decided gram affinity, otherwise it will be decolorized with the host tissue and rendered virtually invisible. The Hotchkiss-McManus and Bauer technics use the same basic principle of oxidizing adjacent hydroxy groups in the mucopolysaccharide components of the fungal cell wall and then visualizing the released aldehyde groups with Schiff reagent. Other tissue elements are also oxidized to an extent, especially glycogen, starch, cellulose, glycolipids, mucin, and glycoproteins, and this may tend to obscure the fungus form. The Gridley and Grocott technics are discussed later. See Table 13-1 for a listing of staining technics for commonly found pathogenic fungi.

Table 13-1. Staining technics for pathogenic fungi*

Fungus	Stains	Additional comments
Actinomyces bovis		
Vary in size from 1 to 300 μm. Appear as "sulfur granules" or as small tangled masses of gram-positive branching filaments.	Grocott and Gram stains best for demonstration. PAS and Gridley technics are not suggested.	Paraffin sections should be cut at many levels to ensure that the characteristic granules are found.
Aspergillus fumigatus		
Appears as broken fragments of hyphae 3 to 12 μm thick.	PAS, Gridley, and Grocott best for demonstration. Gram stain also satisfactory.	
Blastomyces dermatitidis		
Appear as spherical cells 8 to 15 μm thick. Refractile wall gives double contoured appearance. No mycelium; single budding.	PAS and Grocott best for demonstration. Gridley also good.	With Congo red, the cell wall is stained red.
Candida albicans		
2 to 4 μm thin-walled oval yeastlike cells. May be budding; mycelial forms may also be found.	Gridley, PAS, and Grocott are all excellent for demonstration. Gram stain good.	
Coccidioides immitis		
Nonbudding, thick-walled structure (20 to 60 μm in diameter) filled with numerous small (2 to 5 μm) endospores.	Grocott best for demonstration; PAS and Gridley good; Gram satisfactory.	Endemic in southwestern United States.
Cryptococcus neoformans		
Oval to spherical, single-budding, thick-walled organism (5 to 20 μm in diameter) surrounded by a wide, refractile gelatinous capsule.	Grocott and PAS best for demonstration. Gridley and Gram satisfactory.	Exhibits metachromasia with toluidine blue; mucicarmine excellent stain also. Fungus may occur free in masses or within cytoplasm of giant cells.
Histoplasma capsulatum		
Appears as small (1 to 5 μm) oval bodies in the large mononuclear cells.	Grocott technic best for demonstration, PAS, Gridley, and and Gram are satisfactory.	Rarely found extracellularly in tissue; parasite of the mononuclear phagocytic system. Endemic in central United States.
Sporotrichum schenckii		
Appear as cigar-shaped round, oval, and budding cells 3 to 5 μm.	Grocott best for demonstration. Gridley and PAS good. Gram satisfactory.	

*Courtesy Miss Gerre Wells, University of Tennessee, Memphis, Tennessee.

TECHNICS FOR DEMONSTRATION
Hotchkiss-McManus PAS technic[17]

Principle. The principle underlying this technic is similar to that described in the PAS procedure. Here, 1% periodic acid oxidizes the polysaccharides present in the fungal cell walls to release aldehyde groups. These in turn combine with the Schiff reagent to give magenta-colored fungi. Background staining is green on account of the light green counterstain.

Fixation. 10% formalin, Bouin's, Zenker's.

Embedding. Embed in paraffin and cut 5 μm sections.

Solutions
1% aqueous periodic acid
Schiff reagent (p. 165)
Sulfurous rinse (p. 166)
Light green counterstain (p. 187)

Technic
1. Hydrate sections to distilled water.
2. 1% periodic acid solution for 10 minutes.
3. Wash well in running tap water for 10 minutes.
4. Rinse in distilled water, 3 changes.
5. Schiff reagent for 15 minutes. Filter back.
6. Give sections 3 changes of sulfurous rinse, with 2 minutes on each change. Discard each change after use.
7. Wash sections under running tap water for 10 minutes.
8. Counterstain with working solution of light green for 2 minutes. (If counterstain is too dark, running tap water or ammonia water will decolorize the light green.)
9. Dehydrate, clear, and coverslip, using a synthetic mounting medium.

Results
Fungi—red-purple
Background—green

Grocott's modification of Gomori's methenamine silver method[18]

Principle. The first step in the procedure is the oxidation of the tissue and fungal polysaccharides to aldehyde groups. Chromic acid is the oxidant employed, and in addition to oxidizing tissue structures to the aldehyde stage, it also tends to oxidize the newly released aldehyde groups even further to breakdown products that will not combine with the silver reagent and hence are not demonstrated in the final result. This "further oxidation" characteristic of chromic acid has the advantage of suppressing weaker background reactions of collagen fibers and basement membranes and leave reactive to the silver reagent only those substances that possess large quantities of polysaccharide (such as glycogen, mucins, and fungal cell walls). After the oxidation treatment, slides are placed in a solution of sodium bisulfite, which removes traces of chromic acid left in the tissue. A water wash follows and slides are then exposed to the alkaline silver reagent. This reagent produces a selective blackening of the polysaccharides after the chromic acid oxidation; the aldehyde oxidation products are believed to reduce the silver nitrate to metallic silver, thus rendering them visible. Methenamine is added to the silver reagent to give alkaline properties necessary for proper reaction; sodium borate solution is added to the working solution as a buffer. Gold chloride is used to tone the tissue after the silver treatment and eliminate yellow tones from the section. (See p. 182 for further discussion of toning.) Sodium thiosulfate fixes the silver reaction in the tissue by stopping all previous reactions and removing unreduced silver nitrate. Light green is a commonly used counterstain to color the background tissue, though other counterstains, including the H & E technic, may be employed.

Fixation. 10% formalin; Bouin's.

Embedding. Embed in paraffin and cut 5 μm sections.

Solutions
5% aqueous chromic acid

Chromium trioxide	5 gm
Distilled water	100 ml

Stock methenamine silver nitrate (p. 187)
Working methenamine silver solution

5% sodium borate	4 ml
Distilled water	50 ml

Mix the above two solutions and then add 50 ml of the stock methenamine silver solution. Mix again. Pour or filter into a chemically clean staining dish and allow to preheat for approximately 20 minutes prior to use. A Coplin jar containing distilled water may also be preheated.

1% aqueous sodium bisulfite
0.1% gold chloride

Gold chloride 1% solution	10 ml
Distilled water	90 ml

2% sodium thiosulfate
Light green working solution (p. 187)

Technic
1. Hydrate sections to distilled water. (If previously stained sections are being restained by this method, they may be hydrated and the chromic acid treatment will remove the previous stain.)
2. Oxidize in 5% chromic acid for 1 hour. Discard solution after use.

3. Rinse in tap water.
4. 1% sodium bisulfite for 1 minute. Discard solution.
5. Wash in tap water for 10 minutes.
6. Rinse 4 times in distilled water.
7. Place in working methenamine silver solution in oven at 58° to 60° C for 45 to 60 minutes or until sections turn a yellow-brown. Using paraffin-coated or Teflon forceps, remove a control slide, rinse in the warmed distilled water, and check microscopically for adequate silver impregnation. Fungi should be a dark brown. Rinse in distilled water and return to the silver solution if reaction is too pale.
8. Rinse in 6 changes of distilled water.
9. Tone in 0.1% gold chloride for 2 to 5 minutes. Solution may be refiltered and reused for about 100 slides.
10. Rinse in distilled water.
11. Treat with 2% sodium thiosulfate for 2 to 5 minutes. Discard solution.
12. Wash thoroughly in tap water for 5 minutes.
13. Counterstain in working light green solution for 30 to 45 seconds.
14. Dehydrate, clear in xylene, and coverslip, using a synthetic mounting medium.

Results (Plate 1, *G*)
Fungi—sharply delineated in black
Pneumocystis carinii—black
Mucin—taupe to dark grey
Inner parts of mycelia and hyphae—old rose
Background—pale green

Rapid Grocott's methenamine–silver nitrate method for fungi and Pneumocystis carinii[19]

(Procedure time 30 minutes)
Specimen preparation. Cryostat sections of tissue may be used but should be fixed briefly with 10% neutral buffered formalin. Satisfactory results can be obtained on smears and touch preparations. These should be fixed with 95% ethanol for 3 minutes. The method is also useful with paraffin-embedded tissue sections cut at 5 μm.

Solutions
5% aqueous chromic acid
1% aqueous sodium bisulfite
Working methenamine–silver nitrate solution
Stock methenamine–silver nitrate   25 ml
(p. 187)
Distilled water   25 ml
5% sodium borate   2 ml
Make working solution fresh, and filter before use.
0.2% aqueous gold chloride
2% aqueous sodium thiosulfate
Fast green counterstain

Dissolve 0.2 gm of fast green FCF (C.I. 42053) in 0.2% acetic acid. For use, dilute 10 ml of this solution with 40 ml of distilled water.

Staining procedure
1. Use fixed smears, cryostat sections, or deparaffinized and hydrated sections.
2. Place slides in 5% chromic acid that has been heated to approximately 43° C. (This can be accomplished by placing the Coplin jar containing the solution in a 43° C water bath about 15 minutes before use.) Transfer immediately to a 58° C water bath for 5 minutes.
3. Wash briefly in tap water.
4. Place in 1% sodium bisulfite for 30 seconds.
5. Wash in running tap water for 15 seconds.
6. Rinse in 4 changes of distilled water.
7. Place in freshly mixed methenamine–silver nitrate–sodium borate solution that has been heated to approximately 43° C. (This can be accomplished in the same way as with the chromic acid solution.) Transfer immediately to a 58° C water bath for 20 minutes.
8. Rinse in 4 changes of distilled water.
9. Tone in 0.2% gold chloride for 30 seconds. Filter back.
10. Rinse in 2 changes of distilled water.
11. Place in 2% sodium thiosulfate for 30 seconds.
12. Wash in running tap water for 15 seconds.
13. Counterstain with the fast green solution for 30 seconds.
14. Wash briefly in running tap water and rinse in 2 changes of distilled water.
15. Dehydrate, clear in 2 changes of xylene, and coverslip, using a synthetic mounting medium.

Results
Refer to Grocott's modification of Gomori's methenamine silver method (see left column).
Note: An additional procedure to demonstrate *Pneumocystis carinii* is described on p. 250.

Gridley's stain[20]

Principle. The oxidation to aldehydes and other breakdown products by the chromic acid is similar to that described under the Grocott technic. Aldehyde groups combine with the Schiff reagent as described under the PAS technic. Aldehyde fuchsin acts as an aldehyde and reinforces the depth of the Schiff reagent stain by occupying uninvolved linkages of the Schiff reagent. Metanil yellow is the counterstain and colors the background yellow.

Fixation. Any well-fixed tissue.

Embedding. Embed in paraffin and cut 5 μm sections.

Solutions
4% aqueous chromic acid
Chromium trioxide   4 gm

Distilled water   100 ml
Schiff reagent (p. 165)
Sulfurous rinse (p. 166)
Gomori's aldehyde fuchsin solution (p. 197)
Metanil yellow solution
    Metanil yellow   0.25 gm
    Distilled water   100 ml
    Glacial acetic acid   0.25 ml

Technic

1. Hydrate sections to distilled water.
2. Oxidize in 4% chromic acid for 1 hour. Discard solution.
3. Wash in running tap water for 5 minutes.
4. Place in Schiff's reagent for 15 minutes. Filter back.
5. Rinse in 3 changes of sulfurous rinse, with 2 minutes on each change. Discard each change.
6. Wash for 15 minutes in running tap water.
7. Place slides in aldehyde fuchsin solution for 30 minutes. This solution may be filtered back and reused.
8. Remove excess aldehyde fuchsin with a quick rinse in 95% alcohol, followed by several changes of distilled water.
9. Counterstain for 30 seconds with metanil yellow. Overstaining tends to obscure the primary stain colors.
10. Dehydrate, clear, and coverslip, using a synthetic mounting medium.

Results (Plate 1, *H*)

Hyphae—purple and magenta
Conidia—rose to purple
Elastin and mucin—purple
Yeast capsules—deep purple
Background—yellow
Note: Filaments of *Nocardia* and *Actinomyces* are not stained with this method.

VIRAL INCLUSION BODIES

Viruses are a diverse group of extremely small organisms, most visible only with electron microscopic observation. Viruses have been described as obligate intracellular parasites, since they can reproduce only inside host cells and cannot grow on artificial media. Host cells supply enzymes and building materials for the infecting virus to synthesize new viruses. In its simple form, a virus consists of an outer protein coat and an inner core of nucleic acid, either DNA or RNA but not both. Electron microscopic technics have shown that the appearance of a virus may vary. Some of the shapes observed are like spheres (poliovirus), long rods (tobacco mosaic virus), large loaves (vaccinia virus), and tadpoles (bacterial viruses or bacteriophages).

By light microscopy, it is possible to detect aggregates of virus particles inside host cells, and these particles are called "viral inclusion bodies." The single particles comprising the inclusion bodies have been termed "elementary bodies." The inclusion bodies are known by various names; frequently the name given is that of the researcher who described the inclusions.

The inclusions may be found in the cytoplasm (for example, Guarnieri bodies of smallpox [variola], Negri bodies of rabies, molluscum bodies of molluscum contagiosum, and HBsAg of hepatitis B virus) or in the nucleus (for example, in herpes simplex, chicken pox [varicella], and herpes zoster), or they may occur in both nucleus and cytoplasm (for example, in cytomegalic inclusion disease, measles [rubeola], and yellow fever).

Chemical composition and staining reactions of the inclusions vary. Some viral inclusions may be easily seen with an H & E stain, particularly those of cytomegalovirus and the molluscum contagiosum virus. Lendrum's phloxine-tartrazine is good for demonstrating viral inclusions of measles. The inclusions of rabies (Negri bodies) may be shown on formalin-fixed tissue with Parson's stain or on Zenker's fixed tissue with Schleifstein's technic.

Viral hepatitis is a term that refers to an inflammation of the liver caused by any of three viruses, none completely characterized at present. The three viral forms are hepatitis A (also called infectious hepatitis [IH or MS-1], epidemic type or short-incubation type; commonly acquired by an oral route); hepatitis B (serum hepatitis [SH or MS-2], long-incubation type; usually transmitted by parenteral injection); and hepatitis C (many cases of posttransfusion hepatitis are caused by infection with this virus). These types produce similar microscopic pathologic conditions in the liver.

A hepatitis-associated antigen (HAA, or Australia antigen) that is specifically associated with hepatitis B virus has been described. It is now usually called "hepatitis B surface antigen" (HBsAg) since it may actually lie on the virus particle. HBsAg may be stained in paraffin sections by use of either the orcein or the aldehyde fuchsin methods to be described shortly. The HBsAg occurs most frequently as cytoplasmic inclusions in hepatocytes; however, Kupffer cell cytoplasm may occasionally show the antigen's presence, presumably acquired by a phagocytic process. The pattern of distribution of the HBsAg on the hepatocyte cytoplasm varies. If many hepatocytes are affected, the antigen appears as fine granules either diffusely spread throughout the cytoplasm or concentrated in the cytoplasm peripheral to the sinusoid space. With occasional single-liver cell involvement, the HBsAg appears as oval, round, or irregularly shaped aggregates in the cytoplasm, especially in the perinuclear region.

Orcein method for demonstration of HBsAg[21]

Fixation. Formol-saline
Embedding. Cut paraffin sections at 4 μm.

Solutions

Potassium permanganate solution

Potassium permanganate	0.15 gm
Distilled water	100 ml
Concentrated sulfuric acid	0.15 ml

or

5% aqueous potassium permanganate	9.5 ml
3% sulfuric acid	5 ml
Distilled water to	100 ml

2% aqueous oxalic acid
Orcein solution

Orcein (British Drug Houses, Toronto, Ontario)	1 gm
70% ethanol	100 ml
Concentrated hydrochloric acid	1 ml

The pH of this solution should read between 1 and 2. Use additional concentrated hydrochloric acid if necessary. Allow this solution to age at least 48 hours before use, otherwise tissue decolorization will be difficult.
1% hydrochloric acid in 70% ethanol

Technic

1. Hydrate sections to distilled water.
2. Oxidize with the potassium permanganate solution for 10 minutes. Proper oxidation is important for reduced nuclear and cytoplasmic staining and better contrast.
3. Place slides in 2% oxalic acid for 10 minutes (sections should be colorless).
4. Wash in tap water.
5. Stain in orcein solution 4 hours or more at room temperature. Rinse in 70% ethanol.
6. Differentiate with 1% hydrochloric acid in 70% ethanol. Control differentiation by rinsing in 70% ethanol.
7. Dehydrate, clear in xylene, and coverslip, using a synthetic mounting medium.

Results
HBsAg—dark brown

Aldehyde fuchsin method for HBsAg[22]

Fixation. Any well-fixed tissue, preferably 10% neutral buffered formalin.
Embedding. Cut paraffin sections at 5 μm.

Solutions
Potassium permanganate solution (see preceding technic)
1.5% aqueous oxalic acid
Aldehyde fuchsin solution (p. 197)
Nuclear fast red (*Kernechtrot*) counterstain (p. 183)

Technic

1. Hydrate sections to distilled water.
2. Oxidize in potassium permanganate for 5 minutes.
3. Rinse slides in 2 changes of distilled water.
4. Place slides in 1.5% oxalic acid until sections are colorless, usually 10 to 15 seconds.
5. Wash slides gently in tap water for 5 minutes.
6. Transfer slides to distilled water, 2 changes for 1 minute each.
7. Rinse slides in 3 changes of 95% alcohol.
8. Stain slides in aldehyde fuchsin for 1 hour.
9. Remove excess aldehyde fuchsin by rinsing slides in 95% alcohol, 3 times.
10. Counterstain in *Kernechtrot* for 5 minutes. Rinse in several changes of distilled water.
11. Dehydrate in absolute ethanol, 3 changes for 2 minutes each.
12. Clear slides in xylene, 3 changes for 2 minutes each, and coverslip, using a synthetic mounting medium.

Results

HBsAg granules—purple
Lipofuscin granules in hepatocytes and Kupffer cells also stain but should be distinguishable from HBsAg by form and distribution.

Lendrum's phloxine-tartrazine method[23]

Principle. Nuclear staining is the first step and is done with Mayer's hematoxylin solution. Primary cytoplasmic staining is next and is done with phloxine, an acid fluoran dye. Calcium chloride is added to the phloxine solution to intensify the stain. The phloxine staining is differentiated by treatment of the sections with a tartrazine solution. This tartrazine removes the red dye from the collagen and substitutes its own yellow color in it. By prolonged differentiation with the tartrazine solution, certain inclusion bodies possessing strong phloxinophilic tendencies are revealed and, being stained red, are readily identified against the pale yellow background.

Fixation. Preferably in mercuric chloride formalin (9 parts of saturated aqueous mercuric chloride to 1 part formalin); 10% neutral buffered formalin may be used.

Embedding. Embed in paraffin and cut 5 μm sections.

Solutions

Mayer's hematoxylin (p. 142)

Phloxine stain

Phloxine	1 gm
70% ethanol	200 ml
Calcium chloride	1 gm

Tartrazine solution

Tartrazine	2.5 gm
Cellosolve (ethylene glycol mono-ethyl ether)	100 ml

Technic

1. Hydrate sections to distilled water.
2. Stain for 5 to 10 minutes in Mayer's hematoxylin. Filter back.
3. Blue sections in running tap water for 15 minutes.
4. Stain with phloxine solution for 30 minutes.
5. Rinse briefly in distilled water and drain on filter paper.
6. Differentiate with the tartrazine solution until inclusion bodies stand out bright red and the background is yellow.
7. Dehydrate, clear in xylene, and coverslip, using a synthetic mounting medium.

Results

Inclusion bodies—red
Nuclei—blue
Background—yellow

Parson's stain for Negri bodies[24]

Fixation. Formalin.
Embedding. Embed in paraffin and cut 5 μm.

Solutions

Ethyl eosin solution

Solution A

Ethyl eosin	1 gm
95% ethanol	100 ml

Solution B

Acetic acid	0.6 ml
Distilled water	99.4 ml

Working solution

Solution A	22 ml
Solution B	1.25 ml

Sodium borate (borax)–methylene blue solution

Methylene blue	1 gm
Borax	1 gm
Distilled water	100 ml

0.25% aqueous acetic acid

Technic

1. Hydrate sections to distilled water.
2. Stain in working solution of ethyl eosin for 2 minutes.
3. Wash in 95% alcohol.
4. Stain in methylene blue solution for 2 minutes.
5. Rinse in distilled water.
6. Differentiate in 0.25% acetic acid for 2 to 5 minutes.

7. Rinse in 95% ethanol, pass quickly through 2 changes of absolute alcohol, clear in xylene, and coverslip, using a synthetic mounting medium.

Results

Negri bodies—red
Nuclei—blue

Schleifstein's method for Negri bodies[25]

Fixation. Fix blocks not more than 3 mm thick in Zenker's fluid.
Embedding. Embed in paraffin and cut 5 μm sections.

Solutions

Schleifstein's stain

Solution A

Basic fuchsin	1.8 gm
Methylene blue	1 gm
Glycerol	100 ml
Methanol	100 ml

Solution B

Potassium hydroxide	0.01 gm
Tap water	4 liters

Solution should have a slightly alkaline pH.

Working solution

Solution A	10 drops
Solution B	20 ml

Mix immediately before use.

Technic

1. Hydrate sections to distilled water.
2. De-Zenkerize with iodine–sodium thiosulfate sequence (p. 131).
3. Wash well in running water.
4. Place sections on a ring stand and flood with freshly prepared working solution. Gently heat the bottom of the slide until vapor is produced. Allow slide to cool to room temperature.
5. Wash quickly in tap water.
6. Differentiate each slide separately by gently agitating in a jar of 90% ethanol until the section is faint violet in color.
7. Dehydrate, clear, and coverslip, using a synthetic mounting medium.

Results

Negri bodies—deep magenta
Cytoplasm—bluish violet
Erythrocytes—copper red

PROTOZOA AND MISCELLANEOUS PARASITES

Protozoa are single-celled animals. They appear to be simple structurally but are complex functionally, since the single cell functions as a unit to perform all the activities associated with life. Protozoa vary in shape, but all protozoa possess a nucleus and cytoplasm surrounded by a cell membrane. In addition, many protozoa possess special structures, for example, cilia or flagella for movement. The cytoplasm of the trophozoite, or vegetative, stage may contain food reserves in the form of glycogen or chromatoid bodies. Depending on the type of protozoa, there may be a cyst stage. This cyst stage is more resistant than the trophozoite stage to unfavorable conditions because of the tough cyst membrane that protects the organism. In the case of the parasitic amebas, the cyst stage provides a better opportunity for transfer from one host to another.

Some of the diseases caused by organisms in the phylum *Protozoa* include malaria (*Plasmodium* spp.), amebiasis (*Entamoeba histolytica*), sleeping sickness (*Trypanosoma* spp.), leishmaniasis (*Leishmania* spp.), and toxoplasmosis (*Toxoplasma gondii*).

DEMONSTRATION TECHNICS

The Giemsa methods (p. 155) are good for demonstrating malarial parasites, *Trypanosoma*, and *Leishmania*, as well as *Toxoplasma* and *Pneumocystis*. *Pneumocystis carinii* may also be demonstrated by the Grocott (GMS) and rapid Grocott methods (p. 246). Another demonstration method for *Pneumocystis* is described in the next section.

Amebas in tissue sections may be demonstrated, by virtue of their glycogen content, with Best's carmine (p. 167) or the periodic acid–Schiff reaction (p. 166). With phosphotungstic acid–hematoxylin (p. 193), nuclei, chromatoid bars, and fibrils are colored blue. Heidenhain's iron hematoxylin method may be used, especially on smears. With this method, nuclei, chromatoid bars, and fibrils are black. Wheatley's staining procedure may be employed to demonstrate amebas and flagellates in smears.

Worm cuticles may be demonstrated with PAS technic.

Wheatley's stain for intestinal amebas and flagellates [28]

1. Make thin fecal smears, and while they are wet, place in Schaudinn's fixative without acetic acid for 30 minutes to 1 hour.
2. Place in 70% alcohol that contains enough iodine to be an amber color for 2 minutes.
3. 70% ethanol, 2 changes at 2 minutes each change.
4. 50% ethanol for 2 minutes.
5. Place in Gomori's trichrome staining solution for 30 minutes.

Chromotrope 2R	0.6 gm
Light green SF	0.3 gm
Phosphotungstic acid	0.7 gm

Acetic acid	1 ml
Distilled water	100 ml

6. Rinse in 95% ethanol quickly.
7. Absolute ethanol for 1 minute.
8. Clear in 2 changes of xylene for 5 minutes. Coverslip, using a synthetic mounting medium.

Results

Chromatin material—varying shades of red
Cytoplasmic and albuminous material—light green or very pale pink
Diagnostic detail of cysts from *Entamoeba histolytica*, *Entamoeba coli*, *Iodamoeba buetschlii*, and *Giardia lamblia* may be seen. Those from *Entamoeba coli* have a distribution of red stain within their cytoplasm. With the other parasites, the red stain is confined entirely to the nucleus and chromatoid bodies.
Note: Zenker's fixed smears may also be stained. The author recommends 2 minutes of treatment with working Weigert's hematoxylin, followed by tap water, followed by 30 minutes in the staining solution. The results are essentially the same, but the cytoplasm colors gray or gray-green.

Rapid staining procedure for Pneumocystis carinii [29]

Tissue preparation. Paraffin sections, frozen sections, or smears may be used. A variety of fixatives are satisfactory—NBF, formal sublimate, glutaraldehyde, methanol, and ethanol. Smears from sputum, bronchial washings or brushings, and imprints from lung biopsies should be air-dried prior to fixation.

Solutions

Sulfation reagent
Place a Coplin jar containing 30 ml of glacial acetic acid in cold water. *Very slowly,* add 10 ml concentrated sulfuric acid and mix well. *Use mixture within 1 hour.*

Cresyl echt Violett, pH 1.5
A pH 1.5 acid phosphate buffer is prepared by mixing of 60 ml of 0.1 N hydrochloric acid and 40 ml of 0.1 M sodium phosphate monobasic. Add 0.1 gm of *Cresyl echt Violett* to the 100 ml of buffer, mix well, let stand for 24 hours, and filter. The solution is reusable and stable for at least 6 months.

Naphthol yellow S
Dissolve 0.01 gm of naphthol yellow S in 100 ml of 1% acetic acid. The solution is stable and may be reused for several months.

Technic

1. Paraffin sections—deparaffinize in 2 changes of xylene. Wash in 2 changes of absolute ethanol and air-dry. Smears and frozen sections—wash in 2 changes of absolute alcohol and air-dry.
2. Place slides in sulfation reagent for 10 minutes. Agitate occasionally to remove air bubbles.

3. Wash in running water for 3 to 5 minutes.
4. Stain in *Cresyl echt Violett,* pH 1.5, for 10 minutes.
5. Rinse in water and counterstain in naphthol yellow S for 1 minute.
6. Dehydrate in ethanol, clear in xylene, and coverslip, using a synthetic mounting medium.

Results

Cysts of *Pneumocystis carinii,* mucin, and cartilage—rose

Erythrocytes—yellow

Connective tissue—blue to green

REFERENCES

1. Elias, J. M., and Johnsen, T. A.: Positive controls for fungal detection in tissue sections, Am. J. Med. Technol. **42:**277-279, 1976.
2. Taylor, R. D.: Modification of the Brown and Brenn Gram stain for the differential staining of gram-positive and gram-negative bacteria in tissue sections, Am. J. Clin. Pathol. **46:**472-476, 1966.
3. Brown, R. C., and Hopps, H. C.: Staining of bacteria in tissue sections: a reliable gram stain method, Am. J. Clin. Pathol. **60:**234-240, 1973.
4. Lillie, R. D., and Fullmer, H. M.: Histopathological technic and practical histochemistry, ed. 4, New York, 1976, McGraw-Hill Book Co., pp. 726-727.
5. Kinyoun, J. J.: A note on Uhlenhuth's method for sputum examination for tubercle bacilli, Am. J. Public Health **5:**867-870, 1915.
6. Mallory, F. B.: Pathological technique, New York, 1961, Hafner Publishing Co.
7. Thompson, S. W.: Selected histopathological and histochemical methods, Springfield, Ill., 1966, Charles C Thomas, Publisher, pp. 1025-1026.
8. Thompson, S. W., and Luna, L. G.: An atlas of artifacts, Springfield, Ill., 1978, Charles C Thomas, Publisher.
9. Fite, G. L., Cambre, P. J., and Turner, M. H.: Procedure for demonstrating lepra bacilli in paraffin sections, Arch. Pathol. **43:**624-625, 1947, Chicago, The American Medical Association.
10. Fite, G. L., and Honolulu, T. H.: The fuchsin-formaldehyde method of staining acid-fast bacilli in paraffin sections, J. Lab. Clin. Med. **25:**743-744, 1940.
11. Wade, H. W.: Demonstration of acid fast bacilli in tissue sections, Am. J. Pathol. **28:**157-170, 1952.
12. Truant, J. P., Brett, W. A., and Thomas, W., Jr.: Fluorescence microscopy of tubercle bacilli stained with auramine and rhodamine, Henry Ford Hospital Med. Bull. **10:**287-296, 1962.
13. Bridges, C. H., and Luna, L. G.: Kerr's improved Warthin-Starry technic: a study of permissible variations, Lab. Invest. **6:**357-367, 1957, Baltimore, The Williams & Wilkins Co.
14. Kerr, D. A.: Improved Warthin-Starry method of staining spirochetes in tissue sections, Am. J. Clin. Pathol. **8:**63-67, 1938.
15. Dieterle, R. R.: Method for the demonstration of *Spirochaeta pallida* in single microscopic sections, Arch. Neurol. Psychiat. **18:**73-80, 1927.
16. Van Orden, A. E., and Greer, P. W.: Modification of the Dieterle spirochete stain, J. Histotechnol. **1:**51-53, 1977.
17. Kligman, A. M., Mescon, H., and DeLamater, E. D.: The Hotchkiss-McManus stain for the histopathologic diagnosis of fungus diseases, Am. J. Clin. Pathol. **21:**86-91, 1951.
18. Grocott, R. G.: A stain for fungi in tissue sections and smears using Gomori methenamine silver nitrate technic, Am. J. Clin. Pathol. **25:**975-979, 1955.
19. Personal communication, Charles Churkurian, University of Rochester Medical Center, Rochester, N.Y., 1978.
20. Gridley, M. F.: A stain for fungi in tissue sections, Am. J. Clin. Pathol. **23:**303-307, 1953.
21. Deodhar, K. P., Tapp, E., and Scheuer, P. J.: Orcein staining of hepatitis B antigen in paraffin sections of liver biopsies, J. Clin. Pathol. **28:**66-70, 1975.
22. Shikata, T., Uzawa, T., Yoshiwara, N., Akatsuka, T., and Yamazaki, S.: Staining methods of Australia antigen in paraffin section, Jpn. J. Exp. Med. **44:**25-36, 1974 (AFIP modification).
23. Lendrum, A. C.: The phloxine-tartrazine method as a general histological stain for demonstration of inclusion bodies, J. Pathol. Bacteriol. **59:**399-404, 1947.
24. Parsons, R. J.: The staining of Negri bodies in formaldehyde and alcohol fixed tissues, J. Tech. Meth. **19:**104-108, 1939.
25. Schleifstein, J.: A rapid method for demonstrating Negri bodies in tissue sections, Am. J. Public Health **27:**1283-1284, 1937.
26. Wolf, G. L., Cole, C. R., Saslow, S., and Carlisle, H. N.: Staining rickettsiae in sections of formalin fixed tissue: a 12 minute Wright-buffer sequence, Stain Technol. **41:**185-188, 1966, Baltimore, The Williams & Wilkins Co.
27. Simmons, J. S., and Gentzkow, C. J.: Laboratory methods of the United States Army, ed. 5, Philadelphia, 1944, Lea & Febiger.
28. Wheatley, W. B.: A rapid staining procedure for intestinal amoebae and flagellates, Am. J. Clin. Pathol. **21:**990-991, 1951.
29. Bowling, M. C., Smith, I. M., and Wescott, S. L.: A rapid staining procedure for *Pneumocystis carinii,* Am. J. Med. Technol. **39:**267, 1973.
30. Elias, J. M., and Greene, C.: Specific controls for the identification of Gram-positive organisms in tissue sections, Lab. Med. **10:**767-768, 1979.
31. Lambert, C.: Substitution staining for identification of Legionnaires' disease, Lab. Med. **10:**765-766, 1979.
32. Steiner, G., and Steiner, G.: New simple silver stain for demonstration of bacteria, spirochetes, and fungi in sections from paraffin embedded tissue blocks, J. Lab. Clin. Med. **29:**868-871, 1944.

Nerve tissue

FREIDA CARSON

Anatomically the nervous system is divided into the central nervous system (brain and spinal cord) and the peripheral nervous system (cranial and spinal nerves, spinal and autonomic ganglions). Functionally the nervous system is divided into a somatic system (largely voluntary) and an autonomic or visceral system (mostly involuntary). Structurally neural tissue is composed of two main cellular components: neurons with their processes, and neuroglia or supporting cells. Extracellular components are found in peripheral nerves and the meninges (protective covering of the brain and spinal cord).

The choice of fixative for preservation of nervous tissue is governed by the type of studies desired. Ten-percent neutral buffered formalin is probably the most widely used fixative and allows one to perform the majority of special staining technics. Dehydration and embedding are done routinely as a rule, since the majority of special stains can be done on paraffin and celloidin material. It is frequently advantageous to prolong the time in each solution or to use vacuum processing and infiltration. The hematoxylin-and-eosin and azure-eosin methods are the best general stains, but special technics may also be used.

NEURON

A neuron is a complete nerve cell, consisting of a cell body (perikaryon) containing the nucleus and one or more cytoplasmic extensions, or "processes" (axon and dendrites). The cell bodies of neurons vary in size and may reach a diameter of 135 μm. The shape also varies from round or oval to pyramidal. There is usually only one nucleus containing a prominent nucleolus.

Nissl substance

The cytoplasm of the neuron contains several structures including neurofibrils, Golgi apparatus, mitochondria, inclusion bodies, and Nissl substance. These last structures, sometimes referred to as Nissl bodies, chromophil substance or tigroid bodies, are composed primarily of ribonucleic acid (RNA) and protein. Ultrastructurally, they are associated with granular endoplasmic reticulum. The form, size, and distribution of Nissl bodies vary in different types of neurons. They are sharply stained with basic aniline dyes such as thionin, azure A, and Cresyl echt Violett because of the RNA content. By varying the pH and degree of differentiation, one may demonstrate only Nissl substance, or both Nissl substance and the nuclei of other cells. The RNA also may be demonstrated by ribonuclease extraction. (RNA will be present in unextracted sections and absent in extracted sections.)

In neuronal injury the Nissl substance may disappear, first from around the nucleus and then altogether. This loss, called "chromatolysis," is useful in assessing neuronal damage.

Thionin stain for Nissl substance[1]

Fixation. Formalin.
Embedding. Cut paraffin sections at 6 μm.

Solutions

Thionin stain

Thionin	0.5 gm
Distilled water	100 ml
Acetic acid	2 drops

Differentiating solution
Equal parts of absolute alcohol and 1,4-dioxane (histologic)

Technic

1. Xylene.
2. Dioxane.
3. Distilled water.
4. Stain in thionin solution for 5 minutes. Staining solution can be kept and used until exhausted. Filter before using.
5. Differentiate until practically colorless in differentiating solution. Experience determines the time of differentiation. Never place stained sections in water or alcohol before or after differentiation, as both will remove the stain from the cells.
6. Dioxane, 2 changes.
7. Xylene, 2 changes.
8. Mount in synthetic resin.

Results

Nerve cells—bright blue
Background—colorless

Cresyl echt Violett for Nissl substance[2]

Fixation. Formalin-fixed tissues preferred.
Embedding. Cut paraffin sections at 6 μm.

Solutions

Cresyl echt Violett solution
0.5% aqueous solution of *Cresyl echt Violett*
Ripen for 24 to 48 hours. Filter before using.
Balsam xylene solution
Equal parts of Canada balsam and xylene

Technic

1. Xylene.
2. Absolute alcohol.
3. 95% alcohol.
4. Hydrate to distilled water.
5. Stain for 3 to 5 minutes in *Cresyl echt Violett* solution.
6. Rinse in 2 changes of distilled water.
7. 95% alcohol for 30 seconds.
8. Absolute alcohol for 30 seconds.
9. Xylene for 1 minute.

10. Balsam xylene mixture for 2 minutes.
11. Absolute alcohol, 2 changes 10 to 30 seconds each.
12. Xylene, several changes.
13. Steps 10 to 12 may have to be repeated several times.
14. Mount in synthetic resin.

Results (Plate 2, S)

Nissl substance—blue

Gallocyanine stain for Nissl granules[3]

Fixation. Zenker's, Helly's, or 10% formalin.
Embedding. Cut paraffin or celloidin sections at 6 μm.

Solutions

Gallocyanine-chromium staining solution

Chromium potassium sulfate	5 gm
Gallocyanine	0.15 gm
Distilled water	100 ml

Dissolve the chromium potassium sulfate in the distilled water. Add the gallocyanine and shake well. Warm the mixture gradually and boil it for 5 minutes. Cool to room temperature, filter, and add distilled water through the filter to bring the volume again to 100 ml. The solution will keep well for about 1 week.

Technic

1. Xylene.
2. Absolute alcohol.
3. 95% alcohol.
4. Hydrate to distilled water.
5. Place sections in the gallocyanine staining solution for 48 hours at room temperature.
6. Wash in distilled water.
7. 95% alcohol.
8. Absolute alcohol.
9. Absolute alcohol and xylene.
10. Xylene, 2 changes.
11. Mount in synthetic resin.

Results

Nissl substance—blue

Nerve fibers (processes) and neurofibrils

Neurons have two types of processes arising from the cell body—axons and dendrites. Dendrites are usually short, multiple-branching processes that lack myelin sheaths. They may contain both Nissl substance and neurofibrils. Axons (nerve fibers) are neuron processes that carry nerve impulses over long distances. Axons terminate either on the dendrites or cell body of other neurons, forming a synapse, or in a specialized ending associated with an effector organ such as muscle or glands. Some axons are more than a meter in length. They are usually single and originate from a cone-shaped elevation of the cell body known as the axon hillock. The axon and axon hillock contain neurofibrils but no Nissl substance. In older literature, the axon is often referred to as the axis cylinder.

When axons are severed or separated from the cell body, the peripheral segment quickly disintegrates and disappears in a process known as wallerian degeneration.

Neurofibrils are present in the cytoplasm of the cell body, axon, and dentrites. Ultrastructurally they are aggregates of microtubules and neurofilaments and can be demonstrated in light microscopic preparations by gold and silver impregnation techniques. Practically all the silver methods demonstrate both nerve fibers and neurofibrils, but some methods are more suitable than others for demonstrating nerve fibers in the peripheral nervous system because they leave the connective tissue relatively unstained.

Silver technics are capricious and require careful attention to detail. It is important that the glassware be chemically clean. If a black precipitate forms on sections, the most likely cause would be the use of chemically unclean glassware. Doubly or triply distilled water should also be used for the solutions, which should be freshly prepared from reagent-grade chemicals. When handling slides, one should use Teflon or paraffin-coated forceps, never metal forceps.

Gros-Bielschowski technic[4]

Principle. Generally, the Gros-Bielschowski procedure is done on frozen sections. A preliminary silver impregnation with silver nitrate is followed by an ammoniacal silver treatment. Silver is deposited on the neurofibrils and axon and reduced to visible metallic silver (black) by the action of the formaldehyde reducing agent. A solution of gold chloride is used to tone the tissue, and this step eliminates the yellow background caused by the silver impregnation. The section becomes more transparent, the final stain intensity is controlled, and differentiation is improved between the nervous tissue and the other tissue elements. Sodium thiosulfate (hypo) is used to remove the unreacted silver from the tissue and stop the silver impregnation.

Solutions
20% aqueous silver nitrate
20% formalin
Ammoniacal silver
  40% freshly prepared aqueous sodium hydroxide
  10% aqueous silver nitrate

Concentrated ammonium hydroxide
Distilled water
Slowly add 5 drops of the sodium hydroxide to 10 ml of the silver nitrate. This results in the formation of a black-brown precipitate. Dissolve the precipitate by adding concentrated ammonium hydroxide dropwise, shaking it well after each drop. No more than 18 drops should be used. Add 10 ml of distilled water to give a final volume of 20 ml.
Aqueous gold chloride
  Add 3 to 5 drops of 1% gold chloride to 10 ml of distilled water.
Ammonia water
  Add 2 ml of ammonium hydroxide to 8 ml of distilled water.
5% aqueous sodium thiosulfate

Method
1. Place frozen sections in tap water, followed by distilled water for a few minutes.
2. Place in 20% silver nitrate for 1 hour.
3. Pass through several baths of 20% formalin until clouds no longer come off the section. A period of 10 minutes is usually needed.
4. Transfer to ammoniacal silver. Check impregnation and stop when neurofibrils become distinct. (If the neurofibrils color too deeply, begin another section and add an extra drop of ammonium hydroxide to the silver bath.)
5. Transfer for 1 minute to ammonia water and neutralize in very dilute aqueous acetic acid.
6. Wash in water.
7. Tone in gold chloride for 1 hour.
8. Wash in water, and immerse sections in 5% sodium thiosulfate for 5 minutes.
9. Wash in tap water and mount in an aqueous mounting medium (glycerol and egg albumin) or dehydrate in graded alcohols; clear in xylene; and mount in synthetic resin.

Results
Axons—black
Intracellular neurofibrils—black

Bielschowski's method for neurofibrils[4]
Solutions
2% aqueous silver nitrate
Solutions mentioned in preceding section on Gros-Bielschowski technic

Method
1. Formalin-fixed blocks of tissue (3 to 6 weeks in formalin) are cut into thin pieces of tissue and washed in running tap water for 24 hours, followed by several changes of distilled water.
2. Cut thin frozen sections and place in distilled water.
3. Immerse in 2% silver nitrate until brown (16 to 24 hours).
4. Wash rapidly in distilled water and place in am-

moniacal silver solution until deep brown (15 to 20 minutes).

5. Wash in several changes of distilled water.

6. Place in 20% formalin and transfer quickly to fresh formalin solution for about 30 minutes.

7. Follow steps 7 to 9 of the Gros-Bielschowski method.

Results
Intracellular neurofibrils—black

Rio-Hortega method for neurofibrils[4]

Principle. The principle of the technic is similar to that of the Gros-Bielschowski method. Ammoniacal silver carbonate is used instead of ammoniacal silver, however, and gold toning is not recommended unless overimpregnation has occurred. Finest fibrils are not demonstrated, but this technic can be performed on old formalin-fixed material.

Solutions
Any one of the following fixatives may be used:
Fixative mixtures
10% formalin
Formalin–ammonium bromide

Neutral formaldehyde (37% to 40%)	15 ml
Distilled water	85 ml
Ammonium bromide	2 gm

Formalin-uranium

Uranium nitrate	1 gm
Distilled water	85 ml
Formaldehyde (37% to 40%)	15 ml

96% alcohol
1% formalin
10% formalin
Pyridine–silver nitrate mixture

96% alcohol	12 drops
Pyridine	3 drops
2% aqueous silver nitrate	10 ml

Ammoniacal silver carbonate

10% aqueous silver nitrate	10 ml
5% sodium carbonate	5 ml
Ammonium hydroxide	few drops
Pyridine	30 to 45 drops
Distilled water	

Add sodium carbonate slowly to the silver nitrate in a 200 ml cylinder. Add ammonium hydroxide drop by drop to dissolve the precipitate formed. Shake each time an ammonium hydroxide drop is added, and continue until the precipitate is just dissolved. Dilute to 150 ml with distilled water.

Method
1. Fix frozen sections in one of the above fixatives. Formalin is preferable.

2. Warm sections at 50° C in 10% formalin for 10 minutes. Add 2 to 3 drops of ammonium hydroxide to prevent shrinkage.

3. Transfer directly to the pyridine–silver nitrate solution. Warm gently with an alcohol lamp until sections are brownish (5 to 10 minutes).

4. Wash gently in distilled water.

5. Transfer to ammoniacal silver carbonate solution. Warm sections and impregnate for 10 to 15 minutes.

6. Reduce in 10% formalin; rinse in distilled water; complete reduction process in 10% formalin.

7. Mount from tap water in glycerol gelatin.

Results
Neurofibrils—black

Nonidez's method (block method)[5]

Principle. This technic is recommended for the demonstration of axons. Tissue is fixed in chloral hydrate, a chlorinated derivative of acetaldehyde with a somewhat similar chemical relation to formaldehyde. This fixative gives good preservation of the character of the tissues but tends to shrink cytoplasmic structures. Chloral hydrate is often used in nerve tissue fixation, and alcohol is added to the fixative solution, since it aids in giving sharper and more uniform impregnation with the subsequent silver solution. Impregnation is done with aqueous silver nitrate, followed by a reduction process using pyrogallol and formalin. After these steps, tissue is dehydrated and embedded.

Solutions
Fixative solution

50% ethanol	100 ml
Chloral hydrate	25 gm

Dilute ammonia solution

95% ethanol	100 ml
Ammonium hydroxide (concentrated)	0.5 ml

2% aqueous silver nitrate
Reducing mixture

Pyrogallol	3 gm
40% formaldehyde	8 ml
Distilled water	100 ml

Method
1. Fix tissues 1 to 3 days in the above fixative mixture.

2. Blot off excess fluid and transfer to the dilute alcoholic ammonia solution and let remain for another 18 hours in the second change.

3. Wash 5 minutes in distilled water.

4. Place in silver solution at 37° to 40° C for 5 to 6 days. Change solution when it becomes yellow-brown or every 2 days.

5. Wash for 2 to 3 minutes in distilled water.

6. Reduce in reducing mixture for 24 hours.

7. Wash for 2 to 3 hours in several changes of distilled water, dehydrate in alcohols, and clear in amyl acetate (which eliminates tissue harden-

ing caused by some clearing agents such as xylene; butanol or isopropanol may also be substituted). Embed in paraffin. Cut sections to 5 μm, deparaffinize, and mount in synthetic resin.

Results
Nerve endings and nerve fibers—brown black

Bodian's method[6]

Principle. This method uses a silver proteinate compound to impregnate tissue sections. Protargol is the brand name of the silver proteinate most commonly used in the technic, and Protargol is made from partially hydrolyzed protein. (Using this substance, less precipitates are found in sections.) The first step of the procedure is the incubation of the tissue sections in the Protargol solution to which metallic copper has been added. Protargol first impregnates both neural and connective tissue. It is believed that connective tissue is "destained" by the action of the copper, since copper is more reactive than silver and replaces it from the connective fibers. Therefore a greater degree of differentiation between the neural and the connective tissue elements is possible when copper is used. Silver that is deposited on certain tissue structures is subsequently reduced to visible metallic silver by the action of the hydroquinone. Sections are toned in gold chloride, which functions similarly to the way it is used in the ammoniacal silver technics. Oxalic acid may also be used after the toning step to give sections a definite purplish tinge. Oxalic acid also reduces gold chloride and intensifies the stain by increasing the deposit of metallic gold on the section. Oxalic acid treatment should not be prolonged, since overtreatment will ruin the silver proteinate reaction. The function of the sodium thiosulfate has been discussed in the ammoniacal silver section.

Fixation. 10% formalin or alcohol-formalin (9 parts of 95% alcohol to 1 part 40% formaldehyde).

Embedding. Cut paraffin sections at 6 to 8 μm.

Solutions
Protargol solution

Protargol S (Winthrop Laboratories, New York, N.Y.)	1 gm
Distilled water	100 ml

After weighing the Protargol, dust it from the weighing paper over the surface of the water and allow it to dissolve from the surface downward. Do not shake the solution.

Reducing solution

Hydroquinone	1 gm
Sodium sulfite	5 gm
Distilled water	100 ml

Gold chloride solution

Gold chloride (1% aqueous solution) containing 3 drops of glacial acetic acid per 100 ml of solution

Oxalic acid solution

2% aqueous solution of oxalic acid

Sodium thiosulfate solution

5% aqueous solution of sodium thiosulfate

Technic
1. Xylene.
2. Absolute alcohol.
3. 95% alcohol.
4. Distilled water.
5. Place slides in 1% aqueous solution of Protargol containing 4 to 6 gm of clean metallic copper per 100 ml of solution for 12 to 48 hours at 37° C.
6. Wash in distilled water.
7. Reduce in hydroquinone solution for 10 minutes.
8. Wash thoroughly in distilled water.
9. Tone in gold chloride solution for 5 to 10 minutes.
10. Wash in distilled water.
11. If sections do not have a light purple color, place in 2% oxalic acid until sections have a definite purplish tinge (5 to 10 minutes).
12. Wash in distilled water.
13. Remove the residual silver salts with a 5% aqueous solution of sodium thiosulfate for 5 to 10 minutes.
14. Wash thoroughly in distilled water.
15. Dehydrate in 95% alcohol.
16. Absolute alcohol.
17. Xylene, 2 changes.
18. Mount in synthetic resin.

Results (Plate 2, *T*)
Myelinated fibers, the finest nonmyelinated fibers of central and peripheral nervous system, and neurofibrils—black

Holmes' method[2,7]

Principle. This is a modification of Bodian's technic and gives more consistent and reliable results on formalin-fixed material. Attributing the variable results on formalin-fixed material to the fact that the Protargol solution of the Bodian stain never reaches the alkalinity necessary for optimal impregnation, Holmes developed a buffered impregnating solution. The specificity of the stain is determined during impregnation by the effect of the solution pH and the concentration of silver ions. Sections of tissue that have been fixed in the neutral buffered formalin can be stained readily with a 1 in 100,000 silver nitrate solution at pH 8.4. Holmes believes that the primary purpose of the pyridine, which is an alkali, is to modify the electrostatic condition of the tissue. The functions of the reducing solution, gold chloride, oxalic acid, and sodium thiosulfate are discussed under the Bodian technic.

A particularly useful stain is achieved when the Holmes' technic is combined with the Luxol fast blue myelin stain.

Fixation. 10% neutral buffered formalin.

Embedding. Cut paraffin sections at 10 to 15 μm.

Solutions
20% aqueous silver nitrate
1% aqueous silver nitrate
10% pyridine
Boric acid buffer solution

Boric acid	1.24 gm
Distilled water	100 ml

Borax buffer solution

Sodium borate (borax)	1.9 gm
Distilled water	100 ml

Impregnating solution

Boric acid buffer solution	27.5 ml
Borax buffer solution	22.5 ml
Distilled water	257 ml
Silver nitrate, 1%	0.5 ml
Pyridine, 10%	2.5 ml

Reducing solution

Hydroquinone	1 gm
Sodium sulfite crystals	10 gm
Distilled water	100 ml

This solution is stable for only a few days but may be used repeatedly during that time.
0.2% gold chloride solution
2% oxalic acid solution

Technic
1. Xylene.
2. Absolute alcohol.
3. 95% alcohol.
4. Hydrate to distilled water.
5. Place sections in 20% silver nitrate solution for 1 hour.
6. Rinse in distilled water for 10 minutes. Prepare impregnating solution.
7. Place sections in impregnating solution in a covered jar using at least 20 ml of solution per slide. Incubate overnight at 37° C.
8. Remove slides, drain excess solution, and place in reducing solution for at least 2 minutes.
9. Wash in running water for 3 minutes and then rinse in distilled water.
10. Tone in gold chloride 3 minutes.
11. Rinse briefly in distilled water.
12. Place in oxalic acid for 3 to 10 minutes, examining microscopically until the axons are thoroughly blue-black.
13. Rinse in distilled water.
14. Place in sodium thiosulfate 5 minutes and then wash in running water for 5 minutes.
15. 95% alcohol.
16. Absolute alcohol, 2 changes.
17. Xylene, 2 changes.
18. Mount in synthetic resin.

Results
Nerve fibers and neurofibrils—black
Background—gray to rose

Sevier-Munger modification[8]

Principle. Many silver technics used for impregnation of nervous tissue are modifications of Bielschowski's method, introduced in 1902, in which he used a primary silver bath, followed by silver hydroxide and reduction in formalin. Sevier and Munger have adapted a modification introduced by Richardson,[9] to provide a controllable and reproducible technic for use on paraffin sections. The concentration of ammonium hydroxide and formalin and their relative proportions are critical to controlled development of the stain. Sodium thiosulfate is used to remove unreacted silver from the sections.

Fixation. 10% neutral buffered formalin.

Embedding. Cut paraffin sections at 6 to 8 μm.

Solutions
20% silver nitrate
10% silver nitrate
Formalin solution

Formaldehyde (37% to 40%)	2 ml
Tap water	98 ml

5% sodium thiosulfate
Sodium carbonate solution

Sodium carbonate	8 gm
Distilled water	30 ml

Ammoniacal silver (working solution)
To 50 ml of 10% silver, add concentrated ammonium hydroxide drop by drop until the dark brown precipitate that forms has almost disappeared. Shake vigorously between drops and avoid complete decolorization. The end point is a slightly cloudy solution. At this point add 0.5 ml of sodium carbonate solution and shake well. Add 25 drops of ammonium hydroxide and shake well. The solution should now be crystal clear. Filter into a 125 ml Erlenmeyer flask and cover.

Technic
1. Deparaffinize sections and hydrate to distilled water.
2. Preheat 20% silver nitrate to 60° C for 15 minutes. Add slides to warm silver solution and let them remain in the oven for 15 minutes.
3. Rinse one slide at a time in distilled water and place in a clean dry staining jar.

4. While shaking gently, add 10 drops of the formalin solution to the working ammoniacal silver solution. Quickly pour this solution over the slides and let develop for 5 to 30 minutes until golden brown. Check microscopically for completeness of reaction. *Do not wash.* Keep in motion during development to avoid precipitation.
5. Rinse well in 3 changes of fresh tap water.
6. Sodium thiosulfate for 2 minutes.
7. Wash well in tap water.
8. Dehydrate, clear, and mount in synthetic resin.

Results
Nerve endings and neurofibrils—black
Other elements—light brown
Note: This is an argyrophil stain using formalin as a reducing agent and is very useful for demonstrating granules of some carcinoid tumor cells.

NEUROGLIA

"Nerve glue" is an appropriate term for these cells because they provide the internal support of the central nervous system. Connective tissue proper is found only in the meninges covering the brain and in the blood vessels. Glia surround and insulate neurons except where they are in synaptic contact, produce the myelin sheath covering many axons, and function in the regulation of the neuronal microenvironment.

There are four types of glial cells: astrocytes, oligodendroglia, microglia, and ependymal cells. Astrocytes are stellate cells of two configurations: protoplasmic, which occur in the gray matter, and fibrous, which are found in white matter. They provide a support for tracts of nerve fibers and participate in fluid, gas, and metabolite exchange between nervous tissue and the blood and cerebrospinal fluid. Astrocytes participate in scar formation after injury or trauma by proliferation of their processes, forming an area of gliosis. Oligodendroglia are small cells with the primary function in the central nervous system of forming and probably maintaining the myelin sheath. Microglia are fixed phagocytes found throughout the brain and spinal cord.

Ependymal cells line the ventricles and spinal canal and are true epithelial cells. Other than forming a selective barrier between the cerebrospinal fluid and the nervous tissue, their function is not totally understood.

General overview methods

Several methods are particularly useful for studying the general cellular distribution and cytoarchitecture of the tissue. With a scanning objective one may visualize Nissl substance, nuclei, and nucleoli of neurons, as well as the nuclei of the neuroglia. These stains employ basic aniline dyes to stain the DNA of the nucleus and RNA of Nissl substance and nucleoli.

Toluidine blue for nerve cells and glia[10]

Fixation. Alcohol fixation is best; formalin serves well.

Embedding. Cut paraffin sections at 5 to 8 μm.

Solutions
Alcoholic colophonium solution

Colophonium (rosin)	10 gm
95% alcohol	100 ml

Toluidine blue stain

Toluidine blue	0.1 gm
Distilled water	100 ml

Aniline-alcohol solution
10% solution of aniline in 95% alcohol

Technic
1. Xylene.
2. Absolute alcohol.
3. 95% alcohol.
4. Place slides in alcoholic colophonium solution for 3 to 5 minutes.
5. 95% alcohol for 3 minutes.
6. 95% alcohol for 3 minutes.
7. Toluidine blue stain for 30 seconds.
8. Differentiate in aniline-alcohol until the background is clear. Good differentiation shows the smooth muscle in arteries well stained.
9. Oil of cajeput, several changes until clear.
10. Xylene, 2 changes.
11. Mount in synthetic resin.

Results
Nerve cells
Nucleus—pale blue
Nissl bodies—dark blue
Glia
Astrocytes—pale blue
Oligodendroglia—very dark blue

Cresyl echt Violett stain for nerve cells and glia[10]

Fixation. Formalin or Bouin's fixed tissue stains well.

Embedding. Cut paraffin sections at 5 to 8 μm.

Solutions
Cresyl echt Violett acetate

Cresyl echt Violett acetate	1 gm
Distilled water	100 ml

Technic
1. Xylene.
2. Absolute alcohol.

3. Hydrate to distilled water.
4. Stain in *Cresyl echt Violett* acetate solution for 2 minutes.
5. Wash in distilled water.
6. 95% alcohol, 2 changes.
7. Absolute alcohol, 2 changes.
8. Oil of cajeput, several changes until clear.
9. Xylene, 2 changes.
10. Mount in synthetic resin.

Results
Nerve cells
    Nucleus—pale blue
    Nissl bodies—dark blue
Glia
    Astrocytes—pale blue
    Oligodendroglia—very dark blue

Trichrome stain for astrocytes[11]

Fixation. 10% formalin or Elver's fixative.
Embedding. Cut paraffin sections at 5 to 8 μm.

Solutions
Weigert's first mordant

Potassium dichromate	5 gm
Chromium fluoride	2.5 gm
Distilled water	to make 100 ml

Weigert's iron hematoxylin
Solution A

Hematoxylin	1 gm
95% alcohol	100 ml

Solution B

Ferric chloride (29% aqueous solution)	4 ml
Distilled water	95 ml
Hydrochloric acid	1 ml

Working solution
    For use mix equal parts of A and B. The mixture is deep black and is best prepared fresh each time, though it will keep and can be used several days.
Ponceau-azophloxine solution
Solution A

Ponceau 2R	1 gm
Glacial acetic acid	1 ml
Distilled water	100 ml

Solution B

Azophloxine	1 gm
Glacial acetic acid	1 ml
Distilled water	100 ml

Working solution
    Mix 90 ml of 1:500 aqueous solution of glacial acetic acid, and add:
        10 ml of solution A
        10 ml of solution B
Phosphotungstic acid–orange G solution

Phosphotungstic acid	3 gm
Orange G solution	2 gm
Distilled water	100 ml

Technic
1. Xylene.
2. Absolute alcohol.
3. Hydrate to distilled water.
4. Place slides in Weigert's first mordant for 3 to 12 hours.
5. Rinse in 3 changes of tap water.
6. Rinse in distilled water.
7. Stain with Weigert's iron hematoxylin for 2 to 4 minutes.
8. Wash in running tap water.
9. Differentiate in a 0.5% acid alcohol solution for 15 seconds.
10. Wash in tap water.
11. Rinse in a very weak ammonia water solution (1 to 2 drops to 100 ml water).
12. Rinse in distilled water to which a few drops of concentrated acetic acid has been added.
13. Stain with Ponceau-azophloxine solution for 5 minutes.
14. Repeat step 12.
15. Place slides in a 3% solution of phosphomolybdic acid for a few seconds.
16. Repeat step 12.
17. Stain in phosphotungstic acid–orange G for 5 minutes.
18. Wash in tap water several times and repeat step 12.
19. Rinse quickly in one change of distilled water and put into a 0.5% aqueous solution of aniline blue for 1 to 5 minutes.
20. Repeat step 12.
21. 95% alcohol, 2 changes.
22. Absolute alcohol, 2 changes.
23. Xylene, 2 changes.
24. Mount in synthetic resin.

Results
Astrocytes—lavender
Nuclei—pale blue
Nerve cells—blue with a bright red nucleolus

Cajal's gold sublimate method for astrocytes[12]

A delicate procedure that selectively stains astrocytes, Cajal's gold sublimate technic is a gold impregnation method done on frozen sections. It is important to use materials of extreme purity for reagent preparation. Fixation should last no fewer than 2 days and no longer than 25 days in Cajal's formalin ammonium bromide. Prolonged fixation will cause protoplasmic neuroglia to lose stainability. Temperature of the staining solution should not exceed 30° C, and 10° C is best. With old formalin-fixed tissue, frozen sections should be placed in the formalin ammonium bromide fixative for 48 hours before one proceeds with the technic.

Fixation

Formalin ammonium bromide solution

Ammonium bromide	15 gm
40% formaldehyde	100 ml
Distilled water	400 ml

Tissue should be fixed in the above solution for a minimum of 2 days. Tissue will section better if washed in tap water for ½ hour prior to being cut.

Sectioning. Cut frozen sections at 20 to 30 μm.

Solutions

Gold sublimate solution

1% gold chloride (brown gold chloride preferred)	5 ml
1% mercuric chloride	25 ml
Distilled water	5 ml

Note: A mixture of the two chlorides is essential, since either chloride used alone is ineffective for impregnating the neuroglia.

5% aqueous solution of sodium thiosulfate

Technic

1. Wash sections well in distilled water.
2. Stain for 4 hours, keeping them in a dark place, in the gold sublimate solution.
3. Wash in distilled water.
4. Fix for 2 minutes in 5% solution of sodium thiosulfate.
5. Wash thoroughly in distilled water.
6. Mount on slide, blot with bibulous paper, and dehydrate in 95% and absolute alcohol. The blotting prevents the section from curling and shrinking in alcohol.
7. Clear in xylene.
8. Mount in synthetic resin.

Holzer's stain for glia fibers[13]

Fixation. Fix in 10% formalin or formalin alcohol.

Embedding. Cut paraffin sections at 5 to 8 μm.

Solutions

Phosphomolybdic alcohol

0.5% aqueous phosphomolybdic acid (fresh)	10 ml
95% alcohol	20 ml

Absolute alcohol–chloroform mixture

Absolute alcohol	20 ml
Chloroform	80 ml

Crystal violet stain

Crystal violet	5 gm
Absolute alcohol	20 ml
Chloroform	80 ml

Potassium bromide solution

Potassium bromide	10 gm
Distilled water	100 ml

Differentiating solution

Aniline oil	30 ml
Chloroform	45 ml
Concentrated ammonium hydroxide	5 drops

Technic

1. Xylene.
2. Absolute alcohol.
3. Hydrate to distilled water.
4. Place sections in fresh phosphomolybdic alcohol for 3 minutes.
5. Drain off fluid and cover section with absolute alcohol–chloroform mixture.
6. While they are still wet, cover sections with crystal violet stain and allow to remain for 30 seconds.
7. Replace stain with 10% potassium bromide. Wash for 1 minute in this solution.
8. Blot dry.
9. Differentiate for 30 seconds in the differentiating solution.
10. Wash in xylene, several changes.
11. Mount in synthetic resin.

Results

Glia fibers—blue

Phosphotungstic acid–hematoxylin[2]

Described in the chapter on connective tissue, this technic stains glial fibers more satisfactorily when slightly modified. Sodium thiosulfate is not used for decolorization of the iodine because it tends to impair staining. The principle has already been described.

Fixation. Fix in 10% neutral buffered formalin.

Embedding. Cut paraffin sections at 5 to 8 μm.

Solutions

1% potassium permanganate

5% oxalic acid

Phosphotungstic acid–hematoxylin (PTAH)

Hematoxylin	1 gm
Phosphotungstic acid	20 gm
Distilled water	1 liter

Dissolve the solid ingredients in separate portions of the water; dissolve the hematoxylin with the aid of gentle heat. When cool, combine. No preservative is necessary. Ripening requires several weeks, but the addition of 0.2 gm of potassium permanganate will cause the stain to ripen at once.

Technic

1. Xylene.
2. Absolute alcohol.
3. Hydrate to distilled water.
4. Mordant sections in Zenker's with acetic acid overnight at room temperature or 1 hour at 50° C.

5. Wash in running water 15 minutes.
6. Place in Lugol's iodine 15 minutes.
7. Decolorize in 95% alcohol for a minimum of 1 hour. Do *not* take slides through sodium thiosulfate.
8. Distilled water, 3 rapid changes.
9. Oxidize for 5 minutes in potassium permanganate.
10. Decolorize in oxalic acid for 5 minutes.
11. Wash in running water for 10 minutes.
12. Place in PTAH solution for 24 hours.
13. Dip quickly in 95% alcohol.
14. Dehydrate quickly in 2 changes of absolute alcohol.
15. Clear in xylene.
16. Mount in synthetic resin.

Results

Glial fibers—blue
Nuclei—blue
Neurons—salmon
Myelin—blue

MYELIN

Myelin is the white fatty nonliving material forming an insulating and protective sheath around nerve fibers. It is a complex material containing protein, cholesterol, phospholipids, and cerebrosides. Most of the myelin is lost during routine paraffin processing, leaving behind a resistant proteolipid, neurokeratin. The myelin sheath is formed by Schwann cells in the peripheral nervous system and oligodendroglia in the central nervous system.

In wallerian degeneration, myelin covering the disintegrating axon also undergoes a breakdown into simpler lipids, which are eventually removed. This lipid becomes increasingly more sudanophilic and less anisotrophic.

Methods for demonstrating myelin, with the exception of Luxol fast blue, are similar in mechanism. Mordant-hematoxylin solutions attach to the phospholipid component of the myelin sheath, which has an affinity for the basic-charged dye lake. Unsaturation of lipid components may give additional binding sites for the dye lakes. Differentiation is usually accomplished in two steps. The first differentiation removes gross amounts of excess dye lake; the second confines the lake to the desired area.

Weil's method[14]

Principle. Weil's method is a regressive staining technic, and the staining solution consists of hematoxylin and the mordant ferric alum. Myelin has a special affinity for this lake. The sections are overstained, and the excess dye must be removed from undesired areas. A dilute solution of ferric alum is used as the first differentiator, and here the dye distributes itself partly as a soluble lake with the free mordant and partly as a component of the insoluble complex. Since the amount of mordant in the complex is small in comparison with the amount in the differentiating fluid, nearly all the dye will associate itself with the dilute mordant, giving a gross differentiation of the tissue. A borax ferricyanide solution is used to complete the differentiation. The borax is used to give the desired pH to the solution, and the ferricyanide acts as an oxidizing agent to remove any nonspecifically bound hematoxylin lake and form a colorless oxidation product and, by doing so, restrict the stain to myelin sheaths and red blood cells.

Fixation. Fix tissue in 10% formalin solution.

Embedding. Embed in paraffin and cut at 15 μm or embed in celloidin and cut at 25 to 30 μm.

Solutions

Ferric ammonium sulfate solution
    4% aqueous solution of ferric ammonium sulfate
Hematoxylin solution
    1% solution of hematoxylin is made up by the adding of 90 ml of distilled water to 10 ml of a 10% solution of hematoxylin in absolute alcohol. The hematoxylin should be ripened at least 6 months before use.
Staining solution
    Mix equal parts of 4% ferric ammonium sulfate and 1% hematoxylin immediately before use. Do not filter this stain. Do not use it more than once.
Differentiating solution

Borax (sodium borate)	10 gm
Potassium ferricyanide	12.5 gm
Distilled water	1 liter

Technic

1. Xylene.
2. Absolute alcohol.
3. Hydrate to distilled water.
4. Stain for 10 to 30 minutes at 55° C in staining solution.
5. Wash twice in tap water.
6. Differentiate in 4% ferric ammonium sulfate until gray matter can just be distinguished or until stain is removed from the back of the paraffin sections.
7. Wash 3 times in tap water.
8. Complete differentiation in borax ferricyanide solution and control differentiation under the microscope.

9. Wash twice in tap water.
10. Wash sections in dilute ammonia water. Prepare by adding 6 drops of ammonium hydroxide to 100 ml of water.
11. Wash in distilled water.
12. 95% alcohol.
13. Absolute alcohol, 2 changes.
14. Xylene, 2 changes.
15. Mount in synthetic resin.

Results (Plate 2, *R*)

Myelin sheath—blue to blue-black
Red blood cells—very black
This stain can be used to demonstrate hemorrhage.

Pal-Weigert method[15]

Principle. The staining solution for this technic is composed of lithium carbonate and hematoxylin, a mixture that forms a dye lake with tissue components; the attachment is especially strong in the case of myelin sheaths. Potassium permanganate is used for the first differentiator and, by oxidation, aids in restricting the dye lake to the myelin and red cells. The second differentiator is Pal's bleach, which further oxidizes and completes the differentiating procedure. Oxalic acid is used to remove excess permanganate from the section.

Fixation. 10% formalin satisfactory.

Embedding. Celloidin, paraffin, or frozen sections may be used.

Solutions

Mordanting solution
    4% aqueous ferric ammonium sulfate,
        $FeNH_4(SO_4)_2 \cdot 12H_2O$
Staining solution
    Solution A
        Saturated aqueous lithium carbonate   7 ml
        Distilled water   93 ml
    Solution B
        Hematoxylin   1 gm
        Absolute alcohol   10 ml
    The hematoxylin solution does not require ripening.
    For use, add 1 volume of solution A to 9 volumes of solution B
Differentiators
    0.4% aqueous potassium permanganate
    Decolorization solution (prepare just before use)
        Oxalic acid   1 gm
        Sodium sulfite (or potassium sulfite)   1 gm
        Distilled water   to 1 liter

Technic

1. Place sections in the mordanting solution for 2 to 24 hours.
2. Wash in tap water.
3. Place in staining solution for 1 to 2 hours.
4. Wash for 2 to 3 minutes in tap water.
5. Partially decolorize in the mordanting solution until the gray and white matter are barely distinguishable. The time of this initial decolorization varies with the amount of staining.
6. Wash 2 to 3 minutes in tap water.
7. Differentiate in 0.4% potassium permanganate until the gray and white matter are clearly distinguishable when sections are held up to the light. (Sections will be colored brown by the permanganate.)
8. Rinse quickly in tap water.
9. Complete decolorization by treating sections with the decolorizing solution. Gray matter should become completely clear and colorless, except where it contains some myelinated fibers.
10. Wash 2 to 3 minutes in tap water.
11. Wash 5 minutes or more in solution A to restore the blue color lost in decolorizing.
12. Wash thoroughly in tap water.
13. Counterstain if desired.
14. Dehydrate, clear, and mount in synthetic resin.

Results

Myelin sheaths—dark blue
Other structures—unstained (unless a counterstain has been used)

Marchi's method for degenerating myelin[16]

Principle. This technic is used to demonstrate degenerating myelin in tissue sections. The method uses osmium tetroxide, and ordinarily the lipid components present in the myelin would reduce the osmium to a black reduction compound. The normal reduction process is prevented in normal myelin by the addition of an oxidizing agent, such as potassium dichromate or potassium chlorate, to the osmium solution. Since the oxidizing reaction prevents the usual reduction, normal myelin is said to be marchi-negative. The reduction of the osmium by degenerating myelin is not inhibited by the presence of oxidizers and is said to be marchi-positive. There are a number of theories as to why degenerating myelin is not affected by the oxidizers. One postulates that normal myelin lipids are hydrophilic and readily absorb both the osmium and the water-soluble oxidizer, and the reduction is prevented by the simultaneous oxidizing action of the oxidizing agent. In contrast to the normal myelin, it is believed that degenerating myelin is hydrophobic and will therefore not absorb the water-soluble oxidizing agent. It

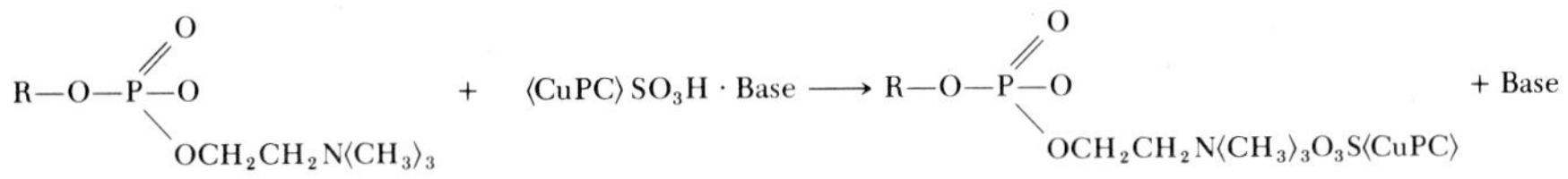

$$R—O—\overset{\displaystyle O}{\overset{\|}{P}}—O \quad + \quad \langle CuPC \rangle\, SO_3H \cdot Base \longrightarrow R—O—\overset{\displaystyle O}{\overset{\|}{P}}—O \qquad + \text{ Base}$$

Choline-containing compound   Luxol fast blue dye type

Fig. 14-1. Acid-base reaction of the Luxol fast blue dye with choline-containing compounds results in the latter being colored blue.

will, however, absorb the osmium, and a black reduction compound is formed by a mechanism similar to that described for the osmic acid method for unsaturated lipids.

Solutions

2.5% potassium dichromate
1% osmium tetroxide
Acetone, petroleum ether, chloroform, and chloroform balsam

Method

1. Fix tissues 2 days in Orth's fluid or 10% formalin.
2. Mordant 7 days in 2.5% potassium dichromate (change solution on third and fifth day).
3. Immerse 14 days in a mixture of the following:

   2.5% potassium dichromate   2 parts
   1% osmium tetroxide   1 part
   Change solution every 7 days and keep in the dark.
4. Wash 24 hours in running water.
5. Dehydrate with acetone, 4 changes at 45 minutes each change.
6. Clear in petroleum ether, 2 changes at 30 minutes each change.
7. Infiltrate with paraffin, 3 changes at 30 minutes each.
8. Embed, section at 5 μm, deparaffinize with chloroform, and mount in chloroform balsam.

Results

Degenerating myelin—black
Background—brown-yellow

Luxol fast blue method[17]

Principle. The dye Luxol fast blue is of the sulfonated copper phthalocyanine type and is the alcohol-soluble counterpart of the water-soluble alcian blue. Dyes of this type are usually represented by the following symbols: (CuPC)SO$_3$H · base. Since this technic is usually done on paraffin sections, lipoproteins, rather than simple lipids, are responsible for the staining. The mechanism is one of an acid-base reaction with salt formation, because the base of the lipoprotein replaces the base of the dye. Studies have shown that the formation of the dark blue precipitates is confined to choline-

containing compounds, and the equation of staining in alcoholic solutions in Fig. 14-1 may apply.

Fixation. 10% formalin.

Embedding. Cut paraffin sections at 10 μm.

Solutions

Solution A
Make up a 0.1% solution of Luxol fast blue MBSN by dissolving 1 gm of the substance in 1 liter of 95% alcohol. Add 5 ml of 10% acetic acid. Filter before using. (This solution is very stable and may be used even after 1 year.)

Solution B
Make up a 0.1% solution of Grubler's *Cresyl echt Violett*, or, if not available, a 0.25% solution of Coleman and Bell's cresyl violet. Before using, add 5 drops of 10% acetic acid to every 30 ml of solution and filter. (When using Coleman and Bell products, heat before filtering.) Dr. Klüver also suggests that Bayer's cresyl violet is satisfactory for use.

Technic

1. Remove paraffin and run sections through absolute alcohol and several changes of 95% alcohol.
2. Stain overnight (16 to 24 hours) in solution A at 57° to 60° C.
3. Immerse in 95% alcohol and wash off excess stain.
4. Wash in distilled water.
5. Begin differentiation by quick immersion in 0.05% lithium carbonate (10 to 20 seconds).
6. Continue differentiation in several changes of 70% alcohol until gray and white matter can be distinguished. Care should be taken not to overdifferentiate.
7. Wash in distilled water.
8. Steps 6 and 7 may be repeated if further decolorization is necessary.
9. Wash thoroughly in distilled water.
10. Stain for 5 minutes in solution B.
11. Wash in 95% alcohol.
12. Wash in absolute alcohol to which has been added 3 drops of neutral balsam.
13. Wash in second dish containing absolute alcohol and 3 drops of neutral balsam. (The first wash frequently becomes milky and makes differentiation and clearing difficult.)

14. Clear in 3 changes of xylene and mount in synthetic resin.

Results (Plate 2, Q)
Myelin fibers—blue to greenish blue
Cells—pink to violet.

Luxol fast blue combination methods

These technics are probably the most useful and reliable methods available for the demonstration of pathologic processes in the nervous system. They combine the Luxol fast blue myelin stain with common staining technics found in use in the majority of laboratories. These include the periodic acid–Schiff, oil red O, phosphotungstic acid-hematoxylin, and Holmes' silver nitrate technics.

LUXOL FAST BLUE–PERIODIC ACID SCHIFF–HEMATOXYLIN[18]

This is a particularly useful combination as it allows a correlative study of the cellular elements, fiber pathways, and vascular components of the nervous system. Each stain is sharpened and complemented by the other.

Fixation. 10% neutral buffered formalin.
Embedding. Cut paraffin sections at 10 μm. Celloidin or frozen sections may be used.

Solutions
Solutions are described under the periodic acid–Schiff reaction and the Luxol fast blue method.

Technic
1. Follow Luxol fast blue procedure through step 9.
2. Place in 0.5% periodic acid solution for 5 mines.
3. Rinse in 2 changes of distilled water.
4. Place in Schiff's solution 15 to 30 minutes.
5. Wash in tap water for 5 minutes.
6. Stain in Harris's hematoxylin for 1 minute.
7. Wash in tap water for 5 minutes. (If background is not clear, dip one time in acid alcohol and wash. If nuclei are not dark blue, dip in dilute ammonium hydroxide briefly and wash.)
8. Dehydrate, clear, and mount in synthetic resin.

Results
Myelin sheath—blue-green
Capillary basement membranes, fungi, corpora amylacea, senile plaques—rose
Nuclei—purple

LUXOL FAST BLUE–HOLMES' SILVER NITRATE[18]

Fixation. 10% neutral buffered formalin or formalin ammonium bromide.

Embedding. Cut paraffin sections at 10 μm.

Solutions
Luxol fast blue
  Luxol fast blue MBSN   1 gm
  95% alcohol   100 ml
  10% acetic acid   0.5 ml
Other solutions are described under Holmes' silver nitrate technic for nerve fibers.

Technic
1. Follow steps 1 to 14 of the Holmes' silver nitrate method.
2. Dip in 95% alcohol briefly.
3. Stain in 1% Luxol fast blue solution overnight at 60° C.
4. Rinse slides in 95% alcohol, and then place in distilled water.
5. Place in 0.05% aqueous lithium carbonate for 15 seconds.
6. Differentiate in 70% alcohol for 20 to 30 seconds.
7. Rinse in distilled water. Steps 5 and 6 may be repeated if more differentiation is needed.
8. Rinse in distilled water.
9. 95% alcohol, 2 changes.
10. Absolute alcohol, 2 changes.
11. Clear in 3 changes of xylene and mount in synthetic resin.

Results
Myelin sheath—blue to green
Nerve fibers—black

LUXOL FAST BLUE–PHOSPHOTUNGSTIC ACID HEMATOXYLIN[18]

When these two dyes are used together, the selective features of each stain are emphasized. Better contrast is achieved if the Luxol fast blue is differentiated to a lighter color than with other methods.

Fixation. 10% neutral buffered formalin.

Embedding. Cut paraffin sections at 5 to 8 μm. Celloidin sections may be used.

Solutions
0.25% potassium permanganate
Other solutions are described under the Luxol fast blue and phosphotungstic acid–hematoxylin technics.

Technic
1. Deparaffinize and hydrate sections to distilled water.
2. Place sections in 0.25% potassium permanganate for 5 to 10 minutes.
3. Rinse in distilled water.
4. Decolorize for 3 to 5 minutes in 5% oxalic acid.
5. Running tap water for 5 minutes.

6. Place in 95% alcohol.
7. Place in 0.1% Luxol fast blue solution overnight at 60° C.
8. Remove excess stain with 95% alcohol.
9. Rinse in distilled water.
10. Place in lithium carbonate for 10 to 20 seconds.
11. Place in 70% alcohol for 30 seconds.
12. Rinse in distilled water. Steps 10 and 11 may be repeated if more differentiation is desired.
13. Place in PTAH solution for 24 to 48 hours.
14. Rinse in distilled water.
15. Lithium carbonate for 5 seconds.
16. Place in 70% alcohol for 15 seconds.
17. Rinse in distilled water.
18. 95% alcohol.
19. Absolute alcohol, 2 changes.
20. Clear in 3 changes of xylene and mount in synthetic resin.

Results
Myelin—blue
Glial fibers—purple

LUXOL FAST BLUE–OIL RED O[18]

Fixation. 10% neutral buffered formalin.
Embedding. Cut frozen sections at 10 to 20 μm.

Solutions
Luxol fast blue

Luxol fast blue MBSN	1 gm
70% alcohol	100 ml
10% acetic acid	0.5 ml

Oil red O

Oil red O	0.4 gm
Acetone	10 ml

Mix well and then add:

80% alcohol	90 ml

0.005% lithium carbonate in distilled water
0.5% acid alcohol

Hydrochloric acid	0.5 ml
50% alcohol	100 ml

Technic
1. Cut frozen section and place in tap water.
2. Take sections through 50% and 70% alcohols.
3. Stain in Luxol fast blue for 2 to 3 hours at room temperature.
4. Briefly place sections in 70% alcohol.
5. Quickly pass through 50% alcohol.
6. Place sections in distilled water containing a few drops of 95% alcohol to control surface tension.
7. Place in lithium carbonate for 20 to 30 seconds.
8. Place in 70% alcohol for 15 to 20 seconds.
9. Take sections through 50% alcohol to distilled water containing a few drops of 95% alcohol.

Steps 7 and 8 may be repeated if further decolorization is needed.
10. Distilled water for 2 to 3 minutes.
11. 70% alcohol, briefly.
12. Using a glass rod, stain section in oil red O for 15 to 30 seconds.
13. Pass sections briefly through 70% alcohol and then 50% alcohol.
14. Rinse in distilled water.
15. Stain in Harris's hematoxylin for 2 minutes.
16. Rinse in distilled water for 2 minutes.
17. Decolorize briefly in acid alcohol and then dip briefly in 50% alcohol.
18. Wash in distilled water.
19. Blue in lithium carbonate.
20. Dip in 70% alcohol.
21. Dip in 50% alcohol.
22. Rinse in tap water.
23. Mount in glycerol gelatin (without phenol) or other neutral water-soluble mounting media.

Results
Fat—red
Myelin sheath—blue

REFERENCES
Copenhaver, W. M.: Bailey's textbook of histology, ed. 15, Baltimore, 1964, The Williams & Wilkins Co.
Davenport, H. A.: Histological and histochemical technics, Philadelphia, 1964, W. B. Saunders Co.
Lillie, R. D.: Histopathologic technic and practical histochemistry, ed. 3, New York, 1964, McGraw-Hill Book Co.
McManus, J. F. A., and Mowry, R. W.: Staining methods—histologic and histochemical, New York, 1963, Harper & Row, Publishers.
Mallory, F. B.: Pathological technic, New York, 1961, Hafner Publishing Co.
Rhodin, J. A. G.: Histology, New York, 1974, Oxford University Press.

Technic references
1. Fletcher, D. E.: Rapid staining procedures for paraffin sections of formalin fixed nervous tissue, J. Neuropathol. Exp. Neurol. 6:299-305, 1947.
2. Luna, L. G., editor: Manual of histologic staining methods of the Armed Forces Institute of Pathology, ed. 2, New York, 1960, McGraw-Hill Book Co.
3. Einarson, L.: A method for progressive selective staining of Nissl and nuclear substance in nerve cells, Am. J. Pathol. 8:295-307, 1932.
4. McManus, J. F. A., and Mowry, R. W.: Staining methods—histologic and histochemical, New York, 1960, Harper & Row, Publishers.
5. Nonidez, J. F.: Studies on the innervation of the heart, Am. J. Anat. 65:361-413, 1939.
6. Mallory, F. B.: Pathological technique, New York, 1961, Hafner Publishing Co.
7. Holmes, W.: Silver staining of nerve axons in paraffin sections, Anat. Rec. 86:157-187, 1943.

8. Sevier, A. C., and Munger, B. L.: A silver method for paraffin sections of neural tissue, J. Neuropathol. Exp. Neurol. **24:**130-135, 1965.

9. Richardson, K. C.: Studies on the structure of autonomic nerves in small intestine, correlating the silver impregnated image in light microscopy with permanganate-fixed ultrastructure in electron microscopy, J. Anat. **94:**457-472. 1960.

10. Weil, A.: Textbook of neuropathology, New York, 1933, Grune & Stratton. Modified by Elsie Toms, Neurosurgical Pathology Laboratory, University of Pennsylvania.

11. Used in the Laboratory of Neurosurgical Pathology at Hospital of University of Pennsylvania. Original reference not known; it may be considered a modification from Dublin, W. B.: Combined stain method for neurologic tissue, J. Neuropathol. Exp. Neurol. **2:**205-206, 1943.

12. McManus, J. F. A., and Mowry, R. W.: Staining methods—histologic and histochemical, New York, 1960, Harper & Row, Publishers. (Original reference: Cajal, W. R.: Quelques méthodes simples pour la coloration de la névroglie, Schweiz. Arch. Neurol. Psychiat. **13:**187-193, 1923.)

13. McManus, J. F. A., and Mowry, R. W.: Staining methods—histologic and histochemical, New York, 1960, Harper & Row, Publishers. (Original reference: Holzer, W.: Über eine neue Methode der gliafaser Färbung, Z. Ges. Neurol. Psychiat. **69:**354-357, 1921.)

14. Weil, A.: A rapid method for staining myelin sheaths, Arch. Neurol. Psychiat. **20:**392-393, 1928.

15. Conn, H. J., Darrow, M. A., and Emmel, V. M.: Staining procedures, ed. 2, Baltimore, 1960, The Williams & Wilkins Co.

16. Lillie, R. D.: Histopathologic technique and practical histochemistry, ed. 3, New York, 1964, McGraw-Hill Book Co.

17. Klüver, H., and Barrera, E.: A method for the combined staining of cells and fibers in the nervous system, J. Neuropathol. Exp. Neurol. **12:** 400-403, 1953.

18. Margolis, G., and Pickett, J. P.: New applications for the Luxol fast blue myelin stain, Lab Invest. **5:**459-474, 1956.

CHAPTER 15

Special cells and tissues

PITUITARY

The pituitary gland (hypophysis cerebri), considered the most complex of the endocrine glands, lies immediately below the base of the brain in a bony prominence (called the "sella turcica") of the sphenoid bone. The gland is connected to the brain by the pituitary stalk, or infundibulum.

The pituitary gland may be divided into four parts:

Pars anterior—main body of the gland
Pars tuberalis—a projection of the pars anterior and
  extending along the anterior and lateral aspects
  of the pituitary stalk
Pars intermedia—a narrow band of glandular tissue
  that lies along the posterior border
Pars nervosa—posterior to the pars intermedia

The pars nervosa and infundibulum have a histologic appearance similar to the nervous tissue from which they are derived, and these structures are sometimes called the neurohypophysis. Two pituitary hormones, oxytocin and antidiuretic hormone, are released from storage sites in the neurohypophysis.

The pars anterior is well-developed and associated with numerous specific hormonal secretions. The pars intermedia is comparatively undeveloped in man, and the pars tuberalis has not been associated with specific endocrine functions. Collectively, these three parts may be referred to as the adenohypophysis and have a microscopic structure that is typical for endocrine glands. Most of the special stains for the pituitary are designed to demonstrate the cell types of the adenohypophysis, chiefly the pars anterior.

The glandular cells of the adenohypophysis may be broadly classified as chromophilic or chromophobic based on their affinity (or lack thereof) for the dyes used in routine staining. Chromophilic cells, in turn, may be subdivided

Table 15-1. Cell types of adenohypophysis

Cell name	Type of cell	Secretion	Action of secretion	Some staining characteristics
Somatotroph	Alpha$_1$ acidophil	Somatotropin or growth hormone (STH)	Proper body growth, protein synthesis, carbohydrate metabolism, etc.	Acidophilic; granules stain orange with orange G–erythrosin
Mammotroph	Alpha$_2$ acidophil	Prolactin or luteotropic hormone (LTH)	Stimulates milk secretion	Acidophilic; granules stain red-orange with orange G–erythrosin
Corticotroph	Beta$_1$ basophil	Adrenocorticotropic hormone (ACTH) and possibly melanocyte-stimulating hormone (MSH)	Acts on zona fasciculata and zona reticularis of the adrenal cortex to stimulate release of glucocorticoids and 17-ketosteroids, respectively	Basophilic, PAS-positive; stains red with aldehyde thionin–PAS reaction
Thyrotroph	Beta$_2$ basophil	Thyroid-stimulating hormone (TSH)	Production and secretion of thyroid hormone	Large cell, irregular shape, basophilic; stains blue-purple with aldehyde thionin–PAS reaction
Gonadotrophs	Delta$_1$ basophil	Luteinizing hormone (LH) (female)	Egg follicle maturation, ovulation, progesterone secretion, some estrogen secretion	Round cells rather than angular, basophilic; granules stain blue-purple-red with aldehyde thionin-PAS reaction
	Delta$_2$ basophil	Interstitial cell–stimulating hormone (ICSH) (male) Follicle-stimulating hormone (FSH)	Stimulates male hormone secretion from the interstitial cells of Leydig *Female:* estrogen secretion; growth and maturation of ovarian follicles *Male:* stimulates sperm production	

into acidophils (30% to 40%) and basophils (5% to 10%) based on the reactions of their specific cell granules with acid or basic dyes. The acidophils and basophils have been further subdivided by their reactions to various special staining techniques, and the cell type of each subdivision has been associated with the secretion of a particular hormone. The chromophobe cells (50%) are believed to represent either precursor cells for the chromophils, or chromophils in various stages of degranulation. Table 15-1 lists additional information about the cell types of the adenohypophysis.

DIAGNOSTIC APPLICATIONS

Primary lesions of the pituitary can cause both mechanical damage because of tumor size (such as increased intracranial pressure) and various hormonal changes. The latter effects may be caused by hyperactivity or hypoactivity. Pituitary hyperfunction can stimulate those secondary endocrine glands dependent on the pituitary (such as thyroid, adrenals, and gonads) to excessive activity. Pituitary hypofunction will result in decreased activity from these glands. In each case, the "target organ" for the secretion from the secondary endocrine glands may also be affected. Because of feedback from the secondary endocrine glands to the pituitary, primary changes in the former can also be reflected in functional and histologic changes in the pituitary. Special stains can serve to identify the cell type comprising the lesion.

The available literature, current and past,

contains numerous methods for staining pituitary granules, which would leave one to believe that none has been completely satisfactory. One of the most meaningful and simplest technics for identification of the cell types is the periodic acid–Schiff reaction by which the granules of basophils can be distinguished by their content of glycoprotein, which is PAS-positive.

Two important facts must be observed in the staining of pituitary granules:

1. Prompt and correct fixation.
2. Fixation should be done in 8 to 12 hours. Overfixation leads to granule depletion.

DEMONSTRATION METHODS
Gomori's chrome alum–hematoxylin–phloxine stain[2]

Principle. This stain distinguishes the alpha and beta cells of the pituitary gland, and the alpha and beta cells of the pancreas. The first step in the procedure is refixation of the tissue sections in Bouin's fluid. The picric acid in Bouin's fluid gives the tissues a strong affinity for acid dyes, since it prevents the dissociation of the carboxyl groups present in the tissue and leaves the amino groups free to react with the acid dyes. Potassium permanganate is then used to oxidize tissue structures. This step is not strictly necessary in staining of the pituitary, but if omitted in staining pancreas, the beta cells will not take the stain. In a pituitary section, oxidation will enhance the color contrast and will provide more reactive sites to combine with dyes and dye lakes. Excess permanganate is decolorized by the action of the sodium bisulfite. The two steps of refixation and oxidation aid in making the basic dyes demonstrate beta cells selectively. Chrome alum hematoxylin, a dye lake with a basic charge, stains the basophilic beta cells, and this particular hematoxylin formula gives the clearest color results of the usual hematoxylin formulas. They color a blue-gray, but the exact mechanism of the affinity of the cationic chromium complex for these granules is not known. It has been shown that chrome alum has an affinity for sulfonic acid radicals.[3] Since beta cells do have a high content of glycoprotein in their granules,[18] binding might occur by attraction of the cationic hematoxylin complex for the negatively charged sulfonic acid groups released from the oxidation of the glycoprotein by the potassium permanganate treatment. Excess hematoxylin is removed by the acid alcohol and the section becomes clear blue. Phloxine, an acid dye, penetrates the alpha, or acidophilic, cells and stains them red. Phosphotungstic acid is used as a differentiating agent and removes the phloxine from connective tissue, leaving it largely unstained in the final stage. The phosphotungstic acid also lessens the vivid red color of the phloxine stain, so that both alpha and beta cells stand out clearly.

Fixation. Bouin's fluid preferred; neutral buffered formalin.

An excellent fixative for the pituitary for this technic is Elftman's chrome alum fixative.[4] The fixative contains a final concentration of 5% chrome alum, 5% formalin, and 5% mercuric chloride. Mix just before use by adding concentrated formalin and chrome alum to a stock solution of 5% mercuric chloride.

Embedding. Cut paraffin sections at 5 µm.

Solutions

Potassium permanganate solution

Potassium permanganate	0.3 gm
Distilled water	100 ml
Sulfuric acid	0.3 ml

Sodium bisulfite solution
5% aqueous solution of sodium bisulfite

Chromium hematoxylin solution

1% aqueous solution of hematoxylin	50 ml
3% aqueous solution of chrome alum	50 ml

To 100 ml of the chrome hematoxylin solution, add 2 ml of 5% solution of potassium dichromate and 2 ml of 0.5 N sulfuric acid. The mixture is ripe after 48 hours and may be used as long as a metallic luster film forms on the surface (usually 4 to 6 weeks). Filter before use. *Note:* If stain is needed for immediate use, add 0.1 gm of potassium iodate to the equal-parts mixture of hematoxylin and chrome alum. Boil until deep blue.

Phloxine solution
0.5% aqueous solution of phloxine B

Phosphotungstic acid solution
5% aqueous solution of phosphotungstic acid

Method

1. Hydrate sections.
2. Refix in Bouin's solution for 12 to 24 hours.
3. Wash thoroughly in tap water to remove picric acid.
4. Treat sections with potassium permanganate solution for 1 minute.
5. Decolorize with 5% solution of sodium bisulfite.
6. Wash well in running tap water about 10 to 15 minutes.
7. Stain in chrome hematoxylin solution about 10 to 15 minutes. Check under microscope until beta cells are deep blue.

8. Differentiate in 1% hydrochloric acid in 70% alcohol for 1 minute.
9. Wash in tap water until the section is a clear blue.
10. Counterstain in phloxine solution for 5 minutes.
11. Rinse in distilled water.
12. Immerse in 5% phosphotungstic acid solution for 1 minute.
13. Wash under tap water for 5 minutes. The section should retain its red color.
14. Differentiate in 95% alcohol. If the section is too red and the alpha cells are not clearly seen, rinse in 80% alcohol for 15 to 20 seconds.
15. Transfer to absolute alcohol, clear in xylene, and coverslip, using a synthetic mounting medium.

Results (Plate 1, *M*)
Alpha cells—red
Beta cells—blue
Delta cells—pink to red

Aldehyde fuchsin and aldehyde thionin

Although aldehyde fuchsin is commonly used as an elastic fiber stain, the solution also may be used to demonstrate the beta cells of pancreatic islets and of the pituitary gland. Beta cells are stained a deep purple. Mechanism, solutions, and method are discussed under the section dealing with elastic fibers. Dichromate fixatives should be avoided, as this will result in murky shades in the final section. The aldehyde fuchsin solution should be fresh.

An aldehyde thionin solution[5] may also be employed in selective staining of certain cells of the anterior pituitary; this solution has staining properties similar to aldehyde fuchsin. However, aldehyde thionin may be used after tissue fixation in a chromate fixative; the significant background staining that would occur if aldehyde fuchsin were used after chromate fixation is not observed. The use of aldehyde thionin in a sequence procedure for cells of the anterior pituitary is described in the following method.

Aldehyde thionin–Luxol fast blue–periodic acid Schiff method for cells of adenohypophysis[6]

Principle. The iodine–sodium thiosulfate procedure used after hydration functions to remove the mercury precipitate caused by the fixative treatment. The acidified potassium permanganate is an oxidizing agent, and its use is necessary for subsequent staining with the aldehyde thionin to occur. The potassium sulfite

functions to remove excess permanganate from the tissue section. Tissues are next treated with an aldehyde thionin solution. The exact mechanism of staining of any tissue component with aldehyde thionin is not known, but it is believed to be similar to aldehyde fuchsin; that is, combinations can occur by salt linkages with acid radicals or various proteins and mucopolysaccharides as well as by nonpolar additions with aldehydes. Luxol fast blue, a copper phthalocyanin dye, colors the acidophil granules a blue to blue-green.[7] There is no evidence that phospholipid or acid mucopolysaccharide content of the acidophil cells accounts for the positive staining with the Luxol blue. It is possible that the reactive protein-bound sulfhydryl groups, arginine, and small quantities of histidine present in the acidophil cells may have an affinity for the copper component of the Luxol blue, and this would account for the positive staining seen. The staining mechanisms that result in a positive periodic acid–Schiff reaction are discussed in Chapter 9.

Fixation. Saturated solution of mercuric chloride in 10% formalin (1 gm of mercuric chloride is soluble in 13.5 ml of water).

Embedding. Cut paraffin sections at 5 μm.

Solutions
2% potassium permanganate and 0.5% sulfuric acid—equal parts mixture
2% potassium sulfite ($KHSO_3$)
Aldehyde-thionin solution

Thionin	0.5 gm
70% ethanol	91.5 ml
Paraldehyde	7.5 ml
Concentrated hydrochloric acid	1 ml

Ripen in a *tightly covered* container for 3 to 4 days. If kept tightly stoppered, the solution is usable for 10 to 14 days.
Note:
a. Use as pure a thionin dye as possible when preparing this solution.
b. It is important that ripening and staining be done in a tightly stoppered container; otherwise, specific staining will not occur.
c. For pituitary staining, best results are obtained with slightly longer ripening. If the aldehyde thionin used is not fully ripe, some nuclear staining will occur.

Luxol fast blue solution
0.1% of the dye dissolved in 95% ethanol. Add acetic acid to a 0.5% concentration. This solution is stable.
0.05% lithium carbonate
1% periodic acid
Schiff reagent (p. 165)

Technic

1. Hydrate sections.
2. Remove mercury deposits with the iodine–sodium thiosulfate sequence (p. 131).
3. Treat slides with the equal parts potassium permanganate–sulfuric acid mixture for 2 minutes.
4. Treat with 2% potassium sulfite for 1 minute. (Do not use oxalic acid as a substitute.)
5. Wash in distilled water.
6. Stain in a covered vessel containing well-ripened aldehyde thionin for 10 minutes.
7. Rinse in distilled water.
8. Dehydrate in 70% ethanol and then in 95% ethanol.
9. Stain in the Luxol fast blue solution for 30 minutes at 57° C.
10. Rinse in 95% ethanol.
11. Clear in distilled water and differentiate in 0.05% lithium carbonate until acidophils are blue-green and the chromophobes either unstained or very lightly stained. Control microscopically.
12. Give slides 4 changes of 70% ethanol.
13. Wash in distilled water.
14. Oxidize in 1% periodic acid for 10 minutes.
15. Rinse in distilled water.
16. Treat with Schiff reagent for 30 minutes.
17. Wash in running tap water for 10 minutes.
18. Dehydrate, clear in xylene, and coverslip, using a synthetic mounting medium.

Results

Thyrotrophs—blue-black with aldehyde-thionin
Gonadotrophs and basement membrane—PAS-positive
Acidophils—intense blue-green
Chromophobes—unstained or very lightly stained by the Luxol fast blue

Safranin O–eriocyanine A[8]

Principle. This technic may be used to demonstrate alpha and beta cells of both pituitary and pancreas. Safranin O is a basic dye and will color the nuclei and basophilic beta cells of both organs a red color. Eriocyanine A is an acid dye and stains the alpha cells blue. Sections should be cut very thin for this technic, preferably 3 to 4 μm.

Solutions

Staining solution

1% safranin O (C.I. 50240)	2 ml
1% eriocyanine A (C.I. 42576)	2 ml
0.1 M citric acid	1.3 ml
0.2 M disodium phosphate	0.7 ml
Distilled water	34 ml

Method

1. Hydrate sections.
2. Staining solution for 30 minutes.

3. Rinse in water.
4. Dehydrate in acetone; clear in acetone-xylene 50:50, followed by 2 changes of xylene. Coverslip, using a synthetic mounting medium.

Results

Nuclei—red
Beta cells—red
Alpha cells—blue
Red blood cells—blue

Periodic acid Schiff–orange G technic for pituitary[9]

Principle. This technic is a combination of a Hotchkiss alcoholic periodic acid–Schiff reaction followed by an acid dye to stain the alpha cells. Periodic acid oxidizes 1,2-glycol groupings (see PAS reaction for list of other chemical groupings attacked by periodic acid) to the aldehyde stage. An acid-reducing rinse follows the oxidation step and is believed to partially block the PAS coloration of collagen and reticular fibers. 70% alcohol is used as the solvent in the procedure on the theoretical grounds that mucoproteins and their oxidation products are soluble in water and might be dissolved by aqueous solutions. Since beta cells are assumed to contain mucoproteins or glycoproteins, alcoholic solutions are used so that staining can take place. Schiff reagent combines with the aldehydes formed to give magenta addition products. Beta cells are colored by the Schiff reagent, but alpha cells are not. Nuclei are then stained and are colored blue-black by the celestine blue–hematoxylin treatment. Differentiation is accomplished through the use of acid-alcohol. Orange G, an acid dye, renders the alpha cells a bright orange. Red blood cells, also acidophilic, are colored orange.

Fixation. Helly's fluid, Zenker's fluid, formol-saline solution.

Embedding. Cut paraffin sections at 5 μm.

Solutions

Alcoholic periodic acid

Periodic acid	0.8 gm
Distilled water	20 ml
0.2 M sodium acetate	10 ml
Absolute ethanol	70 ml

Acid-reducing rinse

Potassium iodide	1 gm
Sodium thiosulfate ($Na_2S_2O_3 \cdot 5H_2O$)	1 gm
Distilled water	20 ml
Absolute ethanol	30 ml
2N hydrochloric acid	0.5 ml

Schiff reagent (see PAS on p. 165)
0.5% celestine blue in 5% iron alum

Mayer's hematoxylin (p. 142)
2% acid alcohol
2 ml hydrochloric acid in 100 ml 70% ethanol
2% orange G in 5% phosphotungstic acid

Method
1. Deparaffinize sections and hydrate to 70% ethanol.
2. Treat for 5 minutes in alcoholic periodic acid solution.
3. Rinse in 70% alcohol and wash in acid-reducing rinse for 1 minute.
4. Rinse in 70% alcohol and immerse for 15 to 45 minutes in Schiff reagent.
5. Wash in running tap water for 10 to 30 minutes.
6. Stain 30 seconds in celestine blue solution, followed by 30 seconds in Mayer's hematoxylin.
7. Differentiate quickly in 2% acid alcohol.
8. Blue sections in tap water.
9. Stain in orange G solution for 5 to 10 seconds.
10. Wash in running tap water until yellow tinge is just visible in acidophilic areas.
11. Dehydrate in 2 changes each of 95% and absolute ethanol, clear in xylene, and coverslip, using a synthetic mounting medium.

Results (Plate 1, *L*)
Nuclei—blue black
Alpha cells—orange
Beta cells—dark red

Congo red stain for beta cells of pituitary[10]

Fixation. 10% neutral buffered formalin or 10% formalin.
Embedding. Cut paraffin sections at 5 μm.

Method
1. Deparaffinize and hydrate sections.
2. Stain in 1% aqueous Congo red solution for 20 minutes.
3. Immerse in saturated lithium carbonate solution for 1 minute.
4. Wash in running tap water for 10 minutes.
5. Stain in Harris's hematoxylin for 1 to 2 minutes.
6. Differentiate in 1% acid alcohol, controlling by the microscope.
7. Blue in ammonia water (10 drops to 100 ml).
8. Dehydrate, clear in xylene, and coverslip, using a synthetic mounting medium.

Results (Plate 1, *P*)
Granules of beta cells—orange red
Granules of alpha cells—yellow
Nuclei—blue black

PANCREAS

The pancreas is a compound gland located between the stomach and the duodenum. It has both exocrine and endocrine secretions. The exocrine secretions, digestive enzymes, are manufactured by the acinar cells. The numerous coarse zymogen granules seen in the apical portions of the cells are the digestive enzymes "in production." The zymogen granules are destroyed by aqueous and alcoholic acetic formalins and Carnoy's and Bouin's fluids, but are well preserved by neutral buffered formalin, Orth's, Kose's, and Möller's fixatives.

Scattered throughout the exocrine portion of the pancreas are aggregations of capillaries and secreting cells called the islets of Langerhans. The cell types present in the islets are responsible for various endocrine secretions, notably insulin by the beta cells and glucagon by the alpha cells. Both these hormones are important in carbohydrate metabolism. Insulin acts to lower blood glucose levels; glucagon raises blood glucose levels. Decreased insulin production is seen in diabetes mellitus. Delta cells constitute a third cell type present in the islets. These are not found in numerous amounts. The delta cells are relatively few in number and difficult to distinguish. A trichrome-PAS procedure may be used to distinguish the delta cells from the alpha and beta cells.

Common stains for demonstrating the alpha and beta cells include the safranin O–eriocyanine A technic, Gomori's chrome alum–hematoxylin–phloxine, and aldehyde fuchsin. These have been discussed in the preceding section of this chapter. Alpha cell granules may be shown with the Grimelius technic (p. 278). The combined Gomori method listed below may also be used.

Combined Gomori methods for demonstrating pancreatic alpha and beta cells[11]

Principle. Iodine is used to oxidize the tissue and make the overall staining time faster. Sodium thiosulfate is used to remove the excess iodine from the section. Aldehyde fuchsin is the stain used to color the beta cells purple. Phloxine B, an acid dye, stains the alpha cells and zymogen granules of the acinar cells red. Phosphotungstic acid is employed to differentiate the phloxine and remove the vivid red dye from the connective tissue so that the alpha and beta cells will stand out clearly.
Fixation. 10% neutral buffered formalin.
Embedding. Cut paraffin sections at 5 μm.

Solutions
Aldehyde fuchsin solution
    Basic fuchsin   1 gm
    65% ethanol   200 ml

Hydrochloric acid	2 ml
Paraldehyde	2 ml

Let stand at room temperature for 2 or 3 days or until stain is deep purple in color. Store in refrigerator. Purchase paraldehyde in small bottles. Do not use old solutions of paraldehyde.

Iodine solution
Iodine	0.5 gm
95% ethanol	100 ml

Sodium thiosulfate solution
Sodium thiosulfate	0.5 gm
Distilled water	100 ml

Phloxine B
Phloxine B	0.5 gm
Distilled water	100 ml

Phosphotungstic acid solution
Phosphotungstic acid	5 gm
Distilled water	100 ml

Method
1. Deparaffinize slides and hydrate.
2. Wash sections in water.
3. Immerse in 0.5% iodine in 95% ethanol.
4. Rinse in tap water.
5. Rinse in 0.5% sodium thiosulfate to remove iodine.
6. Rinse in tap water.
7. Rinse quickly in 80% ethanol.
8. Stain for 60 minutes in Gomori's aldehyde fuchsin solution.
9. Rinse quickly in 2 changes of 80% ethanol. Spot-check beta cells with microscope. If beta cells are not sufficiently stained, put them back into the aldehyde fuchsin.
10. Rinse in water.
11. Stain for 5 minutes in 0.5% phloxine B.
12. Rinse in water.
13. Differentiate for 1 minute in 5% aqueous phosphotungstic acid.
14. Wash slides in running tap water for 5 minutes. If alpha cells are too red, quickly rinse in 80% ethanol (20 seconds or less).
15. Dehydrate, clear in xylene, and coverslip, using a synthetic mounting medium.

Results
Granules of alpha cells—red
Zymogen granules of acinar cells—red
Granules of beta cells—purple

Trichrome-PAS to demonstrate alpha, beta, and delta cells of pancreas[12]

Fixation. Helly's fluid is preferred; 10% neutral buffered formalin; Bouin's is unsatisfactory unless acetic acid is omitted.

Embedding. Cut paraffin sections at 5 μm.

Solutions
Periodic acid solution
Periodic acid	0.6 gm
Distilled water	100 ml

Schiff reagent (p. 165)

Sulfurous rinse (p. 166)
Weigert's iron hematoxylin (p. 190)
Ponceau–orange G
Ponceau 2R (C.I. 16150)	0.2 gm
Orange G (C.I. 16230)	0.1 gm
Distilled water	100 ml
Glacial acetic acid	1 ml

1% phosphomolybdic acid
0.5% phosphomolybdic acid
Light green solution
Light green SF yellowish (C.I. 42095)	1 gm
Distilled water	100 ml
Glacial acetic acid	1 ml

Method
1. Deparaffinize sections and hydrate.
2. Remove mercury pigment with iodine–sodium thiosulfate sequence (see p. 131).
3. Wash in water and oxidize sections in periodic acid for 20 minutes.
4. Wash in running tap water for 5 minutes.
5. Immerse in Schiff reagent for 20 minutes.
6. Treat sections with sulfurous rinse, 3 changes at 30 seconds each.
7. Wash in running tap water for 10 minutes.
8. Stain in Weigert's iron hematoxylin for 10 minutes.
9. Rinse in 95% alcohol and differentiate in acid alcohol.
10. Wash in running tap water for 10 minutes.
11. Stain in Ponceau–orange G stain for 2 hours.
12. Rinse in distilled water.
13. Differentiate in 1% phosphomolybdic acid until collagen and delta cells are colorless.
14. Rinse in distilled water and stain in light green for 5 to 30 minutes.
15. Wash several times in 1% acetic acid for 1 to 2 minutes.
16. Differentiate in 0.5% phosphomolybdic acid for ½ to 5 minutes.
17. Wash in 1% acetic acid for 20 minutes.
18. Dehydrate in absolute alcohol, 2 changes at 5 minutes each.
19. Clear in xylene and coverslip, using a synthetic mounting medium.

Results
Beta cell granules—pale orange yellow
Beta cell cytoplasm—pale yellow green
Alpha cells—deep orange
Delta cells—translucent green
Glycogen, mucin, glycoproteins—red to purple
Nuclei—black
Collagen—green
Red blood cells—yellow

Sieracki's method for demonstration of beta cells in pancreatic islets and their tumors[13]

Fixation. 10% neutral buffered formalin; Bouin's fluid.

Solutions

Mordant

Chromic chloride (reagent grade)	5 gm
5% acetic acid	100 ml

A light purple color develops on standing. Fairly stable for several months at room temperature.

Staining solution

Solution A

New fuchsin (C.I. 42520)	1 gm
70% ethanol	100 ml

Solution B

Hydrochloric acid	2 ml
Paraldehyde U.S.P. (see note below)	2 ml

Add the paraldehyde–hydrochloric acid mixture to the solution of new fuchsin. Allow the stain to stand at room temperature for 24 hours or until the solution is a deep purple color. Store in the refrigerator. This solution is best used within 1 week but may last several weeks.

Note: The paraldehyde should be used from a freshly opened bottle. (If desired, a separate paraldehyde–hydrochloric acid mixture can be prepared in a separate bottle to act as an indicator. When this solution turns a dark muddy brown, the other bottle containing the stain is ready for use.)

Method (two slides used—one without counterstain and one with counterstain)

1. Deparaffinize sections and hydrate.
2. Mordant in the chromic chloride–acetic acid solution for 72 hours.
3. Rinse well in distilled water.
4. Rinse in 70% alcohol.
5. Stain for 6 hours in the aldehyde–new fuchsin solution.
6. Rinse in 70% alcohol.
7. Wash in running tap water for 10 minutes.
8. Rinse in distilled water.
9. Counterstain one slide in Gomori's trichrome stain (see p. 191 for preparation of this solution); do not counterstain second slide.
10. Rinse in 95% alcohol for 30 seconds.
11. Rinse in absolute alcohol for 30 seconds.
12. Clear in several changes of xylene and coverslip, using a synthetic mounting medium.

Results (Plate 1, Q)

Beta cells—deep purple and stand out clearly on slide without counterstain

Note: We have found this an excellent technic for the demonstration of beta cells in a laboratory where fixation is routinely done with Bouin's fluid or neutral buffered formalin.

Scott's rapid staining of beta cell granules in pancreatic islets[14]

Fixation. Bouin's fluid.

Embedding. Cut paraffin sections at 5 μm.

Solutions

Oxidizing solution

0.5% potassium permanganate	50 ml
0.5% sulfuric acid	50 ml

2% aqueous sodium bisulfite

Gomori's aldehyde fuchsin (p. 272)

Method

1. Deparaffinize sections and hydrate to distilled water.
2. Oxidize in the oxidizing solution for 2 minutes.
3. Rinse in distilled water.
4. Decolorize in 2% sodium bisulfite.
5. Wash in tap water for 2 minutes.
6. Stain in Gomori's aldehyde fuchsin for 30 minutes.
7. Rinse in 3 changes of 95% alcohol.
8. Wash in tap water.
9. Counterstain with 0.2% light green SF for 2 minutes.
10. Dehydrate, clear in xylene, and coverslip, using a synthetic mounting medium.

Results

Beta cell granules—deep purple

Cytoplasmic background of beta cells—light green

Cytoplasm of other cells—light green

ADRENAL GLANDS

The adrenal glands are located over the upper end of each kidney. Each gland is composed of two parts, the medulla and the cortex. Both parts have different embryonic origins and cellular structures and secrete different hormones.

Histologically, the cortex is made up of three zones—the outer zone (zona glomerulosa), which shows no special staining characteristics; the middle zone (zona fasciculata), which contains fat droplets; and the inner zone (zona reticularis), which contains cells possessing much brown pigment. The lipid droplets in the middle zone are, for the most part, doubly refractile, and cholesterol is concentrated mainly in this zone.

Cortex and medulla may be demonstrated by routine stains such as hematoxylin and eosin or Masson trichrome. Prompt fixation of material is the most important step to ensure adequate staining. Lipid present in the middle zone of the cortex may be demonstrated by routine lipid dyes.

The medulla is composed of ovoid cells. The cytoplasm of these cells is filled with minute granules, known as chromaffin granules, since they possess the property of coloring brown when fixed in dichromate fixatives. This brown coloration is known as a *positive chromaffin*

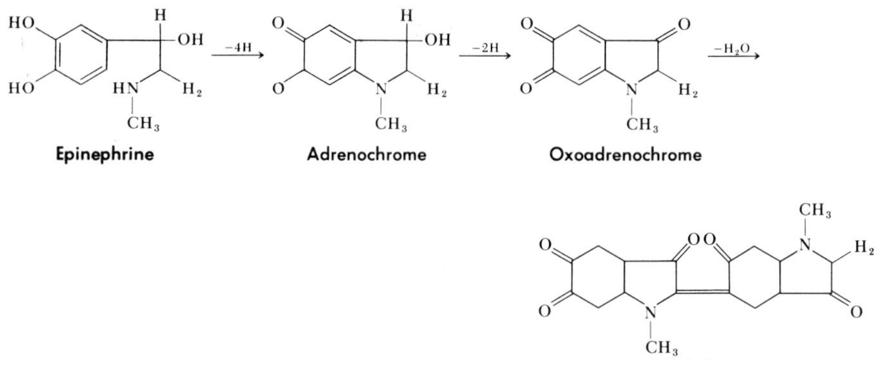

Fig. 15-1. Chromaffin formation in the adrenal.

reaction. The adrenal medulla must be fixed in a primary chromate fixative, Orth's fluid, or Möller's fluid, to demonstrate the chromaffin granules, since even brief fixation in formalin prevents the chromaffin reaction. Chromaffin cell tumors (pheochromocytomas) must likewise be fixed in a primary chromate fixative for adequate demonstration. The presence of acids in the fixatives may also prevent the chromaffin reaction; adrenal chromaffin reactions are most intense when the pH level of the reaction stays about 5 to 6. The current opinion is that substances that give this reaction include catecholamines (epinephrine [adrenaline] and norepinephrine [noradrenaline]), 5-hydroxytryptamine, and dopamine.

In the adrenal, the chromaffin formation is caused by oxidation products of epinephrine and norepinephrine. Lison[15] illustrates this with the equation in Fig. 15-1. Norepinephrine undergoes a similar reaction.

TECHNICS FOR DEMONSTRATING CHROMAFFIN CELLS IN ADRENAL MEDULLA

After fixation in a primary chromate fixative, chromaffin cells may be demonstrated by the Schmorl reducing substance method (p. 223), the periodic acid–Schiff reaction (p. 166), and the Sheehan technic (in the next column).

Chromaffin substance is also argentaffin; that is, it can reduce silver salts to visible metallic silver without the aid of any reducing agent. Although all chromaffin cells are argentaffin, this fact does not imply that all argentaffin substances will give a chromaffin reaction. Melanin, for example, will give a positive argentaffin, but a negative chromaffin reaction.

(Argentaffin methods are detailed on pp. 276 to 278.)

Gomori's chromaffin tissue stain (p. 276) does not require fixation in a primary chromate fixative; however, the reaction is not specific for chromaffin cells.

Sheehan's technic for chromaffin cells[16]

Fixation. Fixation in Orth's fluid is critical.
Embedding. Cut paraffin sections at 5 μm.

Solutions

Aqueous alum hematoxylin

Hematoxylin	1 gm
Aluminum ammonium sulfate or	20 gm
Aluminum potassium sulfate	
Distilled water	400 ml
Thymol	1 gm

Dissolve the hematoxylin crystals in 100 ml of water by the aid of gentle heat. Dissolve the alum in 300 ml of water by the aid of gentle heat. Mix the two solutions together and add the thymol. The combined solution is exposed to air and light in a clear bottle stoppered with a plug of cotton. The solution will be ripened sufficiently for use in about 10 days and will keep for 2 to 3 months. The solution can be ripened at once by adding to it 0.177 gm of potassium permanganate (or 17.7 ml of a 1% aqueous solution of potassium permanganate).

Technic

1. Hydrate sections.
2. Wash sections under running tap water for 10 minutes.
3. Stain in aqueous alum hematoxylin for 3 to 5 minutes.
4. Wash in running tap water for 10 to 15 minutes until nuclear detail is clearly demonstrated in blue.

5. Dehydrate in 2 changes of 95% alcohol and 2 changes of absolute alcohol, clear in several changes of xylene, and coverslip, using a synthetic mounting medium.

Results
Chromaffin granules—yellow to brown
Nuclei—blue

Gomori's chromaffin tissue stain[17]

Fixation. Formalin, Bouin's fluid, or Heidenhain's mercuric chloride formalin (tissues fixed in Orth's fluid do not stain satisfactorily).

Embedding. Cut paraffin sections at 5 μm.

Solutions
Azocarmine G solution
Azocarmine G	0.05 gm
Acetic acid	1 ml
Distilled water	100 ml

Aniline alcohol
Aniline oil	1 ml
95% alcohol	100 ml

3% aqueous phosphotungstic acid
Aniline blue–quinoline yellow solution
Aniline blue	0.5 gm
Quinoline yellow or orange G	2 gm
Phosphotungstic acid	1 gm
Distilled water	100 ml

Technic
1. Hydrate sections to distilled water.
2. Stain in azocarmine G solution for 90 minutes at 58° C.
3. Rinse in tap water and blot until dry with bibulous paper.
4. Differentiate in aniline alcohol by controlling with microscope to the point where chromaffin cells stand out deep pink against much paler cortical cells. This step may be accomplished in 5 minutes, but it may take 1 hour.
5. Rinse *briefly* in tap water.
6. Mordant in phosphotungstic acid solution for 20 minutes. *Do not rinse* after this step but proceed directly with step 7.
7. Stain in the aniline blue–quinoline yellow solution until the connective tissue is deep blue. This step takes from 15 to 40 minutes. (Better contrast is accomplished if quinoline yellow is used instead of orange G.) Control with microscope.
8. Rinse *briefly* in tap water.
9. Dehydrate, clear in xylene, and coverslip, using a synthetic mounting medium.

Results
Cytoplasmic granules in chromaffin cells—purplish red
Alpha cells of pancreatic islets, some cells of the anterior pituitary, neutrophilic leukocytes, myelocytes, and enterochrome cells also possess granules staining deep purplish red to violet by this technic.

SMALL INTESTINE
PANETH CELLS OF SMALL INTESTINE

The crypts of Lieberkühn are simple tubular glands found in the small intestine. These contain Paneth cells, which have large, oval nuclei and coarse, highly refractile granules in the cytoplasm. The granules are intensely acidophilic and stain with acid dyes such as eosin or orange G. They are destroyed by acetic acid fixatives such as aqueous and alcoholic acetic formalin, Bouin's fluid, Gendre's fluid, or Carnoy's fluid but are well preserved by neutral buffered formalin, or mercuric chloride formalin, or by Orth's, Kose's or Möller's dichromate formalin. These granules are sometimes grampositive by the Gram-Weigert technic in human tissue and may be positive or negative with the PAS technic.

Lillie's azure A–eosin B method[8]

Fixation. Neutral buffered formalin, mercuric chloride formalin, Orth's fluid, Kose's fluid, and Möller's fluid; granules destroyed by acetic acid.

Embedding. Cut paraffin sections at 5 μm.

Staining solution
0.1% aqueous solution of azure A	8 ml
0.1% aqueous solution of eosin B	8 ml
0.2 M acetic acid	3.4 ml
0.2 M sodium acetate	0.6 ml
C.P. acetone	10 ml
Distilled water	50 ml

With surgical and fresh animal tissue, pH of staining solution should be 3.74 to 4.1. Autopsy material may stain better at pH 4.5.

Method
1. Deparaffinize sections and hydrate.
2. Stain in the staining solution for 1 hour. Discard after use.
3. Dehydrate in 3 changes of acetone.
4. Clear in 50:50 acetone-xylene mixture.
5. Clear in 2 changes of xylene and coverslip, using a synthetic mounting medium.

Results
Paneth cell granules—pink to red

ARGENTAFFIN AND ARGYROPHIL CELLS
ARGENTAFFIN CELLS

Argentaffin cells usually occur in the surface and glandular epithelia of the stomach and intestines. They are also known as Kulchitsky cells and enterochromaffin cells. Numerous technics may be used to demonstrate argentaffin cells including:

Schmorl's reduction reaction (p. 223)
Chromaffin reaction

Argentaffin technics
Diazo method
Autofluorescence after formalin fixation.

The use of alcohol-containing fixatives must be avoided, since alcohol dissolves argentaffin granules.

The chromaffin reaction is usually not used to demonstrate argentaffin cells, since it is less specific than the other methods listed. Argentaffin cells do *not* need fixation in a primary chromate fixative for the positive chromaffin reaction to occur, however, since the reaction can be observed even after exposure to formalin. The serotonin (5-hydroxytryptamine) content is presumably responsible for the actual chromaffin reaction given by argentaffin cells.

The argentaffin procedures of Fontana-Masson and Gomori-Burtner may be used to demonstrate the argentaffin capacity of the argentaffin cell. A *positive argentaffin reaction* means that these cells can pick up silver and reduce the silver to its visible metallic state without the aid of an extraneous reducing agent. Lillie states that a catechol structure is probably responsible for the reactions of the argentaffin granules, and this diphenol is oxidized to a quinone structure as it reduces the silver.

Fontana-Masson argentaffin reaction[18]

Fixation. Formalin.
Embedding. Cut paraffin sections at 5 μm.

Solutions
Stock silver nitrate solution
  Dissolve 10 gm of silver nitrate in 100 ml of distilled water. To 95 ml of the silver nitrate solution add concentrated ammonium hydroxide until a clear solution with no precipitate is obtained. Add, drop by drop, enough of the remaining 5 ml of silver nitrate solution to cause the clear solution to become slightly cloudy. Let stand overnight before using. Store solution in the dark at room temperature. Stock solution is stable for approximately 1 month.
Working silver nitrate solution
  Just before use, dilute each 25 ml of the stock silver solution with 75 ml of distilled water. Filter.
0.2% gold chloride (p. 182)
5% sodium thiosulfate
Nuclear fast red (p. 183)

Method
1. Hydrate slides.
2. Immerse in silver nitrate working solution for 2 hours at 56° C. Slides may be checked after 1 hour.
3. Rinse in distilled water.
4. Tone in gold chloride for 2 to 3 minutes.
5. Rinse in distilled water.
6. Place in 5% sodium thiosulfate for 1 minute.
7. Rinse in distilled water.
8. Counterstain with nuclear fast red for 5 minutes.
9. Rinse in distilled water twice.
10. Dehydrate, clear, and coverslip, using a synthetic mounting medium.

Results (Plate 1, O)
Argentaffin cell granules—black
Nuclei—pink-red
Cytoplasm—pale pink

Gomori-Burtner method for argentaffin granules[19]

Fixation. Formalin or Bouin's.
Embedding. Cut paraffin sections at 5 μm.

Solutions
Stock methenamine silver solution (p. 187)
Working methenamine silver solution
  To 30 ml of stock methenamine silver solution add 8 ml of Holmes' pH 7.8 borate buffer.
  Holmes' borate buffer, pH 7.8

0.2 M boric acid	80 ml
0.05 M sodium borate	20 ml

Weigert's iodine (p. 131)
5% sodium thiosulfate
0.1% gold chloride
Working light green solution (p. 187)

Technic
1. Deparaffinize sections and hydrate to distilled water.
2. Treat with Weigert's iodine solution for 10 minutes.
3. Bleach with 5% sodium thiosulfate.
4. Wash in running tap water for 10 minutes.
5. Rinse in 3 changes of distilled water.
6. Place sections in Coplin jar containing buffered methenamine silver solution at room temperature and put in a 60° C oven. Check slides microscopically after 1 hour. Check every half hour thereafter until argentaffin cells are well blackened but connective tissue is *not* blackened.
7. Rinse in distilled water.
8. Tone in 0.1% gold chloride for 10 minutes.
9. Rinse in distilled water.
10. Fix in 5% sodium thiosulfate for 2 minutes.
11. Wash 10 minutes in running tap water.
12. Counterstain in working light green solution for 1 minute.
13. Dehydrate, clear in xylene, and coverslip, using a synthetic mounting medium.

Results
Argentaffin granules—black
Background—green

Diazo method for argentaffin cells[20]

Fixation. Neutral buffered formalin or formol-saline.

Embedding. Cut paraffin sections at 5 μm.

Solutions

Staining solution

1% aqueous fast red B salt	5 ml
Saturated aqueous lithium carbonate	2 ml

Add the lithium carbonate solution to the fast red B and mix. Cool at 4° C for 10 minutes prior to use.

Aqueous alum hematoxylin (Harris's or Ehrlich's)

Technic

1. Hydrate slides.
2. Stain in the precooled staining solution for 10 minutes at 4° C.
3. Rinse slides in distilled water.
4. Wash in running tap water for 2 to 3 minutes.
5. Counterstain nuclei with the hematoxylin for 1 to 2 minutes.
6. Blue sections in running tap water for several minutes.
7. Dehydrate, clear in xylene, and coverslip, using a synthetic mounting medium.

Results

Argentaffin cell granules—orange-red
Nuclei—blue

Rapid fixation is important, and this method may not give satisfactory results with autopsy material. Carcinoid tumors of the appendix and small intestine are usually positive; bronchial carcinoids, usually negative.

Detection of argentaffin cells by primary fluorescence (autofluorescence)[21]

Fixation. Neutral buffered formalin or an aqueous formalin mixture.

Embedding. Cut paraffin sections at 5 μm.

Technic

1. Hydrate slides.
2. Coverslip with a nonfluorescent aqueous mounting medium (such as Apathy's).
3. Examine the unstained sections with a fluorescence microscope, using an exciter filter of 300 nm (Schott UG 2) and a barrier filter for colorless ultraviolet light.

Results

Argentaffin cell granules autofluoresce a bright golden yellow color.

Formula for Apathy's mounting medium (R.I. 1.52)

Gum arabic	50 gm
Sucrose	50 gm
Distilled water	50 ml
Thymol	0.05 gm

Dissolve the above using gentle heat. Store in an airtight screw-capped container to prevent evaporation and hardening of the medium.

ARGYROPHIL CELLS

Argyrophil cells are found in larger numbers in the same general locations as the argentaffin cells. These argyrophil cells are capable of being impregnated with silver, but a reducing agent (either chemical or light) is required to reduce the impregnated silver to a metallic visible end product. The Bodian (p. 256), Sevier-Munger (p. 257), and Grimelius (below) procedures may be used to demonstrate these cells.

Argyrophil methods for carcinoid tumors

The Sevier-Munger technic (p. 257) and the Grimelius technic (see below) are both examples of argyrophil procedures that may be used in the differentiation of carcinoid tumors. The Grimelius technic uses a very weak solution of silver nitrate (30 mg/dl) and requires impregnation for 3 to 4 hours at 60° C or overnight at 37° C. The latter produces better staining results in that the cells are shown darker. Reduction is accomplished with a mixture of sodium sulfite and hydroquinone.

The Sevier-Munger technic uses a strong solution of silver nitrate (20 gm/dl) and requires impregnation for only 15 minutes in a 60° C oven. Reduction is accomplished with an ammonical silver solution to which formalin is added.

The two procedures differ in results from each other and also from the Fontana argentaffin technic, though all three methods may be used for carcinoid demonstration. In some cases all three may be positive and in other cases one or both of the argyrophil technics may be positive with a negative Fontana. The Grimelius technic is also useful for demonstrating the alpha cells of the pancreas, whereas the Sevier-Munger stain shows poor demonstration, if any, of these cells.

Grimelius technic[22]

Fixation. 10% neutral buffered formalin.
Embedding. Cut paraffin sections at 5 μm.

Solutions

Silver solution

Silver nitrate ($AgNO_3$)	30 mg
Distilled water	90 ml
0.1 M acetate buffer, pH 5.6 (p. 389)	10 ml

1% aqueous hydroquinone (prepare fresh)
5% aqueous sodium sulfite
Working light green solution (p. 187)

Technic

1. Hydrate slides to distilled water.
2. Place slides in silver solution and put in 37° C oven overnight.
   Note: If procedure cannot be run overnight, the slides can be put in the silver solution for 4 hours in a 60° C oven. Continue with step 3.
3. Make up 1% hydroquinone and 5% sodium sulfite. Place both solutions in a 60° C oven for 1 hour to preheat. At the same time transfer the slides in silver solution from the 37° C oven to a 60° C oven.
4. After the hydroquinone and sodium sulfite have been preheated for 1 hour, combine equal parts of each. Pour silver solution off slides and pour the hydroquinone–sodium sulfite solution onto slides. *Do not wash between these two steps.* Put slides back into the 60° C oven.
5. Slides should remain in hydroquinone–sodium sulfite solution until they turn a light brown (5 minutes or longer). Check slides (control) microscopically for brown staining of alpha cells in pancreas.
6. Rinse slides in distilled water.
7. Counterstain in working light green solution for 3 minutes or longer, until the sections appear green.
8. Rinse in distilled water, dehydrate, clear in xylene, and coverslip, using a synthetic mounting medium.

Results

Granules contained in the following cells stain black:
   Pancreatic alpha cells
   Gastrointestinal enterochromaffin (EC) (argentaffin) cells
   Gastric enterochromaffin-like (ECL) cells
   Thyroid C cells
   Pyloric gastrin (G) cells
   Duodenal small-granule (S) cells
   Adrenal epinephrine- and norepinephrine-producing cells
   Type of pituitary cell perhaps related to ACTH secretion
Note: Cytochemical observations on pancreatic alpha cells indicate that the positive staining is not attributable to glucagon. However, the positive staining seen with argentaffin cells is related to, but probably not caused entirely by the 5-hydroxytryptamine content.

JUXTAGLOMERULAR COMPLEX

The juxtaglomerular complex is not easily recognized with routine stains. The difficulty lies chiefly in the fact that these specific granules cannot be resolved and that the epithelioid cells are not easily distinguished from the smooth muscle cells of the arterioles with which they are in such close association.

Bowie's stain is the classic method for demonstrating juxtaglomerular cells but requires Helly's fixation. The newer technics of Harada may be performed on formalin-fixed tissue. The granules are also PAS-positive.

Bowie's stain for juxtaglomerular granules[23]

Fixation. Fix thin slices of tissue in Helly's fluid for 48 hours.

1. After fixation, wash tissues under running water overnight; start processing in 60% alcohol and routinely embed in paraffin.
2. Cut sections at 4 μm and avoid excessive amount of albumin, since it may interfere with staining.

Method

1. Deparaffinize sections through xylene and alcohols to alcoholic iodine.
2. Immerse for not more than 3 minutes in alcoholic iodine.
3. Remove iodine with 5% sodium thiosulfate for 3 minutes.
4. Wash in running tap water for at least 5 minutes.
5. Mordant in 2.5% potassium dichromate at approximately 40° C overnight.
6. Rinse in distilled water.
7. Immerse sections overnight in 20% ethanol to which 10 to 15 drops of Bowie's stock solution (see below) has been added to each 100 ml of ethanol.
8. Blot sections with bibulous paper.
9. Dip quickly two or three times in 2 changes of acetone to remove excess stain.
10. Differentiate in a 1:1 mixture of xylene and clove oil until sections appear red to reddish purple. Microscopically the renal parenchyma should be red or magenta in contrast to the elastic tissue of the blood vessels, which should be purple-blue. The juxtaglomerular granules, when present, will be the same color as the elastic tissue. RBC's are usually amber as a result of previous dichromate mordanting.
11. Rinse in 2 changes of xylene followed by 2 changes of benzene.
12. Give slides 2 additional changes of xylene and coverslip, using a synthetic mounting medium.

Preparation of Bowie's stock staining solution

1. Dissolve 1 gm of Biebrich scarlet in 250 ml of distilled water and rapidly filter into a beaker.
2. Dissolve 2 gm of ethyl violet in 500 ml of distilled

water and, while shaking the solution, filter a small amount at a time into the beaker that holds the Biebrich scarlet until an abrupt color change (red to violet) occurs. This change indicates the neutralization end point. The addition of excess ethyl violet will cause the neutral precipitate to redissolve and should be avoided.

3. The mixture is filtered and allowed to dry on the filter paper for 24 hours.
4. The stock Bowie solution is made by the dissolving of 0.2 gm of the dried precipitate in 20 ml of 95% alcohol. At least 100 ml of stock solution can be obtained from one batch of the stain if the end point of neutralization is carefully determined.

Note: Stock dye powder can be purchased from Roboz Surgical Instrument Co., 810-18th St., N.W., Washington, DC 20006.

Results (Plate 1, *N*)
Juxtaglomerular granules—purple
Background—lavender

Harada's stain for juxtaglomerular cells[24]

Fixation. Formalin. (Mercuric chloride may be added to a neutral formalin solution for best results.)

Embedding. Cut paraffin sections at 5 μm.

Solutions

0.5% crystal violet in 70% ethanol
Equal parts mixture of aniline oil and xylene

Technic

1. Hydrate sections. Remove mercury precipitate if necessary. Give slides several changes of tap water.
2. Blot sections. Stain in the crystal violet solution for 1 to 3 minutes.
3. Wash briefly in running water. Blot well. (Proper blotting is critical.)
4. With frequent blotting, differentiate in the aniline-xylene solution until all the color has nearly disappeared. This step will take several minutes.
5. Clear sections in xylene, and coverslip, using a synthetic mounting medium.

Results

Juxtaglomerular cell granules—deep purple.
Background—varying shades of faint purple

Modifications[25]

1. After hydration, oxidize sections in an equal-parts mixture of 0.5% potassium permanganate and 0.5% sulfuric acid for 5 minutes.
2. Follow the oxidation with decolorization using 1% oxalic acid for 2 minutes.
3. Rinse in running water, blot, and stain in *either* an acid or an alkaline solution of crystal violet for 1 to 3 minutes.

Acid crystal violet solution
  0.1% crystal violet in
  0.1 N hydrochloric acid
Alkaline crystal violet solution
  0.1% crystal violet in
  0.01 to 0.1 N ammonium hydroxide

4. Proceed with step 3 in the preceding method outline.

Results

Juxtaglomerular cell granules and elastic fibers are deep violet if the acid crystal violet solution is used. Juxtaglomerular cell granules and red cells are deep violet if the alkaline crystal violet solution is used.
Background tissue should appear pale purple.

FIBRIN AND FIBRINOID

Fibrin is a specific protein formed from fibrinogen present in the blood. When present in tissues outside blood vessels, it indicates acute inflammation and damage to the blood vessel wall.

It is homogeneous, strongly PAS-positive, and eosinophilic with the routine hematoxylin and eosin stain. It colors deep blue with Mallory's phosphotungstic acid hematoxylin stain. Weigert's stain for fibrin may also be used to demonstrate the substance. With this technic, the fibrin retains the crystal violet–iodine complex of the stain even after the aniline-xylene differentiation. (If alcohol or acetone is used as the differentiating agent, the fibrin loses the dye lake and is decolorized.) Fibrin is colored dark blue-black with this stain.

More recent technics for fibrin demonstration include immunofluorescent procedures and Carstairs' stain for fibrin and platelets in the same tissue section.

Fibrinoid represents altered collagen and appears as a homogeneous eosinophilic material. It is found in a number of pathologic conditions (rheumatic nodules, walls of blood vessels affected by lupus erythematosus). Staining reactions may be variable because of the presence of altered cytoplasmic substances, but generally fibrinoid and fibrin give the same results.

Weigert's stain for fibrin[8]

Fixation. Absolute alcohol, Carnoy's fluid, or alcoholic formalin.

Embedding. Cut paraffin sections at 5 μm.

Solutions

Lithium carmine solution
Carmine	4 gm
Lithium carbonate, saturated aqueous	100 ml

Thymol   1 gm

Dissolve the carmine in the lithium carbonate solution and boil for 10 to 15 minutes. When solution is cool, add thymol.

Crystal violet solution

Solution A

     Absolute alcohol   33 ml

     Aniline oil   9 ml

     Crystal violet   to saturate in excess

Solution B

     Crystal violet   2 gm

     Distilled water   100 ml

Working solution

     Solution A   3 ml

     Solution B   27 ml

Stock solutions keep well. Working solution keeps about 1 week.

Gram's iodine solution (p. 131)

Method

1. Deparaffinize sections and hydrate to distilled water.
2. Stain nuclei with lithium carmine for 2 to 5 minutes.
3. Wash thoroughly in tap water.
4. Stain for 5 to 10 minutes in crystal violet working solution.
5. Drain and blot with filter paper.
6. Pour Gram's iodine over sections. Allow to stand 5 to 10 minutes.
7. Drain and blot with filter paper.
8. Differentiate with 50:50 xylene-aniline oil from a dropping bottle. Blot and pour on and off until no more purple color comes off.
9. Blot and pour xylene on slide several times to remove aniline.
10. Coverslip, using a synthetic mounting medium.

Results

Fibrin—violet

Gram-positive bacteria—blue black

Keratohyaline—deep violet

Other structures—red or pink

Nuclei—some may be violet

Carstairs' method for fibrin and platelets[26]

Fixation. Formalin-saline for 48 hours or more.

Embedding. Cut paraffin sections at 5 μm.

Solutions

5% ferric alum

Mayer's hematoxylin (p. 142)

Picric acid–orange G solution

     Saturated aqueous picric acid   20 ml

     Saturated picric acid in   80 ml

       isopropanol

     Orange G   0.2 gm

Ponceau-fuchsin solution

     Acid fuchsin   0.5 gm

     Ponceau 2R   0.5 gm

     Acetic acid   1 ml

     Distilled water   to 100 ml

Aniline blue solution

     Aniline blue   1 gm

     1% acetic acid   100 ml

1% phosphotungstic acid

Technic

1. Hydrate sections.
2. Mordant in 5% ferric alum for 5 minutes. Rinse in running tap water.
3. Stain with Mayer's hematoxylin solution for 5 minutes. Rinse in running tap water.
4. Stain in the picric acid–orange G solution for 30 minutes to 1 hour. Rinse once in distilled water.
5. Stain in Ponceau-fuchsin solution for 1 to 5 minutes. Rinse in distilled water.
6. Differentiate with 1% phosphotungstic acid until the muscle is red and background pale pink. Rinse in distilled water.
7. Stain with the aniline blue solution for 30 minutes to 2 hours. Rinse in several changes of distilled water.
8. Dehydrate, clear in xylene, and coverslip, using a synthetic mounting medium.

Results

	Fixation time	
Tissue	48 hours or more	Less than 48 hours
Fibrin	Bright red	Orange to orange-red
Platelets	Gray-blue to navy	Light gray
Collagen	Bright blue	Bright blue
Muscle	Red	Red
Red blood cells	Clear yellow	Red, green, or yellow

SPERMATOZOA
Berg's method for spermatozoa[27]

This staining technic is Putt's modification of the carbol-fuchsin method for acid-fast material. In sections of human testis, spermatozoa are colored a brilliant red, whereas other tissue components, except for pale pink erythrocytes, are blue to purple-blue. The mycolic acid components of the sperm are believed to be responsible for the positive acid-fast reaction. In his article, Berg states that the difference between this technic and other published technics for sperm stems from the changes made by Putt in the Ziehl-Neelsen technic. The previously reported technics use basic fuchsin, whereas Putt reported the much more brilliant color obtained when new fuchsin is substituted. The other change in this technic is the use, after a mordant, of a much weaker differentiating agent than hydrochloric acid–alcohol, which would remove most of the dye from sperm stained with carbol–new fuchsin.

Fixation. 10% neutral buffered formalin.
Embedding. Cut paraffin sections at 5 μm.

Solutions
Putt's carbol-fuchsin solution
New fuchsin	1 gm
Phenol	5 gm
Distilled water	84 ml
Absolute alcohol	10 ml

Saturated lithium carbonate
| Lithium carbonate | 1 gm |
| Distilled water | 100 ml |

Glacial acetic acid alcohol
| Glacial acetic acid | 5 ml |
| Absolute ethanol | 95 ml |

Methylene blue solution
| Methylene blue | 0.5 gm |
| Absolute ethanol | 100 ml |

Method
1. Deparaffinize sections and hydrate to distilled water.
2. Stain for 3 minutes in carbol-fuchsin solution.
3. Place slides directly into saturated lithium carbonate for 3 minutes.
4. Decolorize in glacial acetic acid–alcohol for 5 minutes.
5. Wash in two 1-minute changes of absolute alcohol.
6. Counterstain in methylene blue for 30 to 60 seconds.
7. Rinse rapidly in 2 changes of absolute alcohol.
8. Clear in several changes of xylene and coverslip, using a synthetic mounting medium.

Results (Plate 1, B)
Spermatozoa—brilliant red
Erythrocytes—pale pink
Other tissue elements—blue to purple

MAST CELLS

These cells are found widely distributed in the connective tissue, but their exact function is not yet fully understood. Their cytoplasm contains granules composed of heparin, histamine, and, in some species (such as the rat and mouse), serotonin. These granules are metachromatic, and various metachromatic stains (for example, toluidine blue) will demonstrate their presence. Because of their sulfated mucopolysaccharide content, the cell granules also color with aldehyde fuchsin and alcian blue. Other technics that may be used are described next.

Bujard's acid fuchsin stain for mast cell granules[28]

Fixation. 10% neutral buffered formalin.
Embedding. Cut paraffin sections at 5 μm.

Solutions
1% aqueous acid fuchsin
0.8% bromine water
1% hydrochloric acid in 70% alcohol

Method
1. Deparaffinize sections and hydrate.
2. Stain for 30 seconds in 1% aqueous acid fuchsin.
3. Rinse rapidly in distilled water.
4. Place in bromine water in a closed container for 5 minutes.
5. Wash in distilled water and differentiate in acid alcohol for 1 to 3 minutes, until the sections are a clear mauve color.
6. Dehydrate rapidly, clear in xylene, and coverslip, using a synthetic mounting medium.

Results
Granules of mast cells—deep red to brown

Luna's method for mast cells[29]

Fixation. 10% neutral buffered formalin.
Embedding. Cut paraffin sections at 5 μm.

Solutions
Aldehyde fuchsin (p. 197)
Weigert's iron hematoxylin (p. 190)
Methyl orange solution
| Methyl orange | 0.25 gm |
| 95% ethanol | 100 ml |

Method
1. Deparaffinize and hydrate to 95% alcohol.
2. Stain in aldehyde fuchsin for 30 minutes.
3. Rinse in 95% alcohol.
4. Stain in Weigert's hematoxylin for 1 minute.
5. Wash in running tap water for 10 minutes.
6. Rinse in 95% alcohol.
7. Counterstain in methyl orange solution for 5 minutes or until background is light yellow.
8. Dehydrate in absolute alcohol, clear in xylene, with 2 changes each, and coverslip, using a synthetic mounting medium.

Results
Mast cells—purple
Elastic fibers—purple
Other cellular elements—blue
Background—yellow

EOSINOPHILS
Luna's eosinophil granule stain[29]

Fixation. 10% neutral buffered formalin.
Embedding. Cut paraffin sections at 5 μm.

Solutions

Working Weigert's iron hematoxylin solution (p. 190)

1% aqueous Biebrich scarlet

Working hematoxylin–Biebrich scarlet solution

Weigert's iron hematoxylin solution (working)	45 ml
1% Biebrich scarlet solution	5 ml

1% hydrochloric acid in 70% ethanol

0.5% aqueous lithium carbonate

Technic

1. Hydrate sections to distilled water.
2. Stain in working hematoxylin–Biebrich scarlet solution for 5 minutes.
3. Differentiate in 1% hydrochloric acid in 70% alcohol until desired nuclear detail is achieved (usually 8 dips).
4. Rinse in tap water to remove acid alcohol (3 to 5 minutes).
5. 0.5% lithium carbonate solution until section turns blue and erythrocytes are bright red (usually 5 dips). Wash in running water for 2 minutes.
6. Dehydrate in alcohol, clear, and coverslip, using a synthetic mounting medium.

Results

Eosinophilic granules—red
Erythrocytes—red
Charcot-Leyden crystals—red
Background—blue

REFERENCES

1. Ham, A. W.: Histology, ed. 7, Philadelphia, 1974, J. B. Lippincott Co.
2. Gomori, G.: Observations with differential stains on human islets of Langerhans, Am. J. Pathol. **17:** 395-406, 1941.
3. Hadler, W. A., Ziti, L. M., Patelli, A. S., Vizza, J. A., and DeLucca, O.: Histochemical meaning of the chrome alum hematoxylin and the aldehyde fuchsin staining: an investigation accomplished by a spot-test technique carried on filter paper models, Acta Histochem. **29S:**320-328, 1968.
4. Elftman, H.: A chrome alum fixative for the pituitary, Stain Technol. **32:**25-28, 1957, Baltimore, The Williams & Wilkins Co.
5. Paget, G. E.: Aldehyde-thionin: a stain having similar properties to aldehyde fuchsin, Stain Technol. **34:**223-226, 1959, Baltimore, The Williams & Wilkins Co.
6. Paget, G. E., and Eccleston, E.: Simultaneous specific demonstrations of thyrotroph, gonadotroph and acidophil cells in the anterior hypophysis, Stain Technol. **35:**119-122, 1960, Baltimore, The Williams & Wilkins Co.
7. Shanklin, W. M., Nassar, T. K., and Issidorides, M.: Luxol fast blue as a selective stain for alpha cells in the human pituitary, Stain Technol. **34:** 55-58, 1959, Baltimore, The Williams & Wilkins Co.
8. Lillie, R. D., and Fullmer, H. M.: Histopathologic technic and practical histochemistry, ed. 4, New York, 1976, McGraw-Hill Book Co.
9. Pearse, A. G. E.: The cytochemical demonstration of gonadotropic hormone in the human anterior hypophysis, J. Pathol. Bacteriol. **61:**195-202, 1949.
10. Kerenyi, N.: Congo red as a simple stain for beta cells of the hypophysis, Stain Technol. **34:**343-346, 1959, Baltimore, The Williams & Wilkins Co.
11. Fisher, E. R., and Haskell, E.: Combined methods for demonstrations of pancreatic alpha and beta cells, Am. J. Clin. Pathol. **24:**1433-1434, 1954.
12. McManus, J. F. A., and Mowry, R. W.: Staining methods—histologic and histochemical, New York, 1960, Harper & Row, Publishers.
13. Sieracki, J. C., Michael, J. E., and Clark, D. A.: The demonstration of beta cells in pancreatic islets and their tumors, Stain Technol. **35:**67-69, 1960, Baltimore, The Williams & Wilkins Co.
14. Scott, H. R.: Rapid staining of beta cell granules in pancreatic islets, Stain Technol. **27:**267-268, 1952, Baltimore, The Williams & Wilkins Co.
15. Lison, L.: Histochimie et cytochimie animales, Paris, 1953 (ed. 3, 1960), Gauthier-Villars.
16. Sheehan, D. C.: A comparative study of the histologic techniques for demonstrating chromaffin cells, Am. J. Med. Technol. **30:**237-240, 1960.
17. Gomori, G.: Staining of chromaffin tissue, Am. J. Clin. Pathol. **16:**115-117, 1946.
18. Masson, P.: Carcinoids and nerve hyperplasia of the appendicular mucosa, Am. J. Pathol. **4:**181-211, 1928.
19. Burtner, H. J., and Lillie, R. D.: A five-hour variant of Gomori's methenamine silver method for argentaffin cells, Stain Technol. **24:**225-227, 1949, Baltimore, The Williams & Wilkins Co.
20. Lillie, R. D., Pizzolato, P., Vacca, L. L., Catalano, R. A., and Donaldson, P. T.: The pH range of the diazosafranin reaction of rat and other mast cells, J. Histochem. Cytochem. **21:**441-447, 1973, The Histochemical Society, Baltimore, The Williams & Wilkins Co. (agent).
21. Culling, C. F. A.: Handbook of histopathological and histochemical techniques, ed. 3, London, 1974, Butterworth & Co. (Pub.) Ltd.
22. Vassalo, G., Capella C., and Solcia, E.: Grimelius silver stain for endocrine cell granules, as shown by electron microscopy, Stain Technol. **46:**7-13, 1971, Baltimore, The Williams & Wilkins Co.
23. Smith, C. L.: Rapid demonstration of juxtaglomerular granules in mammals and birds, Stain Technol. **41:**291-294, 1966, Baltimore, The Williams & Wilkins Co.
24. Harada, K.: Rapid demonstration of juxtaglomer-

ular granules with alcoholic crystal violet, Stain Technol. **45:**71-74, 1970, Baltimore, The Williams & Wilkins Co.

25. Harada, K.: An aqueous acid and alkaline crystal violet: a rapid staining sequence for demonstrating juxtaglomerular granules, Anat. Anz. **128:** 431-438, 1971.

26. Carstairs, K. C.: The identification of platelets and platelet antigens in histological sections, J. Pathol. Bacteriol. **90:**225, 1965.

27. Berg, J. W.: Differential staining of spermatozoa in sections of testis, Am. J. Clin. Pathol. **23:**513-515, 1953.

28. McManus, J. F. A., and Mowry, R. W.: Staining methods—histologic and histochemical, New York, 1960, Harper & Row, Publishers (original reference, Bujard, E.: Une coloration strictement élective des granulations basophiles des mastocytes, Bull. Histol. Appl. Microscop. **7:**264, 1930).

29. Luna, L. G., editor: Manual of histologic staining methods of the Armed Forces Institute of Pathology, ed. 3, New York, 1968, McGraw-Hill Book Co.

CHAPTER 16

Eye technics

ROUTINE PROCESSING OF OPHTHALMIC TISSUE FOR LIGHT MICROSCOPY*

NESTOR G. MENOCAL
DOLORES B. VENTURA
MYRON YANOFF

The technics for processing ophthalmic tissue in our laboratory are described in detail. The procedure for grossing of specimens, and the different time tables for processing are given. We have been able to achieve easily reproducible results using the methods described.

The Laboratory of Ophthalmic Pathology at the Scheie Eye Institute processes globes and other ocular surgical specimens according to a well-defined and easily followed protocol. The purpose of this paper is to present our methods for processing tissue.

Specimens submitted to the ophthalmic pathology laboratory can be divided into four general groups: enucleated globes (surgical and autopsy), products of evisceration, biopsies (skin, conjunctival, orbital, etc.), and exenterations. All specimens are immediately placed in glutaraldehyde-formalin fixative[3] (Table 16-1).

Globes and exenteration specimens are fixed whole and for no more than 24 hours. They are then washed for 6 to 24 hours in running tap water and processed, or they may be stored in 10% neutral buffered formalin[4] for future processing. Other surgical specimens are fixed from 4 to 24 hours before processing.

After fixation, the globe is measured in the following axes: anterioposterior, horizontal, and vertical. The length of the attached optic nerve stump is also noted.

The globe is transilluminated (Fig. 16-1) like candling eggs, by a bright light in a specially constructed black view box. The rectangular box measures $1 \times 1 \times 1\frac{3}{4}$ feet. The front panel has an oval viewing hole, $1\frac{1}{2} \times 4$ inches placed about 5 inches from the top. The back panel has a circular hole, 1 inch in diameter, through which a bright source of illumination* is inserted. The two side panels each have a round hole, about $5\frac{1}{2}$ inches in diameter, placed in the upper half of the panel slightly toward the front, for insertion of the examiner's two arms while the globe is transilluminated. The outside and

*Barkan Light, Parson's Optical Service, Inc., San Francisco, California 94102.

Table 16-1. Glutaraldehyde-formalin fixative*

A. Glutaraldehyde (1% solution)†		
Glutaraldehyde (25% in H_2O)	40	ml
Distilled water	960	ml
Monobasic sodium phosphate	1.67	gm
Dibasic sodium phosphate ($Na_2HPO_4 \cdot 7H_2O$)	16.90	gm
B. 10% neutral buffered formalin†		
Formaldehyde (38% to 40% solution)	100	ml
Distilled water	900	ml
Monobasic sodium phosphate ($NaH_2PO_4 \cdot H_2O$)‡	4.0	gm
Dibasic sodium phosphate (anhydrous) (Na_2HPO_4)‡	6.5	gm

*From Yanoff, M.: Am. J. Ophthalmol. **76**:303-304, 1973.
†Mix equal volumes of stock solution A (1% glutaraldehyde) and B (10% neutral bufferd formalin) and use as a routine fixative. May be stored at room temperature for at least 2 months, and probably much longer.
‡Dissolve salt in distilled water before adding glutaraldehyde or formaldehyde. Although glutaraldehyde may be stored at room temperature in quantity, flocculation (which does not impair its fixative properties) is retarded by storage in the refrigerator.

*Slightly modified from Am. J. Med. Technol. **43**(2):156, 1977; copyright 1977, American Society for Medical Technology. This project was supported in part by an unrestricted grant from Research to Prevent Blindness, Inc.

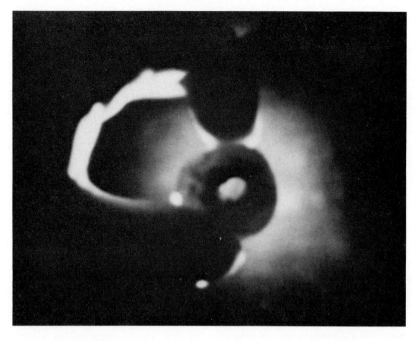

Fig. 16-1. Eye within black box. Light coming from hole in back of box allows easy transillumination.

inside of the box are painted black. Notation is made of any shadows or dark areas, such as tumors and old hemorrhages.

All details of surface topography are recorded. The optic nerve is severed flush with the globe. In the case of clinical diagnosis of tumors the optic nerve and vortex veins are removed before the eye is opened, and each is processed separately to avoid contamination by intraocular contents. The globe is then opened as diagrammed in Fig. 16-2. The globe is cut with a sharp blade* from back to front and about 1 to 2 mm on either side of the optic nerve. The first cut should end through sclera about 1 mm from the corneal-scleral junction. The second cut should end through clear cornea about 1 mm from the scleral-corneal junction, to allow a good view of the anterior chamber and its angle.

If calcium deposits or new bone formation are present within the globe, the globe must be decalcified to facilitate opening of the eye and to prevent damage to the microtome knife. Specimens with calcified areas are placed in a decalcifying fluid (Table 16-2), usually for 1 to 3 days. When the eye is completely decalcified, it is washed in running tap water overnight to remove all traces of acid; then it is placed back in

Table 16-2. Decalcifying fluid

Solution A	
Sodium citrate	50 gm
Distilled water	250 ml
Solution B	
Formic acid, 90%	125 ml
Distilled water	125 ml

Mix equal parts of solutions A and B before use.

10% neutral buffered formalin before macroscopic examination. The decalcifying process does not affect the final results on sections.

A detailed description of the opened eye is recorded. The section is then placed in a metal capsule (cassette) and kept in a jar containing 10% neutral buffered formalin until ready to be processed. Smaller specimens, such as lid biopsies and conjunctival biopsies, are handled in a similar manner after a detailed macroscopic description.

The cassettes are placed in a metal basket and it is attached to the vacuum head of the Autotechnicon Ultra.* Small biopsies are processed overnight on an "8-hour" schedule (Table 16-3). The timer is set so that the Autotechnicon will start to move at 12:00 midnight. Alternately,

---

*Durham Duplex, Durham Enders Razor Co., Mystic, Connecticut 06355.

*Technicon Corporation, Tarrytown, New York 10591.

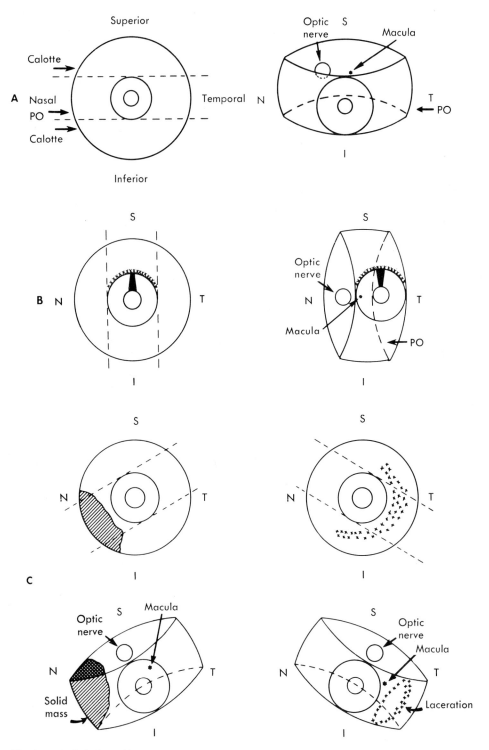

Fig. 16-2. A, *Left,* Dotted lines represent horizontal cuts in eye to be opened in routine fashion. *Right,* Eye opened horizontally. Pupil, optic nerve, and macula all in same plane in specimen. **B** and **C,** Eyes cut open in vertical and oblique planes, respectively, to incorporate areas of interest into main block (cataract scar and superior sector iridectomy in **B,** and solid mass or scleral laceration in **C**). *S,* Superior; *T,* temporal; *I,* inferior; *N,* nasal; *PO,* section through eye containing pupil and optic nerve.

Table 16-3. Autotechnicon Ultra processing schedules

	2 hours	4 hours	8 hours	14 hours
10% formalin alcohol*		30 minutes	30 minutes	1 hour
95% alcohol	5 minutes	10 minutes	30 minutes	1 hour
95% alcohol	10 minutes	10 minutes	30 minutes	1 hour
95% alcohol	10 minutes	10 minutes	30 minutes	1 hour
Absolute alcohol	5 minutes	20 minutes	30 minutes	1 hour
Absolute alcohol	10 minutes	20 minutes	30 minutes	1 hour
Absolute alcohol	10 minutes	20 minutes	30 minutes	1 hour
Clearing agent†	10 minutes	20 minutes	30 minutes	1 hour
Clearing agent	10 minutes	20 minutes	30 minutes	1 hour
Clearing agent	10 minutes	20 minutes	30 minutes	1 hour
Paraffin‡	20 minutes	30 minutes	1½ hours	2 hours
Paraffin	20 minutes	30 minutes	1½ hours	2 hours

*10% neutral formalin in 80% alcohol.
†Clearing Agent, UC-670, Technicon Corporation, Tarrytown, New York 10591.
‡Bioloid—Tissue Embedding Medium, Van Water & Roger Scientific, Rochester, New York 14603.

Table 16-4. Hand processing for exenterations and eyes with necrotic tumors or blood

80% alcohol	Leave for the weekend
95% alcohol	8:00 AM (Monday)
95% alcohol	12:00 noon
95% alcohol	4:00 PM (overnight)
Absolute alcohol	8:00 AM
Absolute alcohol	12:00 noon
Absolute alcohol	4:00 PM (overnight)
Dioxane*	8:00 AM
Dioxane	4:00 PM (overnight)
Paraffin (vacuum)	8:00 AM
Paraffin (vacuum)	10:00 AM
Paraffin	12:00 noon
Embed	2:00 PM

*Dioxane is very toxic and should be used in a well-ventilated area. It is both a dehydrant and a clearing agent and tissues can be left in it for a longer period without excessive hardening.

Table 16-5. Hand processing of minute biopsies*

50 ml of 80% alcohol with 5 ml of stock alcoholic eosin	15 minutes
95% alcohol	15 minutes
95% alcohol	15 minutes
Absolute alcohol	15 minutes
Absolute alcohol	15 minutes
Absolute alcohol	15 minutes
Xylene	15 minutes
Xylene	30 minutes
Paraffin	30 minutes
Paraffin	1 hour

*Agitate periodically to facilitate dehydration.

they can be processed during the day on a 4-hour schedule (Table 16-3). Orbital biopsies, eviscerations, and globes are processed on a 14-hour schedule (Table 16-3). Exenterations and globes containing extensive tumor, exudate, debris, or clotted blood are processed by hand before being embedded (Table 16-4). The density of these tissues requires extended time for fixation, dehydration, clearing, and paraffin infiltration to take place. Minute conjunctival and corneal biopsies are carefully wrapped in filter or lens paper before being placed in a cassette and are either processed by hand (Table 16-5) or processed by the Autotechnicon Ultra on a 2-hour schedule (Table 16-3).

If tissue is not completely dehydrated, the paraffin will not infiltrate. Blocks of poorly processed tissues are easily recognized by a depression in the paraffin that forms over the poorly infiltrated area. It is impossible to cut good sections of such tissues; any section cut from such a block disintegrates when spread on the warm water bath.

One can recycle improperly processed blocks by trimming off excess paraffin and then melting the paraffin in which the tissue is embedded at a 60° to 65° C temperature. The tissue is then taken back through the clearing agent to remove the infiltrated paraffin. It is then passed through three changes of absolute alcohol, and three changes of 95% alcohol. After this, the tissue should be slowly dehydrated through a series of 70% alcohol to absolute alcohol, cleared, reinfiltrated with paraffin, and reembedded.

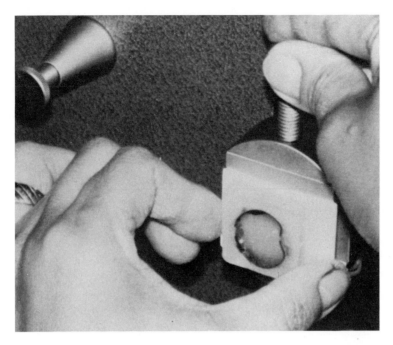

Fig. 16-3. Plastic embedding ring, containing framed paraffin block, fits into object clamp of rotary microtome. Note easily visualized cross section of eye in paraffin block.

After the tissues are processed, the metal basket is transferred to a third container of paraffin from which the tissues are embedded. Bioloid* with a melting point of 56° to 58° C is the most satisfactory paraffin for infiltrating and embedding biopsies and globes. Its elasticity aids in making wrinkle-free sections.

The most convenient and simplified method for embedding is the use of Tissue-Tek† metal molds and plastic embedding rings. The stainless steel base molds are dipped in hot water and inverted to drain on a paper towel, prior to embedding. The molds are available in four different sizes, and those with greatest depth are used for embedding eyes.

To embed, the base mold is filled with paraffin. The tissue is oriented and then is placed in the desired position and pressed gently against the bottom of the base mold with warmed forceps. Do not allow a layer of paraffin to solidify around the specimen, as this will cause separation of tissue and the embedding medium. The accession number is written on one side of the embedding ring, the ring is

pressed firmly into the mold, and the mold is filled to the top with paraffin. The temperature of the embedding paraffin should not exceed 5° C above the melting point. When the paraffin has cooled, a firm film forms across the top of the block; the block is then placed in a pan of cold water. Ice cubes for rapid cooling and hardening cause the block to crack.

For large eyes and exenterations, hand-folded paper boxes or "boats" are used for blocking the specimens. Boats made from a stiff writing paper can be shaped to any size. To embed in paper boats, first fill the boat with paraffin. The eye is then placed in the desired position with the side from which sections are to be cut facing down. The accession number is written on one flap of the paper boat and the identifying label is attached to the opposite flap. This provides a double check and accurately identifies the specimen. When the paraffin has formed a heavy film on the surface of the boat, the block is cooled by floating it in a pan of cold running tap water for approximately 30 minutes. After the paraffin is hard enough, the paper is peeled away. With the aid of a heated knife and melted paraffin the identifying label is attached to one side of the block.

Prior to sectioning, two flotation baths are readied: one of distilled water at room tempera-

*Bioloid, Van Water & Roger Scientific, Rochester, New York 14603.
†Lab Tek Products, Division of Miles Laboratories, Inc., Westmont, Illinois 60559.

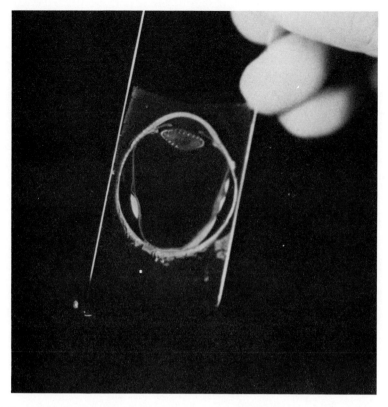

Fig. 16-4. Section of eye, embedded in paraffin, cut at 7 μm, floated, and stretched onto glass slide in hot water bath.

ture to float the cut ribbon of sections, and the other with 0.5 gm of gelatin added to 2 liters of distilled water and heated 57° to 58° C. A thermometer is kept in the hot water bath while cutting is being done, in order to obtain a continuous, accurate check on the temperature.

The Tissue-Tek embedding ring is very convenient because the framed paraffin block fits right into the object clamp of the rotary microtome (Fig. 16-3). Biopsies for routine sections are cut at 5 to 6 μm; eyes are cut at 7 μm. Eyes with thin scleras, such as those with high myopia, are cut at 8 μm. The paraffin block is clamped to the holder with the scleral sides parallel to the knife, the cornea on the left side, and the nerve on the right. The block is "rough cut" until the tissue of interest is exposed. The exposed tissue is soaked with a piece of wet cotton for no less than 10 minutes. With the wet cotton still covering the surface of the block, an ice cube is placed over the cotton for 1 to 2 minutes. The cotton and ice are removed, and a ribbon of sections is cut with a slow even turn of the flywheel of the microtome. During cut-

ting, the free end of the ribbon is gently lifted with the fingers. The other end is handled with a fine-eye forceps when it is removed from the microtome knife. The ribbon is floated in the pan of distilled water at room temperature, and the sections are separated (for large sections such as of globes) or kept in a ribbon of two to eight sections (for small specimens such as most biopsies). Each section is picked up with a glass slide and floated on the other previously prepared hot-water bath (57° to 58° C) to stretch the tissue or tissues to the original size and shape of the blocked tissue (Fig. 16-4). Some cases, such as suspected *Toxocara canis* infestation, may require serial sections of the globe. After sections have been cut, the paraffin blocks are dipped in melted paraffin to seal the tissue.

The slides with mounted tissues are dried in a 58° C oven for 2 to 3 hours or at 55° C overnight. When dry, the sections are stained with hematoxylin and eosin. In addition, we routinely stain one slide of each globe, and often one slide of most other specimens, with the periodic acid–Schiff stain.[2] Other special stains, such as for collagen, elastic tissue, reticulum, and acid mucopolysaccharides, are performed as indicated.

REFERENCES

1. Luna, L. G., editor: Manual of histologic staining methods of the Armed Forces Institute of Pathology, ed. 3, New York, 1960, McGraw-Hill Book Co., p. 8.

2. Menocal, N. G., and Yanoff, M.: Comparative study of periodic acid–Schiff techniques used in ophthalmic pathology, Am. J. Ophthalmol. **87:**525-530, 1972.

3. Yanoff, M.: Formaldehyde-glutaraldehyde fixation, Am. J. Ophthalmol. **76:**303-304, 1973.

4. Yanoff, M., Zimmerman, L. E., and Fine, B. S.: Glutaraldehyde fixation of whole eyes, Am. J. Clin. Pathol. **44:**167-171, 1965.

CHAPTER 17

Enzyme histochemistry

BASIC INFORMATION
Aim of enzyme histochemistry

Histochemistry, the science that encompasses both biochemistry and histology, seeks to identify chemical substances and determine their significance at the cellular level. Enzyme histochemistry is one subclass of histochemistry in general; the specific chemical substances under study are, of course, enzymes.

This chapter includes some general information concerning enzymes as well as specific procedural details for some diagnostically important enzymes. The use of enzymes (notably horseradish peroxidase) as an alternative to fluorescein for labeling antibodies is described in Chapter 18.

Definition of catalyst, enzyme, and substrate

Catalysts are compounds that accelerate chemical reactions. Although a catalyst is a participant in a reaction, it is recoverable in its original state when the reaction is completed. *Enzymes* are proteins that serve as catalysts in the reactions that occur in biologic systems; most of the reactions that living cells undergo would occur very slowly were it not for the catalytic action of enzymes. Enzymes not only speed

reactions but are highly specific, and this specificity may be absolute or relative with regard to the substrate. A *substrate* is defined as the substance that an enzyme acts upon. Enzymes that display relative specificity act on more than one specific reactive group or on different but related groups. The enzyme recognizes its substrate not only by the chemical groups on the substrate, but also by the arrangement of these groups in space; this latter characteristic is called stereochemical specificity.

Location of enzymes

Many enzymes are simply dissolved in cell cytoplasm, and these are called "soluble enzymes." Others are tightly bound to certain cell organelles, notably mitochondria and lysosomes.

Classification of enzymes

According to the nomenclature, enzymes may be classified into six major groups, which are listed as follows:

Oxidoreductases—catalyze transfer of *either* electrons *or* hydrogen ion; subclasses:
  a. Dehydrogenases—catalyze removal of hydrogens

b. Oxidases—catalyze acceptance of electrons by oxygen either directly (aerobically) or indirectly (anaerobically)

Transferases—catalyze transfer of radicals of two compounds without loss or uptake of water

Hydrolases—catalyze introduction of water or its elements into specific substrate bonds; subclasses:

a. Esterases—catalyze hydrolysis of ester linkages

Phosphatases—hydrolyze esters of phosphoric acid and may be considered an esterase subclass

b. Peptidases—hydrolases that attack peptide bonds

Lyases—remove groups from their substrates and leave behind double bonds

Isomerases—catalyze molecular rearrangement

Ligases or synthetases—catalyze formation of new molecules by joining together two other molecules

Factors influencing enzyme demonstration

To be able to identify enzymes at their source and determine their significance, one should understand the chemical nature of the substance, determine the effects of each step in the procedure, and keep in mind the limitations of the method. The following factors all influence enzyme demonstration:

1. *Temperature.* Optimal temperature is that temperature at which maximal enzyme activity may be demonstrated. Most enzymes require incubation at 25° to 37° C for this. Exposure to temperature greater than 56° C destroys enzyme activity.

2. *pH.* There is an optimal pH value for an enzyme at which activity is maximal. In many cases, this pH is near the neutral point on the pH scale, though there are exceptions to this, for example, with the demonstrations for acid and alkaline phosphatases.

3. *Concentration.* The speed of an enzyme reaction is affected by the amount (concentration) of the enzyme, of the substrate, and of reaction products and by any inhibitors or activators that may be present.

4. *Inhibitors.* Enzyme activity may be decreased or abolished by agents called "inhibitors." The inhibitor may be nonspecific, that is, one that acts on all enzymes. Examples of nonspecific inhibitors include heat, agitation, and exposure to acids or certain fixative solutions. Specific inhibitors also exist. These affect a particular enzyme molecule or may act to prevent the formation of a specific enzyme-substrate complex.

5. *Activators.* These are substances that promote enzyme activity. Some commonly used activators include the divalent cations of magnesium, manganese, and calcium.

6. *Circadian rhythms.* The daily or seasonal variation in amounts of enzyme also affects overall activity.

GENERAL TYPES OF ENZYMATIC HISTOCHEMICAL REACTIONS

Azo dye methods. These methods are widely used for many determinations and employ substrates containing one of a number of various naphthol compounds. Enzyme activity frees the naphthol moiety and the naphthol either simultaneously ("simultaneous coupling"), or later ("postincubation coupling"), joins with a diazonium salt. Diazonium salts are reaction products of primary aromatic amines with nitrous acid and are formed by a process called "diazotization." The diazonium salts form reaction products with some aromatic compounds (notably naphthols in histochemistry) to produce insoluble azo dyes marking the site of enzymatic activity.

Indoxyl methods. Procedures employing indoxyl substrates have also been described. The enzyme activity in these cases releases indoxyl radicals that are then rapidly oxidized to insoluble indigo blue end products.

Metal salt methods. These methods may be used when one of the products of the enzyme activity on the substrate is an acid. The released acid is captured by a metal ion in the incubation medium and thereby precipitated. With the use of additional reagents, a series of ionic substitutions take place, and ultimately an insoluble colored salt is formed at the site of enzymatic activity.

Oxidation-reduction reactions. In redox reactions, hydrogen is removed from one substance (oxidation) and transferred to another substance (reduction). Most of the oxidative enzymes are demonstrated by the methods that involve hydrogen transfers from the substrate to a tetrazolium salt. Upon accepting the transferred hydrogen, the tetrazolium salt is reduced to a water-insoluble, purple formazan pigment marking the site of enzyme activity.

SPECIMEN PREPARATION FOR ENZYME HISTOCHEMISTRY

Each enzyme reacts differently to fixative and processing methods, and a single, optimal procedure of tissue preparation for subsequent enzyme demonstration does not exist. Some methods require the use of fresh tissue; other procedures may be performed on tissue that has been fixed.

Fresh-tissue considerations

Since many enzymes are totally inactivated by heat and exposure to conventional fixative and processing solutions, numerous enzyme methods require the use of fresh frozen tissue sections. The use of fresh unfixed tissue has certain disadvantages, however, including the diffusion of enzymes or cofactors and activators from their initial site in the tissue.

Tissue may be frozen by the cryostat freezer plate method, the liquid nitrogen immersion technic or the prechilled isopentane method. Specimens may be more quickly frozen when this last method is used because of the heat-conducting nature of the isopentane. The isopentane method is particularly suitable for muscle tissue and the description of the method follows.

Freezing by use of an isopentane solution (recommended for muscle tissue)

Muscle tissue should be suitably obtained and frozen within 30 minutes after excision. The usual method of freezing is to first mount a transverse section of the muscle on a chuck using 10% tragacanth gum as the adhesive. The chuck with the mounted specimen is then immersed in *prechilled* isopentane until frozen. Isopentane is precooled when a container of the substance is placed into liquid nitrogen. At a temperature of $-160°$ C the isopentane has a slightly syrupy consistency. Care should be taken to remove the muscle sample when freezing is complete, usually after 25 to 30 seconds. Too short a freezing time produces artifacts; prolonged freezing can produce cracking of the block.

Storage of unfixed frozen tissue

If the sample cannot be sectioned immediately after freezing, it may be wrapped in foil and placed in a plastic-lidded container along with a small amount of ice for moisture. Appropriate labels should be used to identify the sample. Specimens may be stored at $-60°$ C until sectioned.

Fixed-tissue considerations

For the demonstration of certain soluble enzymes, some fixation is required in order that sufficient amounts of the enzyme be retained for demonstration. Fixed tissue tends to show fewer diffusion artifacts and, once fixation is complete, there is little progressive enzyme loss. The major disadvantages of the use of fixed tissue include variable degrees of enzyme inactivation and dissolution of certain enzymes into the fixative solution.

Fixatives that have been employed for small tissue pieces include cold ($3°$ to $4°$ C) formalin or cold formol-calcium. Tissue may fix for up to 48 hours in the cold. After fixation, some methods suggest that the tissue be immersed for 2 to 24 hours in a gum-sucrose solution (30% sucrose containing 1% gum acacia). The sucrose solution is believed to assist in membrane stabilization, especially those of mitochondria. (Tissue may be stored in this sucrose solution for indefinite periods at $4°$ C.) After either the fixative treatment or the sucrose treatment, frozen sections may be prepared and stained.

An alternate method to fixing a piece of tissue is postfixing the cryostat sections for 10 to 30 minutes using either cold formalin, formol-calcium, or acetone. After fixation is completed, the tissue sections may be rinsed with distilled water and transferred to the incubation medium.

Cover-slip versus slide staining

The frozen sections may be mounted on slides and stained in Coplin jars. In this case, approximately 50 ml of the incubation solution will be needed. Alternatively, sections may be affixed to cover slips (the 22×22 mm size is usually satisfactory) and incubated in Columbia staining dishes. These "mini-Coplin jars" hold 10 ml of solution, and their use is an excellent way to reduce the amount of solution and therefore the cost of reagents needed. A disadvantage of using the cover slips is that they are too fragile to be etched with an identifying number; therefore, it is essential that the technologist employ some other means to keep cases from getting mixed.

Fixed-smear preparation considerations

Once dry, smear specimens of blood or bone marrow should be fixed promptly, otherwise enzyme activity will decrease. Two fixation procedures follow.

Formalin-methanol method

Immerse smear for 30 seconds at $0°$ to $10°$ C in a formalin-methanol solution. Prepare this solution by mixing 50 ml of 37% to 40% formalin with 450 ml of absolute methanol. Store in a tightly capped container (or containers) below 0° C.

Citrate-buffered acetone

Immerse smear for 30 seconds at 25° C in a citrate-buffered acetone solution. Prepare this solution by adding 105 ml of acetone to 100 ml of a 0.03 M solution of sodium citrate. Store at room temperature.

After immersion in the fixative solution, rinse in distilled or gently running tap water for 10 to 20 seconds and proceed with staining. If staining is to follow *immediately,* air-drying is not necessary. If staining is to be delayed by more than a few hours, allow the fixed specimens to air-dry and then store below 0° C in individual envelopes or other suitable containers.

CONTROLS

Various factors may be involved in the production of false-negative or false-positive results. False-negative reactions may be caused by any or all of the following: insufficient amounts of enzyme, nonoptimal incubation conditions, substrate degeneration, and solubility or diffusion of either the enzyme or the final product of the enzyme activity. False-positive results may be attributable to a nonenzymatic splitting of the substrate, diffusion of the enzyme or final product of enzyme activity away from the initially positive site, nonspecific affinity of tissue components for reagents used in the procedure, and confusion of natural pigments with the colored end product of the reaction.

The use of known positive and negative controls can assist in determining whether the procedure results are satisfactory, and these controls should be stained at the same time and in the same manner as the test slides. Results from the positive control will indicate whether the reagents are working. Positive staining observed in the known negative control indicates that a positive result seen in the test slide is open to question. Negative controls may be prepared by immersion of either a section of a known positive or an alternate test section in boiling water for 15 minutes. Specific inhibitors may also be employed. Frequently a negative control is incubated in a separate medium that lacks only the substrate for the same time that the test section is incubating in a medium that contains the substrate. Positive results seen in the section that was incubated without the substrate indicate that the positive result was not caused by enzymatic activity.

DEMONSTRATION METHODS FOR SPECIFIC ENZYMES

The next section details procedures and theoretical considerations of demonstrations for the following enzymes: alkaline phosphatase (tissue and smears), acid phosphatase, esterase (tissue and smears), Mg^{+2}-activated ATPase, Ca^{+2}-activated ATPase, aminopeptidase, phosphorylase, succinic dehydrogenase, glucose-6-phosphate dehydrogenase, NADPH (TPNH) diaphorase, NADH (DPNH) diaphorase, and peroxidase (smears).

Alkaline and acid phosphomonoesterases

The phosphomonoesterases contain those enzymes that hydrolyze orthophosphate (orthophosphoric acid) from their particular substrates. Phosphomonoesterases are in turn divided into two groups: (1) the acid phosphatases, which liberate orthophosphate at an acid pH, and (2) the alkaline phosphatases, which hydrolyze orthophosphate at an alkaline pH.

Alkaline phosphatases are widely distributed enzymes, and the optimal pH for their activity lies between 9.0 and 9.6. These enzymes are usually activated by magnesium, manganese, zinc, and cobalt ions and are inhibited by cysteine, cyanides, and arsenates. The presence of alkaline phosphatase has been reported for many areas, including the brush borders of the proximal convoluted tubular cells of the kidney and the brush borders of the jejunum, as well as blood and bone marrow, bladder, adrenal glands, breast, ovary, and liver.

Intensely positive reactions for alkaline phosphatase have been reported to occur in certain bone tumors (Ewing's sarcoma, osteogenic sarcoma), synoviosarcoma, acute monocytic leukemia, and leukemoid reaction. Reactions are decreased in granulocytic leukemia and negative in malignant hepatoma, lymphoblastoma, and neuroblastoma.

The acid phosphatases are also widespread; however, cells with a high level of alkaline phosphatase usually have low levels of acid phosphatase. The optimal pH for the reactivity of the acid phosphatases varies from 4.5 to 6.0. There are several kinds of acid phosphatases that may be differentiated by pH optima and sensitivity to various inhibitors. For example, acid phosphatase of prostatic origin is inhibited by low concentrations (0.01 M) of tartrate and fluoride and is unaffected by a formalin (0.5%) inhibitor. Acid phosphatase of liver origin is sensitive to the three inhibitors just mentioned, and an approximate 50% reduction in enzyme reactivity is seen. Erythrocytic acid phosphatase is not affected by tartrate, only slightly affected by fluoride, and totally sensitive to formalin treatment.

Specific areas of the body from which acid phosphatases have been reported to occur include prostate, adrenal cortex and medulla, liver, erythrocytes, brush border of jejunum, and brush border of proximal convoluted tubular cells of the kidney. Intensely positive reactions occur in Reed-Sternberg cells of Hodgkin's disease, gastric carcinoma, prostatic carcinoma and its metastatic lesions, ganglioneuroma, carcinoma of lung and breast, and epidermoid carcinoma of the tongue. Negative reactions are seen in cases of Ewing's sarcoma and osteogenic sarcoma.

Numerous procedures are available for the determination of acid phosphatase and alkaline phosphatase in tissue. Some methods indicate that fresh tissue may be used; some methods may be performed on tissue that has been suitably fixed. The most commonly used procedures are the azo dye methods, though indoxyl methods have also been described.

Naphthol AS-BI phosphate–stabilized diazonium salt method for alkaline phosphatase[1]

Tissue preparation. Either fresh or fixed tissue may be used. Cut cryostat sections at 6 to 8 μm.

Stain mechanism. The naphthol AS-BI phosphate substrate is hydrolyzed by the alkaline phosphatase present in the tissue to release orthophosphate plus a naphthol derivative. The newly released naphthol combines immediately with the diazonium salt present in the incubation medium. This combination results in the formation of an azo dye that marks the site of enzyme activity.

The following diazonium salts have been employed in the detection of the naphthols released by the enzyme action: fast red violet LB, fast blue BB, fast blue RR, and fast red TR.

Reagents
TRIS (tris[hydroxymethyl]aminomethane)–hydrochloric acid buffer, pH 8.74

0.2 M TRIS (24.2 gm/liter)	10 ml
0.1 M hydrochloric acid (HCl)	4 ml
Distilled water	26 ml

Incubation medium (approximately 50 ml for total volume)

Naphthol AS-BI phosphate	5 mg
Dimethylformamide	0.1-0.25 ml
TRIS buffer	25 ml
Distilled water	25 ml
Stabilized diazonium salt (See choices listed in stain mechanism in the previous column.)	30 mg

Procedure
1. Dissolve the naphthol AS-BI phosphate in the dimethylformamide.
2. Add remaining reagents to the dissolved substrate. Mix gently. Filter into a Coplin jar.
3. Incubate sections in filtered medium at 25° C for 30 to 60 minutes.
4. Rinse sections in distilled water.
5. Counterstain, if desired. If the fast red violet or fast red TR was used, counterstain in Harris's hematoxylin for 30 seconds to 1 minute; follow with a 10-minute water wash. If the fast blue BB or fast blue RR was used, counterstain for 10 to 30 seconds in 0.5% aqueous safranin; follow with several changes of distilled water.
6. Coverslip sections in an aqueous mounting medium such as glycerol gelatin or polyvinyl pyrrolidone (PVP).

Results
If the fast red violet LB or fast red TR was used, sites of enzyme activity will be pink-red to red. If the fast blue BB or fast blue RR was used, sites of enzyme activity will be blue to blue-purple. Nuclei will be blue if the hematoxylin counterstain was used; red if the safranin was used.

Controls
Use kidney or jejunum for positive control. For negative control, eliminate the substrate from the incubating solution.

Naphthol AS phosphate–fast blue BB method for alkaline phosphatase[2]

Tissue preparation. Either fresh or fixed tissue may be used. Cut cryostat sections at 6 to 8 μm.

Stain mechanism. Alkaline phosphatase activity releases orthophosphate and naphthol derivatives from the substrate. The naphthol derivatives are simultaneously coupled with the diazonium salt present in the incubating medium to form a deep blue azo dye marking the location of enzyme activity.

Reagents
Stock solution of substrate
1. Weigh out 0.03 gm of naphthol AS phosphate (free acid) and dissolve this amount in 0.5 ml N,N-dimethylformamide.
2. Prepare 100 ml of a TRIS buffer pH 9.1 by combining 25 ml of TRIS, 5 ml of 0.1 N hydrochloric acid and diluting to a 100 ml volume with distilled, deionized water. Adjust pH to 9.1.

3. Add this buffer to the dissolved naphthol AS phosphate, mix, and store at 3° to 4° C.
Fast blue BB

Procedure

1. Weigh 0.01 gm of fast blue BB.
2. Add 10 ml of the prepared stock substrate solution to the diazonium salt. Mix gently. Filtering optional.
3. Incubate sections 15 to 30 minutes at 37° C.
4. Rinse sections well in distilled water.
5. Counterstain, if desired, in 0.5% safranin O for 30 seconds. Rinse sections thoroughly in distilled water after counterstaining.
6. Coverslip, using an aqueous medium such as glycerol gelatin or polyvinylpyrrolidone (PVP). Alternatively, sections may be dried and coverslipped in a synthetic resin.

Results

Sites of alkaline phosphatase activity—deep blue precipitate
Nuclei—red, if safranin counterstain was used

Controls

Use kidney or jejunum for positive control. For negative control, eliminate specific substrate from the incubating medium.

Indoxyl method for alkaline phosphatase[3]

Tissue preparation. Either fresh or fixed tissue may be used. Cut cryostat sections at 6 to 8 μm.

Stain mechanism. Sections are incubated in a buffered medium containing either iodoindoxyl phosphate or bromoindoxyl phosphate as the substrate. Alkaline phosphatase activity releases orthophosphate and an indoxyl derivative from the substrate. The indoxyl derivative is oxidized to insoluble indigo blue to indicate the location of enzyme activity.

Reagents

2 M sodium chloride
Barbital (Veronal)–hydrochloric acid buffer, pH 9.0

0.2 N hydrochloric acid	0.21 ml
0.04 M barbital (Veronal) sodium	12.5 ml

5-iodoindoxyl phosphate or 5-bromoindoxyl phosphate

Procedure

1. Weigh 0.00192 gm of 5-iodoindoxyl phosphate or 5-bromoindoxyl phosphate and place in tube 1.
2. To tube 2 add in the following order:

2 M sodium chloride	5 ml
Distilled deionized water	3 ml
Barbital (Veronal)–hydrochloric acid buffer	2 ml

Mix the contents of tube 2 well and add to the tube 1. Mix again and add to sections.

3. Incubate 30 to 60 minutes at 37° C. (Routine incubation time is 60 minutes.)
4. Rinse cover slips in distilled water when incubation time is completed.
5. Counterstain, if desired, in 0.5% safranin O for 30 seconds. Rinse sections thoroughly in distilled water after counterstaining.
6. Coverslip, using an aqueous mounting medium. Alternatively, sections may be dried and coverslipped in a synthetic resin.

Results

Sites of enzyme activity—fine precipitate of indigo blue
Nuclei—red, if the safranin counterstain was used

Controls

Use kidney or jejunum for a positive control. For a negative control, eliminate substrate from the incubating solution.

Demonstration of alkaline phosphatase in blood smears—naphthol AS-MX phosphate method[4]

Smear preparation and fixation. Prepare thin smears from venous or capillary blood. If venous blood is used, collect in heparin. Avoid EDTA because of its inhibitory effects on the enzyme. Use smears on the day they are made, unless proper fixation and storage procedures have been followed. (See Fixed-Smear Preparation Considerations, p. 294.)

Stain mechanism. At an alkaline pH, alkaline phosphatase releases orthophosphate and a naphthol derivative from the substrate naphthol AS-MX phosphate. The released naphthol combines with the fast blue RR diazonium salt to produce an azo dye, which indicates enzyme activity. Colors range in intensity from pale blue to deep blue, depending on the amount of enzyme present.

Reagents

0.2 M TRIS–hydrochloric acid buffer, pH 8.3

TRIS	2.42 gm
1 N hydrochloric acid	10 ml
Distilled water	100 ml

Stock substrate solution
12.5 mg of the substrate (naphthol AS-MX phosphate) is dissolved in 5 ml of washed dimethylformamide (dimethylformamide is shaken with activated charcoal and passed through a Linde molecular filter).
To the above reagents, add 150 ml of water and enough 1 M sodium carbonate to adjust solution pH to exactly 8.
To this mixture, add 95 ml of the 0.2 M TRIS

buffer, pH 8.3. This solution is stable for several weeks when stored in the refrigerator.
Other substituted naphthol AS phosphate derivatives may be substituted for naphthol AS-MX phosphate (such as naphthol AS-TR or AS-BI).
Fast blue RR
1% aqueous magnesium sulfate
Incubation medium
Just before use, add 1 mg of fast blue RR and 0.1 ml of 1% aqueous magnesium sulfate ($MgSO_4$) for each milliliter of stock solution used. Filter.

Procedure

1. Fix air-dried slides in a Coplin jar filled with cold formalin-methanol solution for 30 seconds.
2. Wash slides in tap water for 10 seconds. Air-dry.
3. Incubate in the freshly prepared and filtered stock substrate solution for 60 minutes at room temperature.
4. Wash in distilled water and dry.
5. Counterstain air-dried slides in a Coplin jar filled with 1% aqueous safranin for 30 seconds.
6. Rinse with distilled water, gently blot dry, and mount immediately with 1% aqueous glycerol.

Results—scoring criteria for rating neutrophils:

The alkaline phosphatase activity is demonstrated in mature and band-form neutrophils by dark blue cytoplasmic granules. It is absent in immature granulocytes, lymphocytes, and monocytes under oil immersion. Count 100 consecutive neutrophils (segmented and band form only). Rate each from 0 to 4 on the basis of the presence and intensity of dye in the cytoplasm. The sum of the ratings of 100 cells is the score.
  0 Colorless, no cytoplasmic staining
  1 Diffuse, pale blue staining
  2 Small distinct blue-black granules
  3 Uniform distribution of medium-sized, blue-black granules
  4 Heavy blue staining granules
  Normal range: 83 to 135 units (OSU)
The activity of the enzyme is altered by various disease states. An increase in activity is seen in myelofibrosis, physiologic leukocytosis, leukemoid reactions, polycythemia vera, and hemolytic anemia. A decrease in activity is seen in chronic myelogenous leukemia, paroxysmal nocturnal hemoglobinuria, and acute myeloblastic leukemia.

Controls

One may prepare a positive control by using blood from a pregnant woman. For a negative control, inactivate a previously fixed smear by immersion in boiling water for 1 minute. Stain the controls along with the test smears.

Naphthol AS-BI phosphate–stabilized diazonium salt method for acid phosphatase[5]

Tissue preparation. Cut cryostat sections of fresh or fixed tissue at 6 to 8 μm. Postfix the sections of fresh tissue in cold acetone for 5 to 10 minutes and allow to air-dry before proceeding with the technic.

Stain mechanism. At an acid pH, the activity of the acid phosphatase releases orthophosphate and naphthol derivatives from the naphthol AS-BI phosphate that serves as the substrate. The released naphthol combines with the diazonium salt to result in the formation of an azo dye indicating sites of enzyme activity. The color of the azo dye will vary depending on the specific diazonium salt used; fast red violet LB, fast blue BB, and fast blue RR have all been employed.

Reagents
  0.2 M acetate buffer, pH 5.2
0.2 M sodium acetate	39.5 ml
0.2 M acetic acid	10.5 ml

  Incubation medium (preparation for approximately 50 ml)
Naphthol AS-BI phosphate	5 mg
Dimethylformamide	0.1-0.25 ml
Distilled water	25 ml
Acetate buffer, pH 5.2	25 ml
Stabilized diazonium salt (See choices listed above in stain mechanism.)	30 mg

  10% manganese chloride ($MnCl_2$)

Procedure

1. Dissolve the naphthol AS-BI phosphate in the dimethylformamide. Add the remaining reagents listed under "incubation medium" (see above) to the dissolved substrate.
2. Mix all reagents gently and filter. Add 2 drops of 10% manganese chloride and mix again before adding to sections.
3. Incubate sections at 25° C for 60 minutes.
4. Rinse sections well in distilled water after incubation is complete.
5. Counterstain, if desired. If the fast red violet was used, counterstain in Harris's hematoxylin for 30 seconds to 1 minute; follow with a 10-minute water wash. If the fast blue BB or fast blue RR was used, counterstain for 10 to 30 seconds in 0.5% aqueous safranin; follow with several changes of distilled water.
6. Coverslip sections, using an aqueous medium such as glycerol gelatin or PVP.

Results

If the fast red violet was used, sites of enzyme activity will be pink-red. If the fast blue BB or fast blue RR was used, sites of enzyme activity will be blue to blue-purple. Nuclei will be blue if the hematoxylin counterstain was used; red if the safranin was employed.

Controls

Sections of kidney, liver, or prostate may be used for a positive control. Eliminate substrate from solution for a negative control.

Additional comments. To distinguish acid phosphatase of prostatic origin, a minimum of three consecutive sections should be cut and mounted on three different slides or cover slips. A triple volume of the incubating solution previously described should be prepared, and one of the three sections incubated in the regular incubating medium. The second sample should be incubated in the following solution:

Tartrate incubating solution
| Regular incubating solution | 9 ml |
| 0.2 M tartrate solution | 1 ml |

To prepare the 0.2 M tartrate:

1. Dissolve 3.002 gm of tartaric acid in 50 ml of distilled water.
2. To this add approximately 35 ml of 1 N sodium hydroxide. Mix well.
3. Bring pH of solution to 4.9 and make up to 100 ml with distilled water. Store solution at 3° to 4° C.

The third tissue sample should be incubated in the following:

Formalin incubation solution
| Regular incubation medium | 10 ml |
| 37% to 40% formalin | 0.13 ml |

Staining from acid phosphatase of prostatic origin should be seen in the regular incubating medium and in the formalin incubating medium. Reactions should be negative in the tartrate medium, since acid phosphatase of prostatic origin is inhibited by tartrate.

Indoxyl method for acid phosphatase[6]

Tissue preparation. Either fresh or formol-calcium–fixed tissue may be used. Cut cryostat sections at 6 to 8 μm.

Stain mechanism. Sections are incubated in a buffered medium with 5-iodoindoxyl phosphate or 5-bromoindoxyl phosphate as the substrate. At an acid pH, the acid phosphatase enzymes act to release orthophosphate and indoxyl derivatives from the substrate. By an oxidative process that is aided by the oxidizing action of the potassium ferricyanide and potassium ferrocyanide solution, the indoxyl derivatives are converted to insoluble indigo blue precipitates that mark the sites of enzymatic activity. The additional oxidizing action of the potassium ferrocyanide and ferricyanide also improves enzyme localization.

Reagents

2 M sodium chloride
0.1 M citrate buffer, pH 5.4
| 0.1 M citric acid | 6.4 ml |
| 0.1 M sodium citrate | 13.4 ml |
0.05 M potassium ferrocyanide
0.05 M potassium ferricyanide
5-iodoindoxyl phosphate or 5-bromoindoxyl phosphate (disodium salt)

Procedure

1. To tube 1 add 0.00192 gm of 5-iodoindoxyl phosphate.
2. To tube 2 add in the following order:
2 M sodium chloride	5 ml
Distilled deionized water	2 ml
Citrate buffer, pH 5.4	2 ml
Potassium ferrocyanide	0.5 ml
Potassium ferricyanide	0.5 ml
Mix contents in tube 2 well and add to tube 1. Mix again and add to sections.
3. Incubate 30 to 60 minutes at 37° C. (Routine time is 60 minutes.)
4. Rinse sections in distilled water when incubation time is completed.
5. Counterstain, if desired, in 0.5% safranin O for 30 seconds. Rinse sections thoroughly in distilled water after counterstaining.
6. Coverslip, using an aqueous mounting medium. Alternatively, sections may be dried and coverslipped in a synthetic resin.

Results

Sites of enzyme activity—fine precipitate of indigo blue
Nuclei—red, if the safranin counterstain was used

Controls

Use kidney or jejunum or prostate for a positive control. For a negative control, eliminate substrate from the incubating medium.

Naphthol AS-BI phosphate–hexazonium pararosanilin method for acid phosphatase[18]

Tissue preparation and controls. See preceding technic.

Stain mechanism. The complex naphthol, naphthol AS-BI phosphate, is hydrolyzed by acid phosphatases present in the tissue, and naphthol derivatives are thereby produced. The naphthol derivatives couple with the unstable diazonium salt, hexazonium pararosanilin, to produce a red azo dye to mark the site of enzyme activity.

Reagents
Stock substrate solution

Naphthol AS-BI phosphate	10 mg
N,N-dimethylformamide	1 ml

Store larger volumes at 4° C.

Stock Veronal acetate buffer solution

Sodium acetate (NaC$_2$H$_3$O$_2$ · 3H$_2$O)	9.714 gm
Sodium barbital (sodium barbiturate)	14.714 gm

Using distilled water, dilute the above reagents to a final volume of 500 ml.

If the hydrated acetate is not available, 5.85 gm of the anhydrous salt may be substituted.

4% sodium nitrite (prepared fresh)

Sodium nitrite	0.4 gm
Distilled water	10 ml

Stock pararosanilin solution

Pararosanilin hydrochloride	1 gm
Distilled water	20 ml
Concentrated hydrochloric acid	5 ml

Dissolve the dye in the water, and add the concentrated acid. Heat gently, cool, and filter. Store at 4° C.

Incubation medium

1. In one test tube, prepare the unstable diazonium salt as follows: mix 0.4 ml of stock pararosanilin solution and 0.4 ml of fresh 4% sodium nitrite solution. Allow to stand for 2 minutes before adding to the rest of the incubation medium.
2. In a second test tube, add the following:

Stock substrate solution	0.5 ml
Stock buffer solution	2.5 ml
Diazonium salt from step 1	0.8 ml
Distilled water	6.5 ml

Check the pH of the above solution and adjust to 4.7 to 5.0.

Procedure
1. Incubate sections in the incubating medium for 15 to 60 minutes at 37° C.
2. Wash in distilled water.
3. Counterstain, if desired, for 30 seconds in 2% methyl green (chloroform extracted). Wash in running water for 1 minute after counterstaining.
4. Coverslip, using glycerol gelatin *or* dehydrate rapidly, clear, and coverslip, using a synthetic mounting medium.

Results
A red azo dye indicates sites of acid phosphatase activity. Nuclei are green if the counterstain was used.

Esterases
Esterases hydrolyze ester linkages. A more specific classification of esterases is dependent on the type of acid and the type of alcohol comprising the ester. Generally, esterases may be subdivided into aliesterases and azolesterases. Aliesterases include (1) nonspecific esterases that hydrolyze glyceryl and other esters of short-chain aliphatic acids, and (2) lipases that will hydrolyze esters of long- and short-chain fatty acids. The latter variety are found chiefly in the pancreas. Azolesterases include cholinesterase and acetylcholinesterase, and these hydrolyze fatty acid esters of choline and acetylcholine, respectively. This group may be found in motor end plates, neurons, synaptic points, and erythrocytes.

In addition to those sites mentioned, esterase activity has also been reported in liver, stomach, kidney, and jejunum. The use of inhibitors has assisted in determining certain esterase subtypes. For example, esterases have been classified as A or B esterases according to their reactivity after treatment with a 0.5 M solution of diisopropyl fluorophosphate (DFP). A esterases, found in the kidney, chief cells of the stomach, and other organs are resistant to the action of the DFP inhibitor; B esterases, found in the liver and pancreas, are sensitive. A solution of physostigmine (eserine) has been found to inhibit the cholinesterases but not to affect lipase or A or B esterases.

Gomori has stated that the type of esterase in tumor cells is identical to that produced by the parent tissue, and the use of inhibitor solutions may assist in determining tumor origins. (Details of these inhibitor procedures are listed in Lillie, R. D., and Fullmer, H. M.: Histopathologic technic and practical histochemistry, ed. 4, New York, 1976, McGraw-Hill Book Co.) Esterase reactions may also be useful in determining the progression of cervical carcinoma. The amount of the esterase increases from slight positive in the normal to moderate with carcinoma in situ to intense in infiltrating epidermoid cervical carcinoma.

Naphthol AS-LC acetate–fast blue RR method for esterase[7]

Tissue preparation. Either fresh or fixed tissue may be used. Cut cryostat sections at 6 to 8 μm.

Stain mechanism. Esterase activity hydrolyzes the naphthol AS-LC acetate substrate, and the released naphthol simultaneously combines with the diazonium salt present in the incubation medium to give an azo dye marking the site of enzyme activity.

Reagents

0.1 M phosphate buffer, pH 7.2

0.2 M Na_2HPO_4	72 ml
0.2 M NaH_2PO_4	28 ml

Dilute the above 100 ml to a final volume of 200 ml with distilled water. Mix and check pH.

Incubation medium

Naphthol AS-LC acetate	3 mg
Acetone	0.3 ml
Distilled water	15 ml
0.1 M phosphate buffer, pH 7.2	15 ml
Fast blue RR (or fast garnet GBC)	15 mg

Dissolve the naphthol acetate in the acetone and then add the remaining reagents in the order given. Mix well, filter, and use immediately.

Procedure

1. Incubate sections in the incubation medium at 25° C for 10 to 30 minutes or until sufficient red or blue color develops. Tissues should be allowed to incubate 2 hours before a negative reaction is reported, according to Lillie.
2. Wash sections well in distilled water.
3. Counterstain, if desired. If the fast garnet diazonium salt is used, a hematoxylin counterstain would provide contrasting blue color to the nuclei. If the fast blue RR is used, 0.5% safranin would give a red nuclear color. Rinse well after counterstaining.
4. Coverslip sections in an aqueous mounting medium such as glycerol gelatin or PVP.

Results

Sites of enzyme activity are marked by a blue azo dye if the fast blue RR was the diazonium salt used, or a red azo dye if the fast garnet salt was employed.

Nuclei—either red or blue depending on the counterstain used

Controls

Liver or kidney sections may be used for a positive control. For the negative control, eliminate the specific substrate from the solution.

Demonstration of esterase activity in blood smears [8]—naphthol AS-D chloroacetate esterase method

Smear preparation and fixation. See remarks on pp. 294 and 297.

Stain mechanism. Similar to the preceding method for tissue esterase demonstration.

Reagents

Fixative: Mix 10 ml of 37% formaldehyde with 90 ml of absolute methanol.

Buffer: Michaelis barbital (Veronal) acetate buffer, pH, 7.4

Stock solution A

Sodium acetate, anhydrous	11.074 gm
Sodium diethylbarbiturate (barbital)	29.428 gm
Distilled water, CO_2 free	to make 1 liter

Stock solution B

Hydrochloric acid, concentrated	8.4 ml
Distilled water	to make 1 liter

Note: Add the acid to about 950 ml of the water; mix well; then dilute to 1 liter.

Working buffer

Mix 5 ml of stock solution A, 5 ml of stock solution B, and 13 ml of CO_2-free distilled water. Check pH.

Incubation mixture: Add in the following order:

Distilled water	20 ml
Buffer	20 ml
Propylene glycol	1 ml
Naphthol AS-D chloroacetate	20 mg dissolved in 1.6 ml of acetone
Fast garnet GBC	40 mg

Harris's hematoxylin

Procedure

1. Place air-dried blood or marrow films in fixative for 30 seconds at 4° C. The films can be stored unstained at room temperature for 2 weeks without significant loss of activity. Wash in running tap water for 10 seconds.
2. Place in incubation mixture for 30 to 60 minutes at 25° C. Wash in running tap water after incubation.
3. Counterstain, if desired, with hematoxylin for 6 to 10 minutes. Wash in running tap water for 2 to 3 minutes. (Counterstaining may diminish the histochemical reaction somewhat.)
4. Gently blot dry and coverslip using 1% aqueous glycerol or Kaiser's glycerol gelatin.

Results

Sites of esterase activity—colored red. Granulocytes exhibit a positive reaction; monocytes are slightly reactive; other formed elements are nonreactive. In neutrophils the naphthol AS-D chloroacetate esterase reaction parallels the peroxidase activity and is found in azurophilic granules. However, is some cases, blasts may be peroxidase-positive and naphthol AS-D chloroacetate esterase–negative, indicating that peroxidase appears earlier in development. The esterase reaction may assist in distinguishing the myeloblasts found in acute granulocytic leukemia and in the terminal stages of chronic granulocytic leukemia from the lymphoblasts of acute lymphocytic leukemia.

Indoxyl method for esterase demonstration [3]

Tissue preparation. Either fresh or fixed tissue may be used. Cut cryostat sections at 6 to 8 μm.

Stain mechanism. The indoxyl acetate substrate or its various substituted derivatives are hydrolyzed by esterase activity to free indoxyl. For precise localization of enzyme activity, the transformation of this diffusible product of enzymatic hydrolysis to the insoluble indigo blue dye should take place rapidly. This rapid conversion to indigo blue is facilitated by a mixture of potassium ferrocyanide and potassium ferricyanide oxidizers. An indigo blue end product marks the sites of enzyme activity.

Reagents
2 M sodium chloride
Barbital (Veronal)–hydrochloric acid buffer, pH 7.6
0.04 M Veronal sodium	12.5 ml
0.2 N hydrochloric acid	1.68 ml

0.05 M potassium ferrocyanide
0.05 M potassium ferricyanide
Substrate: 5-bromoindoxyl acetate (5-bromo-4-chloroindoxyl acetate, 5-bromo-4-indoxyl acetate, or 5-iodoindoxyl acetate may also be used.)

Procedure
1. To test tube 1, add 1.51 mg of substrate
2. To test tube 2, add in the following order:
2 M sodium chloride	5 ml
Distilled deionized water	2 ml
Veronal-HCl buffer	2 ml
Potassium ferrocyanide solution	0.5 ml
Potassium ferricyanide	0.5 ml

   Mix these well.
3. Dissolve the substrate in a few drops of absolute alcohol (4 drops are usually sufficient).
4. Add the contents of tube 2 to the dissolved substrate; mix well again before adding to sections.
5. Incubate sections for 30 to 60 minutes at 37° C.
6. Rinse sections well in distilled water after incubation.
7. Counterstaining, if desired, may be done using 0.5% safranin for 30 seconds. After counterstaining, sections should again be rinsed well in distilled water.
8. Coverslip, using an aqueous mounting medium such as glycerol gelatin or PVP. Alternately, sections may be dried and coverslipped in a synthetic medium.

Results
Sites of esterase activity—indigo blue
Nuclei—red, if safranin counterstain was used

Controls
Liver or kidney may be used for a positive control. For a negative control, eliminate the substrate from the incubating solution.

Adenosine triphosphatases (ATPases)

A number of enzymes that can dephosphorylate adenosine triphosphate (ATP) have been described, and the major ones are the ATP phosphohydrolases: (1) myosin ATPase (calcium activated) and (2) mitochondrial ATPase (magnesium activated). These enzymes catalyze the reaction in which ATP is hydrolyzed to adenosine diphosphate (ADP) and orthophosphate. Alkaline phosphatase is also known to catalyze this reaction, and this can represent a source of nonspecific staining in certain ATPase demonstration methods. The pH of the incubating solution may assist in controlling the nonspecific staining attributable to the presence of alkaline phosphatase, since not all ATPase technics require incubation at a pH that is in the alkaline phosphatase activity range. The use of inhibitors could also serve to decrease nonspecific staining.

The two main ATPase types may be distinguished by their response to Mg^{+2} and Ca^{+2} ions. Myosin ATPase is inhibited by Mg^{+2} ions, and mitochondrial ATPase is inhibited by Ca^{+2}. Another ATPase subtype has been described that is Mg^{+2}-dependent and sensitive to the amounts of Na^+ and K^+ ions in solution.

The proportions of the ions and ATP substrate required for maximum activity vary with the pH of the solution. Interestingly, it has been described that the Pb^{+2} ions used in the conventional Wachstein and Meisel procedure may inhibit ATPase activity in both fresh and fixed tissue. It has also been described that the combination of decreasing the concentration of Pb^{+2} and increasing the concentration of ATP alters the location of the reaction product.

The following methods are given even though some authors doubt that the ATPase enzyme is actually demonstrated.

Lead method for demonstration of Mg^{+2} activated ATPase[9]

Tissue preparation. Fresh or fixed tissue may be used. Cut cryostat sections at 6 to 8 μm.

Stain mechanism. ATPase activity releases orthophosphate from the substrate, and this orthophosphate then combines with lead ions (from the lead nitrate solution) to yield a lead phosphate precipitate. This colorless lead phosphate precipitate is transformed to a colored end product of lead sulfide by the action of the ammonium sulfide. Mg^{+2} (from the magnesium sulfate solution) serves as an activator.

Table 17-1. Summary of major histochemical reactions of human muscle fiber types

Histochemical procedure	Type I	Type II		
		IIa	IIb	IIc (rare)
ATPase, pH 9.4	0 to +1	+3	+3	+3
ATPase, pH 4.6, preincubation	+3	0	+3	+3
ATPase, pH 4.2, preincubation	+3	0	0	+1/+2
NADH (DPNH) diaphorase and NADPH (TPNH) diaphorase	+3	+2	+1	+2
Succinic dehydrogenase	+3	+2	+1	+2
Phosphorylase	0 to +1	+3	+3	+3
Periodic acid–Schiff reaction	+1 to +2	+3	+2	+2

From Dubowitz, V., and Brooke, M. H.: Muscle biopsy: a modern approach, Philadelphia, 1973, W. B. Saunders Co.

Reagents

0.2 M TRIS buffer,   total volume 25 ml
  pH 7.2
  0.2 M TRIS   2.5 ml
  0.2 M maleic acid   2.5 ml
  0.1 M sodium hydroxide   5 ml
  Distilled water   15 ml
0.25% magnesium sulfate
2% lead nitrate
1% ammonium sulfide
Substrate: adenosine triphosphate (ATP)

Procedure

1. Prepare the incubating solution as follows (amounts listed will give a 10 ml total volume):
   a. Dissolve 5 mg of ATP in 4 ml of distilled water.
   b. Add
      TRIS buffer   4.4 ml
      Lead nitrate   0.6 ml
      Magnesium sulfate   1 ml
   c. Mix solution gently and filter before use.
2. Incubate sections at 37° C for 1 to 2 hours. No color change will occur during the incubation step.
3. Rinse sections in 4 to 5 changes of distilled water over a 1-minute period.
4. Transfer sections to 1% ammonium sulfide for 3 minutes. Tissue should be a yellow-brown color. *Note:* The working solution of ammonium sulfide should be prepared fresh before use. The stock ammonium sulfide solution should be protected from light and replaced about once a year, since it gradually deteriorates. Use all ammonium sulfide solutions under a fume hood.
5. Wash sections gently in distilled water.
6. Counterstain, if desired, in 0.5% safranin O for 30 seconds. Fixed frozen sections that show a tendency to come off the slide or cover slip are best air-dried prior to the counterstaining step. Rinse sections thoroughly in distilled water after the counterstaining is complete.
7. Coverslip sections in an aqueous mounting medium. Alternatively, sections may be air-dried and coverslipped in a synthetic medium.

Results

Sites of enzyme activity—black-brown precipitate of lead sulfide

Controls

Liver, myocardium, or jejunum may be used for positive controls. For negative controls, eliminate the ATP from the solution.

The preceding lead method has been used to distinguish normal plasma cells from neoplastic plasma cells. Normal plasma cells exhibit moderate activity; neoplastics show a sharp decrease or absence of activity.

Calcium methods for ATPase demonstration

The calcium methods for ATPase demonstration, employing solutions of different pH values, have been used primarily to distinguish muscle fiber types. Human muscles possess a "mosaic" or "checkerboard" distribution of different fiber types. Routine staining methods do not reveal any pattern of distribution; however, histochemical procedures do.

Muscle fibers may be broadly categorized as type I or type II. Physiologically, those belonging to type I ("red muscle") are "slow" fibers (that is, contract at a comparatively slow rate but are capable of sustained activity). They possess more mitochondria and therefore show positive staining with various oxidative histochemical procedures such as succinic dehydrogenase and NADH diaphorase. (These procedures will be described later in this chapter.) Fibers belonging to the type II class ("white muscle") are further subdivided into types IIa, IIb, and IIc. Types IIa and IIb have clinical significance; however, there are comparatively few type IIc muscle fibers, and it may be that the type IIc fibers are precursors for other fiber types. Generally, type II fibers are "fast" fibers (that is, contract rapidly but cannot sustain continuous activity). They possess fewer mitochondria and therefore give a less intense reaction to stains for oxidative enzymes. Histochemical reactions for the fiber types are summarized in Table 17-1.

ATPase for muscle-fiber types — calcium method[10]

Tissue preparation. See isopentane method, p. 294.

Stain mechanism. Sections are incubated in a solution containing adenosine triphosphate (ATP) substrate and calcium. ATPase present in the tissue hydrolyzes the substrate, and the products formed are adenosine diphosphate (ADP) and orthophosphate. The released phosphate combines with the calcium present to form colorless calcium phosphate. When the tissue is exposed to the cobalt chloride solution, the cobalt is exchanged for the calcium and a colorless precipitate of cobaltous phosphate is now present at the sites of enzymatic activity. Upon treatment with ammonium sulfide, a black insoluble precipitate of cobaltous sulfide is formed and permits visualization of the products of enzymatic activity.

Reagents

Stock barbital solution

Sodium barbital	4.124 gm
Calcium chloride (dihydride)	1.998 gm
Distilled water	1 liter

Store at 25° C.

Barbital acetate buffer (0.2 M)

Solution A

Sodium acetate	1.94 gm
Sodium barbiturate	2.94 gm
Distilled water	100 ml

Solution B

0.1 M (or 0.1 N) hydrochloric acid

Buffer mixture

Solution A	5 ml
Solution B	10 ml
Distilled water	8 ml

Solutions A and B may be stored at 25° C. The buffer mixture is made fresh each time it is needed.

2% cobaltous chloride

1% ammonium sulfide

Adenosine triphosphate, disodium salt

Procedure

1. A minimum of 3 sections per individual case should be cut, since the technique requires incubation at 3 different pH points.
2. Prepare the three pre-incubation solutions that will be needed.

   Preincubation solution pH 10.4

   Prepare by bringing the stock barbital solution to pH 10.4 by the addition of 0.25 N sodium hydroxide.

Preincubation solution pH 4.6

Prepare by bringing the needed amounts of barbital acetate buffer to 4.6 with the addition of 0.1 M hydrochloric acid. Mix while changing the pH, using a magnetic stirrer, if available.

Preincubation solution pH 4.2

Prepare by bringing the needed amount of barbital acetate buffer to 4.2, using 0.1 M hydrochloric acid. Mix while changing the pH, preferably using a magnetic stirrer.

3. Prepare the needed volume of *substrate incubation medium*. Use the following proportions:

Sodium barbital stock solution	10 ml
Adenosine triphosphate, disodium salt	15 mg

   Bring the pH of the above *combination* to 9.4. The pH is critical.
4. Preincubate the sections designated for pH 10.4 at 25° C in the preincubation solution of that pH for 10 minutes. At the conclusion of this 10 minutes, do not rinse, but immediately place sections in the *substrate incubation medium* (pH 9.4) for 30 minutes at 37° C.
5. Preincubate the sections designated for pH 4.6 and 4.2 at 25° C in their respective preincubation solution for 5 minutes. At the conclusion of this 5 minutes, rinse the sections in the stock sodium barbital solution for 3 minutes. At the conclusion of the 3 minutes, transfer the sections *without rinsing* to the *substrate incubation medium* for 30 minutes at 37° C.

   Sections will show no color change during the incubation time.
6. After completion of the 30-minute incubation in the substrate incubation medium, do *not* rinse, but immediately transfer sections to cobaltous chloride for 3 minutes.
7. After the cobalt treatment, *wash sections well* in distilled water, with 3 changes at 1 minute each change.
8. Treat with 1% ammonium sulfide for 10 to 30 seconds. (See precautions with this solution listed under the lead method for ATPase, p. 303.)
9. Wash sections in running tap water for 5 minutes. Check microscopically to ensure that all precipitate has been removed.
10. Dehydrate in graded alcohols, clear in xylene, and coverslip, using a synthetic medium.

Results

Refer to Table 17-1.

Aminopeptidases[11]

Aminopeptidases comprise a number of enzymes that act similarly to hydrolyze peptide bonds. Histochemically, aminopeptidases release β-naphthylamine (or other arylamines) from amide combinations with amino acid carboxyl groups. Both leucyl- and alanyl-naphthyl-amides have been used as substrates. Amino-peptidases are found in highest concentrations in kidney and small intestine, but their presence has also been reported in other tissues including muscle, skin, spleen, and lymph node. Positive staining from aminopeptidase has been reported to occur in cases of melanoma, meningioma, and adenocarcinoma of the colon. Gastric carcinoma rapidly gives an intense reaction, and the technic is useful in defining surgical margins and in diagnosing lymph node metastasis of these tumors. Intense reactions have also been reported to occur in gallbladder carcinoma, and the aminopeptidase technic may assist in finding groups of malignant cells not easily discernible with other stains. The technic may also prove useful in distinguishing proliferating bile ducts (intense positive) from small cords of hepatic parenchymal cells (slight positive) in cirrhotic liver scars.

Demonstration of leucine aminopeptidase in tissue

Tissue preparation. Fresh frozen cryostat sections cut at 6 to 8 μm.

Stain mechanism. Sections are incubated with the substrate L-leucyl-4-methoxy-2-naphthylamide hydrochloride. Aminopeptidase activity releases naphthylamide, which in turn combines with the diazonium salt fast blue B, present in the medium, to produce a reddish azo dye marking the site of enzyme activity. The potassium cyanide functions as an activator. After being stained, sections are treated with a solution of cupric sulfate. The cupric ions chelate with the azo dye that has been formed, and this results in a color shift from the reddish ranges to red-purple. The copper chelation also produces a positive charge on azo dye and makes it insoluble in the organic reagents necessary to dehydrate, clear, and coverslip a slide.

Reagents
0.1 M acetate buffer, pH 6.5

0.2 M sodium acetate	9.8 ml
0.2 M acetic acid	0.2 ml

Adjust pH to 6.5 and dilute 1:1 for use.
Incubation medium

L-leucyl-4-methoxy-2-naphthyl-amide hydrochloride (stock 4 mg/ml)	1 ml
0.1 M acetate buffer, pH 6.5	5 ml
0.85% sodium chloride	3.5 ml
0.02 M potassium cyanide	0.5 ml
Fast blue B salt (tetrazotized diorthoanisidine)	5 mg

The stock substrate solution is stable for several months in the refrigerator. The incubation medium, however, should be mixed fresh each time it is needed.
0.1 M cupric sulfate

Anhydrous cupric sulfate	1.59 gm
Distilled water	to make 100 ml

Procedure
1. Incubate sections in the above medium for 30 minutes to 2 hours at 37° C.
2. Rinse in 0.85% saline solution for 2 to 3 minutes.
3. Place in 0.1 M cupric sulfate for 2 minutes.
4. Rinse in 0.85% saline solution.
5. Dehydrate sections through graded alcohols, clear in xylene, and mount in a synthetic resin.

Results
Sites of leucine aminopeptidase activity—reddish purple deposits

Control
Use jejunum for positive control. For negative control, eliminate the substrate from the solution.

Phosphorylases

Phosphorylases are found in highest concentration in the liver and in skeletal and cardiac muscle where they catalyze the breakdown of glycogen by destroying the α-1,4'-glucosidic linkages. These enzymes play an important role in glycogen catabolism, and phosphorylase deficiency results in an excess storage of glycogen reserves.

In the histochemical reaction, phosphorylase acts on the substrate, glucose-1-phosphate and forms, in the presence of a glycogen primer, a polysaccharide composed of α-1,4-glycosyl units. The in vitro reaction of polysaccharide formation is, therefore, the opposite of the in vivo action of glycogen degradation. This happens because the concentration of the substrate is high, and the concentration of the inorganic phosphate is low. The system equilibrium therefore favors glycogen formation. Adenosine-5'-monophosphate functions as an activator.

Exposure of the sections to an iodine solution after incubation results in a varied color formation in the newly formed polysaccharide. A negative reaction is yellow, and it has been shown that unbranched chains of 4 to 6 glucosyl units will give a negative reaction. A polysaccharide of 8 to 12 units gives a reddish color, followed by various transitional colors as the length of the chain increases. Chain lengths of 30 to 35 units give a blue color. The reason the color is blue rather than red-brown is that the polysaccharide formed by the phosphorylase action is not normal glycogen. For glycogen to color a true red-brown, it has to be branched, and branching will only occur if branching enzyme is allowed to act. However, the action of the branching enzyme is eliminated by the inclusion of alcohol in the incubation medium.

Clinical implications. The term "glycogen storage disease" refers to a series of inheritable disturbances of glycogen metabolism resulting in a deposition of normal or abnormal glycogen. They are classified into nine "Cori" types, and these have other names as well. In McArdle's disease (Cori type V) the patients have a deficiency of muscle phosphorylase, but normal liver phosphorylase. In Cori type VI (Hers' disease) muscle phosphorylase is normal, but liver phosphorylase is abnormal. This means large amounts of glycogen are found in the muscle of patients with Cori type V; and large amounts of glycogen are found in the livers of patients with Cori type VI.

Amylophosphorylase reaction[12]

Tissue preparation. Fresh frozen tissue. Cut sections 6 to 8 μm. If muscle tissue is to be stained, follow the isopentane freezing method, p. 294.

Staining mechanism. See preceding discussion.

Reagents

Sodium acetate–hydrochloric acid buffer, pH 5.6
Sodium acetate	13.6 gm
1 N hydrochloric acid	20 ml
Distilled water	480 ml

Weigert's iodine (p. 131)
Dilute Weigert's iodine
Weigert's iodine	1 ml
Distilled water	9 ml

Iodine-glycerol
Weigert's iodine	2 ml
Glycerol	20 ml

Incubation medium
0.2 M sodium acetate buffer	10 ml
Glucose-1-phosphate (potassium salt)	25 mg
Adenosine-5'-monophosphate (AMP)	5 mg
Glycogen (shellfish)	2 mg
95% ethanol	2 ml

Procedure

1. Mix incubation medium thoroughly and adjust pH to 5.6.
2. Incubate sections at 37° C for 1 hour.
3. Remove sections and place directly into dilute Weigert's iodine for 10 to 60 seconds.
4. Remove sections, gently blotting excess iodine. Coverslip, using iodine-glycerol.

Results

Sites of phosphorylase activity—blue or reddish brown deposits of newly synthesized polysaccharide

See Table 17-1 for muscle fiber type of reactions. *Note:* This is not a permanent stain and will fade with time. To restore stain, remove cover slip and place in dilute iodine until color is restored. Again coverslip, using iodine-glycerol.

Control

Use skeletal muscle for a positive control. For a negative control, pretreat sections with diastase (or α-amylase) to ensure that polysaccharide demonstrated has been formed during the reaction. Alternatively, the glucose-1-phosphate may be omitted from the incubating solution.

Oxidative enzyme

Enzymes classified as oxidative include the dehydrogenases, diaphorases, and oxidases. They are important in catalyzing reactions of the Krebs cycle and other related pathways.

Dehydrogenases include a large number of enzymes that activate hydrogen atoms of specific substrates and catalyze the transfer of these hydrogen atoms to hydrogen acceptors. Dehydrogenases represent the first step in the biologic oxidation of a variety of substances. They are divided into the aerobic dehydrogenases, which transfer the hydrogen to molecular oxygen leading to the formation of hydrogen peroxide, and anaerobic dehydrogenases, which function to transfer hydrogen to acceptors other than molecular oxygen.

Procedures for the demonstration of two dehydrogenases, succinic dehydrogenase and glucose-6-phosphate dehydrogenase, are described in the following section.

Succinic dehydrogenase[13]

Tissue preparation. Fresh frozen sections cut at 6 to 8 μm. Fixed tissue cannot be used. If muscle tissue is to be stained, follow the isopentane freezing method, p. 294.

Stain mechanism. Succinic dehydrogenase, an anaerobic dehydrogenase, is a soluble iron flavoprotein that catalyzes the reversible oxidation of succinic acid to fumaric acid. The histochemical demonstration of the activity of this enzyme is achieved by incubation of fresh frozen sections with a succinate substrate in the presence of a tetrazolium compound. Tetrazoliums are colorless water-soluble compounds employed in histochemistry as redox indicators. Under appropriate conditions, tetrazoliums are reduced to formazans which are water-insoluble colored compounds. Commonly used tetrazoliums include nitro blue tetrazolium (nitro BT or NBT) and tetranitro blue tetrazolium (TNBT). Another tetrazolium salt is MTT, which is 3-(4,5-dimethyl-thiazolyl-2)-2,5-diphenyl tetrazolium bromide; however, reaction products using this salt are not so stable as those using NBT or TNBT. Enzymatic activity releases hydrogen from the substrate, and the released hydrogen is transferred to the tetrazolium. With the addition of hydrogen, the tetrazolium is converted to purple-blue formazan pigment marking the site of enzyme activity.

Reagents
0.2 M phosphate buffer, pH 7.6

0.2 M monobasic sodium phosphate (27.8 gm/liter)	13 ml
0.2 M dibasic sodium phosphate (53.65 gm/liter)	87 ml

0.2 M succinic acid
$NaOCOCH_2CH_2COONa \cdot 6H_2O$
(5.4 gm/dl)
Mix fresh each time it is needed.
NBT solution (1 mg/ml)
0.85% saline
Formalin-saline (0.85 gm of sodium chloride per 100 ml of 10% formalin)
15% ethanol

Procedure
1. Prepare the incubation medium as follows:

0.2 M phosphate buffer	5 ml
0.2 M succinic acid	5 ml
NBT solution	10 ml

2. Incubate sections in the above medium for 30 minutes at 37° C.
3. Wash sections in saline.
4. Postfix for 10 minutes in the formalin-saline solution.
5. Rinse sections in 15% ethanol for 5 minutes.
6. Rinse in distilled water.
7. Counterstaining, if desired, may be accomplished by staining with 0.5% safranin O for 30 seconds. Rinse sections thoroughly in distilled water after counterstaining.
8. Coverslip, using an aqueous mounting medium. Alternatively dehydrate in alcohol, clear in xylene, and coverslip, using a synthetic mounting medium.

Results
Sites of enzyme activity—blue-purple deposits of formazan pigment
For results on muscle-fiber types, see Table 17-1.

Controls
Use myocardium for a positive control. For a negative control, eliminate sodium succinate from the incubating medium.

Glucose-6-phosphate dehydrogenase[14]

This enzyme, found in a wide variety of tissues, acts in an alternative pathway of carbohydrate metabolism known as the hexose monophosphate, or HMP, shunt, and catalyzes hydrogen transfer from glucose-6-phosphate to 6-phosphogluconic acid. The hereditary deficiency of glucose-6-phosphate dehydrogenase (G6PD) (and other enzymes of the HMP shunt) have been responsible for the increased susceptibility of red blood cells to hemolysis in the presence of certain drugs (such as primaquine, acetylphenylhydrazine) or other toxic agents.

Tissue preparation. Use fresh frozen tissue cut at 6 to 8 μm. Fixed tissue cannot be used.

Stain mechanism. Glucose-6-phosphate dehydrogenase acts on the glucose-6-phosphate substrate to release hydrogen. NADP (coenzyme II, TPN in older terminology) acts as an intermediate carrier for the released hydrogen and transports the hydrogen from the substrate to the tetrazolium salt (either NBT or TNBT). Once the tetrazolium salt accepts the hydrogen, it is reduced to the water-insoluble formazan pigment marking the site of enzyme activity.

Reagents
Nicotinamide adenine dinucleotide phosphate (NADP)
Glucose-6-phosphate, sodium salt
Nitro blue tetrazolium (NBT) or tetranitro blue tetrazolium (TNBT)
Dimethylformamide (DMF)
Barium chloride
0.1 M manganese chloride
Barbital (Veronal)–hydrochloric acid buffer, pH 7.4

0.2 N hydrochloric acid	1.9 ml
0.04 M barbital (Veronal) sodium	12.5 ml

Procedure
1. To one tube, add 0.168 gm of barium chloride. To another tube, add 0.03 gm of glucose-6-phosphate, and 0.005 gm NADP. To a third tube, add 0.005 gm of TNBT or NBT.
2. To the tube with the barium chloride, add 4.4 ml of the barbital buffer and 6.4 ml of the distilled water. Mix and add this to the second tube with the NADP and the glucose-6-phosphate.
3. Add the mixed reagents to the tetrazolium salt. (If TNBT is used, dissolve it in a few drops of DMF before adding reagent mixture.) Mix all these well and add 1 ml of the activator solution (manganese chloride). Mix and add this to the tissue sections.
4. Incubate 1 hour at 37° C.
5. Remove sections from medium; rinse in distilled water.
6. Counterstain, if desired, using a 0.5% solution of safranin O for 30 seconds. Rinse sections well in distilled water after the counterstaining step.
7. Coverslip, using an aqueous mounting medium.

Results

Sites of glucose-6-phosphate dehydrogenase activity—deposition of blue-purple formazan pigment

Controls

Use liver for a positive control. For a negative control, eliminate the glucose-6-phosphate from the incubating medium.

NADPH diaphorase[15]

"Diaphorase" is a term given to flavoprotein enzymes that have the property of transferring hydrogen from reduced nicotinamide adenine dinucleotide (NADH) (old term: DPNH) and reduced nicotinamide adenine dinucleotide phosphate (NADPH) (old term: TPNH) to various dyes. The hydrogen transfer reduces the dye. Usually tetrazolium compounds function as the hydrogen acceptor when diaphorases are being demonstrated histochemically, and the product of the reduction is the water-insoluble formazan pigment.

Tissue preparation. Cut fresh frozen sections at 6 to 8 μm. If muscle tissue is to be stained, follow the isopentane method, p. 294.

Stain mechanism. The enzyme acts on its substrate, NADPH, and releases hydrogen. The hydrogen combines with the tetrazolium salt, nitro blue tetrazolium, and this results in the deposition of a blue-purple formazan pigment at the site of the enzyme activity.

Reagents

TRIS–hydrochloric acid buffer, pH 7.4

Tris(hydroxymethyl)aminomethane (TRIS)	6.5 gm
Concentrated hydrochloric acid	3.34 ml
Distilled water	1000 ml

Nitro blue tetrazolium
NADPH

Procedure

1. Prepare the incubation medium:

TRIS–hydrochloric acid buffer	10 ml
Nitro blue tetrazolium	10 mg
NADPH	4 mg

Adjust the pH of the incubation medium to 7.4.
2. Incubate sections in the above medium at 37° C for 20 to 30 minutes.
3. Wash sections in distilled water for 1 minute.
4. Optional: Wash sections in a series of 30%, 60%, 90%, 60%, and 30% acetone. This step will remove fat and is said to thereby improve the quality of the stain. It will, however, cause some reduction in stain intensity.
5. Rinse sections in distilled water for 1 minute.
6. Counterstain sections, if desired, in 0.5% safranin for 30 seconds. Rinse sections well in distilled water after counterstaining.
7. Coverslip sections, using an aqueous mounting medium.

Results

For results on muscle fiber type, see Table 17-1. NADPH diaphorase shows an intense reaction in carcinoma of the colon and in malignant polyps, whereas a normal reaction is seen in benign polyps.

Controls

Use kidney or skeletal muscle for a positive control. For a negative control, eliminate the substrate from the incubating medium.

NADH diaphorase[16]

The procedure and rationale for the NADH diaphorase technic is the same as listed for the NADPH technic except that the substrate required is NADH.

Peroxidase demonstration in blood smears[17]

Smear fixation. Freshly prepared smears are fixed in 75% ethanol for 10 minutes, followed by a water wash. Alternatively, smears may be fixed in 10% formalin-alcohol for 1 to 2 minutes, followed by a water wash.

Stain mechanism. The peroxidase enzyme, if present, will act on hydrogen peroxide present in the staining solution to produce water and free oxygen. The free oxygen will, in turn, oxidize the colorless benzidine present in the staining solution to benzidine blue dye. With time, the benzidine blue color can convert to a more stable benzidine brown color. The sodium nitroprusside serves as a catalyst for the reaction.

Reagents

Benzidine-nitroprusside reagent
0.05 gm of sodium nitroprusside is dissolved in 2 ml of distilled water, and 98 ml of absolute ethanol is added. 0.05 gm of benzidine and 0.05 gm of basic fuchsin are added to the solution. This stain will keep for 3 to 6 months at room temperature. *Note:* See p. 322 for precautions to be observed when using benzidine.

Hydrogen peroxide
1 ml of 10% (volume/volume) of hydrogen peroxide is diluted to 200 ml with distilled water. Prepare fresh before use. Be careful when measuring the peroxide. If too much stock is added, the enzyme can be destroyed before oxygen is liberated; if too little is added, or if the solution itself is not fresh, weak or negative reactions will occur.

Procedure

1. A freshly prepared smear is flooded with 1 vol-

ume of the nitroprusside-benzidine reagent and allowed to stain for 1 minute.

2. An equal volume of hydrogen peroxide is then added to the smear and the mixture is allowed to stain for 4 minutes.
3. The smears are washed well in running tap water for 2 to 3 minutes, air-dried, and examined.

Results

The cytoplasm of mature granulocytes, monoblasts, myeloblasts, and promyelocytes possess granules that contain a peroxidase enzyme. These peroxidase-containing granules are stained deep blue.

Cell nuclei—red

Cytoplasm—pink

Red cells—buff color

Since cells of the lymphocytic series are negative for the peroxidase enzyme, the technic may be used to distinguish the myeloblasts found in acute granulocytic leukemia and in the terminal stages of chronic granulocytic leukemia from the lymphoblasts of acute lymphocytic leukemia.

Controls

For a negative control, eliminate hydrogen peroxide from the incubating medium.

REFERENCES

1. Burstone, M. S.: Histochemical comparison of naphthol AS phosphates for the demonstration of phosphatases, J. Natl. Cancer Inst. **20**:601-615, 1958.
2. Burstone, M. S.: Histochemical comparison of naphthol AS phosphates for the demonstration of phosphatases, J. Natl. Cancer Inst. **20**:601-615, 1958 (modification).
3. Czernobilsky, B., and Tsou, K.-C.: Adenocarcinoma, adenomas and polyps of the colon: a histochemical study, Cancer **21**:165-177, 1968.
4. Ackerman, G. A.: Substituted naphthol AS phosphate derivatives for the localization of leukocyte alkaline phosphatase activity, Lab. Invest. **2**:563-567, 1962, U.S.-Canadian Division of the International Academy of Pathology, Baltimore, The Williams & Wilkins Co. (agent).
5. Burstone, M. S.: Histochemical demonstration of acid phosphatase activity in osteoclasts, J. Histochem. Cytochem. **7**:39-41, 1959, The Histochemical Society, Baltimore, The Williams & Wilkins Co. (agent).
6. Evans, G. W., Whinney, C. L., and Tsou, K.-C.: A new histochemical method for acid phosphatase by the use of 5-iodoindoxyl phosphate, J. Histochem. **14**:171-176, 1966, The Histochemical Society, Baltimore, The Williams & Wilkins Co. (agent).
7. Burstone, M. S.: The cytochemical localization of esterase, J. Natl. Cancer Inst. **18**:167-172, 1957.
8. Moloney, W. C., McPherson, K., and Fliegelman, L.: Esterase activity in leukocytes demonstrated by the use of naphthol AS-D chloroacetate substrate, J. Histochem. Cytochem. **8**:200-207, 1960, The Histochemical Society, Baltimore, The Williams & Wilkins Co. (agent).
9. Wachstein, M., and Meisel, E.: Histochemistry of hepatic phosphatases at a physiologic pH with special reference to the demonstration of bile canaliculi, Am. J. Clin. Pathol. **27**:13-23, 1957.
10. Dubowitz, V., and Brooke, M. H.: Muscle biopsy: a modern approach, Philadelphia, 1973, W. B. Saunders Co., p. 32 (modification).
11. Nachlas, M. M., and Monis, B., Rosenblatt, D., and Seligman, A. M.: Improvement in the histochemical localization of leucine aminopeptidase with a new substrate L-leucyl-4-methoxy-2-naphthylamide, J. Biophys. Biochem. Cytol. **7**:261-264, 1960.
12. Eränkö, O., and Palkama, A.: Improved localization of phosphorylase by the use of polyvinylpyrrolidone and high substrate concentration, J. Histochem. Cytochem. **9**:585, 1961 (modification), The Histochemical Society, Baltimore, The Williams & Wilkins Co. (agent).
13. Nachlas, M. M., Tsou, K.-C., de Souza, E., Chang, C. S., and Seligman, A. M.: Cytochemical demonstration of succinic dehydrogenase by use of a new p-nitrophenyl substituted ditetrazole, J. Histochem. Cytochem. **5**:420-436, 1957, The Histochemical Society, Baltimore, The Williams & Wilkins Co. (agent).
14. Cohen, S., and Way, S.: Histochemical demonstration of pentose shunt activity in smears from the uterine cervix, Br. Med. J. **1**:88-89, 1966 (modification).
15. Nachlas, M. M., Walker, D. G., and Seligman, A. M.: A histochemical method for the demonstration of diphosphopyridine nucleotide diaphorase, J. Biophys. Biochem. Cytol. **4**:29-38, 1958.
16. Nachlas, M. M., Walker, D. G., and Seligman, A. M.: The histochemical localization of triphosphopyridine nucleotide diaphorase, J. Biophys. Biochem. Cytol. **4**:467-474, 1958.
17. Beacom, D. N.: A modification of Goodpasture's technic for the peroxidase reaction in blood smears, J. Lab. Clin. Med. **11**:1092, 1926.
18. Barka, T., and Anderson, P. J.: Histochemical methods using hexazonium pararosanilin as coupler, J. Histochem. Cytochem. **10**:741-753, 1962, The Histochemical Society, Baltimore, Williams and Wilkins Co. (agent).

Immunohistochemistry

ROBERT J. HRAPCHAK

To demonstrate an antigen or antibody in a histologic section, one of the reactants (usually the antibody) may be labeled with a substance such as a radioisotope, fluorochrome, or enzyme. The label then may be detected after formation of an immune complex between the antigen and the specific antibody. The labels themselves have various advantages and disadvantages. Although radioisotopes can be detected in very small amounts, their use in histology requires autoradiographic procedures that are time consuming and may produce poor results. However, histologic labels such as fluorochromes, with subsequent detection by fluorescence methods, or enzymes, with detection by use of specific substrates in light or electron microscopy, produce excellent localizations of the sites of antigen-antibody reactions. In this chapter, after reviewing simple fluorescence methods, we will consider immunologic procedures that use either fluorescence detection systems (immunofluorescence procedures) or enzymic detection systems (immunoenzymic procedures).

FLUORESCENCE PROCEDURES[1-5]

Certain substances are described as being fluorescent. What does this mean? Normally, the electrons of fluorescent compounds are unexcited or said to be in the "ground state." However, fluorescent compounds can absorb light (usually in the ultraviolet [UV] range), and when they do, their electrons enter an energy-rich "excited state." The electrons do not stay in this excited state, but return to the ground state, and in this process release the extra energy. In fluorescence, most of the extra energy is emitted as light of a longer wavelength than the original excitation light. More specifically, the duration of light emission determines whether a substance is classified as fluorescent or otherwise. In fluorescence, the emitted light is given off only during the time of exposure to the excitation light or for a short period of time thereafter. (This distinguishes fluorescence from phosphorescence, in which the emission of light persists for a considerable time after the excitation light is no longer acting.)

Fluorescence may be classified further. If the fluorescence phenomenon is observed in samples that have not been stained with a fluorescent dye, it is termed *primary fluorescence,* or autofluorescence; *secondary fluorescence,* on the other hand, involves the use of special dyes called *fluorochromes.*

Primary fluorescence (autofluorescence)

There are many compounds that can fluoresce naturally without the use of fluorochrome dyes; some of these substances are listed in Table 18-1. Yellow or orange filters usually absorb most of the blue autofluorescence that is characteristic of tissue.

Table 18-1. Examples of autofluorescent substances

Substance	Fluorescent color
Tissue	Bright blue
Collagen fibers	Blue-green
Elastic fibers	Brilliant blue
Lipid droplets	Shades of yellow
Nissl substance	Bright yellow
Ceroid	Shades of yellow
Lipofuscin	Orange
Porphyrin	Intense red
Vitamins	Shades of yellow, red, green, or blue
5-Hydroxytryptamine	Golden yellow after formalin fixation
Tetracycline	Bright yellow

Tissue preparations for primary fluorescence

Usually unfixed smears or fresh frozen cryostat sections are used for the study of primary fluorescence. *Samples should not be mounted on green glass slides.* Postfixation, if desired, may be done by a brief immersion in 95% ethanol. Formalin is not usually used for postfixation since it tends to increase the background tissue fluorescence. An exception is if 5-hydroxytryptamine is to be demonstrated since granules containing this substance fluoresce gold yellow after formalin fixation. See p. 278 for details of this procedure.

It should be noted that in many cases, autofluorescence can mimic specific secondary fluorescence. This can possibly make it difficult to distinguish between the two reactions depending on the particular fluorescent color and structure of the substances stained. *Controls for autofluorescence* should be used in any secondary fluorescence reaction. This is accomplished by including an additional tissue section (or smear) that has been treated similar to the test sample in all respects except actual staining.

Secondary fluorescence

Secondary fluorescence is produced when substances that are not naturally fluorescent interact with a fluorochrome dye. A fluorochrome dye is a special kind of dye that can fluoresce when excited with ultraviolet light. A major advantage of secondary fluorescence technics is

Table 18-2. Commonly used fluorescent dyes and their applications

Dye	Substance stained	Color produced
Acridine orange (C.I. 46005)	DNA RNA	Green Red
Auramine O (C.I. 41000) Rhodamine B (C.I. 45170)	Acid-fast bacilli	Yellow
Phosphine 3R (C.I. 46045)	All lipids except fatty acids, soaps, and cholesterol	Silver white
Fluorescein isothiocyanate (FITC) (fluorescein)	"General tagger" used primarily in immunofluorescence	Apple green
Tetramethyl rhodamine isothiocyanate (TRITC)	"General tagger" but more labile than FITC; can be used in immunofluorescence	Red
Morin (C.I. 75660)	Metal detection, especially aluminum	Greenish white
Rhodamine B sulfonyl chloride (lissamine rhodamine B200) (acid rhodamine B) (C.I. 45100)	May be used (for tagging one antigen) when two antigens are to be identified in the same sample	Orange
Thioflavin T (C.I. 49005)	Amyloid	Bright yellow

Table 18-3. Definitions of some terms used in immunofluorescence and immunoenzymic methods

Antigen	A substance that stimulates the formation of a specific antibody.
Antibody	Complex protein molecules formed in response to an antigenic stimulus—they combine with antigens like a key to a lock. Antibodies are produced by plasma cells and some lymphocytes, and although they resemble each other in overall shape, each antibody has unique features that make it fit to one antigen and not to another.
Antiserum	A serum containing antibodies—antiserums are usually purchased commercially and should be of known *specificity* for a certain antigen. Some antiserums contain additional antibodies, and these additional antibodies may cross-react and confuse interpretation.
Conjugated antiserum	Antiserum containing the specific antibody is conjugated or joined with fluorescein (or some other fluorochrome) or with enzymes.
Immunoglobulin (Ig)	Immunoglobulins are specific types of antibodies and are divided into different classes: IgM, IgG, IgA, IgD, and IgE. Ig molecules are basically composed of 2 heavy and 2 light polypeptide chains and have sites for binding antigens and complement. Immunofluorescent stains are usually performed for IgM, IgG, and IgA.
Complement (C′)	Complement is a factor found in fresh serum and is composed of 9 major components. It is related to the immune system and often may be localized in tissue sections containing immune complexes that were previously deposited in response to certain pathologic conditions. Much tissue injury can result from immune complex and complement interaction.
Fibrin	Fibrin is a specific protein formed as a result of the clotting process. Fibrin deposition and platelet aggregation are prominent features of renal transplant rejections. There are immunofluorescence procedures for staining fibrin.
Granular immunofluorescence *versus* linear immunofluorescence	Deposition of immune complexes may be visualized as clumps or in a comparatively smooth pattern. Certain renal diseases have characteristic deposition patterns when immunofluorescence is done.
	For example, a smooth linear pattern of IgG staining is seen along the glomerular basement membrane in cases of Goodpasture's syndrome. Other renal diseases will give positive staining in a granular pattern. Interpretation of these patterns may be diagnostic.

their ability to demonstrate low concentrations of particular components. The methods also give good contrast, and a low-power magnification can be used for screening purposes. A disadvantage of fluorescence methods is that the localization of the stained substance appears somewhat imprecise because the fluorescence is given off in all directions. Some commonly used fluorescent dyes and their applications are listed in Table 18-2. Details of tissue preparation and staining procedures for these methods are listed in the appropriate chapters.

Immunofluorescence procedures

Immunofluorescence methods are used most frequently to demonstrate sites of immune complexes in smear or tissue samples. Localization is revealed by labeling one of the components of the staining reaction with a fluorochrome dye, and fluorescein isothiocyanate is the most commonly used dye for this purpose. Table 18-3

summarizes definitions of some of the terms that are encountered with immunofluorescence (and immunoenzymic) technics.

The general steps for performing most immunofluorescence methods include the following:

1. Preparation of an antiserum, including animal injections, bleedings, and serum characterization
2. Conjugation of the antiserum with a fluorochrome dye
3. Purification of the conjugated dye
4. Preparation and staining of the test samples

Johnson et al.[6] give information on the preparation, purification, and evaluation of conjugates. In many cases, tagged antiserums can be purchased from commercial sources. It is wise to check the purity of commercial preparations before use by immunoelectrophoresis. Commercial antiserums usually should be diluted before use. One can determine the extent of the

Table 18-4. Common methods of immunofluorescent staining

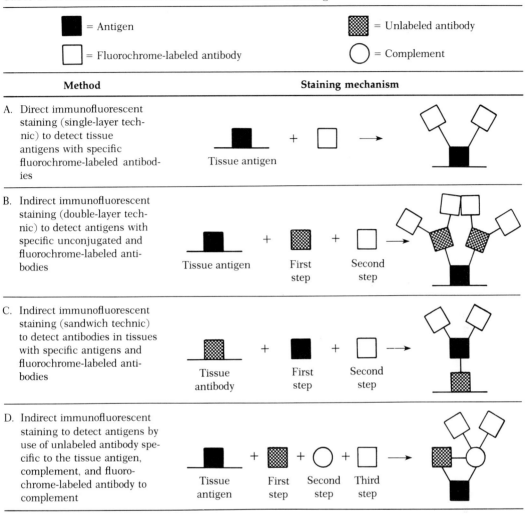

Method	Staining mechanism
A. Direct immunofluorescent staining (single-layer technic) to detect tissue antigens with specific fluorochrome-labeled antibodies	
B. Indirect immunofluorescent staining (double-layer technic) to detect antigens with specific unconjugated and fluorochrome-labeled antibodies	
C. Indirect immunofluorescent staining (sandwich technic) to detect antibodies in tissues with specific antigens and fluorochrome-labeled antibodies	
D. Indirect immunofluorescent staining to detect antigens by use of unlabeled antibody specific to the tissue antigen, complement, and fluorochrome-labeled antibody to complement	

dilution by testing a number of dilutions of the antiserum on a known positive control.

Attachment procedures in immunofluorescence procedures

There are two major types of attachment procedures used in immunofluorescence methods: *direct staining* and *indirect staining*. *Direct methods* permit direct visualization of antigens or antibodies (considered as antigens) in tissue sections by treatment of the sample with a solution containing a fluorochrome-labeled antibody that is specific for the substance to be demonstrated (Table 18-4, *A*). Because the antibody used in detection is fluorochrome-labeled, sites of attachment to the desired antigen can be visualized by using a fluorescence microscope. To perform the direct method, a fluorochrome-la-

beled antibody specific for each antigen studied is needed.

Indirect procedures also may be used to demonstrate either antigen or antibody localized in a tissue section. With the indirect localization of antigen by the double-layer technic, the antigen is in the tissue. Samples are first treated with an unlabeled antibody specific for the particular antigen, followed by treatment of the samples with a fluorochrome-labeled antibody specific to the gamma globulin of the first antibody. This last reagent attaches to sites of the specific antibody that has attached to the antigen sites in tissue. The sites of tissue antigen thereby fluoresce and can be detected by fluorescence examination (Table 18-4, *B*). *Sandwich* technics may be used for an *indirect* localization of antibody in tissue (Table 18-4, *C*).

The sample is treated first with an unlabeled dilute solution of an antigen that is specific for the antibody present in the tissue and therefore combines with it. The sample then is treated with a fluorochrome-labeled antibody corresponding to the antigen used. The fluorochrome-labeled antibody attaches to the antigen that has, in turn, attached to the antibody present in the tissue. Fluorescence should therefore appear at the sites of the original antibody location. Another indirect immunofluorescence technic that uses complement also is possible (Table 18-4, *D*).

Sample preparation for immunofluorescence methods

1. The tissue must be *fresh* and *unfixed*. Embed the tissue on Lab Tek OCT and mount on the metal object disc supplied with the cryostat. The tissue should be frozen promptly (snap-frozen) by liquid nitrogen, cooled isopentane, or any other suitable rapid-freezing method. Some cryostats are equipped with freezing attachments. It is very important to freeze the specimen as soon as possible after it is removed from the patient.
2. Usually 5 or 6 tissue sections (4 μm thick) are cut on the cryostat and picked up with room-temperature slides. *Slides made of green glass should not be used in fluorescence work.*
3. Wash the slides in 3 changes of phosphate-buffered saline for a total of 10 minutes at room temperature.
4. Fix the tissue by placing the slides in acetone for 5 to 10 minutes at room temperature *or* in cold 95% ethanol for 10 to 30 minutes at 4° C. The fixation process prevents antigen (or antibody) diffusion, thereby improving localization.

Other fixatives, such as formalin, have been used but are not considered satisfactory. Glutaraldehyde is itself fluorescent and should be avoided when immunofluorescence methods are performed. Paraffin sections have been used in certain studies[7] but are not satisfactory for many antigens.

General staining procedure considerations for immunofluorescence methods

Tissue sections. The staining procedure should be performed immediately, if possible, but usually not later than 24 hours after the sections are cut and fixed. If the staining cannot be performed immediately, store the fixed and dried sections at 0° C or below. Sections that will be kept unstained for prolonged periods should be stored at $-40°$ to $-60°$ C. Long storage of unstained sections causes unwanted autofluorescence, may produce antigen diffusion, and may lessen antigen reactivity.

Tissue blocks. If staining cannot be performed for *very long* periods of time, frozen blocks of tissue should be stored at the lowest available temperature. The frozen blocks of tissue may be cut away from the metal object disc for storage and then remounted on the disc when the sections are to be cut. When frozen blocks of tissue are stored for any length of time, precautions must be taken to avoid desiccation of the tissue and the embedding medium. Wrap the frozen tissue block in Saran Wrap or aluminum foil. Place the frozen wrapped block in a plastic cup that contains a small amount of ice. Seal the cup and store at $-40°$ to $-60°$ C. Tissue blocks may be stored in this manner for months before sectioning and staining.

Staining procedure considerations for direct immunofluorescence methods[8]

Procedural details will vary somewhat depending on the exact stain being performed.

1. Before beginning the procedure, encircle the tissue with a diamond marking pencil to facilitate location of the tissue after the sections are coverslipped.
2. Rehydrate the tissue by placing the slides in 3 changes of phosphate-buffered saline over a 10-minute period at room temperature. This step facilitates subsequent staining.
3. Remove excess fluid from the slide with cotton gauze to prevent dilution of the antiserum in the subsequent step. Remove all the fluid except that contained within the encircled area. The tissue itself *must not be allowed to dry* from this step onward. Drying produces artifacts, primarily because of salt precipitation.
4. Place a few drops of fluorescein-conjugated monospecific antiserum directly on top of the tissue. Place the slides in a moist chamber for 30 minutes to 2 hours at room temperature. (Petri dishes with dampened filter paper in the bottom of the dishes are convenient moist chambers.)
5. Wash the slides with 3 changes of phosphate-buffered saline over a 10-minute period at room temperature. *Thorough washing is critical*, otherwise nonspecific fluorescence will remain in the tissue and the inter-

pretation of the slides will be confused. A minimum of 3 changes of phosphate-buffered saline solution for 10 to 15 minutes each is considered necessary by some labs.

6. Coverslipping. Several mounting media have been used. In all cases, the mounting media should not dissolve fluorescent material and should not be fluorescent. For proper coverslipping, three methods are used commonly:

Method A. Wipe off excess saline from each slide and coverslip by using a buffered glycerol mounting medium. Gelvatrol may also be used and provides a more permanent mount than does the glycerol. Fading does occur in the slides, but storage of the slides in the dark at refrigerator temperature will prolong preservation of the slides.

Method B. Air-dry slides after the last buffer wash and mount in Fluoromount or DPX.

Method C. Rinse slides in distilled water, blot dry, clear in xylene, and mount in New Unimount.[3]

7. Examination of sections. Ideally, slides should be examined almost immediately after coverslipping. If this is not possible, keep the slides cold and away from light until they can be examined. Examine slides by using appropriate exciter and barrier filters. Culling[3] recommends either a Schott BG 12 or a Schott BG 12 and Schott UG 1 combined exciter filter, along with a barrier filter such as Euphos, Zeiss 44, or yellow green GG 9. Antigen-antibody complex sites appear apple green if FITC is the conjugate dye or orange if rhodamine B is the conjugate dye.

Solutions

Phosphate-buffered saline (PBS)

Sodium chloride	55.3 gm
Na_2HPO_4	10.7 gm
$NaH_2PO_4 \cdot H_2O$	4.1 gm
Distilled water	7 liters

pH should be 7.0 to 7.2.

Buffered glycerol mounting medium

Glycerol	9 parts
Phosphate-buffered saline	1 part

pH should be about 8.6; an acid medium will lessen fluorescent staining.

Gelvatrol mounting medium

Gelvatrol (Monsanto, St. Louis)	20 gm
0.14 M saline solution buffered with 0.01 M KH_2PO_4-$Na_2HPO_4 \cdot 12H_2O$ (pH 7.2)	80 ml
Glycerol	40 ml

Agitate for 16 hours. Autoclave for 15 minutes at pressure of 15 pounds.
pH should be between 6 and 7.

Controls for staining specificity

Staining should occur with preparations that contain the desired antigen, and staining should be located at the antigenic sites only. Appropriate *known positive controls* should be included with test cases. In addition, the following controls may be used:

Autofluorescence control. This is an unstained slide that has been treated like the test slide except that it has not been exposed to the antiserum conjugate. Only autofluorescent sites should be visible when viewed with the fluorescence microscope.

Antiserum absorption. Antiserum may be absorbed either *specifically* or *nonspecifically*. In the former case, the conjugated antiserum is absorbed (twice) with its specific antigen and centrifuged. This specifically absorbed antiserum then is used to stain a known positive control slide containing the specific antigen. No fluorescent staining should be seen since there should be no specific antibody in the conjugate to react with the specific antigen in the tissue. Nonspecific absorption means the antiserum is absorbed with an antigen for which the antibody is *not* specific; no antigen-antibody reaction should take place. Normal staining should occur when nonspecifically absorbed antiserum is used to stain the known positive control.

Use of conjugated control serum. There should be no staining if the section is treated with conjugated control antiserum because this antiserum lacks the specific antibody to react with the antigen. If treatment with unconjugated control serum is followed by specific conjugated antiserum, however, staining should then take place.

Blocking test. This test involves pretreating the section with unlabeled antiserum that is specific for the antigen. An antigen-antibody reaction should occur, and all available antigen binding sites should be filled at this step. The second part of the procedure involves staining the treated section with the fluorescent dye–labeled specific antiserum, and, because all antigen sites have been occupied theoretically, no staining should occur. A similar section may be treated with unconjugated control antiserum that lacks the specific antibody to combine with the antigen. This pretreatment then is followed by exposure of the section to the labeled specific antiserum. Staining should occur, since theoretically no binding should have taken place with the control antiserum and the antigenic sites are free to react with the specific antiserum and thereby be visualized.

Fluorescence difficulties

Fading. All fluorescent preparations will fade upon exposure to strong light, especially ultraviolet light. The rate of fading increases with the increased intensity of irradiation; therefore, excitation at a very short wavelength should be avoided. Some workers believe that a certain amount of recovery from fading can occur if, after fluorescence examination, sections are stored in the dark at a cold temperature.

Decreased stain intensity. Control of the solution pH is important: too alkaline a pH can cause antibody dissociation; too acid a pH, especially in the mounting medium, can cause lessened fluorescence.

Autofluorescence and nonspecific fluorescence. These may be caused by dust, tissue debris, pigments, and background material and create problems by interfering with a clear interpretation of the antigen-antibody reaction. Long storage of sections may produce autofluorescence, and diffuse fluorescence is characteristic for certain organs. Some of the causes of nonspecific staining include the presence of unbound fluorochrome, binding of conjugated serum proteins, or the presence of additional conjugated antibodies in the conjugated antiserum.

Some of the following steps may assist in controlling nonspecific fluorescence:

1. Use of high-quality fluorochromes and specific antiserums.
2. Thorough washing of sections at all washing steps.
3. Dilution of the conjugated antiserum to a point at which there is good specific activity but little or no nonspecific activity. Dilutions needed will vary depending on antiserum strength.
4. Purification of the conjugated antiserum: absorption of the conjugated antiserum with tissue powders can purify the antiserum, since this process removes the nonspecific serum proteins that can cause nonspecific fluorescence.[3] Unreacted fluorescent material in the conjugate can be removed by extraction with activated charcoal or by gel filtration.[1,3]
5. Counterstaining. Counterstains have been used to eliminate nonspecific background fluorescence and enhance cellular detail. Two useful methods for counterstaining slides prepared by the direct and indirect immunofluorescence technics are the methyl green method[9] and the methyl green–Eriochrome black (chromogen black) method.[10] The use of methyl green results

in a red fluorescence of the nuclei, and there is no masking of the specific antigen-antibody fluorescence. It is useful for counterstaining fluorescent preparations of kidney, small intestine, and liver biopsies. The methyl green–Eriochrome black combination counterstain is reported to give excellent elimination of background fluorescence; however, fading occurs more quickly with this counterstain than with the methyl green alone. The Eriochrome black counterstain, used alone, is most useful for counterstaining microorganism preparations, especially smears.

Methyl green counterstain[9]

This counterstain may be used following either the direct or indirect immunofluorescence methods. Counterstain after the final wash, just prior to coverslipping, as follows:

1. Place slides in a working solution of methyl green for 5 minutes.
   Working solution
   0.1% methyl green (C.I. 42590)   4 ml
   Phosphate-buffered saline (pH 7.2)   36 ml
2. Wash in buffer for 5 minutes. (Washing on a shaker with slight-to-moderate agitation is best.)
3. Coverslip in buffered glycerol.

Methyl green–Eriochrome black counterstain[10]

Prepare a working solution of methyl green (see preceding directions) and a 1.65% solution of Eriochrome black (chromogen black ETOO) (C.I. 14645) and proceed as follows:

1. Stain slides in methyl green working solution for 5 minutes.
2. Wash slide in buffer on shaker for 5 minutes.
3. Stain in 1.65% solution of Eriochrome black for 10 minutes.
4. Rinse in 3 changes of buffer.
5. Coverslip by using buffered glycerol.

Fluorescence microscope

In addition to the usual requirements for a microscope, a special light source and special filter system are both needed for fluorescence work. See Fig. 18-1.

Light source

As defined previously, a fluorescent substance is one that, upon being excited with short-wavelength radiation (such as ultraviolet light) will emit light of a longer wavelength (visible light). The light source needed in fluorescence work, therefore, should be one that will give off an appropriate short-wavelength light. The two major

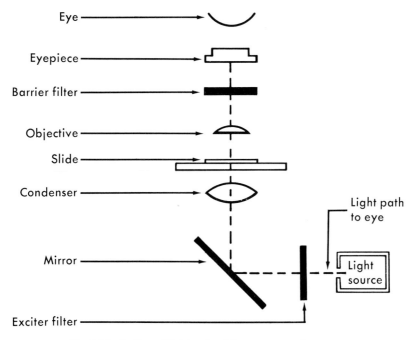

Eye

Eyepiece

Barrier filter

Objective

Slide

Condenser

Light path to eye

Mirror

Light source

Exciter filter

Fig. 18-1. Outline of light path of fluorescence microscope.

Table 18-5. Common illumination sources for transmission fluorescence microscopy

Type	Advantages	Disadvantages
HBO 200 mercury	Intense illumination with over 30% emission at 365 nm; efficient and convenient; does not require water cooling; average life 200 hours; most manufacturers provide this type; good for surface staining of lymphocytes and for immunoglobulin detection	Power unit and replacement burners comparatively expensive; once turned off, lamp cannot be relit until it has cooled; bleaching of fluorescence reaction occurs fairly rapidly because of photochemical destruction of fluorochrome; as lamp gets older, there tends to be a reduction in beam intensity and a resultant decrease in fluorescence excitation
AH4 mercury vapor arc 100 watt (GE)	Adequate for many fluorescent staining methods; average life of bulb 1000 hours	Not good for fluorescent antibody detection
AH6 water-cooled 1000 watt (GE)	Provides the most intense illumination	High internal pressure has to be balanced by a water jacket; this water jacket also cools
Halogen lamps	Convenient and efficient; suitable for most routine applications of fluorescence; control unit and replacement bulbs inexpensive; slow development of photolysis; lamp can be switched on and off and does not need warming-up or cooling-off periods; emits little ultraviolet light; therefore, less autofluorescence of tissue components is apparent	Light emitted may not be bright enough for all immunofluorescence studies

kinds of light sources used are high-pressure mercury vapor lamps and halogen lamps. Some advantages and disadvantages of each are listed in Table 18-5.

Exciter filters

Although the light source used emits short-wavelength light primarily, it does not give off such light entirely, and because of the wavelength variability, an *exciter* filter is needed. This filter is placed between the light source and the reflecting mirror, and its functions are twofold: (1) to allow maximal transmission of the light of the desired wavelength to pass through and to subsequently excite the fluorochrome, and (2) to permit only minimal transmission of undesired wavelength light. The wavelength or wavelengths that are needed are determined by the characteristics of the fluorochrome; for example, with fluorescein conjugates, maximal excitation occurs in the range of 495 nm. The most efficient exciter filters are interference filters, and some are available that transmit 90% of the light up to 490 nm and less than 0.1% of light at 520 nm. Exciter filters can vary in the amount of longer wavelength light that they emit (that is, red end of the spectrum). The undesirable transmission of red light may be controlled by use of a blue glass filter (such as Schott BG 38) of suitable thickness (usually 1 to 2 mm). A further modification to the exciter filter may be useful for examining skin sections. The yellow-green autofluorescence seen when skin sections are stimulated by violet light may be absorbed by interposition of a pale yellow glass Schott GG 475 filter. Heat-absorbing filters (Schott BG 14 [4 mm] or Schott BG 22 [3 mm]) should be placed between the light and other filters to prevent overheating and cracking of the exciter and barrier filters.

Additional exciter filters

2 mm Schott BG 12	Used with dark-ground condenser; transmits 325 to 500 nm; used in many routine fluorescence procedures
4 mm or 6 mm Schott BG 12	Similar to the 2 mm filter above, except used with a bright ground condenser
Schott UG-1	May be used for fluorescent antibody detection when minimal fluorescence is present; transmits 275 to 400 nm
Schott UG-1 with 2 mm Schott BG 12	Combination good for fluorescent antibody work

Balzer FITC	Transmits 90% of light up to 490 nm; less than 0.1% of light at 520 nm; supplement if necessary with Schott BG 38 red-suppression filter

Barrier filters

Fluorescent substances in the specimen become excited by the short-wavelength light that they receive through the exciter filter and emit longer wavelength light. There are now two kinds of light traveling towards the observer's eyes: short-wavelength light from the light source and visible light from the fluorescing specimen. The short-wavelength light (especially if it is ultraviolet light) can cause ocular damage; therefore, another filter, called a *barrier* (or contrast) filter, is needed. These barrier filters are placed in suitable location behind the objective and function to (1) exclude light below a certain wavelength and (2) to allow passage of the longer wavelength light emitted by the fluorescent specimen. In the cases of fluorescein conjugates, the barrier filter should exclude light below 490 nm and maximally transmit light at 525 nm.

Some barrier filters

Yellow Schott OG4; Orange OG5; Zeiss 47 and 50	Use singly or in combination for most fluorescent staining technics
Pale green-yellow Schott GG9; Zeiss 44 or Euphos; Yellow filter Kodak Wratten 12 or Chance 110	Used in fluorescent antibody technics
Schott GG4; Zeiss 41	Used in detection of autofluorescence

Exciter and barrier filters should be combined so that the best excitation range for a particular fluorochrome dye can be chosen and the fluorescence emission selectively transmitted.

Illumination systems

There are presently two systems of illumination that are effective in fluorescence microscopy: dark-field illumination with transmitted light and bright-field epi-illumination. The dark field–transmitted type is most frequently employed, and conventional microscopes can be converted to this type with the proper accessories. The dark-field illumination is accomplished by the use of a cardioid condenser. Enlarging the area for specimen inspection can be accomplished by interposition of a toric lens beneath the condenser. These lenses can be used over a range of objective powers, enable tissue to be inspected and photographed with a low-power objective, and also provide good illumination for critical examination with higher power objectives (40×).

Fluorescence epi-illumination is newer than the transmission type discussed in the previous section. The light source and exciter filter are present and function as they do with the transmission type of fluorescence. The difference with the fluorescence epi-illumination method is that about 80% of the exciting light is reflected by a dichromatic interference filter and passes down the objective to act on the specimen. Emitted light from the specimen passes up the same objective and hits the barrier filter located near the eyepiece. The barrier filter functions as it does in the transmission fluorescence microscope. Fluorescence epi-illumination offers the following advantages: (1) improved excitation efficiency, (2) increased intensity of fluorescence seen with thick specimens, (3) no separate condenser alignments needed since the objective also acts as the condenser, and (4) the technic can be combined with transmitted light technics such as polarization and phase contrast.

Objectives

Initial focusing and scanning are done with a low-power objective (10×). At higher magnifications, fluorescence intensity is enhanced by the use of objectives with a high numerical aperture (n.a.) (for example, 40× apochromat, n.a. 0.90). The increase in apparent brightness can result in doubling titration end points in the fluorescence preparation procedures. These high n.a. objectives can also be fitted with an adjustable iris to minimize flare.

IMMUNOENZYMIC PROCEDURES

As an alternative to fluorescein or other fluorochromes, *enzymes* have also been used for detecting antigens or antibodies. Table 18-6 shows several variations of immunoenzymic staining methods, including enzyme-labeled antibody procedures and unlabeled antibody-enzyme procedures. Although these methods have been studied for some time, they are just now being evaluated for routine use in tissue labs. Consequently, as shown in Table 18-6, there is still confusion concerning terminology of the methods. In addition, such factors as

proper antiserum dilutions, concentrations of enzyme substrates and visualization reagents, and staining times are also quite variable. Several methods are discussed in detail because they show promise for the specific, sensitive localization of antigens (or antibodies) in tissue sections.

Horseradish peroxidase (HRP) is accepted as the most satisfactory enzyme for use, though studies using glucose oxidase, tyrosinase, and acid or alkaline phosphatase also have been described. The enzymic methods offer the following advantages: preparations are permanent, a standard light microscope is used for slide interpretation, and the label is suitable for electron microscopy with modifications in the sample preparation. The major disadvantages include the necessity of an extra step to visualize the enzyme, possibility of false localization because of reaction-product diffusion, and confusion of interpretation because of endogenous enzyme in the sample. Preparation of tissue samples and treatment with conjugate are similar to those procedures described for immunofluorescence methods.

Removal of endogenous peroxidase

The presence of endogenous peroxidase is a problem, especially when fixed tissue is being stained. When frozen sections are used, much of the red cell peroxidase is lost by lysis; its presence in leukocytes is recognizable because of cell morphology. A commonly used method to inactivate endogenous peroxidase requires treatment of the sections with a mixture of methanol and hydrogen peroxide. This procedure does not affect staining of immunoglobulins; however, its effect on the subsequent staining of antigens other than immunoglobulins requires testing.

Method of endogenous peroxidase removal prior to staining of immunoglobulins[11]

1. For paraffin sections, deparaffinize in xylene; rinse in absolute ethanol. Frozen sections should be dried.
2. Treat sections with a fresh 0.5% solution of hydrogen peroxide in methanol for 30 minutes.
3. Rinse sections in methanol.
4. Rinse sections in 3 changes of phosphate-buffered saline to remove all methanol and proceed with the regular demonstration method.

Alternate methods to remove endogenous per-

Table 18-6. Common methods of immunoenzymic staining

1. Enzyme-labeled antibody methods

A. *Direct immunoenzymic staining* with enzyme-labeled specific antibodies

■ = Tissue antigen of species A

□ = Enzyme-labeled antibody from species B specific to antigen of species A

B. *Indirect immunoenzymic staining* with unlabeled and enzyme-labeled specific antibodies (also called "sandwich method")

■ = Tissue antigen of species A

▨ = Antibody from species B specific to antigen of species A

□ = Enzyme-labeled antibody from species C specific to antibody from species B

2. Unlabeled antibody-enzyme methods

A. *Hybrid antibody method* with antibody specific to both antigen and enzyme

■ = Tissue antigen of species A

○ = Enzyme

□ = Hybrid antibody from species B specific to both antigen of species A and enzyme

B. *Indirect immunoenzymic staining* (mixed antibody method; double-antibody method) with specific antibodies and enzyme

■ = Tissue antigen (immunoglobulin) of species A

□ = Antibody from species A specific to enzyme

▨ = Antibody from species B specific to immunoglobulin of species A and antibody of species A specific to enzyme

○ = Enzyme

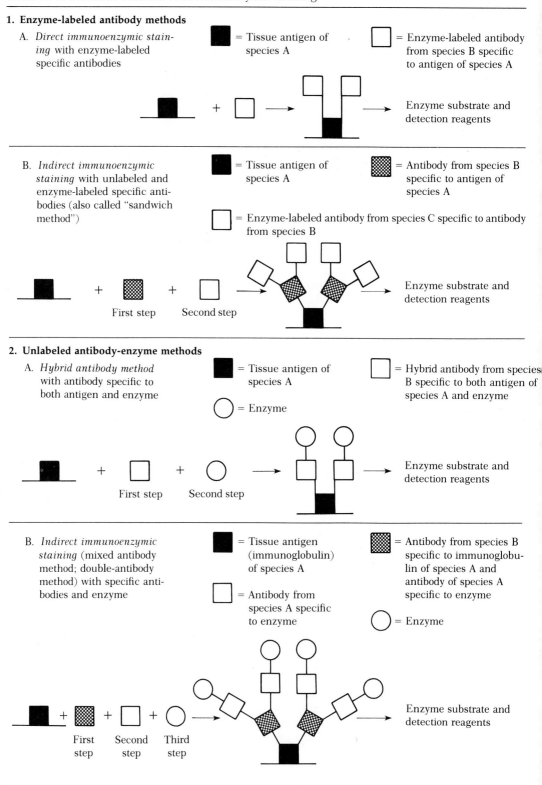

Table 18-6. Common methods of immunoenzymic staining—cont'd

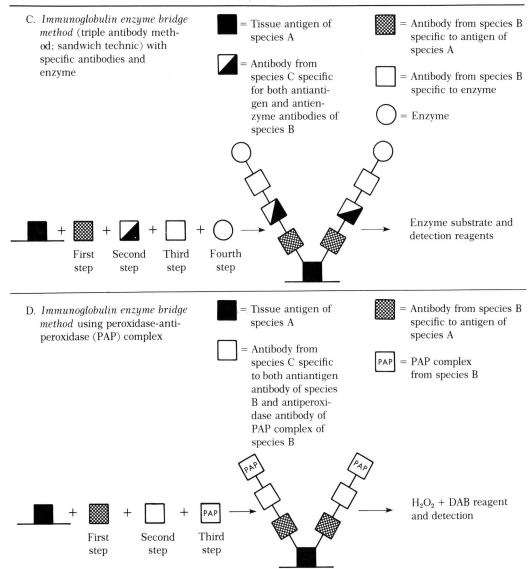

C. *Immunoglobulin enzyme bridge method* (triple antibody method; sandwich technic) with specific antibodies and enzyme

■ = Tissue antigen of species A

◩ = Antibody from species C specific for both antiantigen and antienzyme antibodies of species B

▦ = Antibody from species B specific to antigen of species A

☐ = Antibody from species B specific to enzyme

◯ = Enzyme

First step   Second step   Third step   Fourth step

Enzyme substrate and detection reagents

D. *Immunoglobulin enzyme bridge method* using peroxidase-antiperoxidase (PAP) complex

■ = Tissue antigen of species A

☐ = Antibody from species C specific to both antiantigen antibody of species B and antiperoxidase antibody of PAP complex of species B

▦ = Antibody from species B specific to antigen of species A

PAP = PAP complex from species B

First step   Second step   Third step

H_2O_2 + DAB reagent and detection

oxidase include the use of 0.074% ethanolic hydrochloric acid solution as a fixative (0.2 ml of concentrated hydrochloric acid in 100 ml of ethanol),[12] fixation in 1% sodium nitroferricyanide and 1% acetic acid in methanol.[13] With either of these procedures tissues are treated for 15 minutes at room temperature. Another removal procedure involves room temperature treatment with absolute methanol for 20 minutes followed by 20 minutes in either 0.006% hydrogen peroxide in PBS (unfixed tissue) or 0.0125% hydrogen peroxide in PBS (formalin-fixed tissue).[14] Another method is staining the

endogenous peroxidase prior to the immunostaining; this can produce a reaction product that is a different color from that produced by the benzidine reaction.[15]

Direct immunoenzymic staining method with enzyme-labeled antibody

HRP may be used either as a conjugate with an antibody or as the free enzyme in various direct or indirect immunoenzymic methods. The theory for the direct HRP-labeled antibody immunoenzymic method is as follows (see Table 18-6, *1A*).

1. HRP is covalently linked to the appropriate antibody, and an HRP conjugate is thereby formed.
2. This conjugate is used to stain the tissue or smear sample. If the corresponding antigen is present in the sample, it will form a complex with the antibody to which the HRP is attached.
3. The sample is then treated with a substrate reagent consisting of hydrogen peroxide and 3,3'-diaminobenzidine (DAB). Peroxidase present as part of the antigen-antibody-peroxidase complex will act on its substrate, hydrogen peroxide, to produce water and free oxygen. The free oxygen produced then oxidizes the colorless DAB to give a stable brown reaction product, and positive staining is reported when this brown coloration is observed. The sensitivity of this direct immunoenzymic method is considered to be comparable to fluorescence technics.

Preparation of peroxidase conjugate

A widely used conjugation method is the one-stage glutaraldehyde method[16]; however, this method results in a conjugate of uncertain composition in terms of amount actually conjugated versus amount of unconjugated antibody and enzyme. An additional method for control of the labeling ratio has been described.[17]

Localization of antigens and antibodies in fresh frozen tissue sections or smears by direct immunoenzymic method with HRP-labeled antibody[16]

1. Fix fresh frozen sections or smears for 45 minutes in ethanol-ether (60:40) at 22° C. Alternatively, samples may be fixed for 10 minutes at 4° C with acetone, 95% ethanol, or absolute methanol.
2. Wash slides for 15 minutes in 0.1 M phosphate-buffered saline (PBS), pH 7.2, at 22° C.
3. Incubate samples at 22° C for 3 hours with the HRP conjugate. The optimal working dilution of the conjugate is determined by block titration.
4. Give slides 2 changes of PBS, pH 7.2, for 3 minutes each change.
5. Treat sections with the substrate reagent for 5 to 30 minutes. (Check actual reaction end point by light microscopy, since all tissues may not need this long incubation time.) After the appropriate incubation time, sections are rinsed in distilled water with agitation for 5 minutes, dehydrated, cleared in xylene, and coverslipped with a synthetic mounting medium.

Solutions (based on reference 27)

3,3'-diaminobenzidine (DAB) tetrahydrochloride (Sigma Chemicals or Polysciences, Inc.)
Store this reagent desiccated below 0° C. This reagent is carcinogenic—*handle carefully!* (See below.)

0.05 TRIS–hydrochloric acid buffer, pH 7.6

0.2 M TRIS (tris[hydroxymethyl]-aminomethane)	250 ml
0.1 M hydrochloric acid	325 ml
Distilled water	425 ml

3% hydrogen peroxide

Substrate solution

DAB tetrahydrochloride	25 mg
0.05 M TRIS-hydrochloric acid buffer, pH 7.6	50 ml
3% hydrogen peroxide	0.15 ml

Before use, dissolve the DAB reagent in the buffer. *Immediately* before staining, add the hydrogen peroxide and mix.

Results
Positive staining is brown.

Controls
To detect endogenous peroxidase, another test section should be treated only with the substrate solution. Additional controls include staining with (1) conjugate adsorbed with the corresponding antigen and (2) an unrelated antibody-peroxidase conjugate. No staining should be seen with the latter two solutions.

Precautions and disposal of benzidine solutions

3,3'-diaminobenzidine, like other benzidine-containing compounds, is carcinogenic and should be handled with appropriate care.* Material contaminated with benzidine, such as plastic gloves, should be placed in an approved waste disposal container labeled to indicate the presence of carcinogen. *Do not pour benzidine-containing solutions down the drain.* Solutions of benzidine that are to be discarded should be collected in a sturdy container that has a good closure. An empty 5-gallon alcohol can is suggested. The can must be labeled as containing carcinogens and transported to a company specializing in the disposal of carcinogens. The can is not returnable. Alternatively, contact your safety department for appropriate disposal.

---

*A new *noncarcinogenic* reagent system for demonstrating peroxidase was developed by Hanker, J. S., et al.: Histochem. J. **9**:789, 1977. This new "Hanker-Yates reagent" contains *p*-phenylenediamine and pyrocatechol and may be obtained from Polysciences, Inc., Paul Valley Industrial Park, Warrington, PA 18976. Another *noncarcinogenic* reagent of potential usefulness is 3-amino-9-ethylcarbazole, which was described by Graham, R. C., Jr., et al.: J. Histochem. Cytochem. **13**:150, 1965.

General procedure for indirect immunoenzymic staining of immunoglobulins in paraffin sections of formalin-fixed tissue with HRP-labeled antibody (based on reference 15) (Table 18-6, *1B*)

It has been shown that immunoglobulins in formalin-fixed tissues retain their ability to combine with specific anti-immunoglobulins and that this reactivity lasts for at least 20 years in paraffin-embedded tissue.

Tissue preparation. Fix tissues in 10% formol-saline or 10% neutral buffered formalin. Cut sections 3 to 6 mm in thickness. The thinner the section, the better the results.

Reagents

Monospecific rabbit antiserums to human immunoglobulin IgM, IgG, IgA, kappa and lambda
HRP-labeled anti–rabbit IgG conjugate
Substrate solution (see preceding method)
Mayer's hematoxylin (p. 142)
Determine optimal dilution for use of reagents 1 and 2 by block titrations on positive control human tissue.

Procedure

1. Deparaffinize and hydrate sections to distilled water.
2. Wash in phosphate-buffered saline (PBS) for 3 to 5 minutes.
3. Treat sections with properly diluted rabbit anti–human globulin serum. Allow one section per test case to remain unstained as a control for endogenous peroxidase.
4. Wash in 2 changes of PBS for 5 minutes each change. Use agitation during the washing.
5. Treat sections with properly diluted conjugate (HRP-labeled anti–rabbit IgG conjugate) for 30 minutes.
6. Over a 30-minute period, give slides 3 changes of PBS.
7. Stain for HRP by using the substrate solution described in the previous method. At this point, stain the control slide for endogenous peroxidase.
8. Give slides several changes of distilled water.
9. Counterstain nuclei by using Mayer's hematoxylin (p. 142) for 1 minute.
10. Blue slides in running tap water for 10 to 15 minutes.
11. Dehydrate, clear, and coverslip slides by using a synthetic mounting medium.

Results

Immunoglobulin locations—brown
Endogenous peroxidase sites—brown
Nuclei—blue
The staining of a plasma cell with more than one type of heavy- or light-chain antibody is indication of nonspecific staining, since any one plasma cell synthesizes only one type of immunoglobulin.[15]
Note: Background staining, especially near the edges of the section, may be observed; however, the cause is unknown. This can be reduced or eliminated by treatment of the section with normal serum of the species in which the anti–rabbit IgG was made. Dilute this normal serum 1:5 with PBS for use. This treatment is done after step 2 (previous column) is completed. Drain, but do not wash it off the slides, and proceed with step 3.[11]

Immunoglobulin bridge methods (Table 18-6, *2C*)

These methods with free unconjugated enzymes have been used to demonstrate various tissue antigens including human chorionic gonadotropin,[18] thyroid-stimulating hormone,[19] ACTH-producing cells,[20] and alpha fetoprotein in human fetal liver cells.[21]

HRP is itself antigenic and may be attached to antigen in tissue by specific antigen-antibody reactions. Immunoperoxidase bridge methods to demonstrate an antigen (Ag) in the tissue of species A follow a general staining sequence as below:

1. Solution of anti-antigen (made in species B)
2. Anti–species B antibody (made in species C)
3. Anti-HRP (made in species B)
   Note: Reagent 2 forms an immunoglobulin bridge between reagents 1 and 3
4. HRP antigen

The HRP antigen is bound specifically by the anti-HRP. The presence of the HRP is subsequently demonstrated with the usual substrate solution, and sites containing HRP are colored brown.

Immunoglobulin bridge technic for detection of human chorionic gonadotropin[18]

In this procedure, three immunoglobulin preparations are used, followed by addition of a demonstrable enzyme (HRP) and substrate solution; these components are as follows:

a. Rabbit anti–human chorionic gonadotropin (1:10)
b. Goat anti–rabbit gamma globulin (undiluted)
c. Rabbit antiperoxidase (undiluted)
d. HRP (1.25 mg/dl; type VII in phosphate-buffered saline PBS)
e. Substrate solution: freshly prepared solution containing 30 mg/dl of 3,3'-diaminobenzidine tetrahydrochloride in TRIS-buffered PBS. Immediately before use, 3 drops of 3% hydrogen peroxide are added to 5 ml of the solution.

Procedure

1. Tissues fixed in 10% neutral buffered formalin are dehydrated through graded alcohols, embedded in paraffin, and sectioned serially at 3 μm.
2. Deparaffinize the sections and bring to water.
3. Incubate the rehydrated sections with 2 drops (to cover tissue) of antiserum a for 30 minutes in a moist chamber on a shaker; then drain off excess serum and wash sections for 30 minutes in at least 3 changes of PBS.
4. Incubate the washed sections with 2 drops of antiserum b for 30 minutes in the moist chamber with shaking and wash sections as in step 3.
5. Incubate the washed sections with 2 drops of antiserum c for 30 minutes in the moist chamber with shaking and wash sections as in step 3.
6. Incubate the washed sections with 2 drops of HRP solution d for 30 minutes in the moist chamber with shaking and wash as in step 3.
7. Incubate sections with substrate solution e for 5 minutes at room temperature.
8. Wash the tissue for 10 minutes in PBS, rinse briefly in distilled water, and osmicate for 5 minutes with a few drops of 2% osmium tetroxide (OsO_4) solution. (Osmium serves to stain the reaction product and to counterstain.)
9. Dehydrate the sections, clear, and coverslip in Permount. Reactive cells appear finely granular dark brown–black.

Peroxidase-antiperoxidase methods (PAP methods) (Table 18-6, *2D*)

If whole serum containing anti-HRP is mixed with HRP, a complex is precipitated that can subsequently be dissolved to form a soluble peroxidase-antiperoxidase (PAP) complex. This PAP contains purified anti-HRP. The PAP complex can be used in place of reagents 3 and 4 listed in the general procedures for the immunoglobulin bridge method. Using the PAP complex, the general staining sequence for antigen (Ag) in species A tissue is as follows:

1. Anti-Ag (this reagent made in species B)
2. Anti–species B antibody (made in species C)
3. PAP complex (antiperoxidase raised in species B)

The PAP complex can be prepared by use of animal species other than rabbit (see reference 22 for details). The presence of the HRP is detected with the usual substrate solution, and positive areas appear brown.

A principle advantage of the PAP methods is the increased sensitivity of antigen detection, exceeding that of the direct conjugated method and fluorescence. PAP methods have been used in a number of techniques including those to detect spirochetes,[22] ACTH-secreting cells,[23] prolactin-containing cells,[24] and, lysozyme in Paneth cells.[25]

A more detailed method is as follows:

PAP procedure for solid tissue specimens (based on reference 26)

Reagents

a. 0.2 M TRIS buffer, pH 7.6 (6.6 gm of TRIS, 393 ml of 0.1 M hydrochloric acid, distilled water to 1 liter)
b. TRIS-buffered saline (1 part TRIS buffer added to 9 parts of 0.85% saline)
c. 1% hydrogen peroxide in absolute methanol (freshly prepared)
d. Rabbit antiserum against the antigen to be detected
e. Normal pig serum
f. Pig anti–rabbit IgG
g. Rabbit PAP complex
h. Substrate solution containing 6 mg of 3,3'-diaminobenzidine (DAB) in 10 ml of 0.2 M TRIS buffer (pH 7.6) to which 1 drop of 1% hydrogen peroxide in methanol is added before use.
i. Endogenous peroxidase blocking solution: 0.5% hydrogen peroxide in methanol

Procedure

1. Deparaffinize paraffin sections, rinse in absolute ethanol, and rinse in absolute methanol.
2. Block endogenous peroxidase with fresh solution i for 30 minutes.
3. Rinse sections in solution b for 3 changes, at 2 minutes each change.
4. Reduce nonspecific absorption of pig anti–rabbit IgG by treating sections for 15 minutes with a 1:20 dilution of normal pig serum in TRIS buffer.
5. Drain the diluted normal pig serum from the slide. Do not wash the slide, but treat with the rabbit anti–tissue antigen serum diluted with normal pig serum in TRIS buffer. Stain for 15 to 30 minutes.
6. Repeat step 3 above.
7. Treat with pig anti–rabbit IgG serum diluted 1:20 in normal pig serum in TRIS-buffered saline solution and stain for 15 to 30 minutes.
8. Repeat step 3 above.
9. Treat sections with rabbit PAP complex optimally diluted 1:20 in normal pig serum in TRIS-buffered saline. Stain 15 to 30 minutes.
10. Repeat step 3 above.
11. Add the substrate solution h and treat slides for 4 minutes. Check microscopically.
12. Rinse once in TRIS-buffered saline; wash in tap water for 2 minutes.
13. Counterstain in hematoxylin for 1 minute, differentiate in acid alcohol if necessary, and blue in tap water.
14. Dehydrate, clear, and coverslip slides by using a synthetic mounting medium.

REFERENCES

1. Lillie, R. D., and Fullmer, H. M.: Histopathological technic and practical histochemistry, ed. 4, New York, 1976, McGraw-Hill Book Co.
2. Wilson, M. B.: The science and art of basic microscopy, Bellaire, Texas, 1976, American Society for Medical Technologists, Inc.
3. Culling, C. F. A.: Handbook of histopathological and histochemical techniques, ed. 3, London, 1974, Butterworth & Co. (Pub.), Ltd.
4. Zugibe, F. T.: Diagnostic histochemistry, St. Louis, 1970, The C. V. Mosby Co.
5. Faulk, W. P., and Hitmans, W.: Recent developments in immunofluorescence, Progr. Allergy **16:**9-39, 1972.
6. Johnson, G. D., et al.: Immunofluorescence and immunoenzyme techniques. In Weir, D. M., editor: Handbook of experimental immunology, ed. 3, Chap. 15, Blackwell Scientific Publications. Great Britain. 1978.
7. Dorsett, B. H., and Ioachim, H. L.: A method for the use of immunofluorescence on paraffin-embedded tissues, Am. J. Clin. Pathol. **69:**66-72, 1978.
8. General procedure used at the Department of Pathologic Anatomy, Hospital of the University of Pennsylvania, Philadelphia, Pa.
9. Elbadawi, A., and Schenk, E. A.: Histochemical methods for separate, consecutive, and simultaneous demonstration of acetylcholinesterase and norepinephrine in cryostat sections, J. Histochem. Cytochem. **15:**580-588, 1967, The Histochemical Society, Baltimore, The Williams & Wilkins Co. (agent).
10. Schenk, E. A., and Churukian, C. J.: Immunofluorescence counterstains, J. Histochem. Cytochem. **22:**962-966, 1974, The Histochemical Society, Baltimore, The Williams & Wilkins Co. (agent).
11. Burns, J.: Background staining and sensitivity of the unlabeled antibody-enzyme (PAP) method. Comparison with the peroxidase labeled antibody sandwich method using formalin fixed paraffin embedded material, Histochemistry **43:**291, 1975.
12. Weir, E. E., Pretlow, T. G., Pitts, A., and Williams, E. E.: Destruction of endogenous peroxidase activity in order to locate cellular antigens by peroxidase-labeled antibodies, J. Histochem. Cytochem. **22:**51-54, 1974, The Histochemical Society, Baltimore, The Williams & Wilkins Co. (agent).
13. Straus, W.: Inhibition of peroxidase by methanol and by methanol-nitroferricyanide for use in immunoperoxidase procedures. J. Histochem. Cytochem. **19:**682-688, 1971, The Histochemical Society, Baltimore, The Williams & Wilkins Co. (agent).
14. Streefkerk, J. G. Inhibition of erythrocyte pseudoperoxidase activity by treatment with hydrogen peroxide following methanol, J. Histochem. Cytochem. **20:**829-831, 1972, The Histochemical Society, Baltimore, The Williams & Wilkins Co. (agent).
15. Taylor, C. R., and Burns, J.: The demonstration of plasma cells and other immunoglobulin-containing cells in formalin-fixed, paraffin-embedded tissues using peroxidase labeled antibody, J. Clin. Pathol. **27:**14, 1974.
16. Avrameas, S.: Coupling of enzymes to proteins with glutaraldehyde. Use of the conjugates for the detection of antigens and antibodies, Immunochemistry **6:**43, 1969.
17. Nakane, P. K., and Kawaoi, A.: Peroxidase-labeled antibody: a new method of conjugation, J. Histochem. Cytochem. **22:**1084, 1974, The Histochemical Society, Baltimore, The Williams & Wilkins Co. (agent).
18. Mason, T. E., Phifer, R. F., Spicer, S. S., Swallow, R. A., and Dreskin, R. B.: An immunoglobulin-enzyme bridge method for localizing tissue antigens, J. Histochem. Cytochem. **17:**563-569, 1969, The Histochemical Society, Baltimore, The Williams & Wilkins Co. (agent).
19. Phifer, R. F., and Spicer, S. S.: Immunohistochemical and histologic demonstration of thyrotropic cells in the human adenohypophysis, J. Clin. Endocrinol. Metab. **36:**1210-1221, 1973.
20. Phifer, R. F., and Spicer, S. S.: Immunohistologic and immunopathologic demonstration of adrenocorticotropic hormone in the pars intermedia of the adenohypophysis, Lab. Invest. **23:**543-550, 1970.
21. Nayak, N. C., Das, P. K., Bhuyan, U. N., and Mittal, A.: Localization of α-fetoprotein in human fetal livers: an immunohistochemical method using horseradish peroxidase, J. Histochem. Cytochem. **22:**414-418, 1974, The Histochemical Society, Baltimore, The Williams & Wilkins Co. (agent).
22. Sternberger, L. A., Hardy, P. H., Cuculis, T. J., and Meyer, H. G.: The unlabeled antibody enzyme method of immunohistochemistry. Preparation and properties of soluble antigen-antibody complex (horseradish peroxidase–anti-horseradish peroxidase) and its use in identification of spirochetes, J. Histochem. Cytochem. **18:**315-333, 1970, The Histochemical Society, Baltimore, The Williams & Wilkins Co. (agent).
23. Moriarty, G. C., and Halmi, N. S.: Electron microscopic study of the adrenocorticotropin-producing cell with the use of unlabeled antibody and the soluble peroxidase–antiperoxidase complex, J. Histochem. Cytochem. **20:**590-603, 1972, The Histochemical Society, Baltimore, The Williams & Wilkins Co. (agent).
24. Parsons, J. A., and Erlandsen, S. L.: Ultrastructural immunocytochemical localization of prolactin in rat anterior pituitary by use of the unlabeled antibody enzyme method, J. Histochem. Cytochem. **22:**340-351, 1974, The Histochemical Society, Baltimore, The Williams & Wilkins Co. (agent).

25. Erlandsen, S. L., Parsons, J. A., and Taylor, T. D.: Ultrastructural immunocytochemical localization of lysozyme in the Paneth cells of man, J. Histochem. Cytochem. **22:**401-413, 1974, The Histochemical Society, Baltimore, The Williams & Wilkins Co. (agent).

26. Waller, C. A., and MacLennen, I. C. M.: Analysis of lymphocytes in blood and tissue. In Thompson, R. A., editor: Techniques in clinical immunology, London, 1977, Blackwell Scientific Publications, pp. 170-195.

27. Johnson, G. D., and Dorling, J.: Immunofluorescence and immunoperoxidase techniques. In Thompson, R. A., editor: Techniques in clinical immunology, London, 1977, Blackwell Scientific Publications, pp. 85-115.

CHAPTER 19

Electron microscopy

NAN PILLSBURY

It is difficult in one chapter to cover all the technics required for transmission electron microscopy (TEM) by the electron microscope (EM) histotechnician. The following information will, however, give general information and several specific examples of technics, equipment, and reagents for each step of "normal" processing for specimens from surgical pathology tissues, cells, and fluids. References are cited wherein additional detailed technics and theory may be found for those desiring a more in-depth study and information.

TEM is not considered a speedy method of diagnosis, since it requires several days minimum for results as opposed to frozen section work (an hour or less) or general histology (overnight to 24 hours). It is useful, though, for long-term diseases involving the kidneys, lungs, and tumors among others. Electron photomicrographs offer information and answers to questions such as, Are the basement membranes intact in lungs and kidneys? Are there "blebs" from glomerular loops, and size and type? Are there glomerular deposits present in the basement membrane (as in the case of *lupus erythematosus*)? In tumors it is important to note the presence of tight junctions (desmosomes), tonofibrils, possible virus-like particles (VLP), granular inclusions and types, and whether rings of ribosomes surround larger granules.

Information from TEM in most cases complements that of light microscopy, histochemistry and immunology, and radioautography. It can indicate whether a tumor is malignant. When diagnosis cannot be made from histology by light microscopy alone, electron photomicrographs often can provide the missing piece to the puzzle in order to start therapy and the type of therapy, or to help make the decision whether to operate.

In a small electron microscope laboratory where one to four persons work, results are usually able to be obtained within a week or slightly longer when the number of specimen requests is reasonable. When there is a "rush," and the regular work schedule is abandoned, pictures can be given to the pathologist in 3 days (day 1, fixing and embedding; cure overnight; day 2, thick sections AM, thin sections PM; day 3, scan and take pictures AM, make prints PM).

The methods described present optimal results, that is, cell membranes intact, cytoplasmic structures not displaced and not altered, such as mitochondria with intact cristae, endoplasmic reticulum intact and in place (as are granules and most background substance), and nucleolus and nucleolar material and membranes intact. Fixation times and dehydration procedures are those used where tissue preservation is 90% to 95% that of "research" material but may be completed within 1 day. Where these technics are applied to research, as opposed to clinical tissues, and speed of results is not so crucial, the percent gradation of alcohols may be more gradual over longer periods of time, and curing of the embedding medium may be much slower by use of lower temperatures, even down to room temperature. But, where time is of the essence for diagnosis, the luxury of more time-consuming processing cannot be used. Also, the longer processing time and number of additional solutions may, in themselves, produce artifacts.

FIXATION

Fixation of the sample is the most important step in preparing material for electron microscopy. If more than 15 minutes elapse after excision of a surgical tissue before it is put into fixative, enough autolysis occurs so that an incorrect picture is obtained about the state of the cells in that tissue. Nuclear or cellular membranes may not be intact or are altered, inclusions may break down, mitochondrial cristae may be displaced, blebs may form on the cell surface, ground substance or "background" material may be unevenly dispersed in clumps or destroyed, and many other evidences of cell breakdown that are artifacts of improper fixation.

If it is anticipated that an electron microscope sample is desired, vials containing fixative can be kept in the operating room, or at least in the adjoining utility room. "Zamboni's" fixative[18,20] is stable at room temperature, whereas 2%

glutaraldehyde in phosphate buffer should be kept refrigerated and so should formol-glutaraldehyde combination.[6] Plain formalin (10% formaldehyde of the 37% concentrate) is good for general light histology, but *does not* preserve the tissue so well and is completely unsatisfactory for electron microscopy.

If phosphate-buffered osmium tetroxide is used, a technician must be in a scrub or utility room to mince the tissue in solution immediately after excision. The osmium is not able to penetrate rapidly or a great distance. Hence, if large tissues are placed in osmium tetroxide, only the surface will be fixed and the internal area will have little or no fixation.

The properties of fixatives for electron microscopy are the same as those for light microscopy. These are (1) *speed of penetration* or size of the molecule, (2) *preservation* of tissues and cells, structures, swelling, and shrinkage (carbohydrates, lipids, and proteins must be preserved and intact in situ *without* artifact), and (3) permanent denaturation and stabilization of proteins to make them immobile during further processing but not hardening them.

MORE WIDELY USED FIXATIVES

Zamboni's fixative is a picric acid and paraformaldehyde combination that penetrates fairly rapidly, preserves optimally, and is stable at room temperature for an indefinite period of time.

Paraformaldehyde-glutaraldehyde by Karnovsky (Hayat,[3] p. 340) is sometimes called formaldehyde-glutaraldehyde (F-G) because the paraformaldehyde is dissociated into formaldehyde. The solution seems to penetrate quite rapidly, and little shrinkage of the tissue can be noted. Microtubules are well preserved, but lipid droplets are extracted. It must be kept refrigerated and tends to become too acid if not made up fresh.

2% to 3% glutaraldehyde must be fresh, with pH being checked for acidity. It penetrates slowly but has excellent preservation, particularly of background material. It should not be kept in fixative longer than 2 hours before being postfixed in osmium tetroxide or transferred to gum-sucrose solution, and it must be kept refrigerated. It can be purchased from Polysciences in sealed vials of 8% glutaraldehyde, with pH 7.0 under inert nitrogen to keep stable. Tissues must be washed well in buffer before being postfixed in osmium. Some procedures wash with 13% sucrose overnite and several days with buffer. *Osmium tetroxide, 1% in phosphate buffer,* when once diluted with the buffer, is stable for only a few days in the refrigerator. It is extremely caustic and must be used under fume hood. Heavy metal osmium combines with phospholipids to form a "stain" product. Tissues should be in solution no longer than 1 hour before being washed with buffer.

Ten percent formalin is not satisfactory for electron microscopy work. If tissue has been put into formalin first and electron microscopy work is decided on at a later date, there is little hope of cellular detail if the specimen is left for more than an hour. Even then the morphology and inclusions will most likely be altered beyond satisfactory results for electron microscopy.

Every fixative has properties that make it more desirable than another. You must weigh each in regard to the desirable versus the undesirable properties for your particular laboratory and decide according to the total volume used in a given time, stability of the fixative, general preservation of tissues, whether there is a special interest in lipids, carbohydrates, proteins, and viruses.

FIXATION BY IMMERSION

All tissues taken for electron microscopy samples must be fixed within 15 minutes after excision. Further, they should be minced to 1 ml cubes as soon as possible to ensure proper infiltration and fixation of all portions of the tissue, particularly the slow-penetrating fixatives.

Supplies needed for mincing tissues
Capped, labeled vials containing fixative
  57 × 28 mm for larger tissues, 17 ml capacity, no. 9710-M19 (A. H. Thomas, see Chapter 19 Appendix)
  45 × 15 mm for small samples, 5 ml capacity, no. 9710-D25 (A. H. Thomas)
Sheets of dental wax
One-sided razor or prep blades
Pasteur pipettes with rubber bulbs
Iris forceps (small, thin forceps with fine tips, used for removing tissues from vials and returning after mincing)

Place a large drop of fixative on the dental wax. Remove a piece of tissue from the vial and set into the fixative, making sure that the tissue stays flooded with fixative. While holding the tissue with forceps or pointed bamboo stick, *slice* the tissue into strips from one side to the

other—*do not chop*, because the former way cuts cells apart, whereas the latter forces displacement of fluids and organelles within the cells and tissues. After lengthwise cutting, turn the wax and repeat the procedure crosswise, yielding 1 mm cubed blocks. Return tissue to the fixative in vial. (In case of direct fixation by oxmium tetroxide, the mincing must be done in a fume hood.)

Zamboni's fixative

Zamboni's fixative[18,20] is a good general fixative. It is a picric acid–paraformaldehyde solution that is buffered with phosphate. The solution is stable at room temperature for a year, is not sensitive to light, penetrates rapidly, stabilizes cellular proteins, is not easily destroyed by tissue fluids, and may be used with postosmication.

Besides fixing medium-sized tissues within an hour, it does not cause the tissue material to deteriorate within hours but allows the material to be kept at room temperature indefinitely, and even sent through the mail without the preservation of the surgical specimen being compromised.

Method
Add 20 gm of paraformaldehyde to 150 ml of double-filtered, saturated solution of picric acid. Heat solution to 60° C (waterbath or oven) for 2 hours to dissociate paraformaldehyde into formaldehyde.

Add 2.52% sodium hydroxide (in water) dropwise to alkalize. The solution should be clear.

Filter and allow to cool.

Bring solution to a volume of 1 liter with phosphate buffer. The PAF fixative should have a final pH of 7.3 and an osmolarity of 900 mOsm. (The range of osmolarity can be adjusted from 600 to 900 to give satisfactory results with tissue fixation. Tests should be made to determine what is satisfactory for your particular work.)

Phosphate buffer for Zamboni's fixative

3.31 gm of $NaH_2PO_4 \cdot H_2O$ (monobasic sodium phosphate)
33.77 gm of $Na_2HPO_4 \cdot 7H_2O$ (dibasic sodium phosphate)
or
17.88 gm of Na_2HPO_4
Dissolve salts in 1 liter of distilled water.

Procedure for Zamboni's fixation
1. Place tissue in vial containing Zamboni's fixative. Must be fixed within 15 minutes after removal from patient.
2. Mince specimen into 1 mm cubes as described.
3. Fix in solution for 1 hour minimum before post-

osmication and embedment. (May be left indefinitely at room temperature with little tissue deterioration.)

4. Rinse for 15 minutes in phosphate-buffered saline solution (PBS).

5. Postfix for 1 hour in osmium tetroxide, using procedure under osmium fixation, prefixed specimens.

6. Follow schedule for embedding procedure for Epon.

Glutaraldehyde

Glutaraldehyde by itself is an unstable substance. Upon standing, the pH decreases because of breakdown by oxidation. It is recommended, therefore, that vials in either 8%, 25%, or 70% concentration sealed under inert nitrogen be used. They are convenient; simply make up as much as you need and the pH 7.0 is maintained. The purification of glutaraldehyde can be done, but it is long and tedious. For a small laboratory, time is one of the most important ingredients in an efficiently run department. The solutions in the vials can be diluted easily a short while before use by the phosphate buffer (commonly Millonig's).

The percent concentration of working glutaraldehyde varies with the needs of the laboratory. More commonly, the range is 2% to 4%, with 3% being adequate in most cases, though Hayat[3] prefers higher concentrations.

The time of fixation varies from 0.5 hr for small specimens, to 2 hours maximum. The specimen vials are kept refrigerated during the fixation process. The solution may be changed several times during fixation, and swirl the vials to make sure that fresh solution is in contact with the tissue specimen at all times.

Millonig's buffer[10]

Solutions

A. 13.56 gm of $NaH_2PO_4 \cdot H_2O$ 300 ml
(monobasic)

B. 15.36 gm of NaOH in distilled   300 ml
water

C. 32.4 gm of sucrose   300 ml

D. In a 500 ml volumetric flask make working solution D: 207.5 ml of solution A and 42.5 ml of solution B

Discard 25 ml of solution D. Add 25 ml of solution C. Bring total volume to 500 ml. with distilled water; pH should be between 7.2 and 7.4. Use this solution to dilute concentrated glutaraldehyde.

Procedure for glutaraldehyde fixation

1. Place tissue sample in refrigerated vial containing 2% to 3% glutaraldehyde (or layer over cellular pellet in centrifuge tube for isolated cell

sample). Must be fixed within 15 minutes after removal from patient.

2. Mince specimen into 1 mm cubes as previously described. Glutaraldehyde penetrates rather slowly, and blocks must be small to ensure thorough fixation.

3. Fix for one half to 2 hours in the refrigerator. Change solution 2 to 4 times and swirl vials to ensure fresh fixative being near the tissue.

4. Rinse in Millonig's buffer, pour off (decant), and leave in buffer at 3 changes of 15 minutes each (some laboratories prefer longer washes). (If you do not wish to embed immediately, you may transfer the tissues to gum sucrose after using the buffer. Store in the refrigerator. Good results have been reported from tissues stored several months.)

5. Postfix for 1 hour in osmium tetroxide (OsO_4) using procedure for osmium tetroxide fixation, prefixed specimens (p. 332).

6. Follow embedding procedure for Epon.

Gum sucrose

This solution is used for storage of electron microscopy samples as well as those for histochemistry. The volume that is prepared depends on the amount used in the laboratory. A minimal volume would be 100 ml. The base is 1% gum arabic; the sucrose concentration depends on the use.

Storage: 0.88 M (30%) sucrose with 1% gum arabic

Additive for incubation medium: 0.25 M (8.5%) sucrose with 1% gum arabic

Heat distilled water on stirrer hot plate. Add sucrose. Leave until crystals have dissolved. Slowly add gum arabic and continue to heat and stir until gum arabic has dissolved. Cool and store in refrigerator.

Formol-glutaraldehyde

Since formaldehyde penetrates rather rapidly but does not preserve the tissue well, and glutaraldehyde fixes well but does not penetrate very fast, combinations of these fixatives have been used, using a buffer for their diluent. One of the more popular F-G fixatives is that of Karnovsky.[6]

Stock solution

Paraformaldehyde   2 gm

1 M sodium hydroxide (NaOH)   2 to 4 drops

50% or 10 ml of 25% glutaraldehyde   5 ml
(Check pH, which should be between pH 6.8 and 7.5.)

0.2 M cacodylate buffer, pH 7.4   20 ml

Sodium cacodylate buffers

0. 1 M

Sodium cacodylate   4.28 gm

Calcium chloride (CaCl$_2$)   25 mg
0.2 N hydrochloric acid   2.5 ml
Dilute to 200 ml with distilled water, pH 7.4.
0. 2 M
Sodium cacodylate   8.56 gm
Mix as above. Adjust pH to 7.4 with hydrochloric acid.

The original formula also uses 0.025 gm of calcium chloride, but in our laboratory the solution is more satisfactory without the calcium.

Preparation

Mix the paraformaldehyde with 25 ml of distilled water in a 125 ml Erlenmeyer flask. Heat at 60° C on a stir plate to dissociate the paraformaldehyde to formaldehyde. When moisture forms on the sides of the flask, add sodium hydroxide and stir until the solution clears. Cool solution under the faucet. Filter and add glutaraldehyde and 0.2 M cacodylate buffer. The pH should be 7.2 to 7.4.

Working solution

Dilute 1 : 4 with 0.1 M sodium cacodylate buffer to obtain an osmolarity of over 500 mOsm.
Dilute 1 : 2 for osmolarity over 700 mOsm.

Procedure for formol-glutaraldehyde fixation

1. Place tissue sample in refrigerated vial with formol-glutaraldehyde solution. Must be fixed within 15 minutes after removal from patient.
2. Mince specimen into 1 mm cubes as described, and return vial to refrigerator.
3. For general tissues, fix for 1 hour minimum, with 2 to 3 hours being preferable. May be left overnight with few adverse effects.
4. Rinse *well* in 0.1 M sodium cacodylate buffer, 3 changes of 15 minutes each minimum. (Any residual fixative reacts with osmium when postfixing is done.)
5. Postfix for 1 hour in osmium tetroxide, using procedure for osmium tetroxide fixation, prefixed specimens (p. 332).
6. Proceed to embedding procedure for Epon.

Glutaraldehyde purification

If you do not have vials of glutaraldehyde available, and the pH of the solution is less than 3.5, then it must be "purified."

Mix the old glutaraldehyde with activated charcoal (Norit A, or EX). Let it settle for a week at 4° C. Filter through a Buchner funnel with Whatman filter paper no. 50. Filter again through a Millipore filter (Solvinert, 0.25 mm pore size). The pH should have risen to greater than 5.0. A better quality is achieved with 25% glutaraldehyde.

Osmium tetroxide

Osmium tetroxide was first introduced by Palade in 1952. The buffer he used was Michaelis' barbital (Veronal) acetate buffer at pH 7.4.[3] This system cannot be used with formaldehyde because the reaction between sodium barbital and formaldehyde does not allow buffering capacity up in the pH range of 7.2 to 7.5. More commonly, phosphate-buffered saline (PBS) is used for the working solution of osmium tetroxide.

Some laboratories use a uranyl acetate wash after osmication before dehydration for embedding. It is believed to stabilize proteins and seems to be effective in fixation of membranes. It can, however, make glycogen and other components unstainable. For description, see Glauert.[2]

Phosphate-buffered saline

In a 1000 ml volumetric flask or a 1000 ml graduate (smaller if your laboratory uses small amounts), put the following chemicals:
Monobasic sodium phosphate   0.663 gm
  (NaH$_2$PO$_4$ · H$_2$O)
Dibasic sodium phosphate   4.04 gm
  (Na$_2$HPO$_4$ · 7H$_2$O)
Sodium chloride   8.78 gm
  (NaCl)
Add distilled water to make 1000 ml. The pH should be 7.4. Use 1 N hydrochloric acid, if too alkaline, or 1 N sodium hydroxide, if too acid, and adjust the pH to proper value.

Stock osmium tetroxide

1. To make 50 ml of a 2% solution, clean a sealed ampule of 1 gm of OsO$_4$ with soap and water, *rinse well* with distilled water.
2. IN A FUME HOOD, boil osmium ampule for 15 minutes in distilled water (osmium tetroxide melts).
3. Break OsO$_4$ vial after tapping top to make sure all of the chemical is in the base of the vial. Place opened vial with OsO$_4$ in beaker with 50 ml of hot distilled water. Using forceps (preferably Teflon coated), rinse osmium out of vial and discard vial.
4. Transfer to glass-stoppered brown bottle, seal with cover of Parafilm, and store in the refrigerator. To keep fumes from reacting with the interior of the refrigerator, place bottle in paper towel–lined 1000 ml beaker, and seal with cover of Parafilm.

Working osmium tetroxide

Just before osmication of tissue specimens, prepare a 1% solution of OsO$_4$ by mixing equal amounts of PBS and 2% OsO$_4$. Make up only the amount that is needed, since the phosphate in the buffer tends to

COMMONLY USED FIXATIVES FOR ELECTRON MICROSCOPE SPECIMENS RECEIVED FROM SURGICAL PATHOLOGY

Fixative	Advantages	Disadvantages
Zamboni's	Stable at room temperature for up to 1 year Not sensitive to light Penetrates rapidly Stabilizes cellular proteins Not easily destroyed by tissue fluids May be used without postosmication Tissue not destroyed if left in fixative for several days or longer	Some background substances not finely preserved Lysosomes and some granules not always well preserved
2% to 3% glutaraldehyde	Excellent preservative of all protein Preserves organelles and inclusion granules well Histochemical reactions may be performed on postfixed specimens	Tends to cause shrinkage of both cell and nucleus Penetrates quite slowly—faster than osmium but slower than formaldehyde Must be kept refrigerated Breaks down rapidly Becomes too acid on standing Must wash in buffer for from 3 hours to overnight before postfix or embed
Formol-glutaraldehyde	Penetrates quite rapidly Preserves proteins better than formalin alone	Must be kept refrigerated Glutin breaks down easily

Formaldehyde, 10% of concentrated. Not advised for electron microscopy. Although it penetrates rather rapidly, the poor preservation of the fine protein and the breakdown of cellular organelles and membranes make this fixative unsuitable for electron microscopy.

Buffered osmium tetroxide (OsO_4)	Preserves tissue moderately well Still reacts with phospholipids after glutaraldehyde fixation Can be used alone or after other fixatives	Penetrates slowly Fumes *caustic* to membranes; MUST BE USED UNDER HOOD Readily breaks down in buffer; therefore make up stock in distilled water

make the solution deteriorate and form a precipitate. It can be kept up to 3 days in the refrigerator normally, but a longer period is not advisable.

Procedure for osmium tetroxide fixation

Fresh specimens
1. Place tissue sample into vial containing 1% osmium tetroxide in PBS (diluted just prior to use).
2. *Under a hood,* mince tissue into 1 mm cubes as described.
3. Fix for 1 hour in hood.
4. Rinse briefly with PBS and proceed to embedding procedure for Epon.

Prefixed specimens
1. Briefly rinse in phosphate buffer for osmium phosphate and draw off solution.
2. *Under a hood,* add 1% osmium tetroxide in phosphate buffer to vial.
3. Fix for 1 hour in hood.
4. Rinse briefly with PBS and proceed to embedding procedure for Epon.

EMBEDDING

Transmission electron microscopy (TEM) requires very thin sections (50 to 90 nm) in order for the electrons to penetrate and allow photons to reach the fluorescent viewing screen of the electron microscope. Paraffin is much too soft to permit intact ultrathin sections to be cut. The epoxy resins are the choice of a "routine" TEM laboratory. They are relatively easy to handle and are available from a number of manufacturing sources.

There are three basic types of embedding media used in most TEM laboratories. Those with an Araldite base, those with an Epon 812 base, a mixture of the two, and an epoxy plastic ERL 4206. In recent years, the Epon 812 base was most common. In the spring of 1978, however, the major manufacturer of Epon 812 discontinued its production. Laboratories stocked up while experimenting with the other two sub-

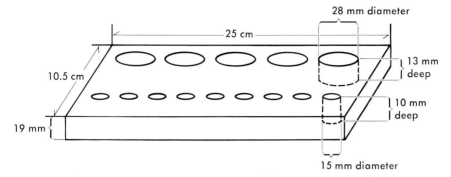

Fig. 19-1. Block for holding vials during dehydration for embedding.

stances to get comparable results. In the fall of 1978, Polysciences, Inc., began making Epon 812. The methods and formulas will be given for all resin mixtures.

VIAL BLOCK USED DURING DEHYDRATION

Vials used for electron microscopy fixation and dehydration are usually quite shallow. Racks for test tubes and other containers are usually too deep, and most often the spaces do not accommodate the size of the vials.

For our laboratory, I have designed an inexpensive and useful device that can be used for our large and small vials during dehydration. The container is made from a board of compressed hardwood strips $10 \times 5 \times 25$ cm (a length of regular wood with the same dimensions can be substituted). One side has a row of 5 wells drilled 13 mm deep with a drill bit 28 mm in diameter. The other side has 10 wells 10 mm deep with a drill bit 15 mm in diameter (Fig. 19-1). Both sized vials fit snugly while at the same time having their caps and openings remaining accessible for changing solutions. The entire block with vials may be placed in the oven during infiltration of the embedding medium and block curing.

EMBEDDING CAPSULES

BEEM capsules are small polyethylene containers used for embedment of electron microscope samples. They have preshaped pyramid tips, which aid in specimen orientation and greatly reduce the time required for block trimming. Most laboratories use the 00 size with caps.

There are BEEM trays that will accommodate 22 of the size 00 capsules per tray. The trays and capsules are available from most general suppliers. A cardboard lid or bottom from a film plate box with punched capsule-sized round holes may be used as a temporary container for capsules.

Conical and bottleneck-shaped tipped BEEM capsules are also available. They allow centrifugation of cell samples right in the capsule. Smaller sizes of BEEM capsules and matching trays with smaller holes, as well as flat embedment molds for specialized samples, can be purchased from several suppliers.

Number 00 gelatin capsules (Lilly) are comparable in size to the 00 BEEM capsules. These contain rounded tips only, and so more initial trimming is needed to prepare the block for sectioning. Varying sizes of gelatin capsules are also available.

Gelatin must be carefully and quickly soaked off in warm water so that the Epon 812 does not soften during soaking. If it softens, it may not return to hardness even after additional curing in the oven. A second pitfall of gelatin capsules is that they sometimes buckle during block curing in the oven.

LABELING

Each block must have its own identifying label, not just a specimen number. When more sections are desired from a particular block, there must be no question about which block was originally used. Many trimmed block tips have a similar size and shape.

Four to 6 mm wide strips can be cut from a piece of typing paper or a 6×9 inch scratch pad, being left attached about 1 cm from the end. The specimen number can be written with a no. 2 pencil within a distance of 25 to 27 mm, or the inside circumference of the capsule. (The number can be typed on uncut sheets also.) Each capsule should have a separate block number, such as 54321-*1*, or 54321-2. Five to nine blocks are usually adequate for routine samples—more for specials. Some laboratories also add the date beneath the number, but that requires a wider strip of paper, which may be bothersome during embedding.

The individual label of 4 × 26 mm can be rolled around the pencil tip with the block number end on the outside. The strip is then inserted into the top of the capsule about 1 to 2 mm from the top. As the paper unrolls, the pressure against the sides of the capsule holds it in place.

EMBEDDING MIXTURES
Araldite formulas

Araldite is a resin that is relatively stable under electron bombardment, is readily soluble in ethanol and acetone, and has replaced the less-stable water-miscible resins such as Durcupan, which gave great difficulty in getting thin sections.[3,7] The two commonly used formulas are those of Glauert and Glauert[2] and Luft.[8]

Glauert and Glauert's formula (1958)

Araldite CY212 (epoxy resin)	10 ml
DDSA (dodecenyl succinic anhydride; another trade name, HY964) (hardener)	10 ml
DMP-30 (2,4,6-tridimethylaminomethyl phenol; also DY064) (accelerator)	0.5 ml
DBP (dibutyl phthalate)	1 ml

In 48 hours mixture sets at 48° C (or overnight, 60° C). If harder blocks are desired, reduce amount of dibutyl phthalate. Amount of accelerator (DY064) is critical—if too much is added, the block becomes hard and brittle.

Luft's Araldite formula (1961)

Araldite 502	27 ml
DDSA	23 ml
DMP-30	0.75 to 1 ml

If the resin and hardener are warmed to 60° C before mixing, their viscosity is decreased. The mixture can be stirred by a glass rod (or Teflon helix on a mechanical rotator) in a warmed graduated cylinder. It can also be shaken in a capped polyvinyl container and placed open in a desiccator under vacuum until the bubbles have dispersed and the resin is clear.

Embedding schedule for Araldite

1. Dehydrate specimens in 2 changes of 70% ethanol of 15 and 5 minutes, respectively. 3 changes of 95% ethanol at 10 minutes each. 3 changes of absolute ethanol at 10 minutes each.
2. Place in propylene oxide for 3 changes at 10 minutes each.
3. Place in a 1:1 mixture of propylene oxide (PO) and Araldite. Swirl gently to be sure mixture surrounds all blocks with no air pockets. Leave 1 hour at room temperature.
4. Add an equal volume of Araldite mixture and leave 3 to 6 hours or overnight at room temperature.
5. Remove propylene oxide and Araldite mixture and replace with Araldite and accelerator only for 24 hours at room temperature.
6. Place small amount of embedding medium into BEEM capsules so that the level is slightly above the bend at the base.
7. Insert specimen block to center and fill capsule to top with Araldite mixture. Be sure there are no bubbles, particularly at the "tip" of the capsule.
8. Capsules may be placed in curing oven overnight at 60° C. (A longer time is preferred by those who believe slower curing produces a more uniform hardness. In this case, the capsules are left at room temperature or 35° C overnight or 24 hours. Then they are placed in a 48° C incubator for 12 to 24 hours and finally 12 hours at 60° C.)

Luft's Epon mixture (1961)
Original formula

Mixture A	
Epon 812	62 ml
DDSA	100 ml
Mixture B	
Epon 812	100 ml
NMA (nadic methyl anhydride)	89 ml

Final or working mixture

70:30 of mixtures of A and B
0.15 ml of DMP-30 for every 10 ml total volume
The hardness may be increased if one uses less of mixture B, and it may be made less hard if one adds mixture B; for example, a 30:70 mixture of A and B would be much less hard than a 70:30 final mixture. The amount of DMP-30 is uniform for all mixtures.

Formula variation

DDSA	43 ml
Epon 812	43 ml
NMA	14 ml
DMP-30	1.5 ml

For any mixture, the ingredients must be mixed *very well*. Two ways are as follows:

Add all ingredients of working mixture to a 100 ml polyethylene cup with sealed cap. Shake vigorously for 5 to 10 minutes until entire mixture is evenly dispersed. The large amount of bubbles generated must be eliminated. If you leave it sitting, the process is relatively slow. A quicker method is to place in a desiccator attached from the lid sleeve to a vacuum outlet. Once the bubbles mostly rise to the top, turn the sleeve for "cutoff" to maintain vacuum, but not so much that the Epon will bubble up and over the top of the polyethylene container.

Once clear, the Epon may be drawn up into 5 and 10 ml disposable plastic syringes with plain tip (*not* Luer lock) for easy dispensing into BEEM capsules during embedment. Epon that is not used may be frozen for later use. Thaw Epon to room temperature before use.

The second mixing method involves a Teflon α-helix attached to the stirring shaft of a small pump. The Epon mixture should be in a wide 100 ml graduate. Let stir at medium speed for 15 to 20 minutes. When stirring is completed, *carefully* pour into a 250 ml beaker (so that there are no bubbles) and draw up into 5 and 10 ml syringes as above.

Embedding procedure for Epon

1. After osmication of tissue blocks, rinse in phosphate buffer used for oxmium tetroxide solution for 5 to 10 minutes.
2. 70% ethanol, 15 and 5 minutes, respectively (Second alcohol may be left overnight in the refrigerator. Rinse briefly in fresh 70% ethanol before continuing dehydration.)
3. 3 changes of 10 minutes each in 95% ethanol.
4. 3 changes of 10 minutes each in absolute ethanol.
5. 3 changes of 10 minutes each (or 2 changes of 20 minutes) in propylene oxide.
6. One hour in 1 : 1 propylene oxide–Epon mixture for 1 hour in 60° C oven. Caps should be off vials to drive off PO and aid in infiltration of the Epon.
7. Embed in BEEM capsules, using Epon mixture. Fill capsules slightly above bend, place specimen in center, and fill with Epon. Recenter specimen with broken applicator stick point if necessary (*careful*—don't puncture capsule tip).
8. Place capsule tray in 60° C oven. Check specimen orientation after 20 minutes and adjust with point of broken orange stick or dissecting needle. Leave 14 to 17 hours, depending on hardness of blocks desired.

Epon 812—Araldite 502 mixture

Stock mixture

Epon 812	31 ml
Araldite 502	25 ml
Dibutyl phthalate	4 ml

Final embedding mixture

Stock	8 ml
DDSA	20 ml
DMP-30	28 drops
	and multiples of this mixture

Mix thoroughly as in plain Epon instructions. If ingredients separate before use, remix just before embedment.

Use the same embedding procedure as in Epon 812.

The Epon-Araldite mixture is believed to be less brittle and harder than the Epon alone.

Spurr's mixture[17] (see Hayat,[3] p. 161)

ERL 4206 was introduced as embedding medium by Spurr for electron microscopy. It possesses the lowest viscosity (7.8 centipoises) of all known plastics in electron microscopy, a property that facilitates rapid penetration into tissues. Since ERL 4206 is miscible with ethanol, it does not require a clearing solvent such as propylene oxide (PO) after ethanol dehydration.

Spurr formula

ERL 4206 (vinyl cyclohexane dioxide)	10 gm
DER 736 (diglycidyl ether of poly-propylene glycol)	6 gm
NSA (nonenyl succinic anhydride)	26 gm
S-1 (dimethylaminoethanol)	0.4 gm

The hardness may be varied by a change in the proportion of the flexibilizer, DER 736. An increase in DER 736 will result in a softer block. An increase in accelerator S-1 will result in increased viscosity and the rate of polymerization.

SECTIONING

Electron microscopy for an anatomic or surgical pathology department makes use of two types of sectioning—thick and thin. The thick (between 0.5 and 2 μm) are used to study the allover picture of the tissue. Also, the area of interest, such as a glomerulus in a kidney biopsy, can be located, and the larger tissue may be subtrimmed to just the area of interest. In this way, more sections may fit on one grid and permit better study without changing grids. These sections are cut with glass knives.

Thin sections run from 50 to 90 nm and from gray to buff in reflected light colors. These are cut with diamond knives if the laboratory can afford them. Fresh (within half a day to overnight at the longest) glass knives may also be used to cut thin sections. If there is only a short while between work processing, however, there is no

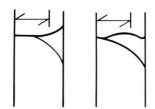

Fig. 19-2. Glass knife-edge shapes indicating optimal cutting area for electron microscope blocks. (After Hayat, M. A.: Principles and techniques of electron microscopy, New York, 1970, Van Nostrand-Reinhold Co.)

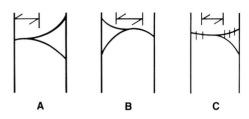

Fig. 19-3. Problem knife-edges with cutting areas too small to be useful. **A,** Curve deflection too extreme, leaving only short cutting area. **B,** Only center portion usable because of double curve. **C,** Large nicks in edge leave narrow distance for sectioning.

time to make fresh glass knives. The diamond knife can easily be mounted, and one can begin cutting immediately for as long as there is time.

PREPARATION OF GLASS KNIVES

The most convenient and time-saving way to produce glass knives is on an *LKB* Knifemaker.* When adjusted properly, this equipment also yields a larger number of more accurate and usable knives. The money saved by less glass being used eventually pays for the machine.

Those needing instructions on making glass knives are referred to (Hayat,[3] p. 190; Kay,[7] p. 220; and Pease,[14] p. 149). These books give specific details, diagrams, and pictures for handbreaking glass knives.

Glass strips may be purchased from LKB in 25 × 400 mm, 6.4 mm thick (30 strips per package); 38 × 400 mm, 6.4 mm thick (20 strips/pkg.); and the 1978 addition of 25 × 400 mm, 10 mm thick (18 strips/pkg.). Polaron* also has glass strips.

Once the glass knives are broken, the edges must be inspected under the microscope at 40× to 50× magnification to check suitability for cutting acceptable sections, both thick and thin. Ideally, the knife has no small nicks along the cutting edge, and only a slight deflection up on the right (Fig. 19-2, *A*) or a slightly convex shape (Fig. 19-2, *B*).

If the deflection is extreme (Fig. 19-3, *A* and *B*) or the edge contains too many nicks (Fig. 19-3, *C*), the cutting area will be very small or unacceptable.

Using a glass knife with large nicks for thick sections may score the block surface so deeply that later thin sections may be difficult or impossible to obtain without slits in them.

*See p. 345.

TROUGHS OR "BOATS"

To use a glass knife for electron microscopy, one must construct a trough around the cutting edge. This provides an area for sections to float on a liquid surface until they are picked up for a slide or grid.

Metal boats made from aluminum, brass, or other metal are available commercially (Fullam* lists Metal Boat No. 5381, 3/pkg.) and may be reused (Fig. 19-4, *A*). Black insulating tape or photographic binding tape cut 8 to 10 mm × 30 mm can be shaped easily to fit around the cutting edge or a glass knife as a "loop trough." The top side of the boat must be a tape edge (from the roll) and must be parallel. If the sides are skewed, the fluid can tilt to one side, making sections aggregate and overlap so that pickup is made difficult or impossible. Cut off excess tape (Fig. 19-4, *B*). Both kinds of boats (troughs) are secured to the knife when a high melting-point wax, such as dental wax, is heated and applied around the bottom edge of the trough. (Paraffin and beeswax can be used also.)

One easy method of application is as follows: Heat the flat end of a weighing spatula over an alcohol lamp, touch a strip of wax to the heated surface, and apply melted wax around the bottom edge of the boat (Fig. 19-4, *C*). Check whether the boat is watertight. If not, heat spatula and touch to the wax on the knife so that it will mold and secure the seal.

KNIFE STORAGE

Once manufactured, the knives with the plastic tape may be stored in a hand-made cardboard box or an LKB knife container. The boxes can be made from empty histology slide boxes of electron microscope plate boxes; the type is the same (Fig. 19-5).

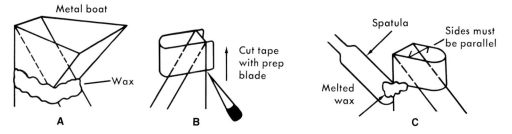

Fig. 19-4. A, Mounted metal boat (trough) on glass knife. **B,** Tape trough on glass knife. Affix tape by pressing one end on left side of knife, turn knife 180 degrees, and press other end to right side, making sure top sides of boat are parallel. **C,** Application of wax for seal.

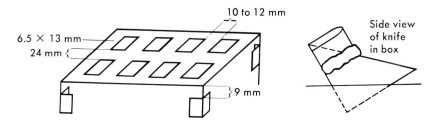

Fig. 19-5. Glass knife storage box. Small cardboard pieces on corner prevent box cover from touching knives.

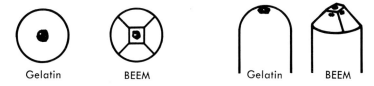

Fig. 19-6. Comparison of gelatin and BEEM capsule shapes with tissue orientation.

TRIMMING BLOCKS

The majority of electron microscope laboratories presently use polyethylene BEEM capsules for embedment. A few still use or prefer gelatin capsules rather than polyethylene.

The pyramidal tip of the BEEM type is easier to use than that of the gelatin since the latter is round bottomed and has to be shaped much more extensively during block trimming. BEEM conical and bottleneck-shaped tips for centrifuged small samples need very little trimming because the blocks are oriented at the tip (Fig. 19-6).

Correct embedment finds the tissue centered at the tip of the block with no surrounding bubbles next to the tissue.

The gelatin can be soaked off in very warm water, but DON'T leave the block in the water—Epon can absorb water and that would ruin the tissue by becoming permanently softened.

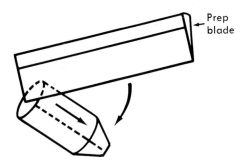

Fig. 19-7. Method of removal of block from BEEM capsule.

BEEM capsules are easily removed by a one-sided razor or prep blade, cutting from top to tip (Fig. 19-7). You must pinch the block tightly while cutting to prevent its slipping and possibly wounding your fingers. You may prefer to hold the top with pliers while making the top-

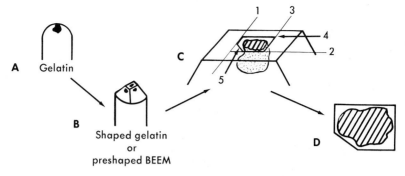

Fig. 19-8. Steps in trimming Epon block.

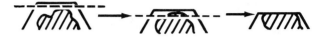

Fig. 19-9. Slide view of "facing" block surface before sectioning.

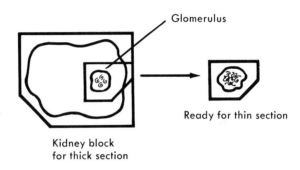

Fig. 19-10. Area from block for thick section subtrimmed for thin sectioning.

to-bottom slit. The cut releases the block from the mould, and the block will pop out when the two sides of the cut are separated.

Since the working area and tissues are so small, a dissecting scope (stereoscopic with variable zoom) should be used for block trimming. Some ultramicrotomes contain a trimming device, but many technicians complain about the lack of preciseness, particularly if the tissues are tilted.

Stands for trimming blocks for electron microscopy are available from DuPont Instruments–Sorvall (Wilmington, Del.). They contain a base that secures a block holder or chuck on a ball joint, tightened by a screw ring. The block per se is held within a collet (ring), available with openings of different diameters to hold varying-sized blocks.

Homogeneous tissues such as liver or muscle may be trimmed to a small size (Fig. 19-8, *A* to

C), and thin sections prepared immediately. Pathologic or specialized tissues such as tumors and kidneys must have thick (1 to 2 μm) sections prepared first for identification of the area of interest. The block is then subtrimmed around that area (Fig. 19-10).

For thick sectioning, a slight collar of Epon should be left around the tissue (Fig. 19-8, *D*). If the area of interest is at the edge, it can remain intact after subtrimming for thin sections. The very edges of thin sections have a tendency to curl or fray during processing and could ruin the quality of the site of interest for photomicrographs, or be destroyed altogether.

After shaping the block, make sure the tissue is exposed in full cross-section. You can tell by visual inspection of the block under the dissecting microscope as well as by the size and shape of the brown-black tissue on the blade as you trim deeper into the block (Fig. 19-9). The

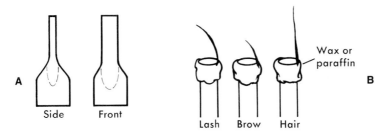

Fig. 19-11. A, Tip of cleaning sticks for knives showing whittled shape from side and front views. **B,** Hair "brushes" for moving sections in knife boat. Held on applicator sticks by wax. It is possible to have ends **A** and **B** on one stick.

edge of the blade must be sharp and have no nicks to assure a plane surface. The base of the pyramid should be a little wider than the tip so that the specimen tip is not long and thin. Thin tips can cause vibration and chatter or even break during sectioning.

THICK SECTIONS

Insert specimen block in ultramicrotome holder, angle corner down. Mount glass knife in holder on the ultramicrotome, using height indicator so that the knife edge is aligned to the middle of the cutting stroke. Set the angle of the knife with the base at an angle +3° setting to begin. If sections are being cut poorly, adjust the angle slightly more or less.

Supplies needed for cutting thick and thin sections

Microscope slides for thick sections. Cleaned, frosted ends with 1½ × 2 cm oval in center made with wax pencil when slide was warmed (ensures no breaks for fluid to escape).

Applicator sticks with whittled tips. Clean knife edge after soaking them in distilled water (Fig. 19-11, *A*).

Hair brushes. For orienting thick and thin sections for pickup and removal of undesirable sections. Use eyelash (best), eyebrow, or cut straight hair (Fig. 19-11, *B*).

Ross lens paper. Cut in quarters. Used for wiping debris from boat surface and drying grids.

2 ml disposable syringe with needle. For filling and adjusting flotation fluid level in knife trough.

Flotation medium. Small container of distilled water or dilute acetone (1 to 2 drops concentrated per 10 ml).

Fill the knife boat with water or dilute acetone by means of the 2 ml syringe with needle. The level should be plane with the sides of the trough. A convex surface sometimes makes cut sections go over the back of the knife as well as

possibly wetting the surface of the block. A concave surface can cause sections to "bunch up," and the color reflections cannot be seen.

If the knife-edge does not "wet," apply a small amount of saliva to a balsa strip that has been soaking in distilled water, and draw the strip across the edge of the knife from left to right. The slight acid in the saliva allows wetting.

Before being cut, a block must be aligned with the knife. Adjust the knife or block so that the perpendicular surfaces are parallel. The shape of the reflected light from the boat surface to the block will look rectangular, not triangular (Fig. 19-12, *A*). In Fig. 19-12, *C*, cut in areas *a* and *b* only, because of large nicks.

Once the block and knife are aligned, slowly manually advance the block toward the knife-edge. Face the surface by cutting sections about 1 μm thick on the right side of the knife. If the block face slopes downward, it must be faced until the full surface *a-b* is exposed, as shown in Fig. 19-12, *B*, in order for the entire cross-section of the tissue to be sectioned.

Once the whole block surface is exposed or faced, you may begin cutting thick sections. First, you must remove debris and unusable sections from the trough surface by drawing a small square of Ross lens paper across the boat surface and then refill the boat to plane level. If you wish to cut thin sections, move the knife to the right so that you may use a fresh knife-edge for cutting.

To cut thick sections, advance the block 1 μm at a time by turning the medium advance wheel one click at a time and pressing the chuck carrier down across the knife-edge. After four to five sections are floating in the boat, pick them up with a special thin loop (Ladd Research Industries[*]), bent perpendicular to the

---

[*]See p. 345.

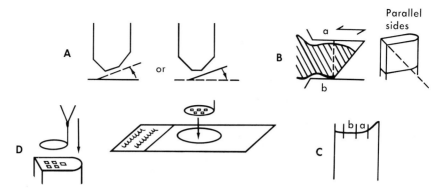

Fig. 19-12. Preparing thick sections. **A,** Aligning knife. **B,** Facing surface. **C,** Cutting locations *a* and *b* are only usable areas of the edge because of nicks. **D,** Pick up sections from boat and set down on slide.

handle, and surround the sections (Fig. 19-12, *D*). Lift the loop up carefully, and sections will be sitting on the drop of water within the loop. (You may need practice to learn picking up the sections on the drop. If you raise the loop either too slow or fast, the sections will remain on the fluid of the boat). Set loop down within wax oval on the slide; sections should remain on slide when you remove the loop.

Staining thick sections

Place slide with floating sections on hot plate prewarmed to 200° F. Leave for 10 to 15 minutes to ensure drying and adhesion to the slide. Keep slide on hot plate, and flood area inside wax circle with 0.1% filtered toluidine blue in 1% sodium tetraborate. Stain for 1 to 3 minutes (pretest time on test tissues to ascertain proper stain intensity). Rinse slide carefully with distilled water from wash bottle (Fig. 19-15, *A*). Since no additional adhesives are used, sections can be washed off with too violent a squirt of water from the bottle. Drain and air-dry. The thick sections are now ready to examine. It is not necessary to mount with a cover slip. (See section on staining for formulas of stain.)

THIN SECTIONS

Once a thick section has been examined and the block subtrimmed (see section on block trimming) (Fig. 19-10), it is ready for thin sectioning. Where glass knives are used, select a fresh one made no longer than half a day before or overnight. Since glass flows, the cutting edge is not sharp enough to produce good uniform "silver sections" if the knife is more than a day old.

Grids for routine section work are copper Athene grids. They are available from all general suppliers. The majority of electron microscopes take 3.2 mm in diameter. (Old Siemens take 2 mm, as do tilt stages for the A.E.I. series E.M.8). The routine mesh size is from 200 to 400. There are slotted and large single-holed grids, but these must have support films such as Formvar to hold the thin sections. (See support film sections in Hayat,[3] Kay,[7] and Pease.[14])

Have precleaned grids ready for use. They should be rinsed in a solvent such as acetone or ethylene dichloride and be air-dried. Half a vial (50 grids) can be poured into a 250 ml beaker with the solvent. Swirl, decant solution, and invert the beaker over a Petri dish with filter paper. Grids will drop onto the surface of the paper when dry and will then be ready to use.

Laboratories possessing diamond knives usually do all thin sectioning on them. Besides more uniform results, the cutting angle and areas of impediments remain the same. Also, if only a few minutes are available for cutting, there may not be time to make fresh glass knives.

If a tissue is known to be hard because the tissue is fibrous or contains calcium deposits or collagen, a glass knife should be used for thin sections. Any of these materials may nick or crack a diamond knife, which is brittle. If a glass knife breaks or nicks, it can be discarded with little financial loss. In 1978, a new 3.5 mm knife cost $1500 from American sources, and more from foreign ones.

Align block and knife and fill boat in the same manner as for thick sections. Make sure to set

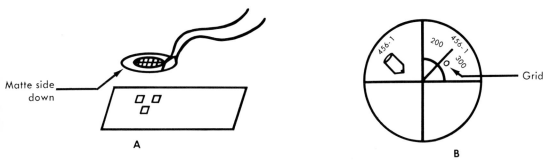

Fig. 19-13. **A,** Picking up thin sections. **B,** Grid with sections in Petri dish.

the cutting angle as suggested by the manufacturer for diamond knives. Manually advance the block till a small piece of surface has been cut. Set thickness for around 100 nm and turn on "automatic" cutting until entire front surface is plane with the knife. Section colors will be gold to purple. For thermal advance microtomes such as LKB, be sure to cool between blocks.

Change the setting to between 500 and 700 Å (50 and 70 nm). Reflected (continuous interference) colors should be silver-gray to silver. If they are still gold (900 Å or more), change to a thinner setting until the color of the sections is correct. If sections are uniform with no holes, nick marks, or chatter (Hayat,[3] p. 225), continue cutting at a rate of 1 to 2 mm/second until a good number of sections are in the boat. Using fine-pointed stainless steel forceps (no. 5 straight and no. 7 curved electron microscope forceps), pick up a clean grid and turn it so that the matte side is facing downward and the rim edge is slightly crimped up (Fig. 19-13, *A*). Touch the grid to the surface of the sections, raise grid, invert while holding small square of Ross lens paper, and draw *slowly* across the surface to remove flotation fluid from the grid (Fig. 19-15, *B*). (If drawn across rapidly, the sections will be forced to the side of the grid or will roll or overlap other sections.) Place grid on no. 1 Whatman filter paper in prelabeled quadrant of Petri dish to dry (Fig. 19-12, *B*).

If grids are noncoated (that is, have no support films), allow to stand for 20 to 30 minutes to ensure adhesion of the sections to the grid before staining. Coated grids (such as Formvar; see Hayat[3] p. 324; Pease[14]; and Kay[7]) should dry at least 15 to 20 minutes, preferably longer.

CLEANING DIAMOND KNIVES

After using a diamond knife, clean it immediately. Balsa strips (from a hobby shop, the kind of balsa used for model airplanes), or orange sticks whittled to long and wide flat tips that have been soaked in distilled water, are the most satisfactory (Fig. 19-11, *A*).

Begin at the left side of the knife and steadily draw the stick across parallel to the cutting edge. Since facing is done on the right-hand side, the cleaning direction is done from best to worst areas of the knife.

Sections that dry on a knife are nearly impossible to remove later, as well as not allowing the knife to wet evenly. If sections have already dried or are difficult to remove, the balsa strip can be soaked in absolute ethanol and drawn across the area of the section. TRY TO STAY AWAY FROM THE CUTTING EDGE. Check the back of the knife also. Concentrated acetone may loosen the mounting cement and should be avoided. Rinse well and remove the remainder of fluid with small pieces of Ross lens paper, a smooth-surfaced tissue. Return the clean knife to the special diamond knife box, and store in a safe place.

STAINING
THICK SECTIONS

A number of stains have been used in the staining of "thick" sections in electron microscopy (0.5 to 2 μm). Basic dyes seem to be most generally effective. Toluidine blue is a most useful stain, since it is metachromatic and accentuates cytoplasmic differentiation. In addition, the recipe is simple and easy to make up as well as being reproducible.

Toluidine blue

Stock solution
0.2% in 2% borax (sodium borate)
Make up about 50 ml at a time for a low-volume laboratory. Let age a few days before use if possible. Store in brown bottle.

Working solution

0.1% to 1% borax

Take 25 ml of stock solution. Dilute 1 : 1 with distilled water (25 ml of toluidine blue plus 25 ml of water). *Filter* into brown bottle. (If you do not filter, stain precipitate will stick to sections and slides.)

Use

Heat slides to 150° to 200° F (65° to 95° C) while drying on a heat-controlled hot plate. With a Pasteur pipette, flood area over and around on sections with stain while slides are *still on* hot plate. Test optimal staining time, which should be between 1 and 2 minutes. If not, increase the concentration of the stock, or dilute the working solution.

Results

Nuclei and chromatin material—dark purple
Red blood cells—deep blue to purple
Fat—gray-green to gray-blue
Cytoplasm—lavender.

Trypan blue

Another stain similar to toluidine blue is 2% trypan blue in 1% sodium borate. The same procedure is used as for toluidine blue. Pretest for optimal time on Epon-embedded sections of tissues similar to those to be used during experimentation.

THIN SECTIONS

The more commonly used stains for thin sections are uranyl and lead stains. Both chemicals contain electron-dense heavy metals, and this factor is essential when proper contrast in cellular components is to be realized for photomicrography.

Uranyl acetate is a nuclear stain and is used first in the double-staining procedure (comparable to hematoxylin in paraffin histology). It specifically binds nuclear proteins.

Lead citrate is a cytoplasmic stain that intensifies the detail of cellular membranes and inclusions, including mitochondria, lysosomes, and ribosomes.

Alkaline lead hydroxide and lead tartrate (Millonig[11]) are additional cytoplasmic stains. The alkaline lead hydroxide is very sensitive to carbon dioxide and can readily form a precipitate upon the sections and show as black spots in the electron microscope.

Preparation of solutions
Uranyl acetate

This "stain" is used in saturated concentration. Its solubility is quite temperature dependent. Uranyl acetate also has a tendency to de-

compose, that is, break down or dissociate; thus the working solution should be made fresh about once a month. The aqueous solution takes longer staining time but allows more control over the intensity. Alcoholic solutions, either ethyl or methyl 25% to 50%, are preferred by some, but they penetrate faster and the staining times run from 1 to 5 minutes. The solubility of uranyl acetate is increased in alcohol, but so does the tendency for the solution to decompose and the necessity of preparing the solution more often (see Hayat,[3] Kay,[7] and Pease[14] about alcoholic solutions).

If it can be noted in the electron microscope that the nuclei and some organelles have lost suitable contrast for photomicrographs, the solutions should be discarded and a fresh one made up. On the other hand, we have used uranyl acetate stock for as long as 3 months in our laboratory with good results. The solution must be kept tightly covered and under refrigeration.

Uranyl acetate

3.75 gm of uranyl acetate, fine-grained salt

If larger crystals only are available, crush them with a mortar and pestle before weighing.

In a 250 ml beaker containing 50 ml of distilled water, add the uranyl acetate.

Place the 250 ml beaker in a 600 ml or larger beaker containing water to the level of that in the smaller beaker. Set both beakers into a sonicator with crushed ice about 2.5 cm deep. The sonicator must also contain water to the level of the fluid in the beakers.

Turn the sonicator setting to the *low* or *1* setting if it has more than one setting, otherwise to *on*. (Make sure you do *not* have the sonicator on while you are stirring with a rod or wish to remove the small beaker by hand. Sonication destroys cells and can do so in your hands as well.)

Leave the uranyl acetate to sonicate for 10 to 15 minutes maximum if no ice is added to the sonicator water (prolonged sonication builds up heat, which will reduce the stainability of the uranyl acetate). Repeat the sonication after a half hour passes, after swirling the small beaker to assure that as much salt as possible is going into the solution. Continue procedure between 1 and 2 hours but no more.

Pour sonicated acetate into a 100 ml capped bottle, including any remaining salt crystals that did not go into solution. Cover cap with Parafilm and place in the refrigerator. Use as *stock solution.*

Before using stain, remove about 10 ml by Pasteur pipette into capped 15 ml conical centrifuge tube. Use this as the *working solution,* only

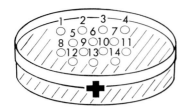 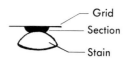

Fig. 19-14. Bottom portion of small Petri dish with wax for staining surface. Rows of stain drops must be even for grid orientation.

keeping it outside refrigerator long enough to put drops on the staining dishes and return.

Before use, it is a good idea to centrifuge in refrigerated equipment at 4° C for 20 minutes at 1800 rpm.

Lead citrate

Method 1

There are two methods of making lead citrate, depending on the availability of chemicals. The easier of the two is with the complete chemical.[16]

Stock solution

Lead citrate	0.25 gm
Distilled water (boiled and cooled)	50 ml
Sodium hydroxide pellet	one

Weigh out lead citrate and place into plastic-stoppered 100 ml graduate. Add distilled water to make 50 ml. Invert a number of times until crystals are mostly dissolved. Add one pellet of sodium hydroxide. Continue inverting a sufficient number of times for solution of chemicals and clearing of reagent. Make sure the stopper is tight and cover with a double layer of Parafilm or equivalent to keep air out. Place in refrigerator overnight before use and for storage.

Working solution

Prior to using, remove 10 ml with Pasteur Pipette into capped 15 ml conical centrifuge tube. Spin 20 minutes in refrigerated centrifuge and spin at 1800 rpm.

If either the stock or working solution container is not tightly capped or covered, carbon dioxide from the air will get in and form lead carbonate, a white precipitate. In the electron microscope this precipitate appears as black blobs on the sections.

Method 2

Lead nitrate, fine crystals	1.33 gm
(If large crystals, crush with mortar and pestle.)	
Sodium citrate	1.76 gm
$(Na_3[C_6H_5O_7]_3 \cdot 2H_2O)$	

Place chemicals in 50 ml volumetric flask.

Add 30 ml of boiled distilled water (cooled 15 minutes while covered). Shake 1 minute and add 8 ml of 1 N sodium hydroxide. The solution should clear after being milky. Add distilled water to make the volume of 50 ml. Store in refrigerator, and use as in method 1.

Staining technics

One of the more common ways to "stain" thin sections is by the use of small glass Petri dishes with a 50 mm inside diameter of bottom part (all over diameter 60 × 15 mm outer diameter). They are convenient to use and easy to store.

Set the bottom parts of two glass Petri dishes on a hot plate heated to 200° to 300° F (95° to 145° C). Melt pink dental wax to a depth of about 4 mm, or about one third of the total depth of the dishes. Set dishes with the melted wax on a flat *untilted* surface until the wax cools and sets. For one dish, cut a fresh piece of dental wax 29 × 37 mm and cut corners to fit into the Petri dish (for lead citrate staining). See Fig. 19-16, *A*.

Uranyl acetate staining

Centrifuge uranyl acetate working solution for 20 minutes at 1800 rpm. Place drops in *even* rows by means of a Pasteur pipette. The drops should be far enough apart to prevent their coalescing. (Some laboratories use alcoholic solutions. Surface tension is less for alcohol and so drops should be farther apart.) A black mark with a felt-tip marking pen can be used at a point in the base to ensure that you note the direction of the dish because there will be no marks indicating the sequence of grids (Fig. 19-14).

Set the grids, section side down, on a uranyl acetate drop. The water base uranyl acetate timing usually runs between 15 and 20 minutes (try 17 minutes on a test grid first). The alcohol base stain reacts faster, that is, between 1 and 5 minutes. Remove grid by gripping the rim with very fine pointed stainless steel forceps (no. 5 or 7), turn section side up and thoroughly wash with distilled water from a wash bottle over a beaker (Fig. 19-15, *A*).

Touch the grid to a small piece of Ross lens paper, and draw off remaining fluid by pulling

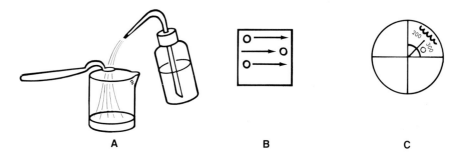

Fig. 19-15. A, Post-stain washing of grid. **B,** Drying grid on Ross lens paper. **C,** Placement of grid in Petri dish.

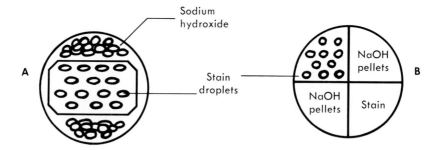

Fig. 19-16. Setups of staining dishes for lead citrate staining.

grid across (Fig. 19-15, *B*). When pulling the grid, you must do it slowly, otherwise the sections will have a tendency to become loose.

Set stained grid on labeled filter paper in a Petri dish, either partitioned polystyrene type of 100 × 15 mm, or smaller 65 × 15 mm. The larger ones can be used for up to four blocks from one case, the smaller one for one block only. If you use more than one size of mesh grid, note that also, as indicated in Fig. 19-15, *C*.

A similar procedure is to place drops of stain on a square of Parafilm and cover with a Petri dish or a culture-dish top. A third procedure is to flood small Petri dishes and place grids on the bottom, section side up. The disadvantage to this last staining method is that any floating debris can be deposited upon the sections while staining and may adhere to them, producing electron-dense blobs or precipitate in the electron microscope.

Special staining dishes are available from Polysciences, Inc. These accommodate a good number of grids, which are placed perpendicularly in a holder with stalled openings in the bottom. The entire staining carrier is immersed in a container of "stain" for optimal staining time. Afterwards, the carrier is washed in several changes of distilled water and placed on a filter paper to dry. The grids dry better if re-

moved from the carrier onto filter paper. One disadvantage of this method is the fact that the grids are on their side, a position possibly allowing the sections to pull off during staining and subsequent washing.

If you do not wish to counterstain, allow grids to dry at least 10 to 15 minutes before inserting into the electron microscope column.

Lead citrate staining

Centrifuge lead citrate working solution for 20 minutes at 1800 rpm in refrigerated centrifuge. (You may spin it at the same time as uranyl acetate, but leave it in the centrifuge to keep cool while using the first stain.)

Use dental waxed–bottom glass Petri dish with an extra wax insert on top. On either side of the wax overlay, place pellets of sodium hydroxide (Fig. 19-16, *A*). Its purpose is to absorb any carbon dioxide from the air. As indicated earlier, carbon dioxide reacting with lead citrate causes a precipitate that will contaminate the sections and appear as black spots on the screen.

A second type of staining dish would be a quadripartite 100 × 15 Petri dish into which dental wax had been poured into the quarters. Two of the areas would contain the sodium hydroxide pellets and two would hold the stain droplets (Fig. 19-16, *B*).

SUPPLIERS OF MATERIALS AND EQUIPMENT FOR ELECTRON MICROSCOPY
(See Glauert[1] and Hayat[3] for extended lists.)

General suppliers in the United States

Electron Microscopy Sciences (EMS)
Box 251
Fort Washington, PA 19034
(215) 646-1566

Ernest F. Fullam, Inc. (EFFA)
P.O. Box 444
Schenectady, NY 12301
(518) 785-5533

Ladd Research Industries (Ladd)
P.O. Box 901 (U.S. Agar Aids)
Burlington, VT 05401
(802) 658-4961

Ted Pella, Inc. (Pelco)
P.O. Box 510
Tustin, CA 92680
(714) 557-9434

Polaron Instruments, Inc.
1202 Bethlehem Pike
Line Lexington, PA 18932
(215) 822-3364

Polysciences, Inc.
Paul Valley Industrial Park
Warrington, PA 18976
(215) 343-6484

Canada

Marivac Ltd.
(agent for Agar Aids)
1872 Garden St.
Halifax, B3H 3R6
Nova Scotia, Canada
(902) 429-0209

England

Agar Aids for Electron Microscopy
(agent for Ladd)
127a Rye St.
Bishop's Stortford
Hertfordshire, England

Polaron Equipment Ltd.
60/62 Greenhill Crescent
Holywell Estate
Watford
Hertfordshire, England

France

Touzart and Matignon
(agent for EFFA)
3, Rue Amyot
75 Paris, France

Vials and Pasteur pipettes

Arthur H. Thomas
3rd and Vine Sts.
Philadelphia, PA 19106
(215) 574-4500 (Gen.)
        574-4555 (Phone order)

Knife breaker, glass strips, stands for block trimming, storage boxes, and grids

LKB Instruments, Inc.
12221 Parklawn Dr.
Rockville, MD 20852
(301) 881-2510

Diamond knives

E. I. DuPont de Nemours and Co., Inc.
Diamond Knife Dept.
Instrument Products Division
Wilmington, DE 19898
(800) 441-7493

Electron Microscopy Sciences (EMS)
Box 251
Fort Washington, PA 19034
(215) 646-1566
(U.S. agents for Diatome, Ltd.)

Epoxy resin and fixation chemicals

EMS, Fullam, Fisher, Ladd, Marivac, Pella, Polaron, and Polysciences

Fisher Scientific Co. is a large organization that has branches in most metropolitan areas of the United States as well as in Canada, Europe, and Mexico. Three of the East Coast branches are listed.

PHILADELPHIA AREA

191 S. Gulph Rd.
King of Prussia, PA 19406
(215) 265-0300

NEW YORK AREA

52 Fadem Rd.
Springfield, NJ 07081
(201) 379-1400

BOSTON AREA

461 Riverside Ave.
P.O. Box 379
Medford, MA 02155
(617) 391-6110

CORPORATE HEADQUARTERS

711 Forbes Ave.
Pittsburgh, PA 15219
(412) 562-8300

Place grids on top of the droplets two at a time, section side down as before, and stain for around 10 minutes. Pretest for proper time.

Remove and wash as before, making sure to not exhale on the grids causing stain precipitate. Set on filter paper in labeled dish and wait about 15 to 20 minutes before placing in the electron microscope column.

Supplies needed to place grids in electron microscope column

Lint-free cloths

Lint-free gloves

No. 5 straight or no. 7 curved electron microscope forceps

Hand lens to observe centering and quality of sections (optional).

Note: For more extensive discussions on stains and staining methods, see Hayat,[3] Kay,[7] and Pease.[14]

REFERENCES

1. Glauert, A. M.: Fixation, dehydration and embedding of biological specimens, New York, 1975, American Elsevier Publishing Co.
2. Glauert, A. M., and Glauert, R. H.: Araldite as an embedding medium for electron microscopy, J. Biophys. Biochem. Cytol. **4:**191, 1958.
3. Hayat, M. A.: Principles and techniques of electron microscopy. Biological application, vol. 1, New York, 1970, Van Nostrand-Reinhold Co.
4. Holt, S. H., and Hicks, R. M.: Studies on formalin fixation for electron microscopy and cytochemical staining purposes, J. Biophys. Biochem. Cytol. **11:**31, 1961.
5. Karnovsky, M. J.: Simple methods for "staining with lead" at high pH in electron microscopy, J. Biophys. Biochem. Cytol. **11:**729, 1961.
6. Karnovsky, M. J.: A formaldehyde-glutaraldehyde fixative of high osmolality for use in electron microscopy, J. Cell Biol. **27:**137A, 1965.
7. Kay, D.: Techniques for electron microscopy, ed. 2, Oxford, 1967, Blackwell Scientific Publications.
8. Luft, J. H.: Improvements in epoxy resin embedding methods, J. Biophys. Biochem. Cytol. **9:**409, 1961.
9. Mercer, E. H.: A scheme for section-staining in electron microscopy, J. Roy. Microscop. Soc. **81:**179, 1963.
10. Millonig, G.: Advantages of a phosphate buffer for osmium tetroxide solutions in fixation, J. Appl. Phys. **32:**1637, 1961.
11. Millonig, G.: A modified procedure for lead staining of thin sections, J. Biophys. Biochem. Cytol. **11:**736, 1961.
12. Palade, G. E.: A study of fixation for electron microscopy, J. Exp. Med. **95:**285, 1952.
13. Pearse, A. G. E.: Histochemistry: theoretical and applied, Boston, 1960, Little, Brown & Co.
14. Pease, D. C.: Histological techniques for electron microscopy, ed. 2, New York, 1964, Academic Press, Inc.
15. Reedy, M. K.: Section staining for electron microscopy, J. Cell Biol. **26:**309, 1965.
16. Reynolds, E. S.: The use of lead citrate at high pH as an electron-opaque stain in electron microscopy, J. Cell Biol. **17:**208, 1963.
17. Spurr, A. R.: A low-viscosity epoxy resin embedding medium for electron microscopy, J. Ultrastruct. Res. **26:**31, 1969.
18. Stefanini, M., DeMartino, C., and Zamboni, L.: Fixation of ejaculated spermatozoa for electron microscopy, Nature **216:**173, 1967.
19. Trump, B. F., Smuckler, E. A., and Benditt, E. P.: A method for staining epoxy resins for light microscopy, J. Ultrastruct. Res. **5:**343, 1961.
20. Zamboni, L., and DeMartino, C.: Buffered picric acid-formaldehyde: a new, rapid fixative for electron microscopy, J. Cell Biol. **35:**148A, 1967.

CHAPTER 20

Inorganic chemistry

ROBERT J. HRAPCHAK

BASIC DEFINITIONS AND CONCEPTS

Simple substances that do not undergo decomposition in any chemical reaction are called *elements*. An *atom* is defined as the basic structural unit of an element. An atom retains its identity through all physical and chemical reactions, and atoms of different elements differ in their chemical and physical properties and have different weights.

Each atom is composed of a central *nucleus* that contains *protons* (positively charged particles) and *neutrons* (electrically neutral particles), around which one or more *electrons* (negatively charged particles) revolve in concentric shells or energy levels. The electrons in the outermost energy level are called *valence* electrons and determine the reactivity of the atom. The number of protons in a neutral atom equals the number of electrons in that atom. The *atomic number* of an atom is defined as the number of protons in the nucleus of that atom.

The *atomic weight* of an element is defined as the atomic weight of an atom of the element relative to the atomic weight of a C (carbon) atom, arbitrarily set equal to 12. The number of neutrons in the nucleus equals the difference between the atomic weight and the atomic number. All the atoms of a given element have the same atomic number but not necessarily the same atomic weight. Varieties of atoms of the same element that have the same atomic numbers but different atomic weights are called *isotopes* of that element. Table 20-1 gives a list of the elements, their symbols (abbreviations used in drawing chemical structures), their atomic numbers, and their atomic weights.

A pure substance that can be broken down chemically into two or more elements is called a *compound*. Water is a familiar compound and can be broken down into the elements hydrogen and oxygen. The smallest part of a compound that has all the properties of the compound is called a *molecule*. Solving lab math problems frequently requires the knowledge of the molecular weight of a compound. The *molecular weight* is the sum of all the atomic weights of the elements comprising the compound. The atomic weights found in Table 20-1 may be used to calculate the molecular weight.

PERIODIC TABLE

The *periodic law* states that the chemical and physical properties of the elements are periodic (repeating) functions of their atomic numbers, and this law is expressed in the *periodic table*, which lists all the elements according to similarities in their chemical and physical properties (Fig. 20-1). Each box in the table gives the following information: an atomic symbol, an atomic number (the number above the symbol), and

Table 20-1. Table of elements

Element	Symbol	Atomic number	Atomic weight	Element	Symbol	Atomic number	Atomic weight
Actinium	Ac	89	227	Mercury	Hg	80	200.59
Aluminum	Al	13	26.9815	Molybdenum	Mo	42	95.94
Americium	Am	95	[243]*	Neodymium	Nd	60	144.24
Antimony	Sb	51	121.75	Neon	Ne	10	20.183
Argon	Ar	18	39.948	Neptunium	Np	93	[237]
Arsenic	As	33	74.9216	Nickel	Ni	28	58.71
Astatine	At	85	[210]	Niobium	Nb	41	92.906
Barium	Ba	56	137.34	Nitrogen	N	7	14.0067
Berkelium	Bk	97	[249]	Nobelium	No	102	[253]
Beryllium	Be	4	9.0122	Osmium	Os	76	190.2
Bismuth	Bi	83	208.980	Oxygen	O	8	15.9994
Boron	B	5	10.811	Palladium	Pd	46	106.4
Bromine	Br	35	79.909	Phosphorus	P	15	30.9738
Cadmium	Cd	48	112.40	Platinum	Pt	78	195.09
Calcium	Ca	20	40.08	Plutonium	Pu	94	[242]
Californium	Cf	98	[249]	Polonium	Po	84	210
Carbon	C	6	12.01115	Potassium	K	19	39.102
Cerium	Ce	58	140.12	Praseodymium	Pr	59	140.907
Cesium	Cs	55	132.905	Promethium	Pm	61	[145]
Chlorine	Cl	17	35.453	Protactinium	Pa	91	231
Chromium	Cr	24	51.996	Radium	Ra	88	226.05
Cobalt	Co	27	58.9332	Radon	Rn	86	222
Copper	Cu	29	63.54	Rhenium	Re	75	186.2
Curium	Cm	96	[247]	Rhodium	Rh	45	102.905
Dysprosium	Dy	66	162.50	Rubidium	Rb	37	85.47
Einsteinium	Es	99	[254]	Ruthenium	Ru	44	101.07
Erbium	Er	68	167.26	Samarium	Sm	62	150.35
Europium	Eu	63	151.96	Scandium	Sc	21	44.956
Fermium	Fm	100	[253]	Selenium	Se	34	78.96
Fluorine	F	9	18.9984	Silicon	Si	14	28.086
Francium	Fr	87	[223]	Silver	Ag	47	107.870
Gadolinium	Gd	64	157.25	Sodium	Na	11	22.9898
Gallium	Ga	31	69.72	Strontium	Sr	38	87.62
Germanium	Ge	32	72.59	Sulfur	S	16	32.064
Gold	Au	79	196.967	Tantalum	Ta	73	180.948
Hafnium	Hf	72	178.49	Technetium	Tc	43	[99]
Helium	He	2	4.0026	Tellurium	Te	52	127.60
Holmium	Ho	67	164.930	Terbium	Tb	65	158.924
Hydrogen	H	1	1.00797	Thallium	Tl	81	204.37
Indium	In	49	114.82	Thorium	Th	90	232.038
Iodine	I	53	126.9044	Thulium	Tm	69	168.934
Iridium	Ir	77	192.2	Tin	Sn	50	118.69
Iron	Fe	26	55.847	Titanium	Ti	22	47.90
Krypton	Kr	36	83.80	Tungsten	W	74	183.85
Lanthanum	La	57	138.91	Uranium	U	92	238.03
Lawrencium	Lw	103	[257]	Vanadium	V	23	50.942
Lead	Pb	82	207.19	Xenon	Xe	54	131.30
Lithium	Li	3	6.939	Ytterbium	Yb	70	173.04
Lutetium	Lu	71	174.97	Yttrium	Y	39	88.905
Magnesium	Mg	12	24.312	Zinc	Zn	30	65.37
Manganese	Mn	25	54.9380	Zirconium	Zr	40	91.22
Mendelevium	Md	101	[256]				

*A value given in brackets denotes the mass number of the longest-lived or best-known isotope. Atomic weights are based on carbon 12.

Fig. 20-1. Periodic table of elements.

the atomic weight (the number beneath the symbol).

Going across a horizontal row (*period*) in this table, the elements are listed according to increasing atomic number. There are 7 periods in the table, corresponding to the number of shells occupied by electrons in the elements.

Going down a vertical column (*group*) in the table, elements with similar properties are listed in families, such as the *alkali metals* (excluding H, in group IA), the *alkaline earth metals* (group IIA), the *transition elements* (groups IIIB through IB), the *halogens* (group VIIA), and the *inert or noble gases* (group 0).

The elements can be broadly divided into two classes, metals and nonmetals. The elements that, in chemical reactions, tend to lose electrons (electron donors) and become positively charged ions are called *metals*. The elements that, in chemical reactions, tend to gain electrons (electron acceptors) and become negatively charged ions are called *nonmetals*. Most of the elements are classified as metals and are found in the white boxes in the table, whereas the elements in the shaded boxes are the nonmetals.

The elements of group 0 are called the inert gases, and they exhibit very low chemical reactivity. Period 6 contains 32 elements, but since 15 of these elements, the *lanthanide series* (La, atomic number 57, through Lu, atomic number 71) have very similar properties, they appear to belong in only one position in the table, and all are listed in a separate row at the bottom of the table. For similar reasons, elements of the *actinide series* are also placed in a separate row. Elements of the lanthanide and actinide series are called the *rare earth elements*. Families with the letter "A" in them have only 1 electron shell in the process of being filled, whereas those with the letter "B" have at least 2 shells being filled. The transition elements, which are indicated in the table, are elements in which inner shells are being filled to capacities of 18 or 32 electrons.

MOLECULAR BONDING

To understand molecular bonding in the formation of molecules from atoms, we must refer to atomic theory. It is known that electrons revolve around the nucleus of an atom in specific shells. These shells, which number 7, represent

Table 20-2. Electron shells of atoms

Shell number	Letter designation	Electron capacity
1	K	2
2	L	8
3	M	18
4	N	32
5	O	32
6	P	18
7	Q	8

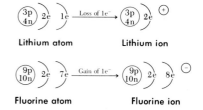

Fig. 20-2. Hydrostatic (ionic) bond formation.

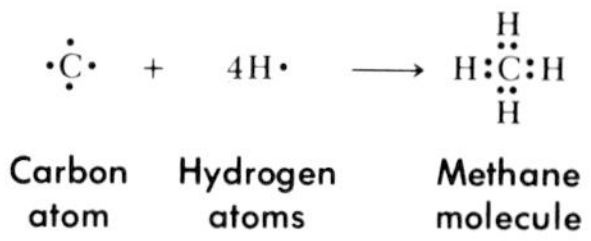

Fig. 20-3. Covalent bond formation.

different energy levels. Only a certain number of electrons can go into each shell, and the electron capacities of the shells are shown in Table 20-2. Since the first shell has a 2-electron maximum, any more than 2 electrons must enter the *second* shell, and any more than 10 must enter the *third* shell, and so on. Atoms have the greatest stability when their outer shells are full, such as in the inert gases, helium (He), neon (Ne), argon (Ar), and so forth. Either electrostatic (ionic) or covalent bonds may be formed based on this tendency of individual atoms to attain this most stable electron arrangement.

Electrostatic (ionic) bonds

Electrostatic (ionic) bonds arise from the actual transfer of an electron from one atom to another to give each of the formed ions the most stable electron configuration. For example, when lithium (Li) and fluorine (F) are brought together, each Li atom (atomic number 3, with outer shell containing 1 electron) loses an electron to the F atom (atomic number 9, with outer shell containing 7 electrons). See Fig. 20-2. By this loss, Li achieves a stable helium (He) configuration (atomic number 2) but now bears a positive charge and is called a Li ion, Li^+; F, by gaining 1 electron, achieves a stable neon (Ne) configuration (atomic number 10, with 8 electrons in the outermost shell) but, because of the added electron, has a net negative charge and is called the fluoride ion, F^-. The two ions, Li^+ and F^-, are then held together by the electrostatic attraction of their opposite charges. Compounds formed in this way are said to be electrostatic or ionic compounds. Electrostatic bonds are formed between elements that lose electrons readily and those that have a strong affinity for electrons.

Covalent bonds

Besides electrostatically bound substances, there is an even larger group of substances whose physical and chemical properties cannot be explained in terms of electrostatic bonds. Molecules of such substances as ammonia, water, and carbon dioxide are bonded nonionically, as are the majority of carbon-containing compounds (see Chapter 21). These molecules are formed by sharing of electron pairs between 2 atoms; that is, they have *covalent (electron-pair)* bonds. Such bonding assures that all the atoms achieve the most stable electron configuration. A simple example of covalent bonding is provided by the compound methane (CH_4). The C atom (atomic number 6), with 4 electrons in its outer shell, requires 4 more electrons to attain the stable Ne (atomic number 10) structure. Each of the H atoms, with 1 electron, needs 1 more electron to attain the stable He (atomic number 2) configuration. These requirements are met when the C atom shares its 4 outer electrons, 1 each with 4 separate H atoms and, in turn, the C atom receives a share in each of the electrons furnished by the 4 H atoms. To illustrate this, electronic symbols will be introduced in which the symbols for C and H represent the nucleus as well as any inner-shell electrons, and the surrounding dots ($\cdot$) represent outer-shell electrons only, that is, the valence electrons (Fig. 20-3). All the bonds in the methane molecule are covalent. It should be noted that the structure for methane is simplified, since methane actually exists as a three-dimensional molecule. Since in this example, the pairs of electrons connecting the 4 H atoms to the C atom are shared equally between the atoms, the molecule as a whole is symmetric with respect to the distribution of electron charge and is, therefore, *nonpolar*.

$$H:\overset{\overset{H}{..}}{\underset{H}{N}:} \quad + \quad H^+ \quad \longrightarrow \quad \left[H:\overset{\overset{H}{..}}{\underset{H}{N}:}H \right]^+$$

| Ammonia molecule | Hydrogen ion | Ammonium ion |

Fig. 20-4. Coordinate covalent bond formation.

Hydrogen
bond

$$H-O-\overset{\downarrow}{\underset{\underset{H}{|}}{\quad}}H-\underset{\underset{H}{|}}{O}$$

Covalent
bond

Fig. 20-5. Hydrogen bond formation.

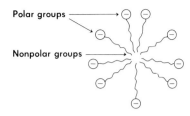

Fig. 20-6. Micelle formation with hydrophobic bonding.

Covalent bond
$$H-Cl$$
Dipole-dipole $\longrightarrow$
interaction
$$Cl-H$$

Fig. 20-7. Dipole-dipole interactions.

If, in forming a molecule, 1 atom (or molecule) supplies both shared electrons, a *coordinate covalent bond* is formed; for example, an ammonium ion is formed by the reaction of an ammonia molecule (NH_3) with a H^+ ion (Fig. 20-4).

Covalent bonds may show *polarity*, which is caused by the unequal sharing of the electron pairs by the 2 bound nuclei; one end of the bond is relatively negative and the other is relatively positive (though the molecule as a whole is electrically neutral), and such a bond is also called a *polar bond*. The greater the *electronegativity* (electron-attraction power) of 1 bonded atom is than that of the other, the more polar will be the bond. A molecule containing a polar bond will itself be polar; such a molecule is called a *dipole*, and an example is $H:F$, in which the highly electronegative F atom attracts the shared electron pair more strongly than does H. (As mentioned before, methane [CH_4] is nonpolar, since the electron pairs are shared approximately equally by the very weakly electronegative atoms C and H.)

Other types of bonds and molecular attractive forces

Hydrogen bonds. In a *hydrogen bond*, a H atom that is bonded covalently to 1 strongly electronegative atom (O, N, F) is also electrostatically attracted to another strongly electronegative atom either in another molecule (*intermolecular hydrogen bond*) or in another portion of the same molecule (*intramolecular hydrogen bond*). A simple example is the hydrogen bond formed between 2 separate water (H_2O) molecules (Fig. 20-5). Although weaker than covalent bonds, hydrogen bonds, in great number, are strong enough to exert significant bonding attractions between molecules capable of forming them. Hydrogen bonds are important in maintaining the structures of proteins and nucleic acids.

Hydrophobic interactions. If molecules containing both highly polar groups as well as water-insoluble, nonpolar (*hydrophobic*) groups are placed in water, the nonpolar groups tend to join together and exclude the water molecules to form a loosely associated structure in which the polar groups are displaced to the surface of the structure. The structure formed is called a *micelle*, and the nonpolar group interactions are called *hydrophobic* (water-fearing) *interactions* (Fig. 20-6). Fatty acids, which contain highly polar, *hydrophilic* (water-loving) carboxyl groups attached to long nonpolar hydrocarbon chains, readily form micelles in this way. Hydrophobic interactions are also important in stabilizing the structures of nucleic acids and proteins and may be *intermolecular* (acting between different molecules) or *intramolecular* (acting between different nonpolar regions in the same molecule).

Dipole-dipole interactions. Molecules also may be held together by *dipole-dipole interactions*. In such interactions, the relatively positive end of 1 dipole attracts the relatively negative end of another dipole in a weak bondlike fashion. For example (Fig. 20-7), the relatively positive H of 1 molecule of HCl (hydrochloric acid) is attracted to the relatively negative Cl atom of another molecule.

Van der Waals forces. Finally, forces that cause attractions between completely nonpolar molecules are called *van der Waals forces*.

These forces are explained by the momentary formation of dipoles, caused by electron movements, which induce oppositely charged dipoles in another molecule. These dipoles change constantly because of electron-distribution changes, but their overall effect is an attraction between the molecules.

OXIDATION-REDUCTION REACTIONS

An oxidation-reduction reaction, taking place in aqueous solution, may be defined as one involving the transfer of electrons from one substance to another. The substance supplying the electrons is the substance oxidized, and the substance acquiring the electrons is the substance reduced. Substances that are used as a source of electrons and that yield them readily are called *reducing agents;* substances that are used because they take up electrons readily are called *oxidizing agents.* The oxidizing agent, which takes up electrons, has a decrease in positive valence or oxidation number, whereas the reducing agent, which loses electrons, has an increase in positive valence or oxidation number.

An oxidation reaction always involves a simultaneous reduction reaction. A general example illustrating this concept is the reaction of potassium dichromate ($K_2Cr_2O_7$) with potassium iodide (KI) in dilute acid (H^+). Here, the orange-red color of the dichromate ion ($Cr_2O_7^{2-}$) changes to the dark green color of the chromic ion (Cr^{3+}) as the Cr^{6+} of the $Cr_2O_7^{2-}$ complex is reduced (reduction in + valance). The colorless I^- of KI changes to the brown atomic iodine (neutral charge), and the acidity of the solution is diminished. I^-, losing an electron, increases its valence and is therefore oxidized. The overall equation (with H^+ being represented by the hydronium ion, H_3O^+) is as follows:

$$6\ I^- + Cr_2O_7^{2-} + 14\ H_3O^+ \rightarrow 3\ I_2 + 2\ Cr^{3+} + 21\ H_2O$$

Another common definition of oxidation is simply the reaction of elements and compounds with oxygen. The element or compound that combines with the oxygen is said to be oxidized, such as with the hematoxylins. Delafield's stain is oxidized by atmospheric oxygen to the oxidation product hematein. Harris's hematoxylin stain uses mercuric oxide to achieve the oxidizing (ripening) effect.

ACIDS, BASES, SALTS, AND AMPHOTERICS
Acids

An *acid,* for our purposes, is defined as a sub-stance that produces H^+ ions (protons) in aqueous solutions (Arrhenius' definition). Acids are important covalent compounds, covalent because they are made up of neutral molecules in which all the atoms, including those of H, are linked by covalent bonds. Many acids, such as sulfuric acid (H_2SO_4) and nitric acid (HNO_3), possess corrosive properties generally associated with the term "acid." Others like citric and tartaric acids, which are organic acids, are constituents of common foods. Aqueous solutions of acids have a sour taste, turn blue litmus paper red, neutralize bases, and react with active metals to give free H. Structurally, the familiar acids all contain the element H, and in the pure anhydrous forms, acids may be liquids, gases, or solids at ordinary temperatures. Pure anhydrous acids in the liquid state are poor conductors of electricity because of the covalent linkages; however, in aqueous solutions, they show electrolytic properties; that is, their solutions conduct an electric current to a greater or lesser degree, depending on the strength of the acid. Obviously, these acids form ions as they dissolve in water. However, the proton (H^+) cannot exist unhydrated in water, but instead it forms a hydronium ion (H_3O^+) by associating with a water molecule. Therefore we can picture the dissociation (ionization) of hydrochloric acid (HCl) in water as follows:

$$HCl + H_2O \rightarrow H_3O^+ + Cl^-$$

According to this, an acid may be defined as a substance that in water solution ionizes with the formation of a hydronium ion as one of the dissociated ions.

Bases

From a functional standpoint, a *base* may be defined as a compound that produces hydroxide (OH^-) ions in aqueous solutions (Arrhenius). Aqueous solutions of a base feel soapy, taste bitter, turn red litmus paper blue, and neutralize acids. Bases are ionically bound solids in the anhydrous form in which the anion (negatively charged ion) is the OH^- ion.

Bases are strong electrolytes; that is, they dissociate (ionize) completely in aqueous solution to form OH^- ions and cations (positively charged ions). Examples are KOH and NaOH. On the other hand, acids may be strong electrolytes (HCl, HNO_3) or weak electrolytes. Acids of the latter type, such as the organic acid, acetic acid, dissociate only partially to H^+ ions and anions.

Other definitions of acids and bases

According to *Brönsted*, an acid is a substance that releases H^+ ions (protons) in solution; that is, an acid is a *proton donor;* and a base is any substance that binds H^+ ions in solution; that is, a base is a *proton acceptor.* By these definitions, such compounds as ammonium ion (NH_4^+) are acids, whereas compounds such as ammonia (NH_3) and sulfate ion (SO_4^{2-}) are bases.

In another system, *Lewis* defined an acid as a substance that can take up an electron pair to form a covalent bond and a base as a substance that can supply an electron pair to form a covalent bond. According to these definitions, such substances as H^+ and aluminum chloride ($AlCl_3$) are acids, whereas OH^-, NH_3, and H_2O are bases. (For routine lab purposes, the Brönsted and Lewis definitions of acids and bases are rarely considered.)

Acids and bases are relative terms only, since many substances can act as acids in certain reactions and as bases in others; these substances are called *amphoteric*. The most familiar amphoteric compound is water, which can act as an acid (proton donor) to ammonia and as a base (proton acceptor) toward HCl.

Neutralization

Neutralization is a reaction between an acid and a base that results in the combination of the H^+ from the acid and OH^- from the base to form water, leaving the metal from the base and the nonmetal or radical from the acid to form a salt, for example:

$$H^+ + Cl^- + K^+ + OH^- \rightarrow H_2O + KCl$$

Since the formation of a salt from an acid and a base leads to the disappearance of the properties of both the acid and the base, they are said to neutralize each other.

Salts

Salts are electrostatically bound compounds that are formed from the reaction of an acid with a base and may be classified as *acidic* (contains replaceable H, such as in $NaHCO_3$ and Na_2HPO_4), *basic* (contains replaceable oxide or hydroxide, such as $Mg[OH]Cl$ and $SbOCl$), or *neutral* (complete replacement of H and OH such as in $NaCl$ and Na_2SO_4).

Simple salts contain a single kind of anion, a single kind of cation, and sometimes H, OH, or oxide ions.

Double salts, such as $KCl \cdot MgCl_2 \cdot 6H_2O$, are formed by the reaction of two simple salts. In solution, a double salt produces only the ions that would be produced in solutions of its two salts, that is, as in the preceding case, K^+, Mg^{2+}, and Cl^-.

Complex salts are formed by the reaction of a simple salt with neutral molecules, such as $CuCl_2 \cdot 4NH_3$. In solution, a complex salt produces a complex ion and an ion of its simple salt, that is, as in the given example, $CuCl_2 \cdot 4NH_3$ produces $Cu(NH_3)_4^{2+}$ and Cl^-.

SOLUTIONS

A homogeneous (similar properties throughout) mixture of two or more substances is a *solution*. Although solutions may be solid, gas, or liquid, liquid solutions are most important for our purposes. In a solution, any small sample retains all the properties of the whole solution, and these properties reflect the properties of its components.

In two-component liquid solutions such as NaCl in water, NaCl is called the *solute*, which is dissolved in the *solvent*, water. In general, the substance with greater amount is considered to be the solvent and that with lesser amount the solute. This general definition applies to cases in which both substances are liquids as well as when one substance is a solid (or gas) and the other is a liquid.

Solubility refers to the amount of a substance that will dissolve in a certain amount of another substance (solvent) at a specified temperature. If a specific solvent is not mentioned, it is assumed to be water; if a specific temperature is not mentioned, it is assumed to be room temperature ($20°$ to $25°$ C).

In general, the attractive forces holding the particles of a solute together must be overcome for solution to result, and if such attractive forces in the solute are strong, the attractive forces between the solute and the solvent also must be strong to result in significant dissolution.

For solutions of liquids in liquids, the general rule is that "like dissolves like"; that is, polar substances will dissolve well in polar solvents, and nonpolar substances will dissolve well in nonpolar solvents.

For solutions of solids in liquids, significant dissolution of the solute occurs only if it or its ions interact strongly with the molecules of the solvent; that is, NaCl dissolves well in water (a polar solvent) but not in a nonpolar solvent, such as xylene.

Besides solute-solvent interactions, pressure and temperature also affect solubility.

With liquid or solid solutes, pressure generally has little effect on solubility, whereas the effect of pressure on gaseous solutes is significant, with increased pressure producing increased solubility of the gas.

With respect to temperature, most solids become more soluble in water with increasing temperature though, for a few solids, solubility is affected little by temperature and in some cases a solid may be less soluble with increasing temperature.

In general, the solubility of gases in liquids decreases with increasing temperature. Temperature usually has only a small effect on the solubility of liquids in liquids.

Types of solutions

A *dilute solution* has little solute in relation to solvent amount.

A *concentrated solution* has a large amount of solute in relation to solvent amount.

A *saturated solution* contains all the solute that a certain solvent can contain under the given conditions.

A *supersaturated solution* contains more solute than is ordinarily soluble under the specified conditions and is very unstable. It is prepared when one dissolves a large amount of solute with heat and then allows the solution to cool.

Colloidal solutions

The solutions mentioned in the preceding paragraphs have all been *"true"* solutions, which are homogeneous mixtures of solvent with solutes that all are less than 1 nanometer (nm) in diameter. One nanometer equals 10^{-9} meter, or 10^{-6} millimeter, or 10 angstroms (Å).

There are solutions, however, that contain particles 1 to 100 nm in diameter; these are called *colloidal solutions*, and their particles are called *colloids*.

Colloids remain dispersed indefinitely in a solvent because of continuous collisions of the colloidal particles with solvent (water) molecules, which is termed *Brownian motion*.

A colloidal dispersion also has the property of scattering light in what is known as the *Tyndall effect;* pure liquids and true solutions do not exhibit this property.

The largest portion of the organic matter of cells and tissues of the body is in the colloidal state.

A special stain for acid mucosubstances involves a colloidal iron dispersion.

Suspensions

Particles larger than about 100 nm also may be mixed in a solvent, but because of their large size, they eventually will settle out of solution if not mixed constantly; such mixtures are called *suspensions*. The particles of suspensions may actually be visible to the eye.

pH AND BUFFERS

pH is a means of easily expressing very low H^+-ion concentrations in solution and is defined as the logarithm of the reciprocal of the H^+-ion concentration (in moles per liter) or the negative of the logarithm of the H^+-ion concentration, that is:

$$pH = \log \frac{1}{[H^+]} = -\log [H^+]$$

A logarithm (log) is the power to which 10 must be raised to give a number; that is, the log of 100 (which is 10^2) is 2, and the log of 0.001 (10^{-3}) is -3. The presence of brackets around the H^+ means that the concentration of H^+ is being considered.

As an example, in pure water or a neutral solution, the $[H^+]$ is 10^{-7} N (0.0000001 N), and the

$$pH = \log \frac{1}{[10^{-7}]} = -\log [10^{-7}] = -(-7) = 7.$$

The pH scale is useful because all H^+ concentrations from 1 N to 0.00000000000001 N (10^{-14} N) can be represented simply by the numbers 0 to 14; therefore, inconvenient decimal notation can be avoided.

pH notation is especially useful in the study of body fluid $[H^+]$, which is critical to health. The approximate pH values of different body fluids are as follows: blood, 7.4; urine, 5 to 8, gastric juice, 1 to 3; saliva, 6 to 7.9; and bile, 7.8 to 8.6.

The greater the pH value, the lower is the acidity. For example, the pH of 10^{-7} N HCl is 7, whereas the pH of 10^{-3} N HCl (a higher H^+ concentration) is 3. One unit of pH represents a tenfold difference in H^+-ion concentration, for example, pH 5 is 0.00001 N H^+, and pH 4 is 0.0001 N H^+. When H^+- and OH^--ion concentrations are equal (10^{-7} N) as in neutral aqueous solutions, the pH is 7. Acid solutions are those whose pH values are less than 7, and basic solutions are those whose pH values are greater than 7. pH measurement is most conveniently done by use of pH meters or color indicators. A *pH meter* is an electrical device that is placed in a solution and directly records the pH value on a scale. An *indicator* is a very weak organic acid or base that undergoes a change of color in the presence of certain concentrations of H^+ and OH^-. Different indicators change color over different specific pH ranges. OH^--ion concentrations may be expressed in an analogous pOH format.

Buffers

A *buffer* resists changes in $[H^+]$ that result from the addition of acids or bases to a solution. Buffers are used for making solutions in which a constant pH is to be maintained and are formed by mixture of a weak (relatively undissociated) acid and its salt or a weak base and its salt in solution.

For example, a buffer may be formed when the weak electrolyte, acetic acid (CH_3COOH, abbreviated as HAc), and its salt, sodium acetate (NaAc), are added to water. The salt, NaAc, is completely dissociated in solution into Na^+ and Ac^-, whereas the acid, HAc, is almost completely undissociated.

Now, if H^+ is added to this buffer system, the H^+ will react with free Ac^- to form undissociated HAc, and if OH^- is added, it will react with undissociated HAc to form free Ac^- and H_2O, that is:

Acid addition: $H^+ + Ac^- \rightarrow HAc$
Base addition: $OH^- + HAc \rightarrow Ac^- + H_2O$

The effect of both reactions is to take up either H^+ or OH^- and lessen their effects on the overall pH of the solution.

The pH of a buffer solution may be determined by the *Henderson-Hasselbalch* equation:

$$pH = pK + \log \frac{[salt]}{[acid]}$$

or for our example,

$$pH = pK + \log \frac{[Ac^-]}{[HAc]}$$

In this equation, the bracketed substances represent concentrations, and pK is a constant that may be found in tables and shows how greatly the acid dissociates.

According to the equation, when H^+ is added to the solution containing buffer and reacts with Ac^- to form HAc, $[Ac^-]$ will decrease and $[HAc]$ will increase, so that $\log \frac{[Ac^-]}{[HAc]}$ decreases, and the pH of the solution decreases slightly. The important thing to remember is that the *pH will decrease only slightly*, whereas if H^+ were added to an unbuffered solution, the pH would decrease ($[H^+]$ would increase) dramatically.

Buffering efficiency is determined by the ratio $[salt]:[acid]$ and is greatest when this ratio is 1. This occurs when the pK of the acid used in the buffer equals the desired pH of the solution.

Buffering capacity is determined by the actual concentrations of $[salt]$ and $[acid]$ and is greater when these concentrations are greater.

Suitable laboratory buffers may be prepared by selection of appropriate weak acid-salt and weak base-salt pairs to cover the desired pH range. (See Chapter 23.)

OTHER PROCESSES

In studying the various mechanisms of staining, several physical properties and processes are important, including adsorption, absorption, capillary action, diffusion, dialysis, and osmosis.

Adsorption

Adsorption is the usually nonchemical adherence of gases, dissolved substances, or liquids on the surface of *adsorbents* such as biologic cells, tissues, and charcoal.

Absorption

Absorption refers to the uptake of a substance by an *absorbent* such as when a sponge or filter paper takes up water.

Capillary action

Capillary action is a force resulting from adhesion, cohesion, and surface tension in liquids that are in contact with a solid (such as a capillary tube). For example, the rise of water in a glass capillary is the result of the strong mutual attraction between water molecules and the strong attraction of water for glass.

Diffusion

Diffusion in a liquid solution is a physical process whereby particles move from regions of higher concentrations to regions of lower concentration and is caused by the continuous motion of the particles, which may be ions, molecules, or colloids. Diffusion of gases also occurs.

Dialysis

Dialysis is a special form of diffusion and refers to the diffusion of solutes through a semipermeable membrane such as cellophane or collodion. A semipermeable membrane is a membrane that allows low molecular weight solutes (such as salts) in a solution but not high molecular weight solutes (such as proteins) to pass through. Dialysis may be used to separate smaller molecules that can pass through the membrane from larger molecules that cannot pass through the membrane.

Osmosis and osmotic pressure

Osmosis refers to the flow of a solvent through a semipermeable membrane from a solution with lower solute concentration into one with higher solute concentration so as to tend to equalize solute concentrations on both sides of the membrane.

Osmotic pressure is the pressure that causes the solvent to pass through the membrane from the solution of lower concentration into the solution of higher concentration and is equal to the pressure that must be applied to the solution of higher concentration to prevent the diffusion of solvent into it through the membrane.

CHAPTER 21

Organic chemistry

ROBERT J. HRAPCHAK

BASIC CONCEPTS

Organic chemistry deals with the chemistry of carbon (C) and its compounds. Although the term "organic" stems from the old idea that C compounds could be formed only from living organisms, today it is known that C compounds may also be synthesized in the lab. Organic chemistry is important because an overwhelming number of all known compounds contain C. Many of these compounds may be extremely large, such as proteins, lipids, and nucleic acids, and are essential to life processes.

The C atom has a total of 6 electrons in 2 orbitals (K and L shells), and its atomic weight is 12; therefore, it has 6 protons and 6 neutrons in its nucleus. Of the 6 electrons in C, 2 are in the inner shell and 4 are in the outer (valence) shell.

If the 2 inner electrons and the nucleus are designated by the atomic symbol, we can draw the C atom as follows:

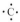

This structure shows only the valence electrons. Similar electronic structures can be drawn for other atoms if all inner-shell electrons and nuclei are indicated by the atomic symbols and only the outer-shell electrons by dots.

C has no tendency to gain or lose electrons but combines with other C atoms (or different atoms) by covalent bonding. C atoms may combine in various numbers to form long- and short-chain structures as well as multiatomic rings. These compounds also may have branches and crosslinks. Atoms other than C also may be pres-

357

ent, such as H, O, N. S, P, and Cl. Two or even three pairs of electrons may be shared between C atoms to form double ($C=C$) and triple ($C\equiv C$) bonds. Although there is free rotation about $C-C$ single bonds, when C atoms are joined by double or triple bonds such rotation is hindered, and the bonded atoms represent planar (flat) structures. Since C has 4 valence electrons, each C atom can have only a maximum of 4 bonds; remember this while studying and drawing the structures mentioned later.

Organic compounds may be designated by *molecular* or *structural* formulas. For the compound ethane, we have:

C_2H_6 Molecular formula, which shows no structural arrangement, but only the type and actual numbers of each atom in a molecule

H H
H:C:C:H Structural formula, with valence electrons being designated by dots
H H

H   H
| |
H—C—C—H Structural formula, with lines indicating shared electron pairs
| |
H   H

An empirical formula may also be used, which is the simplest formula that shows the *relative numbers* of different atoms in a molecule. For ethane, the empirical formula is CH_3. For methane, the empirical and molecular formulas are the same, that is, CH_4.

Although C compounds can be represented by two-dimensional structural formulas, remember that the actual molecules are three-dimensional structures with definite bond lengths and definite bond angles in space.

Isomers

Different compounds that have the same molecular formula (and therefore the same molecular weight) but different properties are called isomers. There are two general types of isomers: *structural isomers* and *stereoisomers*, and each type may be subdivided. Structural isomers have the same molecular formula but different structures and include *chain, position,* or *functional isomers*.

Structural isomers. Simple examples of *chain structural isomers* are butane and isobutane, both alkanes with the molecular formula C_4H_{10} but with differences in arrangement of the C atoms in the chain (Table 21-1, *A, 1*).

An example of *position structural isomers* is the pair propanol and isopropanol, both alcohols with the molecular formula C_3H_8O, in which the C chains are the same but the positions of the OH groups are different (Table 21-1, *A, 2*).

In *functional structural isomers,* such as ethanol and dimethyl ether, both compounds have the same molecular formula, C_2H_6O, but different functional groups and therefore belong to different families of organic compounds (Table 21-1, *A, 3*).

Stereoisomers. Stereoisomers are compounds that have the same molecular formulas and structures but have different configurations (arrangement of atoms in space) and include *geometric and optical isomers.* Examples of geometric isomers are *trans*-2-butene and *cis*-2-butene (Table 21-1, *B, 1*). In these two compounds with double bonds, in which there is hindered rotation about the doubly bonded C atoms, the methyl groups may be on opposite sides of the double bond (*trans*) or on the same side of the double bond (*cis*).

The other type of stereoisomerism involves *optical isomers (enantiomers),* which have the same molecular and structural formulas but different effects on plane-polarized light. When plane-polarized light passes through a solution containing an optically active compound, the plane of light is rotated either to the right (clockwise, indicated by + sign or small *d*) or to the left (counterclockwise, indicated by − sign or small *l*). (*Note:* Do not confuse *d* and *l* with D and L, which are discussed in the section on carbohydrates.) To be optical isomers, molecules must contain asymmetric C atoms (a C atom attached to four different groups), and their mirror images must not be superimposable. Examples of optical isomers are given in Table 21-1, *B, 2*.

When these molecules are viewed in three dimensions, H and OH are considered to project in front of the plane of the page, and CHO and CH_2OH are considered to project behind the plane of the page. The molecules are mirror images that are not superimposable and are, therefore, optical isomers.

We can tell from structural formulas whether two molecules are optical isomers, but we cannot tell whether they give − or + rotation. This can be done only by use of an optical apparatus called a *polarimeter.*

Reactions of organic compounds

Organic compounds undergo many types of reactions depending on their structures. Defini-

Table 21-1. Types of isomers

A. Structural isomers

1. Chain structural isomers

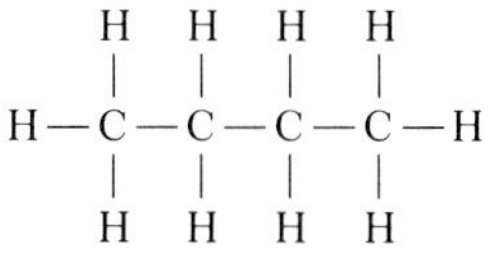

<table>
<tr>
<td>

H   H   H   H
 | | | |
H—C—C—C—C—H
 | | | |
H   H   H   H

(Normal) butane

</td>
<td>

H
|
H   H—C—H   H
 | | |
H—C————C————C—H
 | | |
H   H   H

Isobutane

</td>
</tr>
</table>

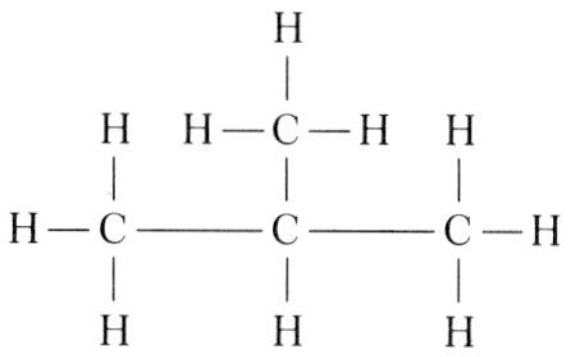

2. Position structural isomers

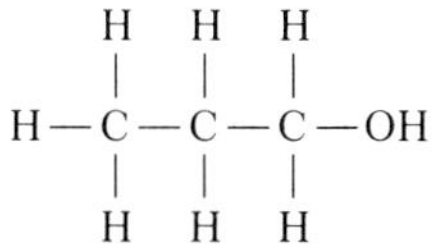

<table>
<tr>
<td>

H   H   H
 | | |
H—C—C—C—OH
 | | |
H   H   H

(Normal) propanol

</td>
<td>

H   OH   H
 | | |
H—C—C—C—H
 | | |
H   H   H

Isopropanol

</td>
</tr>
</table>

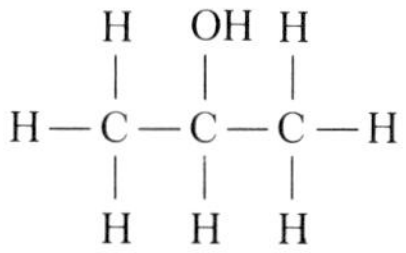

3. Functional structural isomers

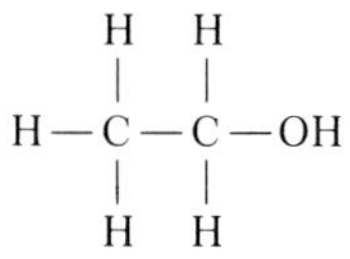

<table>
<tr>
<td>

H   H
 | |
H—C—C—OH
 | |
H   H

Ethanol (an alcohol)

</td>
<td>

H   H
 | |
H—C—O—C—H
 | |
H   H

Dimethyl ether (an ether)

</td>
</tr>
</table>

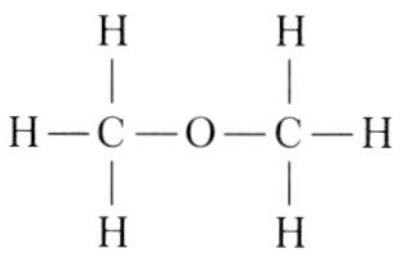

B. Stereoisomers

1. Geometric stereoisomers

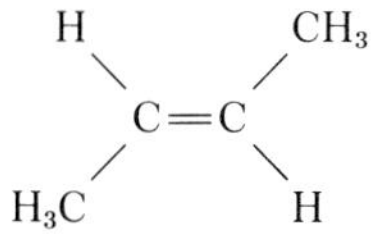

<table>
<tr>
<td>

H   CH₃
 \\   /
  C=C
 /   \\
H₃C   H

trans-2-butene

</td>
<td>

H   H
 \\   /
  C=C
 /   \\
H₃C   CH₃

cis-2-butene

</td>
</tr>
</table>

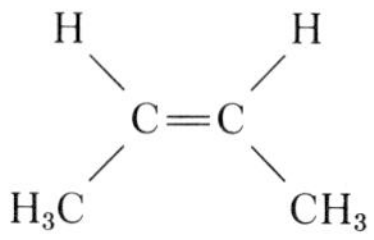

2. Optical stereoisomers

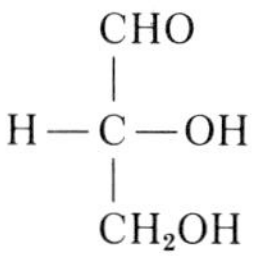

<table>
<tr>
<td>

CHO
|
H—C—OH
|
CH₂OH

(+)-Glyceraldehyde

</td>
<td>

CHO
|
HO—C—H
|
CH₂OH

(−)-Glyceraldehyde

</td>
</tr>
</table>

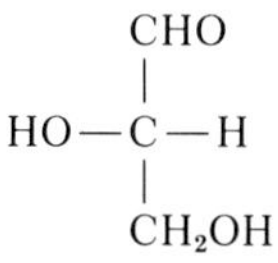

tions of some of these reactions follow, and typical examples are shown in Table 21-2.

addition A reaction in which one molecule combines with another molecule to yield a single molecule.

combustion The reaction of an organic compound with O_2 to produce CO_2, H_2O, and heat.

elimination A reaction in which 2 atoms or groups of atoms are removed from an organic compound to form a less saturated bond.

esterification The reaction of an alcohol with an acid to form esters.

oxidation A reaction in which H atoms are removed or O atoms are added (or both) to an organic compound.

ozonolysis A reaction in which a compound with a multiple bond is cleaved at the bond to produce smaller molecules.

pyrolysis Decomposition of a compound into smaller compounds by high temperatures.

reduction A reaction in which H atoms are added to or O atoms are removed from an organic compound, or both processes occur simultaneously.

Continued on p. 364.

Table 21-2. Reactions of organic compounds

A. Reactions of alkanes
1. Halogenation (substitution)

$$-\overset{\displaystyle |}{\underset{\displaystyle |}{C}}- \quad + \quad Cl_2 \quad \longrightarrow \quad -\overset{\displaystyle |}{\underset{\displaystyle |}{C}}-Cl$$

Alkane   **Alkyl chloride**

2. Combustion

$$R-\overset{\displaystyle H}{\underset{\displaystyle H}{\overset{\displaystyle |}{\underset{\displaystyle |}{C}}}}-H \quad \xrightarrow{O_2 \text{ plus heat}} \quad CO_2 \quad + \quad H_2O$$

Alkane

3. Pyrolysis

$$\text{Alkane} \quad \xrightarrow{\text{High heat}} \quad \text{Smaller alkanes} \quad + \quad H_2 \quad + \quad \text{Alkenes}$$

B. Reactions of alkenes
1. Hydrogenation (addition)

$$-\overset{\displaystyle |}{C}=\overset{\displaystyle |}{C}- \quad + \quad H_2 \quad \xrightarrow{\text{Catalyst}} \quad -\overset{\displaystyle |}{\underset{\displaystyle |}{C}}-\overset{\displaystyle |}{\underset{\displaystyle |}{C}}-$$

Alkene   **Alkane**

2. Halogen addition

$$-\overset{\displaystyle |}{C}=\overset{\displaystyle |}{C}- \quad + \quad Cl_2 \quad \longrightarrow \quad -\overset{\displaystyle |}{\underset{\displaystyle |}{C}}-\overset{\displaystyle |}{\underset{\displaystyle |}{C}}-$$
$$\qquad\qquad\qquad\qquad\qquad\qquad Cl \quad Cl$$

Alkene   **Dichloroalkane**

3. Halogenation (substitution)

$$-\overset{\displaystyle |}{C}=\overset{\displaystyle |}{C}-\overset{\displaystyle |}{\underset{\displaystyle |}{C}}- \quad + \quad Cl_2 \quad \xrightarrow{\text{Heat}} \quad -\overset{\displaystyle |}{C}=\overset{\displaystyle |}{C}-\overset{\displaystyle |}{\underset{\displaystyle |}{C}}-Cl$$

Alkene   **Chloroalkene**

4. Hydration (addition)

$$-\overset{\displaystyle |}{C}=\overset{\displaystyle |}{C}- \quad + \quad H_2O \quad \longrightarrow \quad -\overset{\displaystyle |}{\underset{\displaystyle |}{C}}-\overset{\displaystyle |}{\underset{\displaystyle |}{C}}-$$
$$\qquad\qquad\qquad\qquad\qquad\qquad\qquad OH$$

Alkene   **Alcohol**

5. Ozonolysis

$$R_1-\overset{\displaystyle |}{C}=\overset{\displaystyle \overset{\displaystyle R_2}{|}}{C}-R_3 \quad + \quad O_3 \quad \longrightarrow \quad R_1-\overset{\displaystyle \overset{\displaystyle H}{|}}{C}=O \quad + \quad O=\overset{\displaystyle \overset{\displaystyle R_2}{|}}{C}-R_3$$

Alkene   **Aldehyde**   **Ketone**

Table 21-2. Reactions of organic compounds—cont'd

C. Reactions of alkynes
1. Hydrogenation (addition)

$$-C\equiv C- \xrightarrow{H_2\ catalyst} -C=C- \xrightarrow{H_2\ catalyst} -C-C-$$

Alkyne   **Alkene**   **Alkane**

2. Halogen addition

$$-C\equiv C- \xrightarrow{Cl_2} -C=C- \xrightarrow{Cl_2} -C-C-$$

Alkyne   **Dichloroalkene**   **Tetrachloroalkane**

3. Hydration (addition)

Alkyne + $H_2O \longrightarrow$ Aldehydes or ketones

D. Reactions of benzene
1. Halogenation (substitution)

Benzene + $Cl_2 \rightarrow$ Chlorobenzene + HCl

Benzene   **Chlorobenzene**

2. Alkylation (substitution)

Benzene + $CH_3CH_2Br \xrightarrow{Lewis\ acid}$ Ethylbenzene (CH_2CH_3) + HBr

Benzene **Ethyl bromide**   **Ethylbenzene**

E. Reactions of alcohols
1. Dehydration (elimination)

$$R_1-C-C-R_2 \xrightarrow{Acid} R_1-C=C-R_2 + H_2O$$
$$OH$$

Alcohol   **Alkene**

2. Esterification

$$R_1-OH + R_2C\!\!\begin{smallmatrix}O\\OH\end{smallmatrix} \longrightarrow R_2C\!\!\begin{smallmatrix}O\\OR_1\end{smallmatrix} + H_2O$$

Alcohol **Carboxylic acid**   **Ester**

3. Reaction with halogen halides (substitution)

$$ROH + HCl \longrightarrow RCl + H_2O$$

Alcohol   **Alkyl chloride**

Continued.

Table 21-2. Reactions of organic compounds—cont'd

4. Oxidation

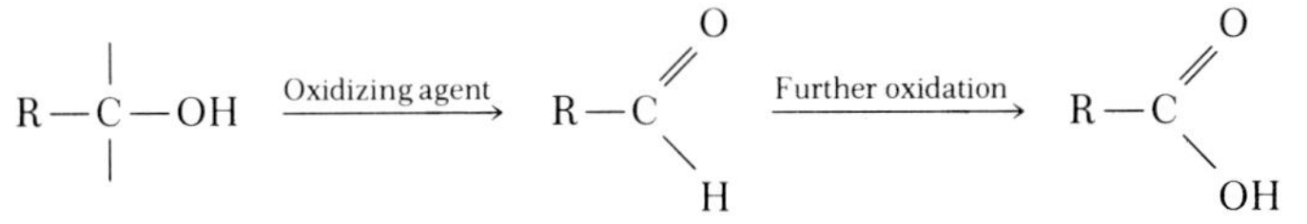

Primary alcohol   Aldehyde   Carboxylic acid

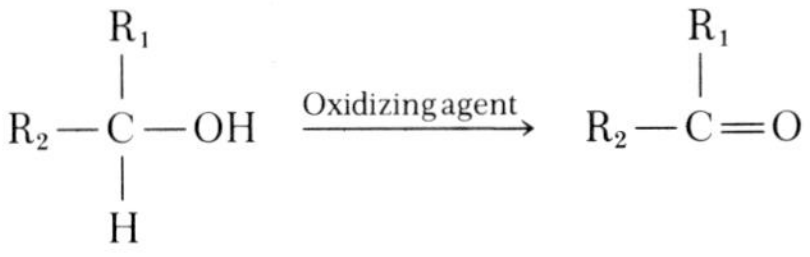

Secondary alcohol   Ketone

Tertiary alcohols are not oxidized easily.

F. **Reactions of aldehydes**
   1. Oxidation

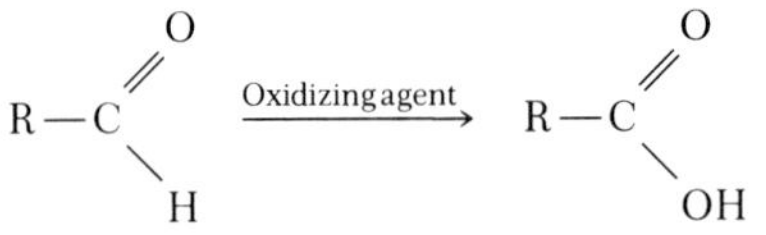

Aldehyde   Carboxylic acid

   2. Reduction

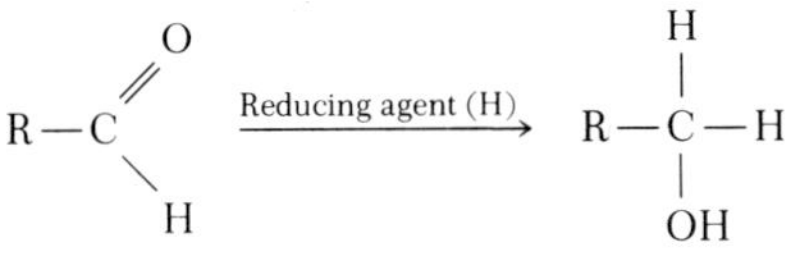

Aldehyde   Primary alcohol

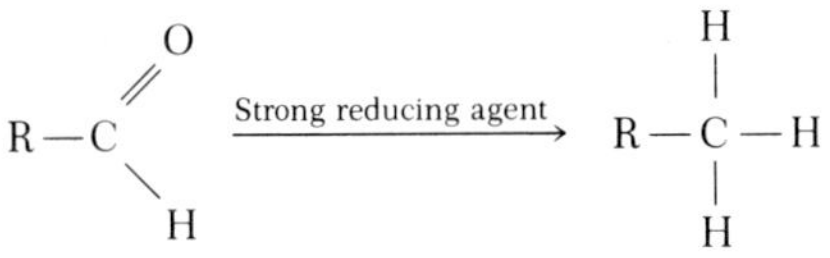

Aldehyde   Hydrocarbon

G. **Reactions of carboxylic acids**
   1. Salt formation

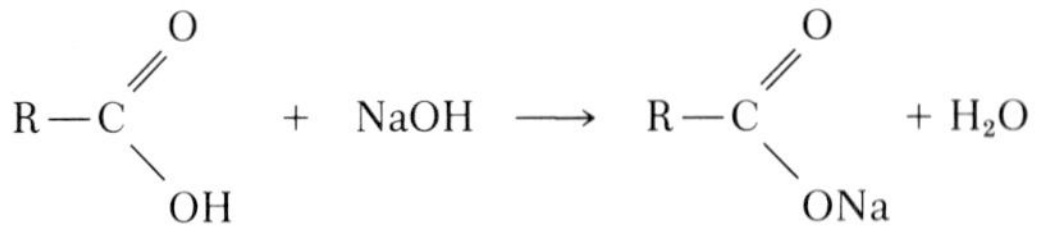

Carboxylic acid   Sodium carboxylate

   2. Esterification

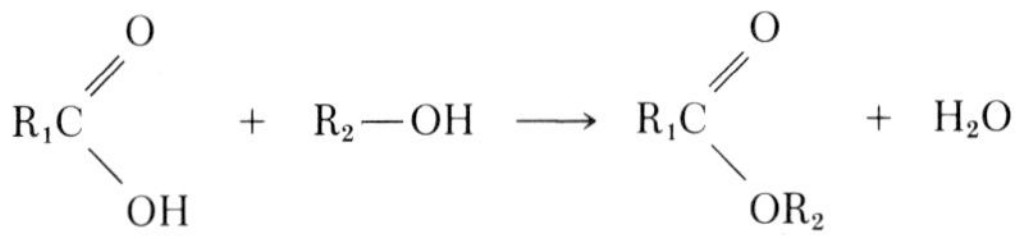

Carboxylic acid   Alcohol   Ester

Table 21-2. Reactions of organic compounds—cont'd

3. Reduction

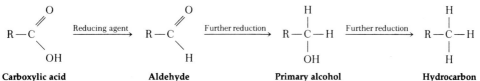

| Carboxylic acid | Aldehyde | Primary alcohol | Hydrocarbon |

H. Reactions of ketones
1. Oxidation

   Ketones are not easily oxidized since they cannot lose H without the rupture of a C—C bond.

2. Reduction

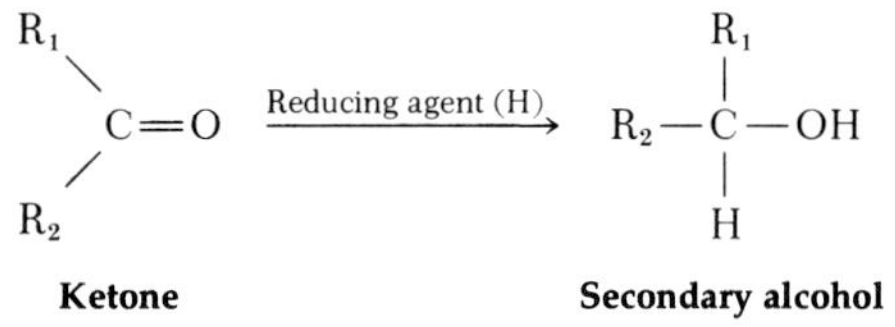

$$
\begin{array}{c}
R_1 \\
\diagdown \\
C{=}O \\
\diagup \\
R_2
\end{array}
\xrightarrow{\text{Reducing agent (H)}}
\begin{array}{c}
R_1 \\
| \\
R_2{-}C{-}OH \\
| \\
H
\end{array}
$$

| Ketone | Secondary alcohol |

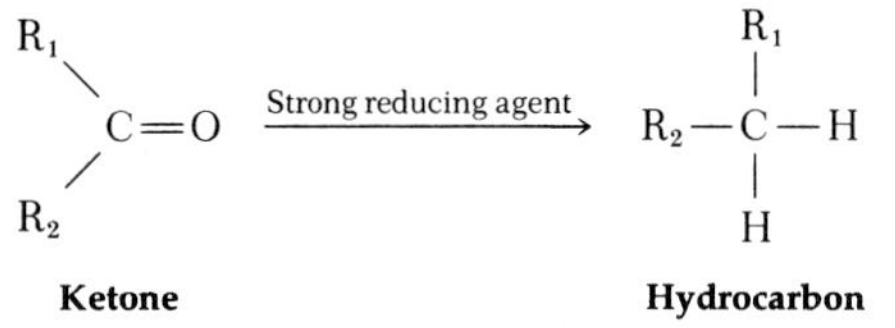

$$
\begin{array}{c}
R_1 \\
\diagdown \\
C{=}O \\
\diagup \\
R_2
\end{array}
\xrightarrow{\text{Strong reducing agent}}
\begin{array}{c}
R_1 \\
| \\
R_2{-}C{-}H \\
| \\
H
\end{array}
$$

| Ketone | Hydrocarbon |

I. Reactions of monosaccharides
1. Oxidation by periodic acid (HIO_4)

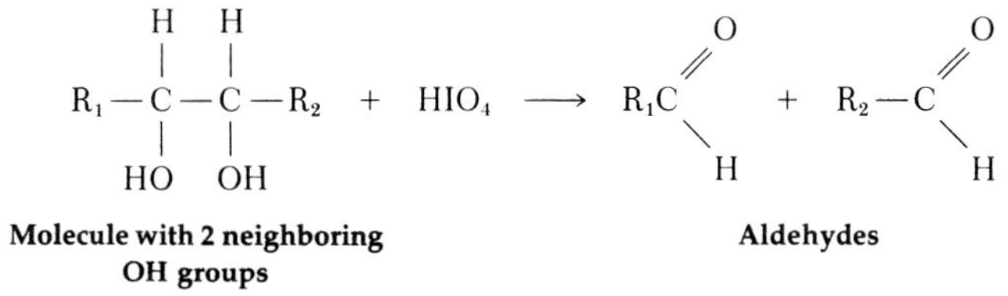

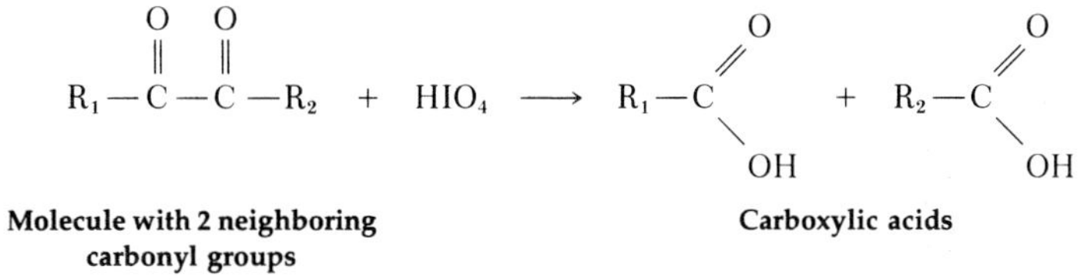

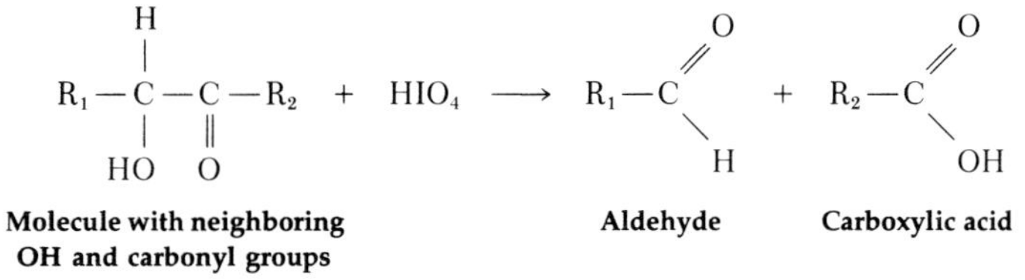

Molecule with 2 neighboring OH groups + HIO_4 → Aldehydes

Molecule with 2 neighboring carbonyl groups + HIO_4 → Carboxylic acids

Molecule with neighboring OH and carbonyl groups + HIO_4 → Aldehyde + Carboxylic acid

Continued.

Table 21-2. Reactions of organic compounds—cont'd

$$R_1-\overset{\overset{\displaystyle H}{|}}{\underset{\underset{\displaystyle OH}{|}}{C}}-\overset{\overset{\displaystyle H}{|}}{\underset{\underset{\displaystyle OH}{|}}{C}}-\overset{\overset{\displaystyle H}{|}}{\underset{\underset{\displaystyle OH}{|}}{C}}-R_2 \; + \; HIO_4 \longrightarrow R_1C\overset{\displaystyle O}{\underset{\displaystyle H}{\Big\langle}} \; + \; R_2C\overset{\displaystyle O}{\underset{\displaystyle H}{\Big\langle}} \; + \; HC\overset{\displaystyle O}{\underset{\displaystyle OH}{\Big\langle}}$$

| Molecule with 3 neighboring OH groups | Aldehydes | Formic acid |

2. Reduction

$$R-C\overset{\displaystyle O}{\underset{\displaystyle H}{\Big\langle}} \xrightarrow{\text{Reducing agent (H)}} R-\overset{\overset{\displaystyle H}{|}}{\underset{\underset{\displaystyle OH}{|}}{C}}-H$$

Aldose   Primary alcohol

$$\overset{\displaystyle CH_2OH}{\underset{\displaystyle R}{\overset{|}{\underset{|}{C}}}}{=}O \xrightarrow{\text{Reducing agent (H)}} H-\overset{\overset{\displaystyle CH_2OH}{|}}{\underset{\underset{\displaystyle R}{|}}{C}}-OH$$

Ketose   Secondary alcohol

Reduction of monosaccharides produces the corresponding alcohols; thus glucose gives sorbitol, and mannose gives mannitol.

salt formation The formation of an ionic compound from a metallic cation and an anion.

substitution A reaction in which an atom or group of atoms in an organic compound is replaced by another atom or group with the breakage and formation of single bonds.

HYDROCARBONS

Organic compounds that contain only covalently bonded C and H atoms are called hydrocarbons. Hydrocarbons include two main classes, aliphatic and aromatic compounds. Aliphatic hydrocarbons include various families, such as alkanes, alkenes, alkynes, and their cyclic analogs (cycloalkanes, cycloalkenes, and cycloalkynes). Aromatics include benzene and similar compounds. In addition, hydrocarbons that contain both aliphatic and aromatic units are called *arenes*, but they are defined as being aromatic hydrocarbons. The various classes and families of hydrocarbons are given in Table 21-3 and discussed below.

Aliphatic hydrocarbons

Alkanes. The alkanes have single $C-C$ covalent bonds and are nonpolar because C atoms of the same very low electronegativity are joined symmetrically. The general formula of alkanes is C_nH_{2n+2}, and examples include methane (CH_4), ethane (C_2H_6), propane (C_3H_8), butane (C_4H_{10}), and pentane (C_5H_{12}) (Table 21-3). In alkanes, the boiling points and melting points increase as the number of C atoms increases because of the stronger intermolecular forces (van der Waals forces) that must be overcome in larger molecules before they boil or melt. Alkanes dissolve in solvents of low polarity (benzene, diethyl ether, chloroform) and undergo very few reactions, which, if they do occur, occur only under rigorous conditions; these include halogenation, combustion, and pyrolysis. For reactions, see Table 21-2, A.

A group that contains one less H than its parent alkane is called an alkyl group, such as methyl, ethyl, propyl, butyl, and pentyl groups, and names of derivatives of organic compounds use such designations.

Alkenes. Alkenes are aliphatic hydrocarbons that contain double-bonded C atoms ($C=C$), and since they have less than the maximum amount of H, they are also called unsaturated hydrocarbons. They may be converted to alkanes by addition of H to the double bonds in a reaction called hydrogenation.

The general formula of alkenes is C_nH_{2n}, and examples include ethene (C_2H_4), propene (C_3H_6), and 1-butene (C_4H_8) (Table 21-3).

Table 21-3. Hydrocarbons

Family	General formula (n = Whole number)	Examples	Structures*
Aliphatic hydrocarbons			
Alkane (C single bond)	C_nH_{2n+2}	Methane	$-\overset{\mid}{\underset{\mid}{C}}-$
		Ethane	$-\overset{\mid}{\underset{\mid}{C}}-\overset{\mid}{\underset{\mid}{C}}-$
		Propane	$-\overset{\mid}{\underset{\mid}{C}}-\overset{\mid}{\underset{\mid}{C}}-\overset{\mid}{\underset{\mid}{C}}-$
		Butane	$-\overset{\mid}{\underset{\mid}{C}}-\overset{\mid}{\underset{\mid}{C}}-\overset{\mid}{\underset{\mid}{C}}-\overset{\mid}{\underset{\mid}{C}}-$
		Pentane	$-\overset{\mid}{\underset{\mid}{C}}-\overset{\mid}{\underset{\mid}{C}}-\overset{\mid}{\underset{\mid}{C}}-\overset{\mid}{\underset{\mid}{C}}-\overset{\mid}{\underset{\mid}{C}}-$
Alkene (C=C double bond)	C_nH_{2n}	Ethene	$-\overset{\mid}{C}=\overset{\mid}{C}-$
		Propene	$\overset{\mid}{C}=\overset{\mid}{\underset{\mid}{C}}-\overset{\mid}{\underset{\mid}{C}}-$
		1-Butene	$\overset{\mid}{C}=\overset{\mid}{\underset{\mid}{C}}-\overset{\mid}{\underset{\mid}{C}}-\overset{\mid}{\underset{\mid}{C}}-$
Alkyne (C≡C triple bond)	C_nH_{2n-2}	Acetylene	$-C\equiv C-$
		Propyne	$-C\equiv C-\overset{\mid}{\underset{\mid}{C}}-$
		1-Butyne	$-C\equiv C-\overset{\mid}{\underset{\mid}{C}}-\overset{\mid}{\underset{\mid}{C}}-$
Diene (2 C=C)	C_nH_{2n-2}	1,3-Butadiene (conjugated bonds)	$\overset{\mid}{C}=\overset{\mid}{C}-\overset{\mid}{C}=\overset{\mid}{C}$
		1,4-Pentadiene (isolated bonds)	$\overset{\mid}{C}=\overset{\mid}{C}-\overset{\mid}{\underset{\mid}{C}}-\overset{\mid}{C}=\overset{\mid}{C}$
Cycloalkane	C_nH_{2n}	Cyclopentane	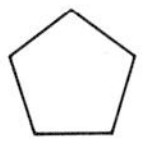 ⬠
Cycloalkene	C_nH_{2n-2}	Cyclopentene	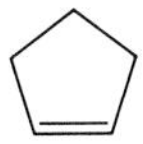 ⬠
Cycloalkyne	C_nH_{2n-4}	Cyclooctyne	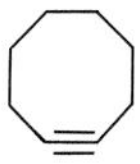 ⯃

Continued.

Table 21-3. Hydrocarbons—cont'd

Family	General formula (n = Whole number)	Examples	Structures*
Aromatic hydrocarbons			
Benzene and related compounds	C_6H_6 (benzene)	Benzene	
Arenes			
Alkylbenzenes (aromatic and alkane parts)	—	Toluene	
		Ortho-xylene	
Alkenylbenzenes (aromatic and alkene parts)	—	Styrene	$CH=CH_2$
Alkynylbenzenes (aromatic and alkyne parts)	—	Phenylacetylene	$C≡CH$

*When no atom is indicated at the end of a C bond, that is, C—, it is understood that H is present.
When no C or H atoms are shown in a cyclic aliphatic structure, C is understood to be present at the junctions of lines, and each C is attached to 2 H atoms unless other groups are indicated.
When no C or H atoms are shown in an aromatic structure such as benzene, C is understood to be present at the junctions of lines, and each C is attached to 1 H atom unless other groups are indicated.

Typical alkenes are insoluble in water but quite soluble in nonpolar solvents. Their boiling and melting points increase with increasing number of C atoms as in alkanes. Alkenes are more reactive than alkanes because of the double bonds and may undergo several types of reactions, including additions to the double bond or bonds, such as addition of halogens and hydration (Table 21-2, *B*).

Alkynes. Alkynes represent another family of aliphatic hydrocarbons that contain triple-bonded C atoms (C≡C) and thus are more unsaturated than the alkenes. Their general formula is C_nH_{2n-2}, and examples include acetylene (C_2H_2), propyne (C_3H_4), and 1-butyne (C_4H_6) (Table 21-3).

Alkynes have low polarity, and their physical properties are similar to alkanes and alkenes; that is, they are insoluble in water but soluble in organic solvents of low polarity; they are less dense than water; and their melting and boiling points increase with increasing C content. Alkynes undergo many addition reactions in which atoms are added to the triple-bonded C atoms. For typical reactions of alkynes, see Table 21-2, *C*.

Dienes. Dienes are unsaturated hydrocarbons that contain 2 double bonds. They are therefore alkenes but have the same general formula as alkynes, C_nH_{2n-2}. Dienes may contain 2 double bonds separated by only 1 single bond (—C=C—C=C—, conjugated double bonds) or 2 double bonds separated by more than 1 single bond (—C=C—C—C=C—, isolated double bonds) (Table 21-3). Dienes have essentially the same properties as the previously mentioned alkenes.

Cyclic aliphatic hydrocarbons. C atoms may also form rings instead of open-chain compounds; these C ring–containing compounds are called cyclic compounds and include the cycloalkanes, cycloalkenes, and cycloalkynes. Cyclic aliphatics are named by prefixing *cyclo-* to the name of the corresponding open-chain hydrocarbon with the same number of C atoms, and examples are cyclopentane (C_5H_{10}), cyclopentene (C_5H_8), and cyclooctyne (C_8H_{12}) (Table 21-3).

The chemistry of these cyclic hydrocarbons is similar to that of the open-chain analogs, and they undergo reactions similar to the corresponding open-chain compounds.

Aromatic hydrocarbons

The other main class of hydrocarbons besides the aliphatics comprises the aromatic com-

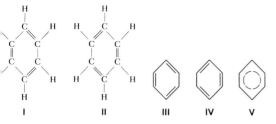

Fig. 21-1. Structural representations of benzene.

pounds, which include benzene (C_6H_6) and compounds resembling benzene in chemical properties. Benzene, though a single molecule, is now known to be a "resonance hybrid" of structures I and II in Fig. 21-1.

By *resonance theory,* which considers molecules that can be represented by two or more structures having the same arrangement of atomic nuclei but differences in electron distribution, benzene is thought of as being intermediate between I and II, that is, a "resonance hybrid" of I and II. This does not mean that benzene is composed of both forms I and II, but rather in benzene all molecules are the same, having a structure intermediate between I and II. With this background, benzene type of compounds can be represented more simply by structures III and IV in Fig. 21-1.

In structures III and IV, C atoms are assumed to be present at each junction of lines, and 1 H atom is assumed to be attached to each C atom.

It is known that although benzene is often represented by structures such as I to IV, all of which indicate 3 C—C single bonds and 3 double bonds, the actual bonds in benzene are all equivalent, each being intermediate between a single and double bond, that is, a hybrid bond. The best structure for benzene, therefore, is V in Fig. 21-1. Structure V shows the overall even distribution of electrons, as depicted by the inner broken circle, over a single benzene molecule. You should remember the significance of structures I to V, since any one may be used to depict benzene in different books.

Although it is easy to see in structures I to IV why benzene has only 6 H atoms (that is, each C atom can have only a total of 4 bonds), this is not clear when structure V is used; therefore, the meaning of structure V should be memorized.

Benzene is a flat, symmetric, stable molecule that undergoes mainly substitution reactions in which it tends to retain its unique aromatic ring system (Table 21-2, *D*).

Aromatic compounds in general have the following properties: they undergo substitution reactions like benzene instead of addition reactions that characterize other unsaturated compounds, thereby retaining their ring systems. In addition, they are very stable, cyclic, and flat molecules.

A group containing one less H than benzene is called the phenyl group (C_6H_5), and "phenyl" will be seen often in the names of organic aromatic compounds.

Arenes. Arenes are hydrocarbons that contain both aliphatic and aromatic constituents, such as the alkylbenzenes (aromatic and alkane parts), alkenylbenzenes (aromatic and alkene parts), and alkynylbenzenes (aromatic and alkyne parts). Examples of these groups are methylbenzene (toluene), vinylbenzene (styrene), and phenylacetylene, respectively (Table 21-3).

The arenes show properties common to both the aliphatic and aromatic units of the molecule, as modified by the other unit. Important solvents in histotechnology are the three isomers of xylene and, as an example, *ortho*-xylene is shown in Table 21-3.

FUNCTIONAL GROUPS

An atom or group of atoms that defines the structure and determines in a large measure the properties of an organic compound bearing it is called a *functional group.* Table 21-4 shows the major functional groups that histotechnologists will encounter. Having discussed organic compounds that have only C—C functional groups, we will now consider types of organic compounds with other kinds of functional groups.

Alcohols

Alcohols are organic compounds that contain the hydroxyl (OH) functional group connected to an alkyl or substituted alkyl group (symbolized by *R*) and have the general formula, ROH. The OH group determines the properties of the alcohols. Alcohols are called primary, secondary, or tertiary according to whether the OH group is attached to a C atom that is attached to one, two, or three other C atoms, respectively. Methanol (CH_3OH) and ethanol (CH_3CH_2OH), both primary alcohols, are common solvents in histotechnology, as are isopropanol (secondary) and *tert*-butanol (tertiary).

The alkyl groups in alcohols may be cyclic, contain unsaturated bonds, contain atoms other than C or H, or even contain aromatic rings.

Table 21-4. Functional groups

Functional group	Structure	Found in
C=C double bond	$-\overset{\|}{C}=\overset{\|}{C}-$	Alkenes
C≡C triple bond	$-C\equiv C-$	Alkynes
Multiple C=C double bonds	$-\overset{\|}{C}=\overset{\|}{C}-\overset{\|}{C}=\overset{\|}{C}-$	Dienes
Amino group	$-NH_2$	Amides Amines Amino acids
Carbonyl group	$-\overset{\overset{O}{\|\|}}{C}-$	Aldehydes Ketones
Carboxyl group	$-\overset{\overset{O}{\|\|}}{C}-OH$	Carboxylic acids
Ether group	$-O-$	Ethers
Hydroxyl group	$-OH$	Alcohols Phenols
Halogen	Br, Cl, F, or I	Alkyl halides Aryl halides Acyl chlorides

Examples of alcohols are shown in Table 21-5, *A*. (*Note:* When the OH group is attached directly to an aromatic ring, the compounds are called phenols, not alcohols.)

Alcohols have both polar and nonpolar characteristics because of the OH and alkyl groups, respectively. Alcohols can form H bonds with each other and other molecules. Alcohols with lower C contents (methanol, ethanol, isopropanol) are soluble in water, but water solubility decreases with increasing C-chain length because of the increasing nonpolar character of the alkyl group. The boiling points of alcohols increase with increasing chain length. Examples of the reactions of alcohols include substitution with replacement of the OH group by a halide; dehydration with formation of a double bond; reaction with an inorganic or organic acid to form an ester; and oxidation of primary and secondary alcohols to carboxylic acids and ketones, respectively. Examples are shown in Table 21-2. *E*.

Aldehydes

Aldehydes are organic compounds that con-

tain the carbonyl functional group (C=O) attached to an aliphatic or aromatic group and a H atom; their general formula is RCHO, and their general structural formula is

$$R-C\overset{\displaystyle O}{\underset{\displaystyle H}{<}}$$

Aldehydes are also called carbonyl compounds, and it is the polar carbonyl group that determines the chemistry of aldehydes.

Aldehydes are easily oxidized and commonly undergo nucleophilic addition reactions; that is, they are susceptible to attack by electron-rich nucleophils (bases) at the relatively positive C atom of the polar C=O group.

Because of the polarity of the C=O group, aldehydes are polar and have higher boiling points than do nonpolar compounds of similar molecular weight, but their boiling points are lower than are similar alcohols or carboxylic acids because they cannot form intermolecular H bonds. When present in polar (aqueous) solvents, aldehydes with lower C number are quite soluble because of H bonding between the aldehyde and water molecules. Aldehydes are also soluble in the common organic solvents. Commonly used aldehydes are formaldehyde, acetaldehyde, and benzaldehyde (Table 21-5, *B*). The common oxidation and reduction reactions of aldehydes are shown in Table 21-2, *F*.

Alkyl halides

Alkyl halides have the general formula *RX,* in which *R* is an alkyl or substituted alkyl group and *X* is Cl, Br, F, or I (halide). Alkyl halides important in histotechnology as solvents include chloroform ($CHCl_3$) and carbon tetrachloride (CCl_4) (Table 21-5, *C*).

Amines

Amines are organic compounds in which an alkyl or aromatic group or groups are substituted for the H atoms of ammonia (NH_3). Amines are called primary, secondary, or tertiary depending on whether one, two, or three non-H groups, respectively, are attached to the N. Amines are polar compounds, and the smaller amines are soluble in water because of the formation of H bonds. They are also quite soluble in less polar organic solvents such as ether, benzene, and ethanol. Amines can form solid, ion-containing salts, such as trimethylammonium chloride. Examples of common amines are given in Table 21-5, *D*.

Carboxylic acids

Carboxylic acids are organic compounds that contain the carboxyl functional group

$$-C\overset{\displaystyle O}{\underset{\displaystyle OH}{\big\langle}}$$

attached to either alkyl or aromatic groups. Their general formula is RCOOH, and their structural formula is

$$R-C\overset{\displaystyle O}{\underset{\displaystyle OH}{\big\langle}}$$

Carboxylic acids show the greatest acidity of the organic compounds. Carboxylic acids are polar and can form H bonds with themselves and other molecules. The aliphatic carboxylic acids

with lower C number are therefore quite soluble in water, whereas the higher C number forms are quite insoluble. Aromatic carboxylic acids are insoluble in water. Carboxylic acids are soluble in organic solvents such as benzene, ethanol, and ether. The carboxylic acids have higher boiling points than similar alcohols because of increased H bonding. Carboxylic acid salts with metals are crystalline solids composed of positive and negative ions and have variable solubilities in water. Common carboxylic acids are shown in Table 21-5, *E*. Some common reactions of the carboxylic acids are given in Table 21-2, *G*.

Ethers

Ethers are compounds with the general formula R_1-O-R_2, in which R_1 and R_2 may be the same or different aliphatic or aromatic groups. Examples are given in Table 21-5, *F*. Ethers are weakly polar compounds and have boiling points similar to alkanes of like molecular weight, and the smaller ethers are slightly soluble in water. Anhydrous diethyl ether (also commonly called ethyl ether or simply ether) is used in histotechnology and is extremely dangerous because of its high volatility and inflammability. ETHERS CAN FORM HIGHLY EXPLOSIVE PEROXIDES IF ALLOWED TO REMAIN IN CONTACT WITH AIR.

Ketones

Ketones are organic compounds that, like aldehydes, contain the C=O group and are therefore also called carbonyl compounds. In ketones, the C=O group is attached to two aliphatic or aromatic groups. Their general formula is R_1R_2CO, and their structural formula is

$$\overset{\displaystyle R_1}{\underset{\displaystyle R_2}{\big\rangle}}C=O$$

Ketones are not so easily oxidized as aldehydes and are generally less reactive than aldehydes in nucleophilic addition reactions.

The physical properties of ketones (boiling and melting points, solubility in polar and nonpolar solvents) are similar to aldehydes. Common ketones, including acetone (used in histotechnology), methyl ethyl ketone, and acetophenone are shown in Table 21-5, *G*. Reactions of ketones are shown in Table 21-2, *H*.

Table 21-5. Examples of common organic compounds

A. Alcohols

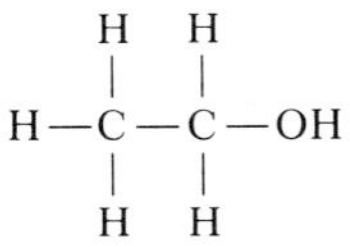

Ethanol
(primary)

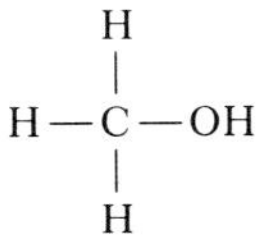

Methanol
(primary)

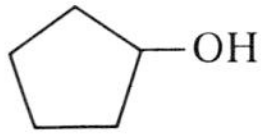

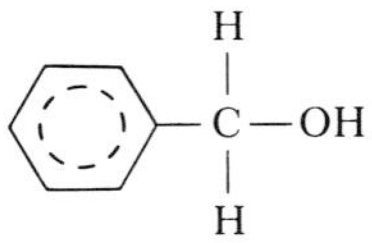

Benzyl alcohol
(primary)

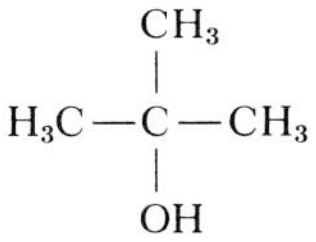

Cyclopentanol
(secondary)

tert-butanol
(tertiary)

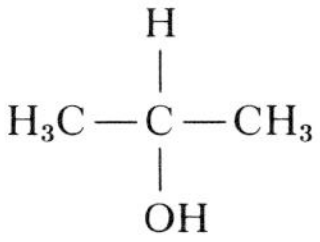

Isopropanol
(secondary)

B. Aldehydes

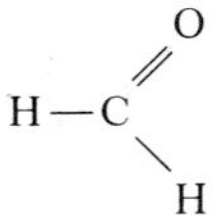

Formaldehyde
(most common aldehyde
in histotechnology)

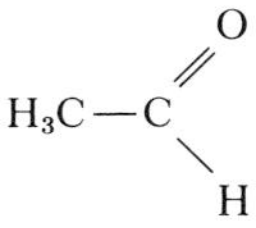

Acetaldehyde

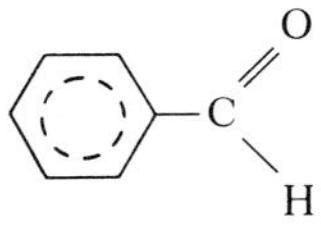

Benzaldehyde

C. Alkyl halides

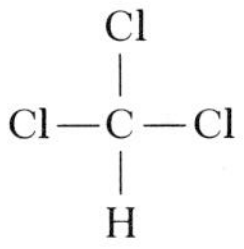

Chloroform

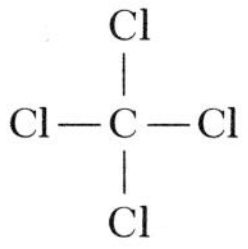

Carbon tetrachloride

D. Amines

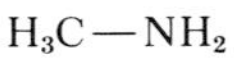

Methylamine
(primary)

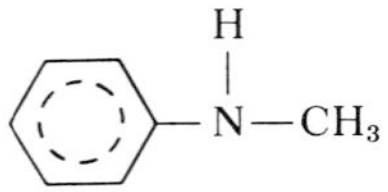

N-Methylaniline
(secondary)

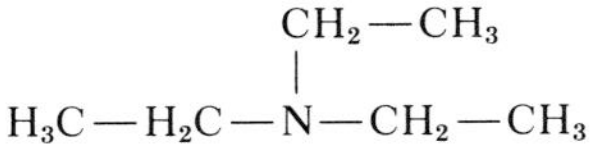

Triethylamine
(tertiary)

E. Carboxylic acids

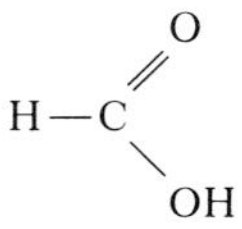

Formic acid

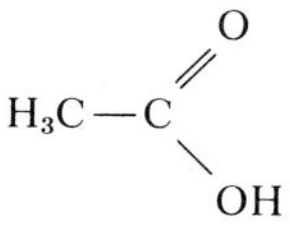

Acetic acid

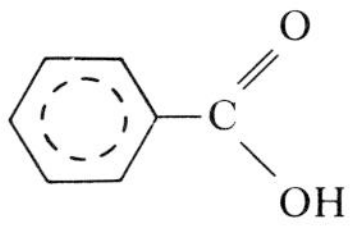

Benzoic acid

F. Ethers

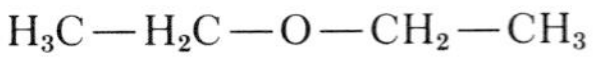

Diethyl ether
(common lab ether)

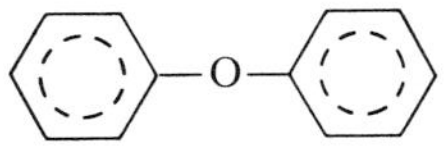

(Di)phenyl ether

G. Ketones

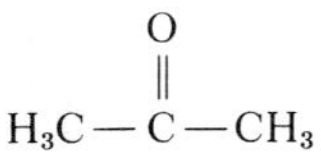

Acetone

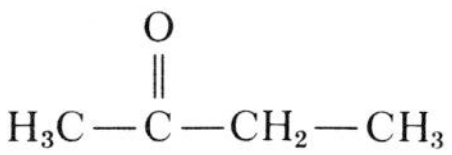

Methyl ethyl ketone

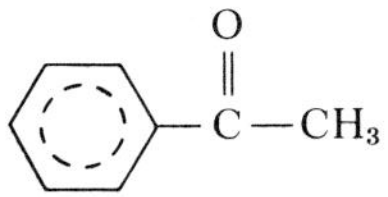

Acetophenone

H. Acid chlorides

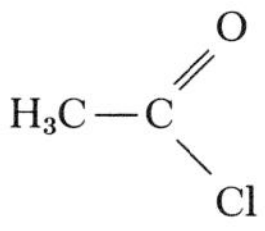

Acetyl chloride

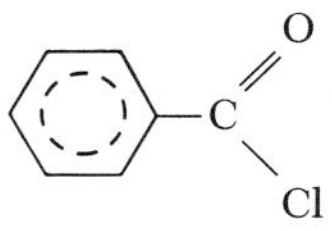

Benzoyl chloride

I. Amides

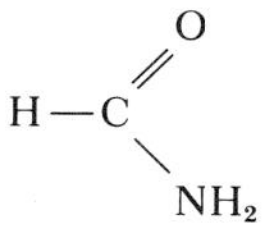

Formamide

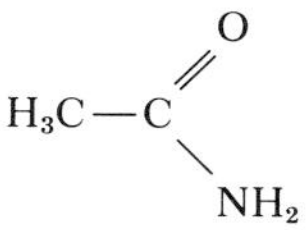

Acetamide

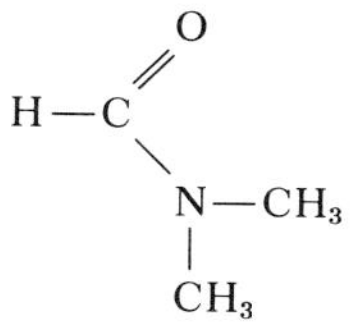

Dimethylformamide

J. Anhydride

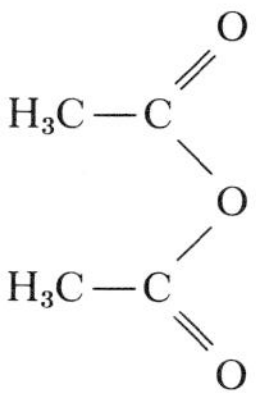

Acetic anhydride

K. Esters

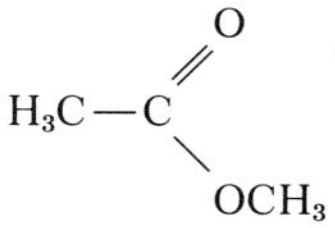

Methyl acetate

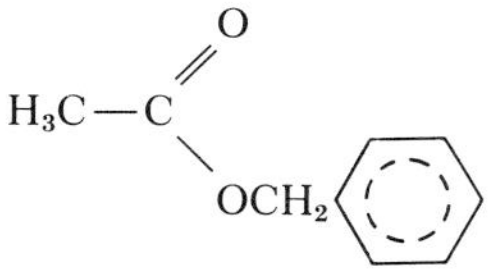

Benzyl acetate

L. Diazonium salt

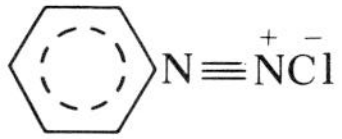

Benzenediazonium chloride

M. Glycols

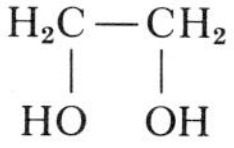

Ethylene glycol

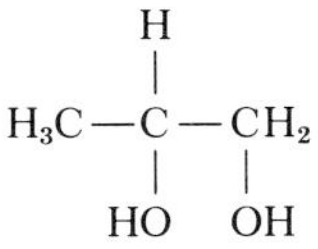

Propylene glycol

N. Heterocyclic compounds

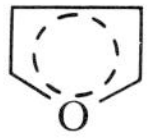

Furan

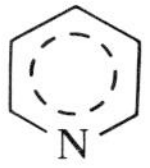

Pyridine

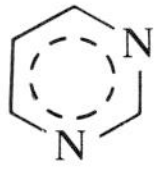

Pyrimidine

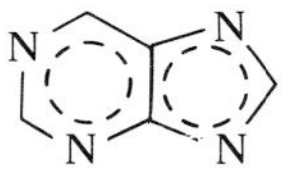

Purine

O. Phenols

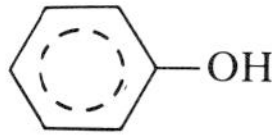

Phenol

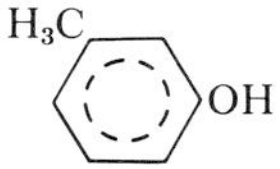

meta-cresol

P. Polynuclear aromatic compounds

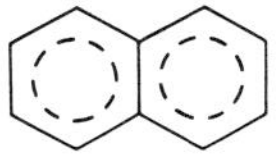

Naphthalene

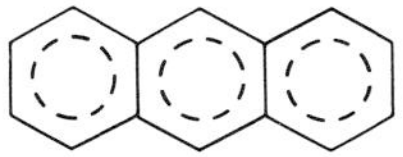

Anthracene

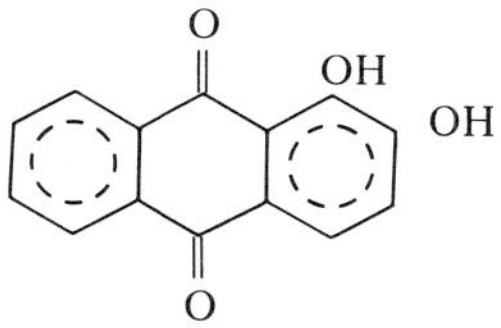

Alizarin

Continued.

Table 21-5. Examples of common organic compounds—cont'd

Q. Monosaccharides

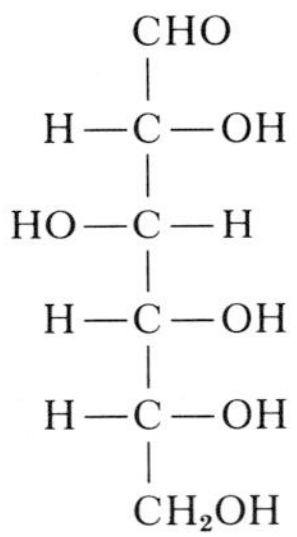

CHO	CH$_2$OH	CHO	CHO
H—C—OH	C=O	H—C—OH	H—C—H
HO—C—H	HO—C—H	H—C—OH	H—C—OH
H—C—OH	H—C—OH	H—C—OH	H—C—OH
H—C—OH	H—C—OH	CH$_2$OH	CH$_2$OH
CH$_2$OH	CH$_2$OH		
D-(+)-glucose (aldohexose)	**Fructose (ketohexose)**	**Ribose (aldopentose, constituent of ribonucleic acids)**	**Deoxyribose (aldopentose, constituent of deoxyribonucleic acids)**

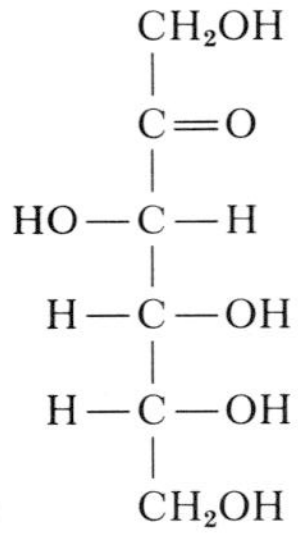

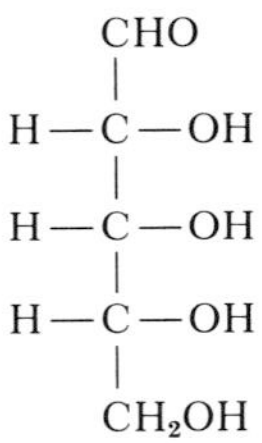

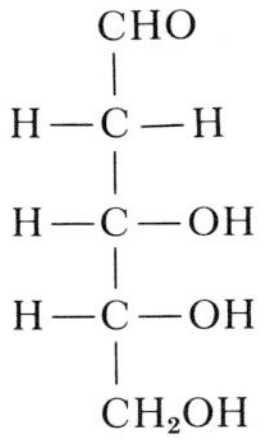

R. Unsaturated fatty acids

H$_3$C—(CH$_2$)$_7$—CH=CH—(CH$_2$)$_7$—COOH   Oleic acid (C$_{18}$H$_{34}$O$_2$)

H$_3$C—(CH$_2$)$_4$—CH=CH—CH$_2$—CH=CH—(CH$_2$)$_7$—COOH   Linoleic acid (C$_{18}$H$_{32}$O$_2$)

H$_3$C—CH$_2$—CH=CH—CH$_2$—CH=CH—CH$_2$—CH=CH—(CH$_2$)$_7$—COOH   Linolenic acid (C$_{18}$H$_{30}$O$_2$)

H$_3$C—(CH$_2$)$_4$—CH=CH—CH$_2$—CH=CH—CH$_2$—CH=CH—CH$_2$—CH=CH—(CH$_2$)$_3$—COOH   Arachidonic acid (C$_{20}$H$_{32}$O$_2$)

S. Steroids and sterols

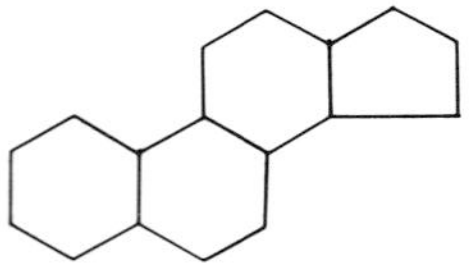

Perhydrocyclopentanophenanthrene ring system

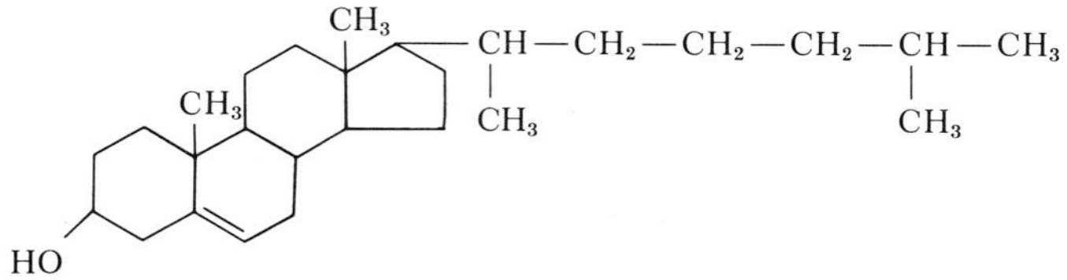

Cholesterol

T. Purine and pyrimidine bases

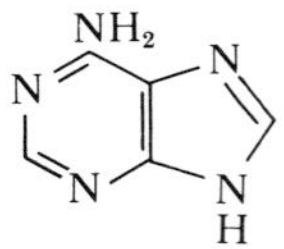

Adenine (purine)

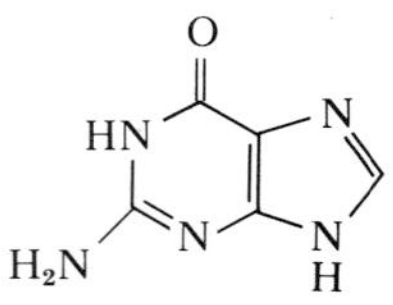

Guanine (purine)

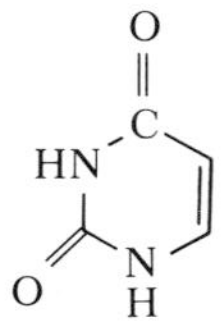

Uracil (pyrimidine)

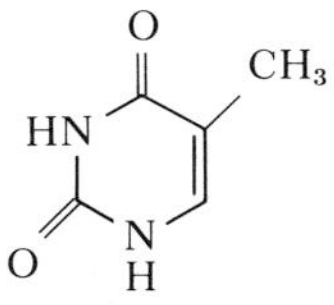

Thymine (pyrimidine)

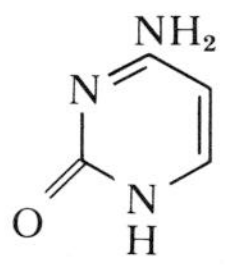

Cytosine (pyrimidine)

Miscellaneous compounds
Carboxylic acid derivatives

In all carboxylic acid derivatives, the OH group of the carboxyl group is removed to form the *acyl* group

$$R-C \overset{\displaystyle O}{\big\backslash}$$

to which various groups may be added. All these derivatives are polar compounds.

Acid chlorides. The structural formula for an acid chloride is

$$R-C \overset{\displaystyle O}{\underset{\displaystyle Cl}{\big\backslash}}$$

in which R may be an alkyl or aromatic group. Common acid chlorides, including acetyl chloride and benzoyl chloride, are shown in Table 21-5, *H*.

Amides. The structural formula for an amide is

$$R-C \overset{\displaystyle O}{\underset{\displaystyle NH_2}{\big\backslash}}$$

in which R may be an aliphatic or aromatic group. Amides, because of the possibility of strong intermolecular H-bonding, have relatively high boiling points. Common amides, including formamide, acetamide, and dimethylformamide (used as a solvent in certain histochemical procedures) are shown in Table 21-5, *I*.

Anhydrides. The structural formula for an anhydride is

$$\begin{array}{c} R_1-C \overset{\displaystyle O}{\big\backslash} \\ O \\ R_2-C \big/ \\ \overset{\displaystyle O}{} \end{array}$$

in which R_1 and R_2 may be the same or different alkyl or aromatic groups. A common anhydride, acetic anhydride, is shown in Table 21-5, *J*.

Esters. The structural formula for an ester is

$$R_1-C \overset{\displaystyle O}{\underset{\displaystyle OR_2}{\big\backslash}}$$

in which R_1 and R_2 may be the same or different alkyl or aromatic groups. Esters are formed by the reaction of an acid (for example, carboxylic acids) with an alcohol. The boiling points of esters are similar to those of aldehydes or ketones of like molecular weight. Esters with up to about five C atoms are soluble in water, and the esters are soluble in common organic solvents. Common esters, including methyl acetate, and benzyl acetate are shown in Table 21-5, *K*.

Diazonium salts

Compounds that are very important in histochemical procedures are the diazonium salts, which contain the $N \equiv N^+$ group attached to an aromatic ring as a cation associated with various anions such as halides (Cl^-, Br^-), nitrate (NO_3^-), and hydrogen sulfate (HSO_4^-).

Diazonium salts are usually unstable solids that are readily soluble in water. They are formed by the reaction of primary aromatic amines with nitrous acid (HNO_2) in a process called *diazotization*. Important dyes are the *azo* compounds, which are formed by the coupling of aromatic compounds with diazonium salts and which contain the group $—N=N—$. An example of a diazonium salt is shown in Table 21-5, *L*.

Glycols

Glycols are alcohols that contain 2 OH groups in either open-chain or cyclic structures. Their properties, such as high boiling points and excellent water solubility, are similar to alcohols with differences expected because of additional functional groups. Ethylene glycol, used in antifreeze formulations, is a common example, as is propylene glycol, which is used as a solvent for certain simple fat stains. See Table 21-5, *M. Compounds such as ethylene glycol are extremely poisonous, especially for cats.*

Heterocyclic compounds

Heterocyclic compounds have rings composed of C as well as N, O, or S. Several of the most important heterocyclics for our purposes are furan, pyridine, pyrimidine, and purine, shown in Table 21-5, *N*. Furan and pyridine are solvents, whereas derivatives of purine and pyrimidine are important constituents of nucleic acids. Compounds containing only C in their rings are called homocyclic or alicyclic compounds.

Peroxides

Peroxides are compounds that contain the —O—O— group, and organic peroxides are formed by the reaction of organic compounds with atmospheric O_2. WHEN UNSTABLE PEROXIDES FORM FROM ETHERS EXPOSED TO AIR, THEY CAN CAUSE EXPLOSIONS.

Phenols

Phenols are organic compounds that contain the OH group attached to an aromatic ring instead of to an alkyl group as in alcohols. The simplest member of this family, which also gives the family its name, is phenol. If a methyl group is also present, the phenols are called cresols as in *meta*-cresol (Table 21-5, *O*). Phenols may be liquids or solids, have high boiling points, and are generally only slightly soluble in water except for phenol itself and a few derivatives. Phenol, also called carbolic acid, is used as one of the components of carbol fuchsin solutions for staining acid-fast substances such as acid-fast bacilli.

Polynuclear aromatic compounds

Organic compounds that contain 2 or more aromatic rings in which 2 C atoms are shared between each 2 rings are called polynuclear aromatic compounds. Examples are naphthalene ($C_{10}H_8$) and anthracene ($C_{14}H_{10}$) (Table 21-5, *P*). Anthraquinoid dyes, related to anthracene, are used in histotechnology. An example is alizarin (Table 21-5, *P*).

BIOLOGICALLY IMPORTANT ORGANIC COMPOUNDS

Having reviewed the basic types of organic compounds and some of their properties and reactions, we will now consider the properties and characteristics of biologically important organic compounds that consist of the types of compounds previously studied, which include the carbohydrates, amino acids, peptides, proteins (including enzymes and some hormones), lipids (including steroid hormones), and nucleic acids.

Carbohydrates

Carbohydrates (sugars, saccharides) are organic compounds composed of C, H, and O that are found in plant and animal tissues. Carbohydrates are either aldehyde derivatives of polyhydroxy alcohols (aldoses) or ketone derivatives of polyhydroxy alcohols (ketoses). There are also carbohydrate derivatives that contain N, P, and S.

A monosaccharide (simple sugar) cannot be hydrolyzed into a simpler form, and its general formula is $C_nH_{2n}O_n$. These simple sugars are also called trioses, tetroses, pentoses, hexoses, and so on, depending on whether they contain three, four, five, six, or more C atoms, respectively. If an aldehyde group is present, these sugars also may be called aldotrioses, aldotetroses, aldopentoses, aldohexoses, and so on, respectively, and if a ketone group is present, they are also called ketotrioses, ketotetroses, ketopentoses, or ketohexoses, respectively. Examples are shown in Table 21-5, *Q*.

A *disaccharide* is a carbohydrate that gives two molecules of the same or a different monosaccharide upon hydrolysis, and its general formula is $C_n(H_2O)_{n-1}$. Examples are sucrose (containing 1 fructose and 1 glucose molecule), lactose (containing 1 glucose and 1 galactose molecule), and maltose (containing 2 glucose molecules).

An *oligosaccharide* is a carbohydrate that gives 2 to 10 monosaccharide units upon hydrolysis.

A *polysaccharide* is a carbohydrate that gives more than 10 monosaccharide units upon hydrolysis. Examples include starches, dextrans, glycogen, and cellulose. Glycogen is the polysaccharide of the animal body and is also called animal starch, whereas cellulose is an important structural component of plants. Polysaccharides may have linear or branched structures, and all monosaccharide units are joined by glycosidic bonds. The most common polysaccharides contain hexose units, and their general formula is $(C_6H_{10}O_5)_n$.

Polysaccharides that contain such monosaccharide derivatives as amino sugars and sugar acids are called *mucopolysaccharides*. Examples are hyaluronic acid, heparin, and chondroitin sulfates.

Mucopolysaccharides may occur in tissues as prosthetic groups of conjugated proteins, such as *mucoproteins*, which contain more than 4% carbohydrate, and *glycoproteins*, which contain less than 4% carbohydrates.

As an example of stereoisomerism in sugars, it is known that the naturally occurring form of the aldohexose glucose is D-(+)-glucose, which is shown as the first structure in Table 21-5, *Q*.

Whereas the (+) indicates the sign of rotation of plane-polarized light, the D indicates the configuration of the OH group at C5 as related to

two standard compounds, D- and L-glyceralde-
hyde. The majority of monosaccharides occurring in nature are also of the D-configuration,
such as D-ribose, D-mannose, and D-galactose.

It is known now that glucose and other sugars exist as cyclic, and not straight-chain compounds; however, these advanced studies are
not important to this discussion. For common
reactions of sugars, see Table 21-2, *I*.

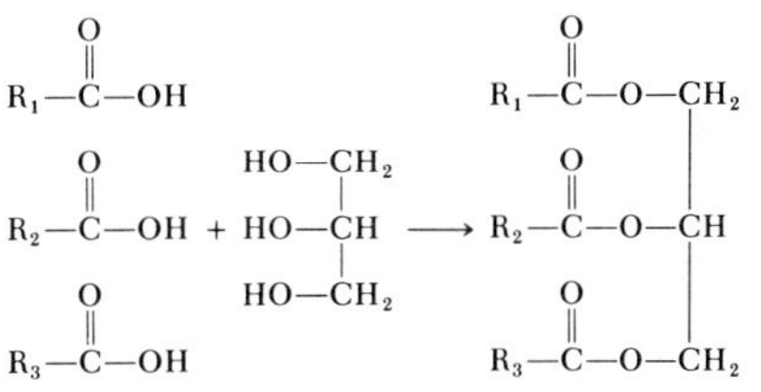

Lipids

Lipids are organic compounds that can be extracted from biologic materials (animal or plant)
with nonpolar "fat" solvents, such as hot alcohol, benzene, chloroform, and ether, and that
are insoluble in water. Of the various types of
lipids, we will discuss fatty acids, triglycerides
(neutral fats), phospholipids, glycolipids, steroids, and sterols.

Fatty acids. Fatty acids are monocarboxylic
acids that usually contain an even number of C
atoms in long, straight, unbranched chains that
may be saturated or unsaturated (with one or
more double bonds). The saturated fatty acids
have the general formula $C_nH_{2n}O_2$. The most
abundant saturated fatty acids of animal origin
are palmitic acid ($C_{16}H_{32}O_2$) and stearic acid
($C_{18}H_{36}O_2$).

Unsaturated fatty acids may contain one or
more $C=C$ double bonds with various formulas depending on the number of double bonds
present. Examples are shown in Table 21-5, *R*.

Oleic acid is the most abundant of all natural
fatty acids. Linoleic, linolenic, and arachidonic
acids are essential fatty acids and must be supplied in the diet for proper nutrition. Because
of the double bonds, geometric structural isomers can exist in the unsaturated fatty acids,
and the most common are the *cis* forms. In addition, various-position structural isomers are
possible. Unsaturated fatty acids oxidize slowly
in air by the process of rancidification.

Triglycerides (neutral fats). Only small
amounts of free fatty acids exist naturally, most
being present as esters with glycerol in the triglycerides. Glycerol is a three-C compound containing three OH groups. See Fig. 21-2.

R_1, R_2, and R_3 may be the same or different,
saturated or unsaturated, or in various combinations of these.

The neutral fats are important in the diet because of their high energy value and since they
are carriers for the "fat-soluble" vitamins. In
addition, the fats serve as heat insulators and
protect against injury in the body. Fats may be

Fig. 21-2. Formation of triglycerides.

hydrolyzed by acids, alkalis, or enzymes to re-
form the fatty acids and glycerol. When alkali
(NaOH, KOH) is used, the process is called
saponification, and the alkali salts of the fatty
acids *(soaps)* are formed. When acid is used,
free fatty acids are formed.

Steroids. Steroids are derivatives of the perhydrocyclopentanophenanthrene ring system,
which comprises four fused rings and contains
additional groups at C positions 3, 10, 13, and
sometimes 17 (Table 21-5, *S*).

Other typical steroid compounds include the
bile acids, sex hormones (androgens and estrogens), and vitamins.

Sterols. A sterol is an alcohol of a steroid and
contains the OH group at position 3 and an
eight- to ten-C side chain at position 17.

Cholesterol, which is important in both normal and pathologic biochemistry is a sterol with
an eight-C side chain at position 17, a OH
group at C3, and a double bond between C
atoms 5 and 6 (Table 21-5, *S*). Cholesterol,
when present in the blood, has been associated
with atherosclerosis. Most of blood cholesterol is
esterified, especially to unsaturated fatty acids.
It is also present in most animal lipid fractions.

Phospholipids (phosphatides). Phospholipids are esters that contain fatty acids and glycerol as well as phosphoric acid groups, N-
containing compounds, and various other substituents. Typical examples of phospholipids
include (1) lecithins (phosphatidylcholines),
which contain fatty acids, glycerol, phosphate,
and choline groups; (2) phosphatidylethanola-
mines, which contain fatty acids, glycerol, phosphate, and ethanolamine groups; and (3) phos-
phatidylserines, which contain fatty acids, glycerol, phosphate, and serine groups.

Glycolipids. Glycolipids are lipids that contain carbohydrate groups (primarily galactose)
instead of phosphoric acid residues as in phospholipids. They include such classes as the
gangliosides and cerebrosides.

Amino acids, peptides, and proteins
Amino acids

Amino acids are carboxylic acids that have an amino (NH_2) group at different positions in the chain. In proteins, the α-amino acids occur; in these compounds, the NH_2 group is located on the C atom in the α-position in the molecule. The α-position is the C atom next to the COOH group. See Fig. 21-3, *A*.

The simplest α-amino acid is glycine (Fig. 21-3, *B*).

Of the more than 20 amino acids present in proteins, 10 are "essential" to vertebrates; that is, they must be supplied in the diet since they cannot be synthesized in the body. The essential amino acids are arginine, histidine, isoleucine, leucine, lysine, methionine, phenylalanine, threonine, tryptophan, and valine.

The amino acids may be classified as neutral, basic, or acidic, depending on the additional groups present in their molecules. Some amino acids contain aromatic rings (tyrosine, phenylalanine), and others contain S (cystine, methionine, cysteine), basic groups (histidine, arginine), hydroxyl groups (threonine, serine), additional carboxyl groups (glutamic acid, aspartic acid), or other substituents.

Amphoteric properties of amino acids. Because they contain both NH_2 and COOH groups, amino acids are amphoteric; that is, they may react as acids or bases in solution, depending on the pH. Therefore, amino acids may exist in any of three forms in solution, depending on pH, as shown in Fig. 21-4.

In acid solution (structure *A*), both NH_2 and COO^- groups are protonated to NH_3^+ and COOH, respectively, producing a molecule with a net charge of +1. In basic solution (structure *C*), both NH_2 and COO^- groups are unprotonated, producing a molecule with a net charge of −1. However, when the pH value is such that the basic NH_2 group is protonated but the acidic COO^- group is not (structure *B*), the negative and positive charges are equal and there is no net charge. The pH at which an amino acid behaves neither as an acid nor as a base and does not move in an electric field is called the *isoelectric point (IEP)*.

The dipolar structure *B* in which though + and − charges are present the molecule has no net charge is called a "zwitterion" (pronounced "tsvitter-ion").

At pH values less than the IEP, as in structure *A*, the amino acid has a net positive charge and will migrate to the negative electrode (cathode) in an electric field, whereas at pH values greater than the IEP, as in structure *C*, the amino acid has a net negative charge and will migrate to the positive electrode (anode) in an electric field.

Peptides and peptide bonds

α-Amino acids may be linked by peptide bonds

$$\begin{array}{cc} O & H \\ \| & | \\ -C & - N- \end{array}$$

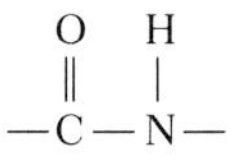

by which the COOH group of one amino acid is bound to the α-NH_2 group of another amino acid with the elimination of water (Fig. 21-5).

The remainders of the amino acid molecules (R_1, R_2) form side chains. Peptides contain two or more amino acids linked by peptide bonds. Peptides with small numbers of amino acids, such as two, three, and four, are called di-,tri-, and tetrapeptides and so on. Fig. 21-5 shows a *dipeptide*. *Polypeptides* contain large numbers of bonded amino acids. Proteins are composed of one or more polypeptides, each having many hundreds of amino acids.

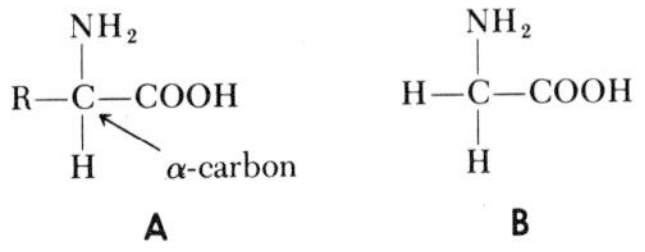

Fig. 21-3. A, General formula of α-amino acids. **B,** Glycine.

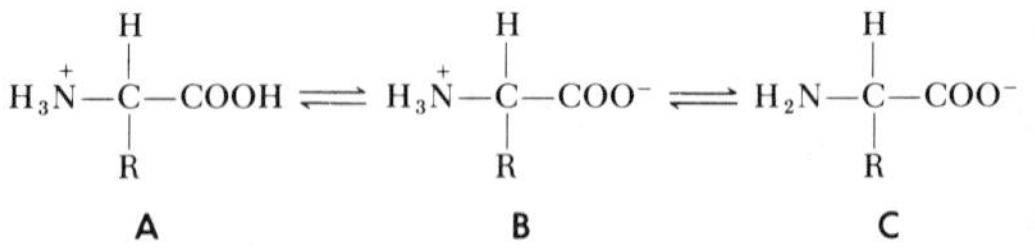

Fig. 21-4. Amphoteric properties of an amino acid

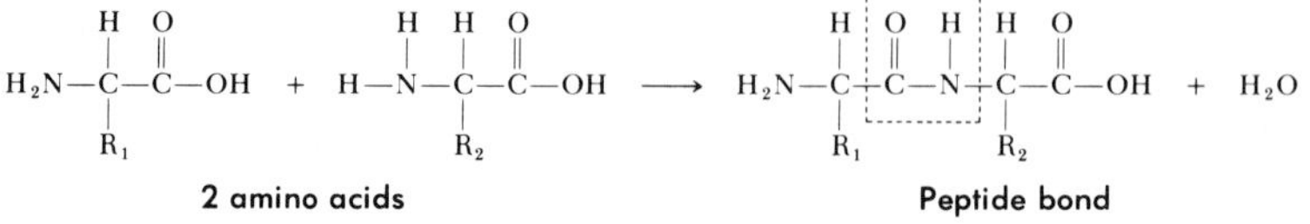

Fig. 21-5. Peptide bond formation.

Proteins

Proteins, which have numerous functions in living organisms, are high-molecular-weight organic compounds composed of one or more polypeptide chains, each of which, in turn, is composed of hundreds of amino acids. Besides C, H, O, and N, most proteins also contain S; also Cu, Fe, I, P, or Zn may be present. Proteins exhibit various biologic functions and include all enzymes, cell structural components, some hormones, and oxygen transport compounds (hemoglobin). Proteins are amphoteric compounds because of the presence of amphoteric amino acids in them. There are two major classes of proteins: simple and conjugated. *Simple proteins* contain only α-amino acids or their derivatives and include the albumins, globulins, histones, protamines, and several other types. *Conjugated proteins* are proteins joined to nonprotein organic or inorganic substances (prosthetic groups) and include nucleoproteins (proteins combined with nucleic acids), glycoproteins (contain carbohydrates with less than 4% carbohydrate), mucoproteins (contain carbohydrates with greater than 4% carbohydrate), lipoproteins (proteins containing lipids), and metalloproteins (proteins that bind metals such as Fe or Cu), and several other types.

Protein structure. Protein structure may be described on four different levels as primary, secondary, tertiary, and quaternary structure. *Primary structure* of proteins refers to the number and sequence of amino acids in the polypeptide chain or chains of the protein. *Secondary structure* refers to the specific ordering of the polypeptide chain or chains in a protein as determined by H bonds. *Tertiary structure* refers to further ordering of the polypeptide chain or chains of a protein as a result of interactions between side chains of the amino acids, including H bonding, van der Waals forces, and salt links. *Quaternary structure* refers to the relation in space of separate polypeptides in a protein with more than one peptide chain.

Protein reactions. *Precipitation* is a reaction in which previously soluble proteins are made insoluble and, therefore, precipitate from solution. Precipitation may be caused by (1) concentrated mineral acids, (2) heavy metals, (3) trichloroacetic acid, (4) tannic acid, (5) phosphotungstic acid, (6) phosphomolybdic acid, (7) alcohols and other organic solvents, or (8) heat. Acids 3 to 6 cause protein precipitation when the proteins are on the acidic side of their IEP

values, whereas agents 7 and 8 cause precipitation of proteins at their IEP values.

Denaturation is a reaction in which the secondary, tertiary, and quaternary structures of proteins are destroyed, but not their primary structure. Denaturation may be caused by any of the above-mentioned precipitating agents as well as by irradiation (x rays, ultraviolet light) and pH changes.

Finally, by hydrolysis, proteins may be broken down to their component amino acids by use of acids, alkalis, or digestive enzymes.

Nucleoproteins

Nucleoproteins, a type of conjugated protein, contain a nucleic acid attached to simple, usually basic, proteins, such as histones or protamines and are found in all biologic cells. The nucleoproteins constitute a large part of chromatin of cell nuclei and are also found associated with ribosomes (involved in protein synthesis) in the cell cytoplasm. The nucleoproteins may be extracted from biologic tissues and hydrolyzed into their component proteins and nucleic acids.

Nucleosides, nucleotides, and nucleic acids
Nucleosides

Nucleosides are compounds that contain a purine or pyrimidine base and a ribose or deoxyribose unit. Compounds with ribose are called ribonucleosides and those with deoxyribose are called deoxyribonucleosides. The structures of the bases are shown in Table 21-5, *T,* and those of the sugars in Table 21-5, Q.

Nucleotides

The basic structural units of the nucleic acids are called nucleotides, which are composed of a purine or pyrimidine base attached to a sugar (ribose in ribonucleotides or deoxyribose in deoxyribonucleotides) that, in turn, contains an esterified phosphate group. See Table 21-6 for the names of the common nucleosides and nucleotides.

Other nucleotides. The individual nucleotides, containing either ribose or deoxyribose but not bound in nucleic acids, as well as their diphosphate and triphosphate derivatives are also very important in general metabolism. Examples are adenosine diphosphate (ADP) and adenosine triphosphate (ATP).

Nucleic acids

Nucleic acids, which are important in trans-

Table 21-6. Bases, nucleosides, and nucleotides

Base	Ribose derivatives		Deoxyribose derivatives	
	Nucleoside	Nucleotide	Nucleoside	Nucleotide
Adenine	Adenosine	Adenylic acid	Deoxyadenosine	Deoxyadenylic acid
Guanine	Guanosine	Guanylic acid	Deoxyguanosine	Deoxyguanylic acid
Thymine	—	—	Thymidine	Thymidylic acid
Cytosine	Cytidine	Cytidylic acid	Deoxycytidine	Deoxycytidylic acid
Uracil	Uridine	Uridylic acid	—	—

mitting genetic information as well as in metabolism and protein biosynthesis, are high-molecular-weight polynucleotide polymers. The major forms are ribonucleic acid (RNA) and deoxyribonucleic acid (DNA). Hydrolysis of nucleic acids yields components of the nucleotides, that is, purine and pyrimidine bases, a pentose sugar (ribose in RNA) or a deoxypentose sugar (deoxyribose in DNA), and phosphoric acid.

DNA contains the bases adenine, cytosine, guanine, and thymine, whereas RNA contains the first three bases but has uracil in place of thymine.

DNA is known to comprise genes that determine the genetic characteristics of living organisms. A gene is a specific part of a DNA molecule that codes for a single polypeptide. Since DNA molecules can contain thousands of genes, thousands of different polypeptides can conceivably be formed.

DNA molecules are composed of two poly-nucleotide chains with pairing of specific purine and pyrimidine bases between chains to form double-helical structures.

Various types of RNA are important in translating the code carried by DNA, and these are (1) *messenger RNA,* which receives the code from the DNA molecule in the nucleus and carries it to the cytoplasmic ribosomes where specific proteins are synthesized, (2) *transfer RNA,* which combines with amino acids to ensure that they are inserted in the proper sequence in the protein being formed on the ribosomes, and (3) *ribosomal RNA,* which comprises a large portion of the ribosomes.

Enzymes

Enzymes are proteins that catalyze biochemical reactions in living matter. In this process, the enzymes themselves are not used up or changed permanently though they can produce significant changes in the compounds that they act upon, their *substrates.* Enzymes are impor-

tant since they permit reactions to occur at temperatures found in living cells that would otherwise require much higher temperatures. Enzymes may act alone or need other compounds to assist in their action; such compounds are called *cofactors* and they may be either metal ions or organic compounds called *coenzymes.* If the coenzyme is bound tightly to an enzyme, it is then called a *prosthetic group.* Some coenzymes are derived from vitamins. Enzymes may also be inhibited in their action by specific compounds called inhibitors.

Many enzymes are named by adding the suffix *-ase* to the name of the substrate or substrates acted upon: that is, a phosphatase catalyzes the hydrolysis of phosphate esters. A systematic classification divides enzymes into six classes that describe the type of chemical reaction that is catalyzed, as follows: (1) oxidoreductases (oxidation-reduction), (2) transferases (transfer of functional groups), (3) hydrolases (hydrolysis), (4) lyases (additions to double bonds), (5) isomerases (isomerizations), and (6) ligases (formation of bonds with ATP cleavage).

Although some enzymes are quite specific and catalyze only a single reaction, others are relatively nonspecific and act on various substrates.

The activity of enzymes is highly dependent on temperature, the presence of specific ions, and the pH of the reaction medium.

In the simplest form of an enzyme-catalyzed reaction, the enzyme, E, combines with a substrate, S, to first form an intermediate enzyme-substrate, ES, complex in which a chemical change is produced, followed by release of the unchanged enzyme and product P:

$$E + S \rightleftharpoons ES \rightleftharpoons E + P$$

The hypothesis that an ES complex must form before an enzyme can act was developed by L. Michaelis and M. L. Menten in 1913.

Table 21-7. Hormone source, structure, and class

Endocrine gland	Hormone produced	Structure and organic class
Thyroid gland	Thyroxine	**Amino acid derivative**
Ovary	Estradiol	**Steroid**
Adrenal medulla	Epinephrine	**Catecholamine**
Pancreas	Insulin	A protein (with two linked peptide chains) with a molecular weight of about 5700
Neurohypophysis	Vasopressin	A nonapeptide amide containing 6 amino acids and 3 amino acid amides

A basic equation in enzyme studies is the Michaelis-Menten equation:

$$v = \frac{V_{\max}[S]}{K_M + [S]}$$

in which v is the velocity of the reaction, $V_{\max}$ is the maximum velocity possible when all enzyme is combined with substrate, $[S]$ is the substrate concentration in moles per liter, and K_M (Michaelis-Menten constant) equals the $[S]$ concentration at which the velocity of the reaction is one half that of the maximum velocity.

Hormones

Hormones are compounds synthesized by the endocrine glands and carried by the circulation to tissues in which the hormones specifically initiate various metabolic processes. Hormones include many different types of organic compounds such as proteins, polypeptides, catecholamines, steroids, and iodinated amino acids. Typical examples are given in Table 21-7.

CHAPTER 22

Medical terminology

Medical terminology is the professional language of those who are either directly or indirectly engaged in the medical field. Records of medical terminology and its usage extend as far back as 400 B.C., when Hippocrates coined many words relating to anatomy and disease processes. Although the majority of medical terms claim Greek and Latin ancestry, some have been adopted from modern languages, especially German and French. Theoretically, in word formation one should safeguard the purity of the language by joining Greek roots to Greek prefixes and suffixes and Latin roots to Latin combining forms, but in reality, many terms are bilingual in their derivation. In medical terminology, one will frequently find that the name of the organ descends from Latin or Old English or another language, whereas the name of the disease affecting that organ descends from Greek. For example, the term "marrow" has an English and Germanic origin, whereas the inflammation of the marrow "myelitis" stems from Greek *myelos*. Compare unrelated Latin *medulla*, which in Latin means 'marrow.'

The best way to learn the meaning of unknown medical terms is to break the word into its component parts of suffixes, roots, and prefixes and analyse them. Analyzing in this manner may reveal the complete meaning of the word. For example, when "appendectomy" is analyzed "ectomy" means 'removal' and "append" refers to 'appendix,' hence 'removal of the appendix.' Some terms, when analyzed, only imply the meaning, which in turn requires a more precise definition. An example of such a case would be the term "anemia." Analysis of the component parts gives the impression of total lack of blood, whereas more precisely, it refers only to a decreased red cell count and decreased hemoglobin content.

There are three main elements of medical terms: prefixes, roots, and suffixes. Prefixes consist of one or two syllables placed before a word to modify its meaning. Roots are the main body of the word and are usually modified by prefixes, suffixes, or both. Suffixes are syllables attached to the end of a word or root to modify the meaning, and these may be subdivided into diagnostic, operative, or symptomatic.

The diagnostic affixes and terms are drawn from Sister Mary Agnes Clare Frenay, S.S.M.: Understanding medical terminology, ed. 3, St. Louis, 1964, Catholic Hospital Association Publishers.

DIAGNOSTIC AFFIXES (G—Greek derivation, L—Latin derivation)

Affix	Meaning	Affix	Meaning
Diagnostic suffix		-desis (G)	binding, fixation
-cele (G)	hernia, tumor, protrusion	-lithotomy (G)	incision for and removal of stones
-emia (G)	blood, blood condition		
-ectasis (G)	expansion, dilatation	-pexy (G)	suspension, fixation
-iasis (G)	condition, formation of, presence of	-plasty (G)	surgical correction, plastic repair of
-itis (G)	inflammation	-rhaphy (G)	suture
-malacia (G)	softening	-scopy (G)	inspection, examination
-megaly (G)	enlargement	-stomy (G)	creation of a more or less permanent opening
-oma (G)	tumor		
-osis (G)	disease process or condition	-tomy (G)	incision into
-pathy (G)	disease	-tripsy (G)	crushing, friction
-ptosis (G)	falling		
-rhexis (G)	rupture	**Symptomatic suffix**	
		-algia (G)	pain
Operative suffix		-genic (G)	origin
-centesis (G)	puncture	-lysis (G)	dissolution, breaking down
-ectomy (G)	excision	-oid (G)	like

DIAGNOSTIC AFFIXES (G—Greek derivation, L—Latin derivation)—cont'd

Affix	Meaning	Affix	Meaning
-osis (G)	increase, condition	phago- (G)	eat
-penia (G)	deficiency, decrease	philo- (G)	like
-spasm (G)	involuntary contractions	procto- (G)	rectum
		pseudo- (G)	false
Root		psycho- (G)	soul, mind
adeno- (G)	gland	pyelo- (G)	pelvis
aero- (G)	air	pyloro- (G)	pylorus
angio- (G)	vessel	pyo- (G)	pus
arthro- (G)	joint	radio- (L)	ray
bio- (G)	live, life	spondylo- (G)	vertebra
blepharo- (G)	eyelid	tracheo- (G)	neck
cardio- (G)	heart	tuberculo- (L)	tubercle
cerebro- (L)	brain	viscero- (L)	organ
cephalo- (G)	head		
cervico- (L)	neck	**Prefix**	
cheilo-, cheil-, chil- (G)	lip	ab- (L)	from, away from
		a-, an- (G)	without, not
cheiro-, cheir-, chir- (G)	hand	ad- (L)	adherence, increase, near, toward
chol-, chole- (G)	bile	ana- (G)	upward, excessive, again
		ante- (L)	before
chondro- (G)	cartilage	anti- (G)	against
costo- (L)	rib	bi- (L)	two, both, double
cranio- (L)	skull	circum- (L)	around
cysto- (G)	bladder, sac	co-, con- (L)	together, with
cyto- (G)	cell	contra- (L)	against, opposite
dacryo- (G)	tear	dys- (G)	bad, difficult, painful
dactylo- (G)	finger, toe	ec- (G)	out
dermo- (G)	skin	ecto- (G)	outside
encephalo- (G)	brain	em-, en- (G)	in
entero- (G)	intestine	endo- (G)	within
gastro- (G)	stomach	epi- (G)	upon, at, in addition to
glyco- (G)	sweet	ex- (L) (G)	out, away from, over
hemo-, hemato- (G)	blood	hemi- (G)	half
		hyper- (G)	excessive, above
hepato- (G)	liver	hypo- (G)	under, below, deficient
hyster- (G)	uterus	inter- (L)	between
ileo- (L)	ileum	macro- (G)	big
ilio- (L)	ilium	para-, par- (G)	beside, around, near, abnormal
leuko- (G)	white		
lipo- (G)	fat	peri- (G)	around, about
litho- (G)	stone	post- (L)	after
lyso- (G)	dissolving	pre- (L)	before
meningo- (G)	membrane	pro- (L) (G)	in front of, forward
metro- (G)	uterus	retro- (L)	backward
myelo- (G)	marrow	semi- (L)	half
myo- (G)	muscle	sub- (L)	under, below
nephro- (G)	kidney	super-, supra- (L)	above, beyond
ophthalmo- (G)	eye	sym-, syn- (G)	with, along, beside
osteo- (G)	bone	trans- (L)	across, over
pneumo- (G)	lung, air	tri- (G)	three

DIAGNOSTIC TERMS COMMONLY USED IN THE HISTOPATHOLOGY LABORATORY

Terms	Meaning
Skin	
callositas, keratosis	a circumscribed thickening and hypertrophy of the horny cells of the epidermis
cellulitis	inflammation of the skin and subcutaneous tissue without pus formation
dermatitis	inflammation of the skin; common forms are contact dermatitis, venenata dermatitis (reaction to an irritant or sensitizer, for example, poison ivy) exfoliative dermatitis (scaling off of dead skin associated with crust formation, generalized redness, and edema) dermatitis medicamentosa (this is drug eruption)
gangrene	necrosis of tissue
melanoderma	abnormal brown or black pigmentation of the skin
tinea	any fungus skin disease
tumors of skin growths	basal cell carcinoma (malignant skin ulcer) keloid (new growth of scar tissue) nevus, birthmark (congenital pigmentation of a circumscribed area of the skin) squamous cell epithelioma (malignant skin ulcer affecting areas of chronic irritation)
mastitis	inflammation of breast
frozen section	microscopic study of slides made from fresh tissue of lesion; valuable for rapid diagnosis while patient is on operating table to determine the need for conservative surgery, should the tissue be a benign lesion; or for radical surgery, should a malignant lesion be found
incisional biopsy	tissue of lesion obtained for pathologic verification
Musculoskeletal	
exostosis	hyperplasia of bony surfaces
multiple myeloma	primary malignant tumor of bone marrow
osteitis	inflammation of a bone
osteitis deformans, Paget's disease	disease characterized by progressive bowing and thickening of shafts of long bones, thickening of skull, and cystic bone changes
osteomalacia	softening of bones resulting from loss of calcium from disease
osteomyelitis	inflammation of bone and bone marrow
osteoporosis	acquired disorder characterized by a reduction in amount of bone present in skeleton
periostitis	inflammation of the outer covering of the bone
spondylitis, Pott's disease	tuberculosis of the spine
chondroma	a benign neoplasm composed of cartilage
chondrosarcoma	malignant tumor arising from cartilage
fibrositis, periarthritis, muscular rheumatitis, or periarticular fibrositis	a rheumatoid condition affecting the muscles and tissues around joints
leiomyoma	benign smooth muscle tumor
myasthenia gravis	condition characterized by excessive muscular weakness not caused by muscular atrophy
myosarcoma	malignant muscular tumor
myositis	inflammation of a voluntary muscle
rhabdomyoma	a striated muscle tumor
Nerves	
neuritis, neuropathy	disease of the peripheral nerves commonly associated with degenerative processes
neuroma	tumor of the nerve sheath occurring in solitary or multiple lesions; multiple neuromas are known as von Recklinghausen's disease
brain tumors	
primary gliomas	arising from glial cells that are found in brain and spinal cord
meningiomas	tumors arising from meninges
pituitary adenomas	tumors of the pituitary gland
laminectomy	excision of one or more laminae of vertebrae; method of approach to the spinal cord

DIAGNOSTIC TERMS—cont'd

Terms	Meaning
Cardiovascular	
aneurysm	a dilatation or bulging out of the wall of the heart, aorta, or any other artery
cardiac arrest	cessation of effective heart action, usually caused by asystole or ventricular fibrillation
carditis	inflammation of the heart
endocarditis	inflammation of the membrane lining the cavities of the heart and heart valves
myocarditis	inflammation of the heart muscle that may result in myocardial fibrosis followed by cardiac enlargement and congestive heart failure
pericarditis	inflammation of the membrane lining the cavities of the heart and heart valves
aortic stenosis	narrowing of the aortic valve
arteriosclerosis	a group of processes that have in common thickening and loss of elasticity of arterial walls
atherosclerosis	a type of arteriosclerosis characterized by focal intimal lipid deposits
Lymphatics	
lymph nodes	encapsulated lymphoid tissue scattered along the lymphatics in chains or clusters
lymphatics	thin-walled vessels widely distributed throughout the body and containing many valves
Hodgkin's disease	malignant lymphoma that produces lymph-node enlargement in the neck, enlargement of spleen and liver, and lung and bone involvement
lymphadenitis	inflammation of the lymph nodes
lymphangitis	inflammation of the lymphatics
lymphangioma	tumor composed of lymphatics
lymphoma	tumor composed of lymph tissue
lymphosarcoma	malignant invasive tumor composed of lymphocytes or lymphoblasts
Urogenital	
nephrectomy	excision of kidney
nephrotomy	incision into kidney
pyelotomy	incision into renal pelvis
dilatation and curettage	instrumental expansion of the cervix and scraping of the uterine cavity to remove endometrial tissue for diagnosis; placental tissue in incomplete abortion; fibroids
Respiratory	
anthracosis	disease of lungs caused by prolonged inhalation of fine particles of coal dust
atelectasis	a functionless, airless lung or portion of lung
carcinoma of lung	malignant new growth and most important of the neoplastic diseases of the lung
histoplasmosis	fungus disease caused by *Histoplasma capsulatum*
Digestive	
biopsy of liver	removal of small piece of tissue for microscopic study
hepatic lobectomy	removal of lobe of liver
hepatotomy	incision into liver substance
cholecystectomy	removal of gallbladder
choledocholithotomy	incision into gall duct for removal of gallstones
exploratory laparotomy	surgical opening of abdomen for diagnostic purposes
gastrectomy	partial or complete removal of stomach
Metabolic diseases	
amyloidosis	amyloid deposits in body tissues, especially in kidney, spleen, and liver; primary systemic amyloidosis is a familial type with myocardial and skeletal muscle involvement; secondary parenchymatous amyloidosis is a condition usually associated with infection and multiple myeloma
amyloid	an abnormal complex material, primarily protein, the exact biochemical composition of which is not known; bears a superficial resemblance to starch

CHAPTER 23

Laboratory mathematics and miscellanea

LABORATORY MATHEMATICS
Preparation of percent solutions

Percent is defined as "parts per hundred" and preparation of this type of solution generally falls into the following two categories:

Weight-volume relationship, that is, grams (or milligrams) of solute dissolved in an appropriate solvent to a final solution volume of 100 ml. This type of solution is usually abbreviated *w/v*.

Volume-volume relationship, that is, milliliters of liquid "solute" are added to liquid solvent and the final solution volume is made to 100 ml. This kind of solution may be abbreviated *v/v*.

Examples
1. Preparation of 100 ml of a 5% aqueous solution (w/v) of lithium carbonate would first involve weighing 5 gm of the solid. This is dissolved in some distilled water and when dissolved, the final dilution is made to 100 ml. The solution should be mixed thoroughly before using.
2. The preparation of 2 liters of a 15% solution of sodium chloride (NaCl, $MW = 58.5$) would involve the weighing of how many grams of the substance? This problem may be solved as follows:

The concentration of the solution should be 15%. On a weight/volume basis, this means 15 gm of the substance diluted to a total volume of 100 ml.

A 2000 ml final volume is required. Set up the proportion:

$$\frac{15 \text{ gm}}{100 \text{ ml}} = \frac{X \text{ gm}}{2000 \text{ ml}}$$

$$X = 300 \text{ gm}$$

Note: The molecular weight is not needed when solving a problem of this type.

3. Preparation of 100 ml of 70% ethanol (v/v) would involve measurement of 30 ml of

distilled water and dilution to a final volume of 100 ml with 70 ml of absolute alcohol.

Preparation of molar solutions

The quantity of substance whose weight in grams is numerically equal to its molecular weight is called a gram-molecular weight or "mole" of that substance. A solution that contains 1 mole of a substance in a final volume of 1 liter is called a "molar solution."

Examples
1. Preparation of 1 liter of a 1 M solution of sodium hydroxide would first involve finding the molecular weight of the compound (molecular weight is the sum of the atomic weights). The molecular weight of NaOH is 40; thus in this example, 40 gm would be weighed and dissolved in distilled water, and the final dilution would be made to 1 liter.
2. Prepare 150 ml of a 0.2 M solution of hydrochloric acid (MW = 36.5; specific gravity = 1.19; % by weight = 37%). One of the ways to solve this problem is as follows:

First, look at the concentration that is needed— 0.2 M solution of HCl. You know by definition that a 1 M solution of HCl would contain 36.5 gm per 1000 ml. Figure how many grams would be contained in 0.2 M:

$$\frac{36.5 \text{ gm}}{1 \text{ M}} = \frac{X \text{ gm}}{0.2 \text{ M}}$$

$$X = 7.3 \text{ gm}$$

Second, look at the volume needed in the final result. You need 150 ml of the 0.2 M solution. The preceding proportion gave you the amount required to prepare 1000 ml of a 0.2 M solution. Just set up another proportion:

$$\frac{7.3 \text{ gm}}{1000 \text{ ml}} = \frac{X \text{ gm}}{150 \text{ ml}}$$

$$X = 1.09 \text{ gm}$$

You are, of course, dealing with a concentrated acid solution and, since you cannot weigh out a liquid conveniently on a balance, you want to find the amount you are going to have to pour out in order to achieve the required 1.09 gm.

Each milliliter of the acid you are using weighs 1.19 gm (by definition of specific gravity). Pure HCl accounts for 37% (or 0.37) of that amount. Multiplication of the two numbers shows that each milliliter of the acid really contains 0.44 gm of pure HCl.

Dividing this factor into the 1.09 gm shows that 2.5 ml of the liquid acid is equivalent to weighing out 1.09 gm. Since you need 150 ml total volume and since 2.5 ml of that will be acid, you will need 147.5 ml of distilled water.

As a safety precaution, prevent splashing from adding water to concentrated acid by (in this example) filling your cylinder with about 145 ml of water, adding the 2.5 ml of the concentrated acid, *mixing well,* and then adding water to the final volume of 150 ml.

Preparation of normal solutions

A normal solution may be defined as containing 1 gram-equivalent weight of solute dissolved in 1 liter of solution. A gram-equivalent weight, in turn, is defined as the quantity of substance that will replace or react with 1.008 gm of hydrogen. Convenient formulas that may be used to calculate the equivalent weight are the following:

$$\text{Equivalent weight} = \frac{\text{Molecular weight}}{\text{Total oxidation number of cations}}$$

$$\text{Equivalent weight} = \frac{\text{Molecular weight}}{-(\text{Total oxidation number of anions})}$$

Examples
1. To prepare 1-liter amounts of 1 N solutions of the following compounds, the required amounts in grams would be:

   HCl (hydrochloric acid) 36.5 (because of one replaceable hydrogen)
   H_2SO_4 (sulfuric acid) 49 (because of two replaceable hydrogens, the gram amount is half that required for molarity)
   $Al(OH)_3$ (aluminum hydroxide) 26 (because of three hydroxyls that could react with H^+; the normal solution contains one third the amount of grams required for molarity)

2. How many milliliters of concentrated sulfuric acid (H_2SO_4) are needed to prepare 3 liters of a 0.8 N solution? (MW = 98; sp. gr. = 1.84; % by weight = 98%.) One of the ways to solve the problem is as follows:

You are asked to prepare 3 liters of a 0.8 N solution of sulfuric acid. By definition, a 1 N solution of H_2SO_4 would contain 49 gm/liter. A proportion shows:

$$\frac{49 \text{ gm}}{1 \text{ N}} = \frac{X \text{ gm}}{0.8 \text{ N}}$$

$$X = 39.2 \text{ gm}$$

39.2 gm would be sufficient for 1 liter of a 0.8 N

solution; however, you want 3 liters at that concentration, or 117.6 gm.

You are dealing with a concentrated liquid acid and it will be necessary to find out the amount of pure acid contained in each milliliter of the bottled reagent. Each milliliter of the acid you are using weighs 1.84 gm/ml (by definition of specific gravity). Of that amount, 98% (or 0.98) is pure sulfuric acid. Multiplication of the two factors shows that each milliliter of the bottled reagent really contains 1.8 gm of the acid.

Dividing this factor (1.8) into the total gram amount needed (that is, 117.6) shows that you will need a total volume of 65 ml of the concentrated acid. Since you need 3000 ml total and 65 ml of that to be will be the concentrated acid, the amount of distilled water needed is 2935 ml.

As a safety precaution, prevent acid splashing by adding about 2900 ml of distilled water to the container, add the 65 ml of concentrated acid, *mix well*, and then complete the dilution by adding the rest of the distilled water to a final volume of 3000 ml.

Solution dilution

The preceding three types of solutions all contain a certain amount of solute in a fixed volume of solution; the amount of solute contained in a given volume of solution is equal to the product of the volume, V, times the concentration, C. If it is necessary to dilute a certain-strength solution to a weaker concentration, the total volume will be increased, but the total amount of solute will remain unchanged. The two solutions with different concentrations that contain the same amount of solute may therefore be related to each other according to the following equation:

$$\frac{V \times C}{\text{(Solution 1)}} = \frac{V \times C}{\text{(Solution 2)}}$$

It is extremely important that the *volume units and concentration units on both sides of the equation be the same.*

Examples

1. Find the volume of a stock solution of 15% sodium chloride that would be required to prepare 200 ml of a 3% solution (the above equation may be used):

$$V_1 \times C_1 = V_2 \times C_2$$
$$X \times 15\% = 200 \text{ ml} \times 3\%$$
$$X = 40 \text{ ml}$$

40 ml of a 15% solution are needed and a final dilution is made to 200 ml with 160 ml of distilled water.

2. Prepare 4500 ml of a 15% solution of formalin. For the particular problem under consideration, you want to prepare a total final volume of 4500 ml of 15% formalin. You are using stock formalin, which is really 37% to 40% concentrated. However, for mathematical purposes, a stock solution of formalin is considered to be 100% concentration. The specific equation for this problem is as follows:

$$(X \text{ ml})(100\%) = (4500 \text{ ml})(15\%)$$
$$X = (4500 \text{ ml})(15\%)$$
$$X = 675 \text{ ml of concentrated}$$
$$\text{formalin needed}$$

For the amount of distilled water needed, subtract the amount of stock concentrated formalin from the total volume:

4500 ml (total volume of the 15% solution)
− 675 ml (part of total that is stock formalin)
3825 ml of distilled water

Dilutions expressed as ratios. If a dilution to be made is expressed as a ratio, such as "make a 1:10 dilution," the *1* represents the amount of original material to be diluted and the *10* the total volume amount to which the material is diluted. A 1:10 dilution therefore has one part of the original material diluted with 9 parts of diluent to give a total 10 parts of final volume.

Calculations using dye content. Dye lots may vary in their percentage of contained dye, and when the dye content changes considerably, solutions made from it should be accordingly adjusted by weight. This may be accomplished with use of a gravimetric factor, which is defined as the ratio of two dye contents for the purpose of correcting the weight of stain used in a formula. For example, a stain of 94% dye content is used with good results in a 2% solution. When this lot of stain is used up, new material with 76% dye content is received. A 2% solution of the new dye content would not have the equivalent strength or staining properties of the old solution. To make the two equivalent, therefore, it is necessary to multiply the gravimetric factor by the desired weight being used, that is:

$$\text{Gravimetric factor} = \frac{94 \text{ (dye content lot 1)}}{76 \text{ (dye content lot 2)}} = 1.24$$

1.24 times 2 gm/100 ml (gm/dl) (the desired weight in this example) equals 2.48. So 2.48 gm/dl of the new dye will be equivalent to 2.0 gm/dl of the old dye.

Temperature conversion

Most labs use the Celsius scale for measuring temperature and the fixed points on this scale are 0° as the freezing point and 100° as the boiling point. The other commonly used system is the Fahrenheit scale, and here the freezing point is 32° and the boiling point 212°. Since each degree on the scale is equivalent to $9/5$ that of the Fahrenheit and since the Fahrenheit scale has 32° difference between the freezing point to the 0 point, the following formula for changing Fahrenheit measurement to Celsius applies:

Fahrenheit measurement = (Celsius $\times$ $9/5$) + 32

To change from Fahrenheit to Celsius, the reverse is true. 32 is first subtracted from the number of Fahrenheit degrees, and this result is multiplied by $5/9$ since each degree on the Fahrenheit scale equals $5/9$ of a Celsius degree.

Celsius measurement = (Fahrenheit − 32) $\times$ $5/9$

Conversion tables

Weight units	Grams	Ounces
milligram	0.001	0.0000353
gram	1	0.0352740
kilogram	1000	35.2740
ounce	28.3495	1
pound	453.5924	16

Volume units	Liters	Fluid ounces	Liquid pints	Cubic centimeters
milliliter (cubic centimeter)	0.001	0.0338	0.0021	1
liter	1	33.815	2.113	1000
fluid ounce	0.0296	1	0.0625	29.57
liquid pint	0.4731	16	1	473.17

COMMONLY USED BUFFER REAGENTS

Reagent		Molecular weight
Acetic acid	CH_3COOH	60.03
Barbital sodium (sodium 5,5-diethyl barbiturate)	$C_8H_{11}O_3N_2Na$	206.18
Borax (sodium tetraborate)	$Na_2B_4O_7 \cdot 10H_2O$	381.43
Boric acid	$B(OH)_3$	61.84
Cacodylic acid	$(CH_3)_2AsO_2H$	137.99
Citric acid, anhydrous	$C_3H_4(OH)(COOH)_3$	192.12
Citric acid, crystals	$C_3H_4(OH)(COOH)_3 \cdot H_2O$	210.14
Glycine	NH_2CH_2COOH	75.07
Hydrochloric acid	HCl	36.465
Maleic acid	$HOOCCH{=}CHCOOH$	116.07
Medinal, *see* Barbital sodium		
Potassium acid phosphate (potassium dihydrogen phosphate)	KH_2PO_4	136.09
Potassium hydroxide	KOH	56.104
Sodium acetate (anhydrous)	CH_3COONa	82.04
Sodium acetate crystals	$CH_3COONa \cdot 3H_2O$	136.09
Sodium acid phosphate (sodium dihydrogen phosphate)	$NaH_2PO_4 \cdot H_2O$	138.01
Sodium citrate crystals	$C_3H_4OH(COONa)_3 \cdot 5½H_2O$	357.18
Sodium citrate, granular	$C_3H_4OH(COONa)_3 \cdot 2H_2O$	294.12
Sodium chloride	NaCl	58.46
Sodium hydroxide	NaOH	40.0
Sodium phosphate, dibasic	Na_2HPO_4	141.98
Sulfuric acid	H_2SO_4	98.082
Tris(hydroxymethyl)aminomethane (tromethamine,TRIS,tris buffer)	$H_2NC(CH_2OH)_3$	121.14
Veronal Sodium, *see* Barbital sodium		

PREPARATION OF MOLAR AND NORMAL ACID SOLUTIONS FROM CONCENTRATED ACID SOLUTIONS

For 1-liter amounts that are sufficiently accurate for histologic purposes, measure approximately 900 ml of distilled water into a 1-liter volumetric flask. Add the required amount of acid listed in the last column. Mix well and dilute up to the 1-liter mark. Mix again and store in a properly labeled bottle.

Sulfuric acid*

Specific gravity	% H$_2$SO$_4$ w/w	Grams of H$_2$SO$_4$ per liter	Normality	Milliliter amount needed for 1 liter of a 1 N solution Double volume to prepare 1 liter of a 1 M solution.
1.8337	95	1742	35.51	28.2
1.8355	96	1762	35.93	27.86
1.8364	97	1781	36.31	27.6
1.8361	98	1799	36.68	27.3
1.8342	99	1816	37.03	27.1
1.8305	100	1831	37.34	26.8

Hydrochloric acid*

Specific gravity	% HCl w/w	Grams of HCl per liter	Normality	Milliliter amount needed for 1 liter of a 1 N or a 1 M solution
1.1789	36	424.4	11.64	86.0
1.1837	37	438.0	12.01	83.3
1.1885	38	451.6	12.38	80.8
1.1932	39	465.4	12.75	78.4
1.1980	40	479.2	13.14	76.2

Nitric acid*

Specific gravity	% HNO$_3$ w/w	Grams of HNO$_3$ per liter	Normality	Milliliter amount needed for 1 liter of a 1 N or a 1 M solution
1.4048	68	955.3	15.16	66.0
1.4091	69	972.3	15.43	64.9
1.4134	70	989.4	15.70	63.8
1.4176	71	1006	15.96	62.7
1.4218	72	1024	16.25	61.6

Acetic acid*

Specific gravity	% CH$_3$COOH w/w	Grams of CH$_3$COOH per liter	Normality	Milliliter amount needed for 1 liter of a 1 N or a 1 M solution
1.0700	80	856.0	14.254	70.157
1.0699	81	866.6	14.429	69.298
1.0698	82	877.2	14.607	68.460
1.0696	83	887.8	14.784	67.643
1.0693	84	898.2	14.957	66.860
1.0689	85	908.6	15.130	66.095
1.0685	86	918.9	15.302	65.353
1.0680	87	929.2	15.473	64.630
1.0675	88	939.4	15.643	63.928
1.0668	89	949.5	15.811	63.249
1.0661	90	959.5	15.977	62.590
1.0652	91	969.3	16.141	61.956
1.0643	92	979.2	16.305	61.330
1.0632	93	988.8	16.463	60.734
1.0619	94	998.2	16.620	60.169
1.0605	95	1007	16.799	59.636
1.0588	96	1016	16.918	59.109
1.0570	97	1025	17.068	58.590
1.0549	98	1034	17.218	58.079
1.0524	99	1042	17.351	57.633
1.0498	100	1050	17.484	57.194

*From Lillie, R. D., and Fullmer, H. M.: Histopathologic technic and practical histochemistry, ed. 4, New York, 1976, McGraw-Hill Book Co.

Sodium acetate–acetic acid buffer (0.2 M, pH 3.6 to 5.8)

Sodium acetate · $3H_2O$, MW = 136.09; 0.2 M solution contains 27.22 gm in 1000 ml.

pH at 18° C	0.2 M sodium acetate (ml)	0.2 M acetic acid (ml)
3.6	0.75	9.25
3.8	1.20	8.80
4.0	1.80	8.20
4.2	2.65	7.35
4.4	3.70	6.30
4.6	4.90	5.10
4.8	5.90	4.10
5.0	7.00	3.00
5.2	7.90	2.10
5.4	8.60	1.40
5.6	9.10	0.90
5.8	9.40	0.90

From Walpole, G. S.: J. Chem. Soc. [Org.] **105**:2501, 1914.

Sodium acetate–hydrochloric acid buffer (pH 0.65 to 5.2)

Anhydrous sodium acetate, MW = 82.04; 1 M solution contains 82.04 gm in 1000 ml.
Sodium acetate · $3H_2O$, MW = 136.09; 1 M solution contains 136.09 gm in 1000 ml.

pH	1 N HCl	1 M NaAc	Distilled water
0.65	20	10	20
0.75	18	10	22
0.91	16	10	24
1.07	14	10	26
1.24	13	10	27
1.42	12	10	28
1.71	11	10	29
1.85	10.7	10	29.3
1.99	10.5	10	29.5
2.32	10.2	10	29.8
2.64	10.0	10	30
2.72	9.95	10	30.05
3.09	9.7	10	30.3
3.29	9.5	10	30.5
3.49	9.25	10	30.75
3.61	9.0	10	31
3.79	8.5	10	31.5
3.95	8	10	32
4.19	7	10	33
4.39	6	10	34
4.58	5	10	35
4.76	4	10	36
4.92	3	10	37
5.20	2	10	38

From Walpole, G. S.: J. Chem. Soc. [Org.] **105**:2501, 1914; modified from Pearse, A. G. E.: Histochemistry, ed. 2, Boston, 1960, Little, Brown, & Co., by Lillie, R. D., and Fullmer, H. M.: Histopathologic technic and practical histochemistry, ed. 4, New York, 1976, McGraw Hill Book Co.

Boric acid–borax buffer (0.2 M in terms of borate; pH 7.4 to 9.0)

Borax, $Na_2B_4O_7$ · $10H_2O$, MW = 381.43; 0.05 M solution (= 0.2 M borate) contains 19.07 gm in 1000 ml. Boric acid, MW = 61.84; 0.2 M solution contains 12.37 gm in 1000 ml.
Borax, $Na_2B_4O_7$ · $10H_2O$, may lose water of crystallization and it should be kept in a stoppered bottle.

pH	0.05 M borax (ml)	0.2 M boric acid (ml)
7.4	1.0	9.0
7.6	1.5	8.5
7.8	2.0	8.0
8.0	3.0	7.0
8.2	3.5	6.5
8.4	4.5	5.5
8.7	6.0	4.0
9.0	8.0	2.0

From Holmes, W.: Anat. Rec. **86**:157, 1943.

Citric acid–sodium citrate buffer (0.1 M, pH 3.0 to 6.6)

Citric acid · H_2O, MW = 210.14; 0.1 M solution contains 21.01 gm in 1000 ml.
Na_3 citrate · $2H_2O$, MW = 294.12; 0.1 M solution contains 29.4 gm in 1000 ml.

pH	0.1 M citric acid (ml)	0.1 M Na_3 citrate (ml)
3.0	18.6	1.4
3.2	17.2	2.8
3.4	16.0	4.0
3.6	14.9	5.1
3.8	14.0	6.0
4.0	13.1	6.9
4.2	12.3	7.7
4.4	11.4	8.6
4.6	10.3	9.7
4.8	9.2	10.8
5.0	8.2	11.8
5.2	7.3	12.7
5.4	6.4	13.6
5.6	5.5	14.5
5.8	4.7	15.3
6.0	3.8	16.2
6.2	2.8	17.2
6.4	2.0	18.0
6.6	1.4	18.6

Values taken from a curve constructed from the data of Lillie, R. D.: Histopathological technic and practical histochemistry, New York, 1954, The Blakiston Co., Inc., p. 450.

Dibasic sodium phosphate–citric acid buffer (pH 2.2 to 8.0)

Cannot be used in the presence of Ca^{++} or Mg^{++}.
Na_2HPO_4 · $2H_2O$, MW = 178.05; 0.2 M solution contains 35.61 gm in 1000 ml.

Citric acid · H_2O, MW = 210.14; 0.1 M solution contains 21.01 gm in 1000 ml.

pH	0.2 M Na_2HPO_4 (ml)	0.1 M citric acid (ml)
2.2	0.40	19.60
2.4	1.24	18.76
2.6	2.18	17.82
2.8	3.17	16.83
3.0	4.11	15.89
3.2	4.94	15.06
3.4	5.70	14.30
3.6	6.44	13.56
3.8	7.10	12.90
4.0	7.71	12.29
4.2	8.28	11.72
4.4	8.82	11.18
4.6	9.35	10.65
4.8	9.86	10.14
5.0	10.30	9.70
5.2	10.72	9.28
5.4	11.15	8.85
5.6	11.60	8.40
5.8	12.09	7.91
6.0	12.63	7.37
6.2	13.22	6.78
6.4	13.85	6.15
6.6	14.55	5.45
6.8	15.45	4.55
7.0	16.47	3.53
7.2	17.39	2.61
7.4	18.17	1.83
7.6	18.73	1.27
7.8	19.15	0.85
8.0	19.45	0.55

From McIlvaine, T. C.: J. Biol. Chem. **49**:183, 1921.

Sodium hydrogen maleate–NaOH buffer (0.05 M, pH 5.2 to 6.8)

0.2 M NaH maleate is prepared when 23.2 gm of maleic acid (or 19.6 gm of maleic anhydride) and 8 gm of NaOH are dissolved in water and the volume is made up to 1000 ml.

pH at 25° C	0.2 M NaOH (ml)	0.2 M NaH maleate (ml)	
5.2	7.2	50	
5.4	10.5	50	
5.6	15.3	50	
5.8	20.8	50	Dilute each mixture to 200 ml with H_2O
6.0	26.9	50	
6.2	33.0	50	
6.4	38.0	50	
6.6	41.6	50	
6.8	44.4	50	

From Temple, J. W.: J. Am. Chem. Soc. **51**:1754, 1929.

Na_2HPO_4–NaH_2PO_4 buffer (0.1 M, pH 5.8 to 8.0)

Na_2HPO_4 · $2H_2O$, MW = 178.05; 0.2 M solution contains 35.61 gm in 1000 ml.
Na_2HPO_4 · $12H_2O$, MW = 358.22; 0.2 M solution contains 71.64 gm in 1000 ml.
NaH_2PO_4 · H_2O, MW = 138.0; 0.2 M solution contains 27.6 gm in 1000 ml.
NaH_2PO_4 · $2H_2O$, MW = 156.03; 0.2 M solution contains 31.21 gm in 1000 ml.

pH	0.2 M Na_2HPO_4 (ml)	0.2 M NaH_2PO_4 (ml)	
5.8	8.0	92.0	
6.0	12.3	87.7	
6.2	18.5	81.5	
6.4	26.5	73.5	
6.6	37.5	62.5	
6.8	49.0	51.0	Dilute each mixture to 200 ml with H_2O
7.0	61.0	39.0	
7.2	72.0	28.0	
7.4	81.0	19.0	
7.6	87.0	13.0	
7.8	91.5	8.5	
8.0	94.7	5.3	

From Gomori, G.: Methods in enzymology, New York, 1955, vol. 1, p. 143.

KH_2PO_4–NaOH buffer (0.05 M, pH 5.8 to 8.0)

For sodium-free buffers use KOH.
KH_2PO_4, MW = 136.09; 0.2 M solution contains 27.22 gm in 1000 ml.

pH at 20° C	0.2 M KH_2PO_4 (ml)	0.2 N NaOH (ml)	
5.8	5	0.372	
6.0	5	0.570	
6.2	5	0.860	
6.4	5	1.260	
6.6	5	1.780	Dilute each mixture to 20 ml with H_2O
6.8	5	2.365	
7.0	5	2.963	
7.2	5	3.500	
7.4	5	3.950	
7.6	5	4.280	
7.8	5	4.520	
8.0	5	4.680	

From Clark, W. M., and Lubs, H. A.: J. Biol. Chem. **25**:479, 1916.

Sodium cacodylate–HCl buffer (0.05 M, pH 5.0 to 7.4)

$Na(CH_3)_2$ · AsO_2 · $3H_2O$, MW = 214.02; 0.1 M solution contains 21.40 gm in 1000 ml.

pH at 15° C	0.1 M Na(CH₃)₂ · AsO₂ · 3H₂O (ml)	0.1 N HCl (ml)	
5.0	100	93.5	
5.2	100	90.1	
5.4	100	85.2	
5.6	100	78.4	
5.8	100	69.6	Dilute
6.0	100	59.1	each
6.2	100	47.7	mixture
6.4	100	36.5	to 200
6.6	100	26.6	ml with
6.8	100	18.6	H₂O
7.0	100	12.6	
7.2	100	8.3	
7.4	100	5.4	

From Plumel, M.: Bull. Soc. Chim. Biol. (Paris) **30**:129, 1948.

Sodium carbonate–sodium bicarbonate buffer (0.1 M, pH 9.2 to 10.8)

Cannot be used in the presence of Ca^{++} or Mg^{++}. $Na_2CO_3 \cdot 10H_2O$, MW = 286.2; 0.1 M solution contains 28.62 gm in 1000 ml.
$NaHCO_3$, MW = 84.0; 0.1 M solution contains 8.40 gm in 1000 ml.

pH		0.1 M Na₂CO₃ (ml)	0.1 M NaHCO₃ (ml)
20° C	37° C		
9.16	8.77	1	9
9.40	9.12	2	8
9.51	9.40	3	7
9.78	9.50	4	6
9.90	9.72	5	5
10.14	9.90	6	4
10.28	10.08	7	3
10.53	10.28	8	2
10.83	10.57	9	1

From Delory, G. E., and King, E. J., Jr.: Biochem. J. **39**:245, 1945.

Sodium diethylbarbiturate (Veronal)–HCl buffer (0.04 M, pH 6.8 to 9.6)

Sodium diethylbarbiturate, MW = 206.2; 0.04 M solution contains 8.25 gm in 1000 ml.

pH at 18° C	0.04 M sodium diethylbarbiturate (ml)	0.2 N HCl (ml)
6.8	100	18.4
7.0	100	17.8
7.2	100	16.7
7.4	100	15.3
7.6	100	13.4
7.8	100	11.47
8.0	100	9.39

pH at 18° C	0.04 M sodium diethylbarbiturate (ml)	0.2 N HCl (ml)
8.2	100	7.21
8.4	100	5.21
8.6	100	3.82
8.8	100	2.52
9.0	100	1.65
9.2	100	1.13
9.4	100	0.07
9.6	100	0.35

From Britton, H. T. S., and Robinson, R. A.: J. Chem. Soc. **122**:1456, 1931.

Michaelis's sodium diethylbarbiturate (Veronal)–HCl buffer

Sodium diethylbarbiturate, MW = 206.2; 0.1 M solution contains 20.618 gm in 1000 ml.

pH	0.1 N HCl	0.1 M barbital sodium
6.4	19.6	20.4
6.5	19.5	20.5
6.6	19.4	20.6
6.7	19.3	20.7
6.8	19.1	20.9
6.9	18.8	21.2
7.0	18.6	21.4
7.1	18.2	21.8
7.2	17.8	22.2
7.3	17.3	22.7
7.4	16.8	23.2
7.5	16.1	23.9
7.6	15.4	24.6
7.7	14.5	25.5
7.8	13.5	26.5
7.9	12.4	27.6
8.0	11.4	28.6
8.1	10.3	29.7
8.2	9.2	30.8
8.3	8.2	31.8
8.4	7.1	32.9
8.5	6.1	33.9
8.6	5.2	34.8
8.7	4.4	35.6
8.8	3.7	36.3
8.9	3.1	36.9
9.0	2.6	37.4
9.1	2.2	37.8
9.2	1.9	38.1
9.3	1.5	38.5
9.4	1.0	39.0
9.5	0.8	39.2
9.6	0.6	39.4
9.7	0.4	39.6

Recalculated on a 40 ml volume and interpolated arithmetically from the table on p. 454 on Lillie, R. D.: Histopathologic technic and practical histochemistry, ed. 2, Philadelphia, 1954, The Blakiston Co., Inc.

Tris(hydroxymethyl)aminomethane–maleic acid buffer (pH 5.08 to 8.45)

Tris(hydroxymethyl)aminomethane, MW = 121.14; 1 M solution contains 121.14 gm in 1000 ml.

Maleic acid, MW = 116; 1 M solution contains 116 gm in 1000 ml.
Sodium hydroxide, MW = 40; 0.5 M solution contains 20 gm in 1000 ml.

pH	1 M maleic acid (ml)	1 M tris(hydroxymethyl)- aminomethane (ml)	0.5 M sodium hydroxide (ml)	Distilled water (ml)
5.08	5	5	1	39
5.30	5	5	2	38
5.52	5	5	3	37
5.70	5	5	4	36
5.88	5	5	5	35
6.05	5	5	6	34
6.27	5	5	7	33
6.50	5	5	8	32
6.86	5	5	9	31
7.20	5	5	10	30
7.50	5	5	11	29
7.75	5	5	12	28
7.97	5	5	13	27
8.15	5	5	14	26
8.30	5	5	15	25
8.45	5	5	16	24

From Gomori, G.: Proc. Soc. Exp. Biol. Med. **68:**354, 1948.

Tris(hydroxymethyl)aminomethane–HCl ("TRIS-HCl") buffer (0.05 M, pH 7.2 to 9.1)

Tris(hydroxymethyl)aminomethane, MW = 121.14; 0.2 M solution contains 24.23 gm in 1000 ml.

pH 23° C	pH 37° C	0.2 M TRIS (ml)	0.1 N HCl (ml)	
9.10	8.95	25	5.0	
8.92	8.78	25	7.5	
8.74	8.60	25	10.0	
8.62	8.48	25	12.5	
8.50	8.37	25	15.0	
8.40	8.27	25	17.5	
8.32	8.18	25	20.0	
8.23	8.10	25	22.5	Dilute each
8.14	8.00	25	25.0	mixture to
8.05	7.90	25	27.5	100 ml with
7.96	7.82	25	30.0	H₂O
7.87	7.73	25	32.5	
7.77	7.63	25	35.0	
7.66	7.52	25	37.5	
7.54	7.40	25	40.0	
7.36	7.22	25	42.5	
7.20	7.05	25	45.0	

CYTOLOGY
Sidney Coleman

Preparation of exudates and fluids for sectioning (cell block)

Exudates are fluids that accumulate in tissues and serous cavities as a result of an inflammatory process.

Fluids of various types, but especially those from the serous cavities, often require microscopic examination of the cells they contain. This may be done on a fixed or unfixed specimen. By the procedure that follows, you may section the fluid on a rotary microtome using the paraffin embedding technic. The fluid collected must be sent to the laboratory as soon as possible.

1. Pour the fluid into a large test tube and centrifuge, with tubes balanced, at high to medium speed for 15 to 30 minutes. If blood is seen in the fluid, add 2% by volume of glacial acetic acid to prevent coagulation and to lake red cells.
2. Pour off the supernatant fluid, leaving cell sediment in the bottom of the test tube.
3. If desired, a smear may be made from a portion of this sediment and processed by the Papanicolaou technic for the study of malignant cells (see Papanicolaou staining technic, p. 393).

4. Pour a small amount of 10% formalin directly into the test tube and let stand for 15 to 30 minutes or longer. The formalin will cause the sediment on the bottom to coagulate into a soft mass. You may remove the mass by inverting the tube and tapping or by using a wooden applicator stick.
5. Place the sediment in fine gauze or lens paper (folded) in a tissue capsule or capsules if there is a large amount.
6. Fix the sediment 6 to 24 hours, or 3 hours in warm 10% formalin (at 45° C).
7. The block is now treated as any other piece of tissue by the paraffin technic.
8. If the specimen received is in too small a quantity to spin down, make smears directly for the hematoxylin and eosin and Papanicolaou technics. Or tint the fluid with a drop of eosin and pour directly over very fine gauze or lens paper. Place in a capsule and process as usual.

Preparation of smears for Papanicolaou technic*

Exfoliative cytology is the study of dead cells that have been cast off. The primary purpose is for the cytologic study of possible early detection of cancer. A positive diagnosis is not made from a smear, only by a surgical biopsy from the area.

Most commonly smears are obtained from the

_____
*For additional study, refer to *The Cytologic Diagnosis of Cancer,* Vincent Memorial Hospital, New York, N.Y.

female reproductive tract; the vagina, cervix, endocervix, and the endometrium. Smears are also made from prostatic fluid, urine sediment, pancreatic drainage, spinal fluid, mouth or oral cavities, sputum, gastric and bronchial aspirates, pleural, peritoneal, and acetic fluids, colon washings, and recently blood.

The smears should be fresh and never allowed to dry out. They must be fixed immediately or else the chromatin will be distorted. The smear is made on a clean slide or an albumen-coated slide and appropriately identified. As previously discussed under fluids, some specimens, such as exudates and other washings, might have to be centrifuged before a smear is made. Urine and other acellular fluids are usually put through a Millipore filter and processed on the filter.

Papanicolaou, in his technic, suggests fixation in equal parts 95% alcohol and ether, though excellent results have been obtained with fixation in 95% alcohol only. Spinal fluids yield best results when fixed in 10% formalin and blood films in Carnoy's fixative. Isopropanol is preferred for the Millipore technic.

Some types of smears may fix in 15 minutes, a minimum of 1 hour will permit more complete penetration of the cells. They may stay several days or weeks, if the level of the fixing solution is kept above the smear.

After fixation the slides may be stained routinely with hematoxylin and eosin or other stains. The preferred stain is the Papanicolaou method.

Papanicolaou staining procedure for gynecologic cytology specimens —regressive method (University of Tennessee Cytology Laboratory)

Fix all cytology specimens while the material is still wet. *Do not allow it to dry before fixation.*
The following is from fixative of 95% ethanol to xylene:

Hydration	80% ethanol	3 dips or 10 seconds
	70% ethanol	3 dips
	50% ethanol	3 dips
	Distilled water	3 dips
Chromatin staining	Harris's hematoxylin (p. 142)	45 seconds to 4 minutes (varies with age and dilution because of volume of material stained)
Rinse	Distilled water	3 dips
Differential extraction	0.25% hydrochloric acid	1 dip (quick)
Rinse	Tap water	1 dip
Bluing	Gentle running tap water	6 minutes
Dehydration	50% ethanol	3 dips
	70% ethanol	3 dips
	80% ethanol	3 dips
	95% ethanol	3 dips

Continued.

*Papanicolaou staining procedure for gynecologic cytology specimens —
regressive method —cont'd*

Cytoplasmic counterstaining	*Orange G6	1½ minutes
Rinse	95% ethanol 95% ethanol	3 dips (gently but thoroughly) 3 dips
Cytoplasmic counterstaining	*EA 50	1½ minutes (3 minutes for mailed-in fixed specimens)
Rinse	95% ethanol 95% ethanol 95% ethanol	3 dips 3 dips 3 dips
Complete dehydration	Absolute ethanol (100%) Absolute ethanol and Xylene (1:1)	½ minute ½ minute
Clearing	Xylene Xylene Xylene	½ minute 5 minutes Until coverslipped with a mounting medium (Permount)

*Note: Store stains overnight in well-stoppered *dark glass bottles*. Filter xylene after each group of slides is coverslipped. Filter fixative and reuse as rinses after orange G6 and EA 50. Filter stains every other day.

Automatic staining technic
(Shandon Scientific Co., Inc.)

Station number	Ingredients in staining trough	Time in minutes	Accumulative minutes
1	80% ethanol	1	1
2	70% ethanol	1	2
3	50% ethanol	1	3
4	Distilled water	1	4
5	Dilute hematoxylin in water (3:1)	1½	5½
6	Distilled water	1	6½
7	Distilled water	1	7½
8	0.25% hydrochloric acid	Instant dip	—
9	Running tap water	6	13½
10	Distilled water	1	14½
11	70% ethanol	1	15½
12	80% ethanol	1	16½
13	95% ethanol	1	17½
14	Orange G6	1½	19
15	95% ethanol	1	20
16	95% ethanol	1	21
17	EA 65	1½	22½
18	95% ethanol	1	23½
19	95% ethanol	1	24½
20	Absolute ethanol	1	25½
21	Absolute ethanol	1	26½
22	Absolute ethanol and xylene	1	27½
23	Xylene		

Staining method for undecalcified bone
(Hospital of the University of Pennsylvania)

1. Place slides directly into Delafield's hematoxylin 30 min.
2. Rinse in running tap water.
3. Acid alcohol (1% hydrochloric acid in 70% ethanol). Two quick dips.
4. Rinse twice in clear water.

5. Blue in saturated lithium carbonate in distilled water.
6. Run in tap water.   5 min
7. Stain in eosin (p. 153 for formula).   3 min
8. 95% ethanol.   1 min
9. 95% ethanol.   1 min
10. 95% ethanol.   1 min
11. Absolute ethanol.   1 min
12. Absolute ethanol.   1 min
13. Equal parts absolute ethanol to xylene.   1 min
14. Repeat 13.
15. Xylene.
16. Xylene.
17. Xylene and mount in HSR in xylene.

Morphology of abnormal cells

Shape
  Variation from normal
  Degenerate forms with rough lines
  Serrated
Color
  Usually intensely colored (hyperchromic)
  Uneveness of color
Size of nucleus
  Nucleus not in proportion to cytoplasm
  Large nucleus to small amount of cytoplasm
Morphology
  Nucleus not smooth
  Abnormal clumping of chromatin (outstanding feature)
  Cytoplasm folded and irregular

SAFETY

Helen N. Futch

The excerpts forming this section are from the Joint Commission on Accreditation of Hospitals Program on Hospital Accreditation Standards—Pathology and Medical Laboratory Services. The following safety pages are taken from the revision of the Pathology and Medical Laboratory standards approved by the Board of Commissioners at its April 1978 meeting, published in the 1979 edition of the *Accreditation Manual for Hospitals* and due to be surveyed for accreditation purposes after January 1, 1979.

REGULAR AND CONVENIENT AVAILABILITY

Pathology and medical laboratory services and consultation shall be regularly and conveniently available to meet the needs of patients as determined by the medical staff. Provision must be made, either on the premises or in a reference laboratory, for the prompt performance of adequate examinations in the following fields:
  Anatomic pathology
  Hematology
  Chemistry
  Microbiology
  Clinical microscopy
  Parasitology
  Immunohematology
  Serology
  Virology
  Nuclear medicine, as it relates to the pathology and medical laboratory services
  Note: Such examinations shall be performed in sufficient depth to meet the usual needs of the medical staff.

LABORATORY TECHNOLOGISTS AND SUPPORTIVE PERSONNEL

Standard I. There shall be a sufficient number of qualified laboratory technologists and supportive technical staff to perform, promptly and proficiently, the tests required of the pathology and medical laboratory services. A qualified medical technologist shall:
Be a graduate of a medical technology program approved by a nationally recognized body
or
Have documented equivalent education, training, and/or experience. Meet any current legal requirements of licensure or registration. Be currently competent in the field.

Interpretation I. The director of the pathology and laboratory services shall:
Assure that procedures and tests that are outside the scope of education, training, and experience of the individuals employed to perform technical procedures in the laboratory shall not be performed in the pathology and medical laboratory services.
Maintain documentation of the qualifications of such personnel to perform these procedures.
Assign work that shall be consistent with the qualifications of the employee.

STUDENT TECHNOLOGISTS

The education and in-hospital training of student technologists shall be carried out only in programs approved by the appropriate professional educational organizations recognized by the United States Office of Education. Student technologists shall:

> Be supervised by qualified individuals at all times.
>
> Not be assigned responsible call duty alone.
>
> Not perform emergency laboratory procedures (to be performed only by qualified technologists).

The director, supervisors, and laboratory personnel must comply with applicable federal, state, and local laws and regulations. The director shall be responsible for the qualifications and performance of the staff.

EDUCATION PROGRAMS PROVIDED

There shall be provision for technologists and other technical personnel, including supervisors, to further their knowledge and skills:

> Through hospital-based educational opportunities, such as:
>> On-the-job training
>> In-service education programs
>
> As feasible, at least for supervisory personnel, through attendance at outside workshops, institutes, and local, regional, or national society meetings.

In-service

There shall be in-service education programs that shall:

> Be held at defined intervals that are reasonable for the size and needs of the technological staff.
>
> Be documented with respect to:
>> Program content
>> Extent of participation
>
> Have provision for participation of personnel of all work shifts. Continuing education programs shall be based, at least in part, on:
>> Findings of quality-of-service evaluation studies.
>> The principles of laboratory safety.

Safety—functional safety and sanitation

There shall be a written plan of action for personnel to implement in the event of a serious accident in the laboratory, and the provisions of the plan shall be made known periodically to all laboratory personnel as part of the continuing education program relating to safety.

ORIENTATION

An orientation program shall be provided for each laboratory employee, and participation shall be documented.

SUFFICIENT SPACE, EQUIPMENT, AND SUPPLIES PROVIDED

There shall be sufficient space, equipment, and supplies within the pathology and medical laboratory services to perform the required volume of work with optimal accuracy, precision, efficiency, timeliness, and safety.

The laboratory environment shall be conducive to the optimal performance of:
> Personnel
> Equipment

Ventilation system

The ventilation system:
> Shall provide an adequate amount of fresh air.
>
> Must be able to remove toxic and noxious fumes.

Bench space

There shall be adequate, conveniently located bench space for:
> The efficient handling of specimens
> The housing of:
>> Equipment
>> Reagents

Work areas

Work areas shall be:
> Arranged to minimize problems in:
>> Transportation
>> Communication
> Adequately lighted to facilitate:
>> Accuracy
>> Precision

Utilities

There shall be a sufficient number of properly located utilities. Equipment and instruments shall be appropriate for the services required and shall include:

> A sufficient number of properly grounded electrical outlets with adequately stabilized voltage.
>
> Monitoring and recording of voltage levels at electrical sources to which automated equipment is connected.
>
> An emergency power supply sufficient, in the event of a power failure, to:
>> Permit the performance of essential laboratory studies, including the use of a microscope.
>> Maintain any essential refrigerating or heating elements.

Instruments and equipment

The performance of instruments and equipment must be evaluated frequently enough to assure that they function properly at all times. Appropriate records shall be maintained:

For each piece of equipment, showing:

The date of inspections, validations, or performance evaluations.

Significant actions taken in response to revealed deficiencies.

Of temperatures recorded daily for all temperature-controlled instruments.

Safety precautions taken

Special precautions shall be taken to avoid unnecessary physical, chemical, and biological hazards.

Storage practices
Functional safety and sanitation

Safeguards shall be instituted for a laboratory where flammable gases and liquids frequently are present in bulk storage, for example, propane, hydrogen, methane, ether, acetone, xylene, and alcohol:

Alcohol shall be withdrawn from large drums only with the drum in the upright position and by use of an approved hand pump.

Smoking shall be prohibited in any area where flammable gases or liquids, or oxygen, are in storage or in use.

Note: The preceding two areas shall be identified with "no smoking" signs. Where indicated, the signs shall be multilingual or shall make use of symbols.

Electrical equipment unsafe for use with flammable or combustible liquids shall be so labeled and such use prohibited.

Supplies of flammable gases within the laboratory shall:

To the maximum extent possible, be stored according to the same standards for enclosure as those described for flammable anesthetizing gases.

Not ordinarily exceed 2 days' working needs.

Supplies of flammable liquids shall be:

Limited in the laboratory to 2 days' working needs.

Stored, when in excess of 10 gallons, in an approved storage cabinet containing not more than 60 gallons and vented to the outside.

Other procedures in the laboratory should provide that:

Flammable liquids or gas cylinders shall not be positioned near flame or heat sources.

All refrigerators shall be labeled to identify whether or not they are safe for storage of flammable liquids.

Use of flammable or combustible reagents

Tissue processors and similar automatic equipment employing flammable or combustible reagents shall be:

Well-ventilated

Operated at least 5 feet from storage of combustible materials.

The use of safety cans for compatible flammable liquids is encouraged where the liquid content retains its functional and compositional stability.

The heating of flammable liquids should be performed only in suitable fume hoods.

SPECIAL SAFETY MEASURES

Special safety measures shall be provided for areas of the hospital that present an unusual hazard to personnel or patients, including:

Facilities for flushing the eyes, body, and clothing with large quantities of water shall be provided in or near the areas in which caustic or toxic materials are used.

Rooms in which volatile and/or toxic chemicals are used shall be adequately ventilated and equipped with noncombustible fume hoods.

Refrigerators for the storage of flammable material shall be provided where indicated.

Radiation decontamination facilities shall be provided wherever radioactive isotopes are used.

Biological safety cabinets shall be provided for the protection of laboratory personnel who handle specimens containing known or suspected highly virulent microorganisms.

Bulk storage of concentrated acid shall be located near the floor level, and the storage area appropriately identified.

A fire blanket and self-contained breathing apparatus are recommended for the clinical laboratory.

INFECTION CONTROL MEASURES

Laboratory wastes, such as culture plates, tubes, sputum cups, or swabs, shall be:

Sterilized by autoclaving prior to washing or discarding.

or

Sealed in impervious containers clearly marked for special handling and then incinerated.

QUALITY CONTROL PROGRAM IN EFFECT

Quality control systems and measures of the pathology and medical laboratory services shall be designed to assure the medical reliability of laboratory data.

General quality controls

The laboratory and, as appropriate, each of its components shall be licensed as required. There shall be a documented quality control program in effect for each section of the pathology and medical laboratory services. General quality controls required of and practiced by the pathology and medical laboratory services shall include, but should not necessarily be limited to, the following:

The use of proficiency testing programs for each discipline offered by the clinical laboratory.

Current descriptions of and instructions for all analytic methods and procedures. There shall be a complete written description of each test procedure, including:

Control and calibration procedures.

Pertinent literature references.

Descriptions of test procedures shall be:

Immediately available to the appropriate laboratory analyst.

Current.

Documentation of at least annual review by:

The director of the pathology and medical laboratory services

or

The appropriate supervisor of the organized laboratory component.

Note: The director or supervisor shall approve in writing all changes in the laboratory procedures.

Validation of methods used.

Daily surveillance of results by the director or appropriate supervisor, including results of tests:

Ordered and reported through transmission of information between the laboratory and nurses' stations (including direct computer feed).

Performed on an emergency basis outside of regularly scheduled laboratory staffing periods.

Documentation of remedial action taken for

detected deficiencies or defects as identified through quality control measures or authorized inspections.

Preventive maintenance, periodic inspection, and performance testing of equipment and instruments, with maintenance of appropriate records.

Evaluation of analytical measuring equipment and instruments with respect to all critical operating characteristics.

Evaluation of automated volumetric equipment.

Note: Certification is acceptable for manual volumetric equipment.

Performance of tests and operation of instruments within temperature and humidity required for proper performance.

Documented monitoring of temperature-controlled spaces and equipment.

Convenient location of essential utilities.

Proper preparing, storing, dispensing, and periodic evaluation of all solid and liquid reagents, including water, to assure accuracy and precision of results.

Note: There shall be written guidelines for this requirement.

Labeling of reagents and solutions for:

Identity.

Strength.

Cautionary or accessory information.

Preparation and expiration dates, as appropriate.

Note: There shall be written guidelines for this requirement. Materials of substandard reactivity and deteriorated materials may not be used.

Written procedures for:

The preparation of patients.

Collection, preservation, transportation, receipt of specimens to assure satisfactory specimens for the tests to be performed.

Note: These procedures must also be observed for specimens that are sent to reference laboratories.

The identification of specimens.

The review of the performance of personnel of all laboratory work shifts on a regular basis by the pathologist or appropriate laboratory supervisor.

Quality control records

Quality control records shall be retained for at least 2 years, and equipment maintenance records shall be retained for the life of each instrument used.

WRITTEN PROCEDURES DEVELOPED

Written procedures shall be developed for those who collect specimens, in order to assure that the specimens are satisfactory for the tests to be performed. There shall be evidence that such procedures have been approved by the director of the pathology and medical laboratory services. The procedures shall relate to at least the following:

The ordering of tests.

Standards and special methods used for:

The preparation of patients.

The collection of specimens.

Precautions to be followed for special procedures.

Proper identification, storage, and preservation of specimens.

Requests for tests made in writing or electronically

All requests for laboratory tests shall be made in writing or by electronic means. Orders of requisitions for inpatient and outpatient services must clearly identify:

The patient.

The requesting practitioner.

The tests required.

Any special handling required.

The date and the time (when relevant) the specimen was collected.

The date and the time the request and/or specimen reached the laboratory.

Requests for examinations of surgical specimens shall also contain a concise statement of the reason for the examination.

Records and reports maintained and filed

Required records and reports shall be maintained and, as appropriate, shall be filed in the patient's medical record and in the pathology and medical laboratory services.

Authenticated, dated reports of all examinations performed by the pathology and medical laboratory services shall be made a part of the patient's medical record. The director of the pathology and medical laboratory services shall be responsible for all hospital laboratory reports. *Note:* When tests are performed in a reference laboratory, the name of the laboratory performing the test must be included in the report placed in the patient's medical record.

The pathologist shall be responsible for the preparation of a descriptive diagnostic report of:

Gross specimens received.

Necropsies performed.

Reports of diagnoses

Diagnoses made from surgical specimens and necropsies shall be:

Expressed in acceptable terminology of a recognized disease nomenclature.

Indexed for retrieval.

Reports of tests and examinations

Reports of all anatomic laboratory tests performed shall be:

Readily available to the individual ordering the tests.

Filed promptly in the patient's medical record.

Record of accession

The pathology laboratory shall maintain a record of the daily accession of specimens and an appropriate system for identification of each. The record shall include at least:

Identification of:

The laboratory.

The patient.

The practitioner ordering the test or evaluation.

The date and time (when relevant) of:

Specimen collection.

Specimen receipt.

The reason for any unsatisfactory specimen.

The test or evaluation performed and the result.

The date and time of reporting to the requesting practitioner or patient care unit.

Note: Duplicate copies of all anatomic examinations performed should be retained in the laboratory in a readily retrievable manner.

Retention of records

Requirements for record retention:

Should be determined by:

Applicable local, state, and federal statutes and regulations.

Local needs.

but

Shall be for at least 2 years.

ANATOMIC PATHOLOGY AND SURGICAL PATHOLOGY

Specimens removed during a surgical procedure:

Shall ordinarily be sent to the pathologist for evaluation.

Shall be:

Properly labeled.

Packaged in preservative as designated.

Identified as to patient and source in the operating room or suite at the time of removal.

Must be accompanied by:

Pertinent clinical information.

To the degree known, the preoperative and postoperative surgical diagnoses.

The laboratory receiving surgically removed specimens for examination shall:

Document receipt of such specimens.

Assure the identity of the specimens and patients throughout:

Processing.

Storage.

Microscopic sections

Each microscopic section shall ordinarily be evaluated by a pathologist. The equipment, methods, and stains used in the production of microscopic slides must provide tissue sections from which a pathologist can make diagnoses with reasonable assurance.

If an electron microscopy facility is present in the hospital:

There shall be established and enforced precautions regarding:

Radiation hazards

Electrical hazards

Fluorescence and immunofluorescence procedures should be available to meet indicated diagnostic requirements.

Reports of all electron microscopic studies performed for diagnostic purposes shall be included in the clinical record.

The following controls are to be observed:

Special stains shall be controlled for intended reactivity with positive and negative slides.

Microscopic slides must be:

Adequately and permanently identified.

Properly indexed and stored to maintain their diagnostic value.

Paraffin blocks must be:

Adequately identified.

Properly indexed.

Stored in a cool place.

Protected against damage.

Specimen availability and storage

All tissue sections shall be readily available for:

Reference.

Use in consultations.

Microscopic slides, paraffin blocks, bone marrow aspirates, needle biopsy specimens, and gross tissue specimens shall be stored for as long as they are required:

For patient care purposes.

In accordance with federal and state requirements.

Gross specimens shall be retained in a proper fixative for at least 7 days after:

All required microscopic sections are examined.

The reports are reviewed and signed.

Notice to all laboratory personnel

IN CASE FIRE IS DISCOVERED

1. **KEEP CALM.** Do not excite others.
2. **Remove from immediate danger any patients** who may be in the immediate area, and call the telephone operator to report the fire.
3. **TURN IN ALARM.** Use pull-down alarm.
4. **CLOSE ALL DOORS AND WINDOWS** in the area.
5. **USE THE NEAREST** appropriate **FIRE EXTINGUISHER** to begin fighting the fire.

Type of extinguisher	Type of fire for which appropriate	
CO_2	"B" and "C"	Flammable liquids Flammable chemicals
CO_2	"B" and "C"	Oil and grease
CO_2	"B" and "C"	Electrical equipment
Soda acid	"A"	Wood, paper, rags, glowing embers

PULL-DOWN ALARM IS LOCATED IN HALLWAY ACROSS FROM LABORATORY

OPERATE THE SODA ACID EXTINGUISHER BY TURNING IT UPSIDE DOWN.

OPERATE THE CO_2 EXTINGUISHER BY PULLING SAFETY PIN AND SQUEEZING LEVER.

■ ■ ■

TOTAL EVACUATION: Laboratory employees should go to the ground floor exits and assist in evacuating patients.

DISASTER PROGRAM: The Director of Laboratories will arrange for full-scale operation of Laboratory Service, using all available equipment and personnel.

Director of Laboratories

SAFETY REGULATIONS

In case of burns or splashes from ACIDS, CAUSTICS, OR STRONG TOXINS—RAPID FLUSHING WITH VOLUMES OF WATER is the immediate treatment of choice. Use the most immediately available source of water.

In case of eye splashes or burns, use step-on eye washer or eye-wash bottle for continued flushing, and contact a physician.

MECHANICAL PIPETTING DEVICE MUST BE USED FOR ALL PIPETTING OF ACIDS, CAUSTICS, AND STRONG TOXINS.

PLUGGED DISPOSABLE PIPETS ARE TO BE USED FOR PIPETTING OF JAUNDICED SERUM AND BLOOD AND FOR ANY MATERIALS KNOWN OR SUSPECTED TO BE INFECTIOUS.

_____

Director of Laboratories

HISTOPATHOLOGY LABORATORY INFECTION CONTROL

1. **Double-bag** all waste material.
2. **Rubber gloves** must be worn at grossing area (when handling specimen or cleaning). Scrub hands thoroughly after removal of gloves.
3. **All sharp items** must be placed in metal disposal container.
4. **All dissecting instruments** must be placed in Lysol solution (or other disinfectant).
5. **Water baths** must be washed, rinsed, and dried daily.
6. **Cutting board**—Cover with disinfectant and leave overnight.
7. **Recording equipment**—Wipe with gauze sponge containing disinfecting solution. No need to rinse.
8. **Formalin solutions**—Avoid tap water containing mycobacteria. Rinse bottle often.
9. **Autotechnicon processor**—Detergent-wash, and dry beakers weekly. (More often if large volume is run.)
10. **Tissue cassettes,** soak in solvent to remove wax. Place in detergent bath, wash clean, scald, and towel-dry.
11. **Sink** must be cleaned with Lysol solution daily. All tissue residue, blood, bone, hair, suture, etc. must be removed.
12. **Weighing scale**—Disengage weighing pan, wash with Lysol, and dry.
13. **Wet tissue**—Must be stored in 10% formalin solution in leakproof container. After 6 weeks specimen may be disposed of. Containers must be placed in double plastic bags, sealed, and incinerated at 2000 degrees.
14. **Door knobs, handles of cabinets, lights plates, faucets, paper towel holders,** and **telephones** should be wiped with gauze sponge containing disinfectant solution.
15. **Floor** should be scrubbed daily using double-bucket system.
16. If **lab coats** are worn, they should be removed before leaving laboratory.
17. **Waste baskets** should be emptied daily.
18. **Never place objects in the mouth.**
19. **Aprons** worn during grossing must be washed with Lysol solution.
20. NO SMOKING—NO EATING—NO DRINKING in this area.

SAFETY WITH XYLENE
NIOSH recommended standard for occupational exposure to xylene

A complete document on criteria for occupational exposure to xylene has been prepared by the National Institute for Occupational Safety and Health (NIOSH). NIOSH recommends adherence to the present Federal Standard of 100 ppm as a time-weighted average for up to a 10-hour workday, 40-hour workweek. NIOSH also recommends a ceiling concentration of 200 ppm as determined by a sampling period of 10 minutes.

The recommended standard is part of a continuing series of criterion documents developed by NIOSH in accordance with the Occupational Safety and Health Act of 1970. The document was transmitted to the Occupational Safety and Health Administration in the Department of Labor on May 23, 1975, for review and consideration in the standard setting process.

Xylene, also called dimethylbenzene, or xylol, is produced commercially from both petroleum and coal tar. Total United States xylene production in 1971 was 612,325,000 gallons, and NIOSH estimates that 140,000 workers are potentially exposed. Xylene is an organic solvent for some gums, resins, and oils and is a constituent of paint, lacquers, varnishes, inks, dyes, adhesives, and cleaning fluids. It is also an additive in gasoline. The proposed standard would apply to the processing, manufacture, use, or other occupational exposure to xylene as applicable under the Occupational Safety and Health Act of 1970.

Xylene has an irritant effect on the skin and

mucous membranes and can have variable effects on the liver, kidneys, and gastrointestinal tract. Another major problem of xylene toxicity is its narcotic effect on workers, causing symptoms such as muscular weakness, lack of coordination, and mental confusion, which may pose a risk to the worker and others. Current evidence indicates that xylene is not toxic to the blood and blood-forming organs.

NIOSH recommends comprehensive preplacement medical examinations, with subsequent examinations every 2 years, for workers subject to xylene exposure. It is also recommended that containers of xylene have labels warning of flammability and that personal protective equipment be provided to prevent skin or eye contact. The NIOSH document calls for engineering controls to be used wherever feasible to maintain xylene concentrations below the prescribed limits with respirators used only in certain nonroutine or emergency situations.

The criterion document was reviewed by five consultants, two professional societies, and government agencies having an interest and responsibility for occupational safety and health. The proposed standard is considered appropriate, and no additional information that would affect the recommended standard is now available.

The criterion document may be ordered from:

Office of Technical Publications
National Institute for Occupational Safety
and Health
Post Office Building
Cincinnati, Ohio 45202

LABORATORY PATHWAY FOR BIOPSY SPECIMEN AND RESPONSIBILITIES
Helen N. Futch

Surgical procedure

The patient is biopsied (Fig. 23-1) (sample of suspected abnormal tissue is removed for examination).

Identification of biopsy tissue specimen

1. *Histotechnologist* is responsible for system to ensure proper identification of biopsy tissue specimen.
2. *Pathologist* examines tissue (pathologist's initial contact with biopsy specimen), records the description, and selects representative sections to be made into slides with which the diagnosis is made.
   Pathologist's workup on the patient biopsy

is completed by 5:00 PM on the day of the biopsy operation. Biopsy specimen becomes the responsibility of the *histotechnologist* at this point.

Responsibilities of histotechnologist

These responsibilities require experience, skill, knowledge, and judgment:

1. *Preservation of biopsy tissue sample in proper chemical fluid fixative;* type of fixative depends on type of tissue to be preserved and examined; length of exposure to these chemical fixatives is critical.
2. *Design appropriate processing schedule* for tissue specimen in automated processing machines; normal time is 16 hours. Inadequate processing will result in slides (sections) that are difficult or impossible to diagnose, particularly when one attempts to diagnose neoplastic disease (cancer). Histotechnologist must monitor automated processing equipment at regular intervals, but if some failure occurs, histotechnologist must be able to recognize tissue processing failures and apply corrective measures before continuing the procedures.
   a. *Major steps involved in processing tissue*
      (1) *Fixation* in chemical fluids for preservation of tissue
      (2) *Dehydration,* to remove all water from the tissue
      (3) *Clearing* tissue of all chemicals used in dehydration
      (4) *Infiltration* of tissue with paraffin
      Each step will produce specific tissue characteristics, and these characteristics must be identified independently.
   b. *Corrective measures* for improperly fixed tissue dependent on a number of variables:
      (1) Biopsy tissue type
      (2) Size of biopsy tissue specimen
      (3) Pathologic condition (disease or abnormality) of the tissue specimen
      The skill and knowledge of the histotechnologist are essential in exercising appropriate action to ensure that the final preparation of the tissue is of diagnostic quality.
3. *Embedding of tissue specimen in paraffin block*
   Histotechnologist is responsible for identifying normal tissue components and relationships as well as abnormal lesions in

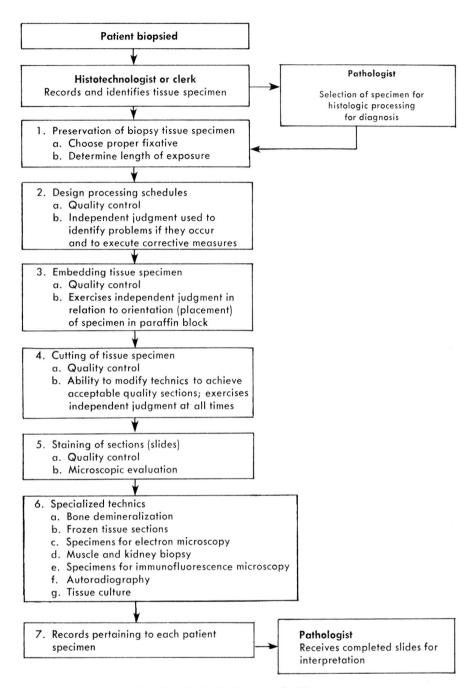

Fig. 23-1. Path of a biopsy in the laboratory.

order to place tissue specimen in proper position for cutting to make slides (sections) for acceptable microscopic evaluation by the pathologist. *Note:* Inadequately trained laboratory personnel can ruin a tissue specimen at this point by placing the specimen in the paraffin block so that:

a. the abnormality (lesion) is cut away and discarded when paraffin sections are being prepared for slides.

b. the lesion is inverted and never seen by the pathologist.

c. the pathologist recognizes inaccurate embedding, but the tissue specimen sample is cut (sliced) too poorly to salvage specimen for proper re-embedding.

All of these situations can cause:

a. delay of the diagnostic report.

b. inaccurate diagnosis, which JEOPARDIZES THE PATIENT'S TREATMENT.

c. insufficient tissue on slide for any diagnosis.

ADDITIONAL TISSUE MAY BE IMPOSSIBLE TO OBTAIN FROM THE PATIENT.

4. *Cutting (slicing) of tissue specimen*

Equipment used for ultrathin slicing of tissue is called a *microtome.*

The tissue specimen must be sliced so thin that the pathologist can accurately evaluate the structure of cells that make up the tissue. Minute and careful examination of cells is critical in the identification of neoplastic disease (cancer). A diagnosis by the pathologist is essential to assist the clinician (surgeon, radiotherapist, internist, and so on) in a choice of therapy, that is, chemotherapy, surgery, radiotherapy, or any combination of all these treatment modalities.

Factors assuring accurate and acceptable sectioned (sliced) tissue specimens are as follows:

a. Proper use and care of scientific equipment (microtomes, and so on)

b. Adequately sharpened microtome knives

c. Recognition by the histotechnologist of variation in tissue specimen components that will affect cutting; modification of technics for each type of tissue to assure a properly sectioned (sliced) specimen for diagnostic examination.

5. *Staining of slides of tissue specimen sections*

Each type of biopsy tissue can be stained with numerous special fluid dyes (stains), depending on which portions of the cells and tissue structures the pathologist wishes to examine under the microscope.

a. The histotechnologist must be able to recognize tissue components and structures, evaluate staining qualities of each tissue sample, and choose the proper stains to reveal the normal and abnormal structures in the tissue section.

b. The histotechnologist must be able to modify technics and stains to ensure proper staining of all tissues, regardless of structural abnormalities.

Factors affecting staining results:

(1) Fixation (whether or not it has been done properly)

(2) Automated processing of specimen

(3) Pathologic condition (abnormality) of specimen

(4) Thickness of section

(5) Staining reagents (dyes)

(6) Staining technic

6. *Specialized selective technics required for diagnostic purposes*

a. Routine staining

(1) Bone demineralization

(2) Frozen tissue sectioning technics

(3) Preservation and processing of tissue specimens for examination by electron microscope

(4) Specialized technics for the following:

(a) Muscle biopsies

(b) Kidney biopsies

(c) Tissue specimens for examination by immunofluorescence microscope

(d) Autoradiography

(e) Tissue culture

The histotechnologist must be able to identify and develop appropriate technics and methodology and conduct these technics when they are requested by the pathologist.

b. *Nonroutine staining*

(1) For specific tissue structures

(2) Metabolic by-products

(3) Specific cellular morphology (structural components)

(4) Infectious microorganisms

(5) Endogenous and exogenous pigments

The histotechnologist must:

(a) establish and exercise proper quality control

(b) be qualified to perform or develop requested technics for slide demonstration of structures or cellular components

(c) be able to select and obtain appropriate control material and apply to appropriate technic

(d) apply independent judgment based on sound theoretical

background to determine microscopically the quality and adequacy of staining; manipulation or modification of the technic for better quality may be required

7. *Maintenance of patient records in department*
   a. The histotechnologist may be responsible for maintaining the following up to date and accurate:
      (1) Accession book (record of each tissue specimen that enters the laboratory)
      (2) Card files
      (3) Diagnostic reports (on each tissue specimen examined by the pathologist)
   b. The histotechnologist is responsible for maintaining permanent files of the following:
      (1) Paraffin blocks (embedded tissue specimens)
      (2) Microscopic slides made from paraffin blocks

Summary

In referring to the flow chart (Fig. 23-1), which represents the sequential steps taken in the pathology department to arrive at a patient diagnosis, one may observe the following:

1. From the time the pathologist selects the unprocessed tissue biopsy specimen, to be prepared for microscopic examination until the completed slides are returned to the pathologist for diagnostic examination, many technical procedures are performed by the histotechnologist.

2. These procedures require the exercise of independent judgment by the histotechnologist, and this judgment is based solely on training, skill, experience, and theoretical knowledge.

3. The performance of all histologic technics involved in the production of completed slides ready for diagnosis by the pathologist is the sole responsibility of the histotechnologist.

4. The improper selection or performance of any of the above described technics may cause disastrous results for the patient, such as the following:
   a. Misdiagnosis, leading to
   b. Inadequate or incorrect treatment
   c. No treatment at all
   d. Delay in treatment

5. The pathologist, in order to make an accurate diagnosis, must rely on the competence, knowledge, and experience of the histotechnologist responsible for the correct management of the patient's tissue specimen. The quality of the diagnosis is directly related to the quality of laboratory preparation.

Quality control

Personnel in all laboratories should carefully study the quality control regulations of those agencies by whom they are inspected, and after doing so, should develop their own quality control program. The laboratory should continuously survey all aspects of the laboratory operations that have an impact upon test results. If this is to be monitored properly, a planned written schedule of the servicing of equipment and instruments must be established. Reagents and stains must be evaluated by testing. The performance of the equipment in the laboratory must be checked by laboratory personnel according to instructions that are specifically established by the director and the laboratory supervisor. If this is done, a problem can become apparent immediately and remedial action can be started. Records of all surveillance of equipment and instruments and the remedial actions taken must be maintained.

The laboratory facilities must be adequate and instruments and equipment must be properly maintained, since laboratory testing that is accurate cannot be achieved in a laboratory that is inadequately equipped and improperly monitored. Work areas, in addition to the space required for equipment and instruments, must have clear work space for the technologist who is performing the work. Adequate storage space in the immediate work area must be provided for the supplies with which the personnel are working, in addition to card files and procedure manuals. The technologist should be supplied with electricity, gas, water, or anything else needed in doing the laboratory work. Containers for disposal should be located so that disposable materials can be transported into them with minimal hazard to the technologist.

Temperatures must be monitored and recorded; maintenance activities, along with repairs and replacements, must be recorded.

REQUIREMENTS FOR REAGENTS

Reagents of good quality must be used in the preparation of microscope slides for patient diagnosis. These reagents must be properly identified, and labels should contain the information for the following:

1. Identification of the reagent or solution
2. Identification of the strength or concentration of the solution
3. Recommended storage requirements
4. Identification of the initials of the person preparing the solution
5. Date of preparation
6. Shelf-life expectancy and date of expiration

7. Potential hazards of the solution

In addition to these labels, all containers in which dry or liquid reagents are purchased should have the date recorded on the outside of the container when they were received in the laboratory and when they were opened for use.

STANDARD OPERATING PROCEDURE MANUAL

A standard operating procedure manual (SOPM) must be prepared to provide detailed instructions to the technologists working in the laboratory. The manual must contain all the methodology used in the laboratory and must be signed by the director and supervisor, either of whom should review any changes in reagents and control procedures and check the documentation of pertinent literature references. Textbooks may not be used in place of a standard operating procedure manual but may be used in addition to the manual.

Card files may be used at the work bench and should be available to technologists at all times.

Procedures outlined in the SOPM cannot be changed without written approval of the laboratory director or supervisor. All quality-control checks and methods must be recorded in the SOPM, and the laboratory must have available records of the dates, inspection, validation, remedial action, monitoring, evaluation, and changes with the dates of the changes in any and all laboratory procedures. The personnel in the laboratory must be kept aware of quality-control requirements so that they can be part of the monitoring requirements.

The procedures for collecting specimens must be compiled in a written form in the SOPM. The methods used must include specimen identification, preservation, and storage of the specimen. Detailed instructions on the use of fixatives, date and time of specimen collection, and pertinent information on the patient must be recorded on requisition forms on specimens coming to the laboratory. The method of reporting the diagnosis on frozen sections and other specimens should be recorded in the SOPM.

QUALITY CONTROL ON FIXATION

It is important that the pH of a solution of formalin not drop below pH 6.0. This drop is attributable to the formation of formic acid and can be prevented by the use of neutral buffered formalin. When the solution is between 5.6 and 6.0 or under pH 5.6, DNA and RNA are poorly preserved, reticulum fibers may be partially hydrolyzed, and acid mucopolysaccharides are more soluble. As a result, special staining technics such as methyl green pyronin, reticulum, or the alcian blue technics are poor.

The standard operating procedure manual should record the data on properly preparing the formalin fixative. This should definitively state the volume of commercial 37% formalin, the volume of water used, as well as the weights of the buffer salts and the final pH of the fixation. If the fixative is prepared in 10- or 20-gallon bottles, the respective data, as formerly stated, should be on the label of each bottle and each batch of fixative should be checked for pH.

The choice of routine fixative in any laboratory is the choice of the pathologist, but the supervisor should know and record correct fixatives for special stains in the SOPM. Some of these are Zenker's for phosphotungstic acid–hematoxylin (PTAH); Carnoy's for methyl green pyronine (see chapter on fixation).

Another area of quality control relative to fixatives is the disposal of any fixative containing mercuric chloride if these are used routinely, since it is important that the toxic material in these fixatives be prevented from entering the sewage system.

QUALITY CONTROL OF DEHYDRANTS AND CLEARING AGENTS AND EMBEDDING MEDIA

The properties of dehydrants and clearing agents and embedding media are well covered in the chapters on these subjects. A word of warning in the quality-control chapter—the use of dirty water or alcohol-contaminated agents to process tissue is poor economy. Reagents used for processing or in the staining sequence should be replaced relative to the work that goes through them. A hydrometer can be used to monitor the specific gravity of the solutions. If everything else is right with proper thickness of the tissue and proper fixation but with contaminated solutions, the processing cannot be good. The SOPM should definitively record the method of processing including time, temperature, and specific gravity of the solutions to assure good-quality material for patient sections.

QUALITY CONTROL OF SPECIAL STAINS

All special staining procedures should be recorded in the SOPM with a quality-control form.

John P. Koski, in his article on "Quality Control in the Histology Laboratory, Qualitative and Quantitative Aspects" (*Laboratory Medicine*, vol. 6, no. 9, September 1975) stated the following rules:

Rule #1 for histologic quality is, therefore: All factors should be constant except for one, the variable, which is to be demonstrated.

Rule #2 for histologic quality control: If any constant factor is changed from the normal procedure, one or more other constants must be checked to compensate for it.

John Koski further states that if the technologist suspects that a particular demonstration fails to show what is expected, the technologist should be able to explain why the method failed, for if he cannot explain why it failed, he will not know what step to change to make the procedure work correctly a second time. For this reason, all information on a technic should be recorded in the SOPM.

Rule #3: Record all quantitative data for reference. For example, a weak PAS reaction may be due to a low concentration of oxidizing agent (check the date on the procedure sheet for the periodic acid solution), an improper pH of Schiff's reagent (measure the pH), incorrect time of exposure to the working reagents (check the SOPM against the recommended method) or an exhausted Schiff's reagent (check when it was made). Each point can be checked if the laboratory has a control log.

Special stains must be controlled for intended reactivity with positive and negative controls. Control sections should be marked with the patient's number and the word "control" written below the identifying technic on the label. These control slides should be filed with the patient's slides for ready reference and consultation. If the patient's tissue on which a special stain is requested is fixed in Bouin's fluid, the control tissue must be fixed in the same fixative. This is true of other fixatives as well.

QUALITY CONTROL ON ROUTINE HEMATOXYLIN AND EOSIN STAINING

The pH of the hematoxylin in which slides are routinely stained should be checked. When slides come out of the bluing agent (lithium carbonate or ammonia water), they should be checked microscopically to be sure the hematoxylin is staining the nuclei and the excess hematoxylin has been removed from those structures it should not stain. After completion

of the H & E stain and mounting of the slide, it should be microscopically checked for good quality control. Are the nuclei and cytoplasm properly stained; have the sections been properly cleared; are there bubbles, dirt, debris, fingerprints, or precipitate on the slide? Are the sections properly labeled.

One should keep a maintenance program for equipment and instruments, listing the model and serial number, dates of services performed, parts installed, and the interval and date of the next service.

A monitoring log or periodic function check sheet should be used where the temperatures of all paraffin baths, paraffin dispensers, warming plates, flotation baths, freezers, cryostats, refrigerators, drying ovens, or any other instruments should be recorded. If the readings are not in the acceptable range, record on the back of the sheet an explanation and corrective measures taken. A calibration record of liquid in glass thermometers should also be done.

There should be a complete equipment inventory, listing the name and make of the instrument, model and serial number, purchased from, installed by, the date, length of warranty, purchase price, and location of the manual of instructions covering the equipment.

Make records on everything you use and date it. When microtomes are cleaned, adjusted, and lubricated and when automatic stainers and paraffin dispensers as well as cryostats are cleaned, oiled, and disinfected, or when the solutions are changed on the automatic tissue changers.

There certainly must be a system for quality of incoming material. The proper request form (printed to fit the particular needs of your laboratory) must be complete with positive identification of tissue. This form must be securely attached to the specimen bag or container. If the tissue is in a container, the lid must be tightly fitted, filled with the appropriate fixative, and the specimen collected or submitted according to the written directions in your SOPM.

What is the quality of safety in your laboratory? Instructions for action in case of fire should be posted and are required reading. The use of fire extinguishers should be taught to all laboratory employees. Fire alarms, fire extinguishers, a fire hose, fire blankets, and asbestos gloves should be provided. An automatic sprinkler, facilities for rapid flushing of caustic and toxic chemicals, emergency overhead shower, foot-operated eye washers, goggles, and mechanical pipetting equipment must be available in the laboratory, and all personnel should be instructed in their proper handling.

Safety hoods should have a minimum air flow of 50 cubic feet per minute across their face opening. All electrical equipment must be grounded. Instruments and contaminated glassware should be placed in a chemical disinfectant after use.

The storage of records must be organized to facilitate retrieval. Paraffin blocks must be clearly and adequately identified and stored in a cool place with adequate fire precautions.

The following charts should help you in setting up the quality control in your laboratory.

Charts for setting up quality control in the laboratory

MICROSCOPE MAINTENANCE CHART

Room number: _____   Microscope serial number: _____   Hospital asset number: _____

C = Cleaned   LA = Light sources adjusted
IN = Inspected   T = Technician who did the quality control

January	February	March	April	May	June
July	August	September	October	November	December

MICROTOME MAINTENANCE PROCEDURE

Model number: _____   Machine serial number: _____

Date	1	2	3	4	5	6	7	8	9	10	11	12	13	14	15	16	17	18	19	20	21	22	23	24	25	26	27	28	29	30	31
Daily																															
Remove all paraffin residue from instrument																															
Oil screws and slideways with light machine oil																															
Technician's initials																															
Weekly																															
Remove protective covering, oil indicated areas with red dots, and oil sliding surfaces with light machine oil																															
Remove, disassemble, and clean, oil, reassemble, and replace knife holder																															
Technician's initials																															

Annually, microtome is to be inspected, cleaned, and adjusted by company service department representative.

Date: _____   Representative's initials: _____

Report malfunctions of equipment using standard "Request for repair form" and notify supervisor immediately.

Temperature to be regulated to $36° \pm 1° C$

HEATED FORMALIN WATER BATH

Month: _____ Year: _____

I = Initial temp. C = Correct temp. T = Technician	Bath I			Bath II			Bath III			Bath IV		
Date	I	C	T	I	C	T	I	C	T	I	C	T
1												
2												
3												
4												
5												
6												
7												
8												
9												
10												
11												
12												
13												
14												
15												
16												
17												
18												
19												
20												
21												
22												
23												
24												
25												
26												
27												
28												
29												
30												
31												

Corrective action: (1) Adjust thermostat on front of water bath to regulate. (2) If unable to regulate, call electrician.

Temperatures to be regulated to 2° to 4° C above melting point of the paraffin used

	Unit I			Unit II			Unit III		
Date	I	C	T	I	C	T	I	C	T
1									
2									
3									
4									
5									
6									
7									
8									
9									
10									
11									
12									
13									
14									
15									
16									
17									
18									
19									
20									
21									
22									
23									
24									
25									
26									
27									
28									
29									
30									
31									

TISSUE-TEK II EMBEDDING UNITS

Month: _____ Year: _____

I = Initial temp.
C = Correct temp.
T = Technician

Corrective action: (1) Measure adjust thermostat on paraffin reservoir. (2) If unable to adjust, call repairman.

FUME-GARD HOOD MAINTENANCE CHART

(Sampling made every 90 days by fire and safety department and filter changed when samples read greater than 100 ppm)

Hood number	Date	Air sample work area	Reading above exhaust	Date filter changed	Technician's initials

Temperatures to be regulated to 2° to 4° C above the melting point of the paraffin used

PARAFFIN-BATH TISSUE PROCESSORS

Month: _____ Year: _____

I = Initial temp. C = Correct temp. T = Technician	Day: _____			Day: _____			Day: _____			Day: _____		
Paraffin bath	**I**	**C**	**T**	**I**	**C**	**T**	**I**	**C**	**T**	**I**	**C**	**T**
1												
2												
3												
4												
5												
6												
7												
8												
9												
10												
11												
12												
13												
14												
15												
16												
17												
18												
19												
20												
21												
22												
23												
24												
25												
26												

Corrective action: (1) Adjust thermostat by turning thermostat screw below handle clockwise to reduce heat, counterclockwise to increase heat. (2) If unable to adjust temperature, remove equipment and call electrician. Replace equipment.

Temperatures to be regulated to 2° to 4° C above the melting point of the paraffin used

PARAFFIN-BATH TISSUE PROCESSORS—cont'd

Month: _____ Year: _____

I = Initial temp. C = Correct temp. T = Technician	Day: ____			Day: ____			Day: ____			Day: ____		
Paraffin bath	I	C	T	I	C	T	I	C	T	I	C	T
27												
28												
29												
30												
31												
32												
33												
34												
35												
36												
37												
38												
39												
40												
41												
42												
43												
44												
45												
46												
47												
48												
49												
50												
Ultra I												
Ultra II												

Corrective action: (1) Adjust thermostat by turning thermostat screw below handle clockwise to reduce heat, counterclockwise to increase heat. (2) If unable to adjust temperature, remove equipment and call electrician. Replace equipment.

PARAFFIN-BATH TEMPERATURES (QUALITY CONTROL)

Regulate at 60° C

Paraffin bath number: _____   Location: _____

Month: _____

Date	Time	Tech.	56	57	58	59	60	61	62	Other
							Temperature °C			
1										
2										
3										
4										
5										
6										
7										
8										
9										
10										
11										
12										
13										
14										
15										
16										
17										
18										
19										
20										
21										
22										
23										
24										
25										
26										
27										
28										
29										
30										
31										

Paraffin bath number: _____   Location: _____

Month: _____

Date	Time	Tech.	56	57	58	59	60	61	62	Other
							Temperature °C			
1										
2										
3										
4										
5										
6										
7										
8										
9										
10										
11										
12										
13										
14										
15										
16										
17										
18										
19										
20										
21										
22										
23										
24										
25										
26										
27										
28										
29										
30										
31										

If the paraffin temperature is consistently above 62° C or below 56° C, report this to the supervisor.

RECORD OF FRESH REAGENTS USED

Tissue processor: _____

Month: _____

Reagent		Day							
Number	Type	1	5	10	15	20	25		31

RECORD OF FRESH REAGENTS USED

Tissue processor: _____   Month: _____

Reagent		Day						
Number	Type	1	5	10	15	20	25	31
1	Bouin's							
2	Bouin's							
3	80% ethanol							
4	95% ethanol							
5	95% ethanol							
6	Absolute ethanol							
7	Absolute ethanol							
8	Chloroform							
9	Chloroform							
10	Paraffin							
11	Paraffin							
12	Paraffin							

RECORD OF FRESH REAGENTS USED

Tissue processor: _____

Month: _____

Reagent		Day							
Number	Type	1	5	10	15	20	25	31	
1	80% ethanol								
2	80% ethanol								
3	95% ethanol								
4	95% ethanol								
5	Absolute ethanol								
6	Absolute ethanol								
7	Absolute ethanol								
8	Chloroform								
9	Chloroform								
10	Paraffin								
11	Paraffin								
12	Paraffin								

RECORD OF FRESH REAGENTS USED

Tissue processor: _____   Month: _____

Reagent		Day																															
Number	Type	1				5					10					15					20					25									31
I	95% ETOH																																		
II	95% ETOH																																		
I	100% ETOH																																		
II	100% ETOH																																		
I	THF																																		
II	THF																																		
III	THF																																		
I	Paraffin																																		
II	Paraffin																																		
III	Paraffin																																		

Temperature to be adjusted to 60° ± 2° C

PARAFFIN-OVEN TEMPERATURE CHART

Month: _____ Year: _____

I = Initial temp. C = Correct temp. T = Technician	Paraffin oven I			Paraffin oven II			Paraffin oven I			Paraffin oven II		
Date	I	C	T	I	C	T	I	C	T	I	C	T
1												
2												
3												
4												
5												
6												
7												
8												
9												
10												
11												
12												
13												
14												
15												
16												
17												
18												
19												
20												
21												
22												
23												
24												
25												
26												
27												
28												
29												
30												
31												

Setting: To set oven temperature, turn indicating dial with pointer at 2½ to register 60° ± 2° C, regulated by thermometer inserted into top of oven.

Corrective action: (1) Adjust thermometer by turning temperature-control dial counterclockwise to reduce heat, clockwise to increase heat. (2) If unable to adjust temperature, call electrician.

PARAFFIN-OVEN TEMPERATURES (QUALITY CONTROL)

Regulate at 60° C

Number: _____

Location: _____

Date last checked against Bureau of Standards Thermometer: _____

If the oven temperature is consistently above 64° C or below 58° C, report this to the supervisor.

Month: _____

Date	Time	Tech.	Temperature °C							Other
			58	59	60	61	62	63	64	
1										
2										
3										
4										
5										
6										
7										
8										
9										
10										
11										
12										
13										
14										
15										
16										
17										
18										
19										
20										
21										
22										
23										
24										
25										
26										
27										
28										
29										
30										
31										

Month: _____

Date	Time	Tech.	Temperature °C							Other
			58	59	60	61	62	63	64	
1										
2										
3										
4										
5										
6										
7										
8										
9										
10										
11										
12										
13										
14										
15										
16										
17										
18										
19										
20										
21										
22										
23										
24										
25										
26										
27										
28										
29										
30										
31										

Temperature to be recorded to 70° ± 2° C

A-SKI STAINER TEMPERATURE CHART

Month: _____   Room: _____

Day	Temperature	Technician's initial
1		
2		
3		
4		
5		
6		
7		
8		
9		
10		
11		
12		
13		
14		
15		
16		
17		
18		
19		
20		
21		
22		
23		
24		
25		
26		
27		
28		
29		
30		
31		

Corrective action: (1) Adjust temperature by turning temperature-control dial to the left to reduce heat, and right to increase heat. (2) If unable to adjust temperature, call electrician or service man.

Corrective action: Adjust by turning thermostat inside stainer. Temperature-control dial located on bottom righthand side of stainer.

SKI STAINER

Month: _____

W.B. = Wash bottle
SMA = 3-liter flat container

*Number of eosin will vary; see supervisor.

Reagents filled	1	2	3	4	5	6	7	8	9	10	11	12	13	14	15	16	17	18	19	20	21	22
W.B. 100% ETOH																						
W.B. 95% ETOH																						
W.B. 80% ETOH																						
W.B. 0.25% acid ETOH																						
W.B. 0.5% alkaline ETOH																						
SMA 0.25% acid ETOH																						
SMA 0.5% alkaline ETOH																						
Stainer maintenance																						
Xylene 1																						
Xylene 2																						
Xylene 3																						
Xylene 4																						
100% ETOH 1																						
100% ETOH 2																						
100% ETOH 3																						
95% ETOH 1																						
95% ETOH 2																						
80% ETOH 1																						
Water																						
Hematoxylin 1																						
Hematoxylin 2																						
Hematoxylin 3																						
Hematoxylin 4																						
Water																						
0.25% acid ETOH																						
H_2O																						
0.5% alkaline ETOH																						
80% ETOH																						
Eosin 1																						
Eosin 2																						
Eosin 3																						
*Eosin 4																						
*Eosin 5																						
95% ETOH 1																						
95% ETOH 2																						
100% ETOH 1																						
100% ETOH 2																						
THF/xylene 50:50																						

Temperature to be recorded to $4° \pm 3°$ C

REFRIGERATOR-TEMPERATURE CHART

Month: _____ Room: _____

Day	Temperature	Technician's initials
1		
2		
3		
4		
5		
6		
7		
8		
9		
10		
11		
12		
13		
14		
15		
16		
17		
18		
19		
20		
21		
22		
23		
24		
25		
26		
27		
28		
29		
30		
31		

Corrective action: (1) Adjust by turning thermostat inside refrigeration. (2) If unable to adjust, call electrician.

REFRIGERATOR TEMPERATURES (QUALITY CONTROL)

Refrigerator number: _____

Location: _____

Date last checked against Bureau of Standards Thermometer: _____

If the refrigerator temperature is consistently above 10° C or below 2° C, report this to the supervisor.

Month: _____

Date	Time	Tech.	Temperature °C											Other
			1	2	3	4	5	6	7	8	9	10	
1													
2													
3													
4													
5													
6													
7													
8													
9													
10													
11													
12													
13													
14													
15													
16													
17													
18													
19													
20													
21													
22													
23													
24													
25													
26													
27													
28													
29													
30													
31													

Month: _____

Date	Time	Tech.	Temperature °C											Other
			1	2	3	4	5	6	7	8	9	10	
1													
2													
3													
4													
5													
6													
7													
8													
9													
10													
11													
12													
13													
14													
15													
16													
17													
18													
19													
20													
21													
22													
23													
24													
25													
26													
27													
28													
29													
30													
31													

PARAFFIN-DISPENSER TEMPERATURES (QUALITY CONTROL)

Regulate at 60° C

Number: _____

Location: _____

Date last checked against Bureau of Standards Thermometer: _____

If the dispenser temperature is consistently above 62° C or below 58° C, report this to the supervisor.

Month: _____

Date	Time	Tech.	Temperature °C						Other
			58	59	60	61	62		
1									
2									
3									
4									
5									
6									
7									
8									
9									
10									
11									
12									
13									
14									
15									
16									
17									
18									
19									
20									
21									
22									
23									
24									
25									
26									
27									
28									
29									
30									
31									

Month: _____

Date	Time	Tech.	Temperature °C						Other
			58	59	60	61	62		
1									
2									
3									
4									
5									
6									
7									
8									
9									
10									
11									
12									
13									
14									
15									
16									
17									
18									
19									
20									
21									
22									
23									
24									
25									
26									
27									
28									
29									
30									
31									

BONE WORK SHEET

Date	Case	Fixative	Decal solution	Date decalcification completed	Neutralization solution	Date bone processed	Comments

SURGICAL SPECIMEN WORK SHEET

Date: Describer: Surgical pathology number: _____	Number of pieces submitted	Remarks	Number of pieces embed- ded in blocks	Number of slides stained

Hospital of the University of Pennsylvania

REPORT OF PATHOLOGIST'S CONSULTATION

Patient's name _____ OR No. _____

Surgeon _____ Date _____

Gross examination and diagnosis only _____

_____

_____

Microscopic diagnosis on rapid section _____

_____

Comment _____

_____

069013   Signed _____

CASE-HELD AND TISSUE-STAINING REQUEST

Date: _____ Case number: _____

This case being held because

☐ Special stains (see below)   ☐ Preliminary report issued (yes, no)
☐ Extra sections/Recutting (see below)   ☐ Clinical history
☐ Fixation   ☐ Decalcification
☐ Addendum report to follow   ☐ Additional material submitted awaiting tissue section
☐ Special processing   ☐ Tissue being reoriented in paraffin block
☐ Reprocessing
☐ Consultation (outside) (specify) _____
☐ Consultation (Univ. of Tenn.) (specify) _____
☐ Other (specify) _____

Tissue-staining request

Rush: _____ Routine: _____ Teaching: _____
Recut: _____ Serial sections: _____ Deeper: _____ Times: _____ Thickness in µm: _____

Special stains:

Alcian blue _____	Kidney battery _____
AB-PASH _____	LFB _____
Acid-fast _____	LFB-PAS-H _____
Amyloid _____	LFB-PTAH _____
Azan _____	Liver battery _____
Best's carmine _____	Lymph node battery _____
Bile _____	Masson _____
Calcium _____	Methyl green pyronine _____
Elastic _____	Mucicarmine _____
Esterase _____	Nissl _____
Fat _____	PASH with digestion _____
Fontana-Masson _____	PASH _____
Giemsa _____	PAS-LG _____
GMS _____	PTAH _____
Gram (Brown/Hopps) _____	Reticulum _____
Iron _____	
Other: 1. _____	2. _____

The pathologist and resident responsible for completing this case are:

_____   _____
Pathologist   Resident

White copy: Surgical Pathology secretary
Yellow copy: Resident
Pink copy: Histopathology Laboratory

If this case is rush,
please bring the slip to Mrs. Sheehan's office.

Slides written by _____ on _____

SPECIAL STAIN REQUEST SLIP

(Attach slide with Scotch Tape and place in Special Stain request box in Mrs. Sheehan's office.)

Pathology number: _____ Date requested: _____ Dr.: _____

Hematoxylin and eosin requests:

☐ Cut at _____ different levels.
☐ Rotate block 90 degrees (2 levels).
☐ Cut _____ slides for _____.

Special stains:

4 ☐ Acid-fast (Kinyoun's) *AF & AR (Cut #1 & 3 AF, 2 & 4 AR serially on surgical cases only.)*
2 ☐ Acid mucopolysaccharides (Alcian blue–Kernechtrot) *AlBlK*
2 ☐ Acid mucopolysaccharides (colloidal iron) *Coll Iron*
3 ☐ Alpha cells, pancreas (Grimelius) *Grim*
2 ☐ Ameba (Wheatley) *Ameba*
2 ☐ Amyloid (Congo red) *CR-10 μm*
2 ☐ Amyloid (crystal violet) *CV-10 μm*
4 ☐ Argentaffin (Fontana-Masson) *2 Font & 2 Schmorl*
3 ☐ Argyrophil (Grimelius) *Grim*
3 ☐ Argyrophil (Sevier-Munger) *Sev Mun*
2 ☐ Australia antigen (aldehyde fuchsin) *Ald Fuch*
2 ☐ Australia antigen (orcein) *Orcein*
2 ☐ Bacteria (Brown-Brenn Gram stain) *Gram*
2 ☐ Basement membranes (periodic acid–methenamine silver) *Meth*
2 ☐ Beta cells (Scott's aldehyde fuchsin) *Scott*
2 ☐ Bile (Hall's) *Bile*
2 ☐ Blood cells (Giemsa-Sheehan modification) *Giem*
2 ☐ Calcium (alizarin red S) *Aliz RS*
2 ☐ Calcium (*von Kossa*)
2 ☐ Carbohydrates (periodic acid–Schiff) *PAS*
2 ☐ Carbohydrates (including AMP) (alcian blue–periodic acid Schiff) *AlBl*
2 ☐ Collagen (Masson trichrome) *Tri*
2 ☐ DNA (Feulgen) *Feul*
2 ☐ DNA and RNA (methyl green pyronine) *MGP*
2 ☐ Eosinophils (Luna stain) *Luna-E*
2 ☐ Elastic (Gomori aldehyde fuchsin) *Ald Fuch*
2 ☐ Elastic (Verhoeff-Van Gieson) *Elas*
☐ Fat (bring tissue to lab in fixative) *(oil red O)*
2 ☐ Fungus (Gridley) *Grid*
2 ☐ Fungus (Grocott) *Gro*
4 ☐ Glycogen (periodic acid–Schiff before and after diastase) *2 PAS-BD, 2 PAS-AD*
4 ☐ Hyaluronic acid (colloidal iron before and after hyaluronidase) *2 Coll BH, 2 Coll AH*
2 ☐ Iron (Gomori technic) *Iron*
6 ☐ Legionnaires' disease (Dieterle) *Diet*
4 ☐ Melanin (silver reduction with and without KMnO$_4$ bleaching) *(2) AgNO$_3$, (2) KMnO-AgNO$_3$*
2 ☐ Metachromasia (toluidine blue) *TolBl*
2 ☐ Mucin (mucicarmine) *Muci*
2 ☐ Muscle (Mallory phosphotungstic acid–hematoxylin) *PTAH*
2 ☐ Myelin sheath (Klüver's luxol fast blue) *LFB-5 μm*
2 ☐ Myocardial infarcts (hematoxlyin–basic fuchsin–picric acid) *HBP*
2 ☐ Nerve fibers (Bodian) *Bod*
2 ☐ Pituitary (alpha and beta cells) *Pearse*
2 ☐ *Pneumocystis carinii* (Grocott for *Pneumocystis*) *Pneum*
2 ☐ Reticulin (Nasser-Shanklin) *Ret*
6 ☐ Spirochetes (Dieterle) *Diet*
2 ☐ Uric acid (fix in absolute alcohol) (Gomori methenamine silver) *Uric*

Other technics: Please bring references to Mrs. Sheehan.

_____
_____
_____

REQUEST FORM FOR EXPERIMENTAL WORK

Date submitted: _____
Date processed: _____

TO: Surgical Pathology Laboratory
Hospital of the University of Pennsylvania, 4th Floor Administration Bldg.

FROM: Dr. _____

_____

_____

Date requested: _____ Date finished: _____

Hematoxylin and eosin requests:

☐ Cut _____ slide(s) and stain with hematoxylin and eosin
☐ Cut _____ slides at different levels and stain with hematoxylin and eosin
☐ Cut *serial sections* and stain with hematoxylin and eosin

Special stains: Names of special stains:

☐ (No. of slides for) _____
☐ (No. of slides for) _____
☐ (No. of slides for) _____
☐ (No. of slides for) _____

Charge information:

(1) slide stained with hematoxylin and eosin $4.00
(1) slide stained with a special stain $5.00
(1) fat stains and decalcification (each slide) $6.00

GRANT NUMBER: _____

BILL TO: _____

_____

_____

_____

CRYOSTAT TEMPERATURES (QUALITY CONTROL)

Regulate at −20° C

If the cryostat temperature is consistently above −17° C or below −23° C, report this to the supervisor.

Number: _____

Location: _____

Month: _____

Date	Time	Tech.	Temperature °C						Other
			−22	−21	−20	−19	−18		
1									
2									
3									
4									
5									
6									
7									
8									
9									
10									
11									
12									
13									
14									
15									
16									
17									
18									
19									
20									
21									
22									
23									
24									
25									
26									
27									
28									
29									
30									
31									

Month: _____

Date	Time	Tech.	Temperature °C						Other
			−22	−21	−20	−19	−18		
1									
2									
3									
4									
5									
6									
7									
8									
9									
10									
11									
12									
13									
14									
15									
16									
17									
18									
19									
20									
21									
22									
23									
24									
25									
26									
27									
28									
29									
30									
31									

CENTRIFUGE MAINTENANCE

International Centrifuge Model HN-S

Serial number: _____
Purchased: _____

Quarterly inspection

Date	Brushes	Condition	Commutator	Condition	Checked by

| | | | | Paraffin dispenser (cleaned) | | Cryostats (cleaned and oiled) | |
Date	Microtome (lubricated)	Automatic stainer (cleaned)	Routine stains	1	2	1	2

EQUIPMENT MAINTENANCE
(as outlined)

MISCELLANEOUS TEMPERATURE RECORD (DAILY RECORDINGS)

LT = Lab-Tek Products
AO = American Optical Corp.

| Date | Water bath | | | Paraffin dispenser | | | Warming plates | | Refrigerator and freezer | | Large oven | Small oven | Freezer | Automatic stainer | Cryostats | | |
	1	2	3	1	2	LT	1	2	Ref.	Fr.					1	2	AO

INVENTORY OF STAIN REAGENTS

Department: _____

Stains and dyes (solutions): _____

Name	Source	Identifying number	Amount	Date received	Date opened or made	Positive contents	Negative contents	Stability period

MAINTENANCE PROCEDURE FOR SMITH-KLINE AUTOMATIC STAINER

Daily AM

1. Turn power switch on.
2. Check and raise solution levels.
3. Check, regulate, and record oven temperature at $70° ± 2°$ C.

To correct drying-chamber temperature

1. Adjust temperature by turning temperature-control dial located on bottom, right-hand side of stainer to the left to reduce heat and to the right to increase heat.
2. If unable to adjust temperature, call an electrician or serviceman.
3. Stain control slide and examine microscopically to assure quality before staining any diagnostic material.

Daily PM

1. Turn power switch off.
2. Change all reagents except hematoxylin and eosin.
3. Wash containers.
4. Set up stainer for following day.
5. Change hematoxylin and eosin as needed.

Weekly (on Fridays)

1. Clean paraffin residue in slide warmer with gauze dipped in xylene.
2. Wash stainer with 1 part chlorine bleach, 9 parts water solution.
3. Clean outside covers with Fantastik cleanser.

Monthly

1. Clean Tygon tubing with suction.
2. Spray WD-40 on conveyor chain.
3. Clean water jets in bottom of strainer with wire pick to remove mineral deposits.

REFERENCES

1. Personal communication with the following:
   Freida Carson, Ph.D., Education Coordinator and Director of Histopathology Laboratory, Baylor University Medical Center, Dallas, Texas.
   Helen N. Futch, Education Coordinator, School of Histotechnology, M. D. Anderson Hospital, Houston, Texas.
   Gerre Wells, Education Coordinator, School of Histotechnology, University of Tennessee, Memphis, Tennessee.
2. Doris S. Castle (Histotechnologist, King's Daughters' Hospital, Ashland, Kentucky): Quality—the endangered species, presented at the ASMT Convention, Chicago, Illinois, 1976.
3. Koski, J. P.: Quality control in the histology laboratory—qualitative and quantitative aspects, Lab. Med., vol. 6, no. 9, Sept. 1975.

Glossary

absorption Property whereby a dye causes the tissue to take up the same color as the dye shown in solution: the physical-solution theory of staining, which is supported by the fact that staining a tissue with a dye causes the tissue to become the same color as the solution of the dye, not the color of the dye in dry form.

accelerator Solution that speeds up the reaction between tissue and stain, such as chloral hydrate in silver impregnation.

accentuator Solution that increases the affinity or selectivity of a stain, such as phenol in carbol-fuchsin.

achromatic Without color, not staining readily.

acid-fast Pertaining to bacteria that are readily decolorized with an acid within a carbol-fuchsin stain.

acidophilic Acid loving, able to be readily stained with acid dyes, such as cytoplasm with eosin.

adsorption The staining theory in which both physical and chemical factors take part in the mechanism of salt formation—the basic action of stains; a physical reaction dependent on the charge on the ionized dye and the material on which the dye is precipitated. In selective absorption certain ions may be adsorbed by certain substances more readily and retained longer than by others.

affinity A liking for or attraction for.

aldehydes An organic compound containing carbon, oxygen, and hydrogen represented by the following group:

$$-RC{\overset{\displaystyle O}{\underset{\displaystyle H}{\Big\langle}}}$$

amphoteric Said of a substance capable of reacting either as an acid or as a base, depending on the pH of the solution.

amyloid Starchlike protein abnormally found as an internal cellular product of the liver, spleen, and kidneys.

anthracotic Characterized by anthracosis, which is an accumulation of carbon from inhaled smoke or coal dust in the lungs or in lymph nodes.

argentaffin Reaction whereby cells can reduce silver solutions to metallic silver without the aid of an extraneous reducer.

argyrophil Cells capable of being impregnated with silver but a reducing agent is required to reduce the silver to a metallic visible end product.

artifact Something produced artificially; modification of the appearance or structure of tissue caused by a chemical of some other exterior agent, such as air bubbles, loose tissue floaters, and autolysis.

autogenous pigment Natural (made within body) melanin, that is, to show difference between pigments that are not artifacts and those that are artifacts, such as formalin pigment.

autolysis Enzymatic digestion of cells by enzymes present within them.

auxochrome Chemical group present within a dye that causes affinity of a chromophore for the tissue similar to a mordantary action. For a compound to be called a dye and possess affinity for tissue, it must have in the molecule not only the chromophore grouping, but also an auxiliary group that gives the compound the property of electrolytic dissociation and it is this salt-forming property that gives the dye an affinity to attach itself to tissue.

bacillus Rod-shaped bacterium.

bacterium In general, any microorganism of the order Eubacteriales; a non–sporeforming, rod-shaped microorganism. A loosely used generic name for any rod-shaped microorganism, especially enteric bacilli and morphologically similar forms.

barrel The objectives on a microscope are found at the lower end of the barrel. The ocular is found at the upper end of the barrel. The barrel is also called the body tube of the microscope.

basophilic Having an affinity for or staining readily with basic dyes.

bevel angle Angle between the cutting facets of the microtome knife. In knives manufactured in America this varies between 27 and 32 degrees.

blastospore Spore formed by budding along a hypha, pseudohypha, or single cell, as in the yeast.

budding Process of asexual reproduction in which the new cell develops as a smaller outgrowth from the *older* parent cell, characteristic of yeasts or yeast-like fungi.

buffer Solution containing acid and alkaline components in desired concentrations to maintain as nearly as possible a given pH when other acid or alkaline ingredients are added.

capsule Colorless, transparent, mucopolysaccharide sheath on the wall of a cell or spore.

chelating agents Agents that are organic compounds having the power of binding certain metals. For decalcification, sodium edetate (EDTA, Sequestrene, Versene) has the power of binding calcium ions.

chromatins Dark, more readily stained portion of nucleus, containing DNA-gene carrier.

chromogens Benzene compounds containing chromophore radicals called chromogens. Although colored by the presence of the chromophore radical, the compound itself possesses no affinity for tissue cells or fibers and is easily removed from tissue by simple mechanical processes.

chromophore Chemical entity that within a dye produces color, that is, a color bearer, having certain definite atomic groupings associated with color.

clearance angle Angle between the knife bevel and the paraffin block.

clearing Process of dealcoholization that renders tissue transparent; Intermediate step in processing to remove the dehydrant and replace it with a clearing agent that is miscible with the parafin.

coagulation Clotting. Cloudiness, flocculation, and clot formation are grades or stages in a single process of coagulation. The more concentrated the protein sol and the more vigorous the fixative, the greater will be the tendency of the coagulated particles to cohere in a single clot.

coccus Bacterium of round, spheroid, or ovoid form, usually less than 1 μm in diameter.

condenser Part of microscope immediately beneath the stage that concentrates light on the tissue.

conidiophore Specialized hyphal structure that serves as a stalk on which *conidia* (spores) are formed. The suffix, *-phore,* means 'carrier' and is added to the combining form that denotes what is being carried: conidium (spore) and *-phore* (carrier, bearer).

cytology Anatomy, physiology, pathology, and chemistry of the cell.

decalcification Process wherein the calcium salts are removed before bone or any calcified tissue can be processed and sectioned with a routine microtome.

decolorization Removal of stain or excess stain from tissue sections; a regressive procedure of staining.

dehydration The process of removal of free water. The use of graded strengths of ethanol to gradually displace the water in the tissue with alcohol.

diaphragm Part of microscope that regulates the amount of light illuminating the object being examined.

diastase Enzyme that specifically digests glycogen.

differentiation Removal of excess stain from tissue until color is retained only by the tissue element to be studied; ability to contrast the tissue element against an unstained background.

elective solubility Ability of stains to dissolve in tissue fluids.

embedding Casting tissue in various agents that harden.

endogenous Said of pigments found within tissue and cells that develop, originate, or arise from causes within and that grow from within.

exogenous Said of pigments that originate or are produced outside the body.

filamentous Long, cylindric, threadlike; hyphaforming.

fixation Primarily the stabilization of protein.

fixative Chemical that must do everything a preservative does and, additionally, must modify tissue constituents in such a way that they retain their form when subjected to treatment that would have damaged them in their initial state.

fixed Word used in relationship to the fixation of tissue; tissue is fixed when protein has been stabilized by subjection of the tissue to a substance that renders proteins insoluble and prevents autolysis.

fungus (pl., fungi) A relatively simple plant that is either filamentous or unicellular, is not differentiated into root, stem, and leaf, and lacks chlorophyll. It does have a true nucleus enclosed in a membrane and has cellulose or chitin, or both, in the cell wall. (From *Medically Important Fungi,* by D. H. Larone.) The following are terms affiliated with fungi: blastospore, budding, capsule, conidiophore, filamentous, hypha, septate, spherule, and spore (see their definitions).

glycogen Colorless carbohydrate cell product related to starch. It is water soluble and found commonly in liver.

hematein Product of oxidation of hematoxylin; the active coloring agent.

hematogenous Pertaining to anything produced from, derived from, or transported by the blood.

hypha (pl., hyphae) Tubular or thread-like structure of the fungi. Many together compose the *mycelium,* a mat of intertwined hyphae making up the colony of fungus.

hypo Sodium thiosulfate.

impregnation Deposition of salts of gold or silver on or around, but not in, the elements demonstrated in tissue.

infiltration Act of passing into or interpenetrating a substance, cell, or tissue. Tissues are infiltrated.

ion-exchange resin Resin added to an acid decalcifying solution to protect the tissue while the calcium is rapidly removed from the solution of formic acid into the resin. The ion-exchange resin method of decalcification gives faster decalcification, preserves cellular detail, and eliminates daily solution changes.

knives, microtome The following are necessary for proper knife usage:
Angle, clearance 3 to 8 degrees
   Bevel 27 to 32 degrees
   Wedge 15 degrees
Celloidin sectioning Use plano-concave knife.
Cryostat sectioning Use a 30-degree angle.
Cutting edge Check at 100$\times$ with 10$\times$ oculars and 10$\times$ objectives.
Paraffin sectioning Use wedge-shaped knife.
Sharpness Ability to cut a ribbon of section at 2 μm with no compression, depending on type of paraffin and of knife.

lake Insoluble compound formed when a substance combines with a dye radical.

lens Glass device that magnifies the image of an object. The compound microscope consists of two separate lens systems—the objective and the ocular.

light source In modern microscopes, the light source is supplied by low-voltage electric bulbs operated by a transformer adjusted to the intensity of light required.

light spectrum Colors from red (about 700 nm from peak to peak of the wavelength) to blue (about 400 nm).

lipid Lipoid, substance resembling fat.

lysochrome Stain that uses elective solubility (dissolves in tissue fluid) or has no affinity except for solution (that is, all Sudan stains, with fat stain being limited).

magnification, final Result from multiplying objective by ocular.

magnification, maximum Capability of the light.

MBE (methylene blue extinction) pH value at which methylene blue will cease to stain.

metachromasia Change of color, a tissue color reaction different from the stain used, such as with toluidine blue, a blue stain that gives a violet color.

metallic impregnation Reduction of a metal or metallic compound by tissue to its elementary state, thus leaving a black deposit.

methylation Artificial reduction of metachromasia with methanol.

microanatomic Pertaining to the branch of anatomy in which the structure of cells, tissues, and organs is studied with the light microscope.

microtome knives See **knives, microtome.**

microtomy Section-cutting; the making of thin sections of tissues for examination under the microscope.

micrometer (formerly **micron**) 1/1000 of a millimeter or 1/25,000 of an inch.

microscopes Instrument using electromagnetic radiation to obtain enlarged image of small objects difficult or impossible to see by the unaided eye; composed mainly of the following parts and concepts: barrel, condenser, diaphragm, lenses, light source, light spectrum, magnification (both final and maximum), nosepiece, objective, ocular, and refraction, which see.

microscopy Investigation of minute objects by means of a microscope.

mineral Any homogenous inorganic material; it may be studied by microincineration to give information on its amount and distribution without the organic elements interfering. Minerals such as calcium, magnesium, silicon, and iron can be identified in an incinerated section.

miscible Capable of mixed.

mordant Substance that is a salt or a hydroxide of a metal and serves to strongly attach dye molecules to tissue, such as alum for hematoxylin, or picric acid in Bouin's fixative for Masson's trichrome stain.

Mycobacterium A genus of gram-positive, acid-fast, slender, straight or slightly curved rods; slender filaments occasionally occur, but branched forms rarely are produced.

noncoagulation Lack of clot formation.

nosepiece On lower end of barrel, part that revolves and can handle multiple objectives. Objectives should remain screwed into the nosepiece to avoid damage.

object stage Platform that sits above the condenser with an opening through which the light passes. A mechanical stage moves the slide slowly in either of two mutually perpendicular directions.

objective Lens at lower end of barrel having a major responsibility for the magnification and resolution of the image; it is the most important component of the microscope. Several objectives may be on a rotatable nosepiece.

ocular Lens at upper end of microscope barrel.

OCT Commercial embedding medium for cutting sections on a cryostat.

orthochromatic Said of a stain that stains tissue in a predictable way, such as blue stain staining tissue a blue color.

oxidation Process of combining with oxygen, or increasing the valence of an atom or ion by the loss from it of hydrogen or of one or more electrons, thus rendering it more electropositive, as when iron is changed from the ferrous $(2+)$ to the ferric $(3+)$ state $(+ =$ electropositive charge, the loss of an electron).

oxidizing agents In Delafield's hematoxylin the oxidizing is accomplished by the atmosphere. Alum hematoxylin may be oxidized in an instant when oxidizing agents such as mercuric oxide, sodium iodate, or potassium permanganate are added. Oxidizing agents such as *ferricyanide, bisulfite,* and *permanganate* may be used as differentiators in staining: *periodic acid* is the oxidizing agent in the PAS technic; *chromic acid* is the oxidizing agent in the Grocott and Gridley technics.

pigments Heterogenous group of substances containing enough natural color to be visible without staining, such as melanin, which is found normally in the skin, hair, and eyes but may occur pathologically anywhere in the body.

plano-concave knife Type of knife for cutting celloidin sections.

polychromatic Said of stain that exhibits many colors on tissue.

polymerization Chemical reaction in which two or more small molecules combine to form larger molecules that contain repeating structural units of the original molecules; for example, metachromasia is believed to be caused by polymerization of the dye molecules in the tissue.

precipitate Substance separated from a solution or suspension by a chemical or physical change usually as an insoluble amorphous or crystalline solid. A precipitate is a product of some process or action.

preservative fluid that will neither shrink or swell tissue, nor dissolve its constituent parts, but will kill bacteria and molds and render enzymes inactive.

preserved Said of a tissue when it has been placed in a preservative fluid.

progressive Staining to the desired intensity without differentiation.

protein-denaturing Baker (1958) states "the word means a non-additive change in a protein during fixation, causing it to become less capable of remaining in intimate relation with water as a sol or gel, and more reactive. The resulting loss of solubility ordinarily mainfests itself in coagulation, if the protein be a sol; a gel is rendered harder and opaque." The chief denaturing fixatives are methanol, ethanol, acetone, nitric acid, and hydrochloric acid.

reduction Loss or removal of oxygen or taking up of hydrogen.

refraction Deviation of light in passing obliquely from one medium to another of different density. Refractive behavior of light brings about the formation of images; therefore refraction is the most important underlying concept in the functioning of the microscope.

regressive Said of staining method by which the section is uniformly stained and then differentiated until the desired staining is reached.

resolution Optical ability to distinguish detail and separate close objects at minimal distance from each other.

ripening Process of preparing hematoxylin by oxidation.

septate Characterized by the presence of partitions; certain fungal mycelia are septate.

spherule Large round structure containing spores.

spore Cell, or unit of several cells, produced by the fungus and capable of functioning like a seed, that is, developing into a mature fungus; unit of dissemination or reproduction.

sulfation Artificial production of metachromasia with sulfuric acid.

universal solvents Chemical reagents that avoid the use of two solutions, a dehydrating and a clearing agent. Dioxane, tertiary butanol, and tetrahydrofuran are universal solvents.

vital staining Uptake of a dye by a living substance, intravital and supravital.

yeast True fungi whose usual growth form is unicellular. The term "yeastlike fungi" include members of the genera *Candida* and *Cryptococcus*.

Appendix A

SUPPLIERS OF SOME MATERIALS AND EQUIPMENT MENTIONED IN TEXT

Autotechnicon: Technicon Instruments Corp., Tarrytown, N.Y.

Bear Brand oil: Norton Co., Troy, N.Y.

Bioloid: VWR Scientific, Inc., San Francisco, Cal.

Bowie's stain: Roboz Surgical Instrument Co., 810 18th St., N.W., Washington, D.C.

Buehler LTD: Buehler Ltd., Evanston, Ill.

Cacodylic acid, sodium salt, superior MCB-1257CX5: Matheson, Coleman & Bell, East Rutherford, N.Y.

Carbowax: Union Carbide Corp., Carbon Products Division, New York, N.Y.

Celloidin: Schering Corp., Port Reading, N.J.

Eukitt mounting media: Calibrated Instrument Co., Ardsley, N.Y.

Fume-Gard (nos. 920 and 929): Lerner Laboratories, Stamford, Conn.

Gillings-Honico: Bronwill Scientific, Rochester, N.Y.

H/1 Bright 5030: Hacker Instruments, Inc., Fairfield, N.J.

Harleco Synthetic Resin, Harleco, Gibbstown, N.J.

Histoclad: Clay Adams Co., Parsippany, N.J.

Honeywell Automatic Stainer: Honeywell Inc., Denver, Col.

Isomet Low Speed Saw: Buehler Ltd., Evanston, Ill.

JB-4 "Porter Blum" microtome: DuPont Instruments–Sorvall, DuPont Co., Newtown, Conn.

Jung knives: American Optical Corp., Buffalo, N.Y.

Kimwipes: Kimberly Clark Corp., Neenah, Wis.

Kleenex: Kimberly Clark Corp., Neenah, Wis.

Knife sharpener: Hacker Instruments, Inc., Fairfield, N.J.

Lab-Line Instruments: See Tims.

Lab-Tek VIP: Lab-Tek Products, Division of Miles Laboratories, Inc., Naperville, Ill.

Leitz Sledge: Scientific Products Div., American Hospital Supply Corp., McGaw Park, Ill.

Lipshaw Automatic Tissue Changer

Lipshaw Histomolds: Lipshaw Manufacturing Corp., Detroit, Mich.

LKB Knifemaker: LKB Instruments, Inc., Rockville, Md.

Micro Tissue Capsule no. 331: Lipshaw Manufacturing Co., Detroit, Mich.

Namount: Matheson, Coleman & Bell, East Rutherford, N.J.

OCT: Ames Co., Division of Miles Laboratories, Inc., Elkhart, Ind.

Paper towels no. 237 Garland: Fort Howard Paper Co., Green Bay, Wis.

Paraformaldehyde, no. 421: Eastman Organic Chemicals Div., Eastman Kodak Co., Rochester, N.Y.

Paraplast: Sherwood Medical Industries, Inc., St. Louis, Mo.

Parlodion: Mallinckrodt Chemical Works, Jersey City, N.J.

Peel-A-Way Disposable Embedding Molds: Lipshaw Manufacturing Corp., Detroit, Mich.

Permount: Fisher Scientific Co., Pittsburgh, Pa.

Scott's Micro Assembly Wipes, No. 5310: Scott Paper Co., Industrial Highway and Tinicum Island Road, Philadelphia, Pa.

Technicon resin: Technicon Instruments Corp., Tarrytown, N.Y.

Tetrahydrofuran: Fisher Scientific Co., Pittsburgh, Pa.

Tims (preassembled): Lab-Line Instruments, Inc., Melrose Park, Ill.

Tissueprep: Fisher Scientific Co., Pittsburgh, Pa.

Tissue Tek III Processor, Tissue Tek Embedding Rings: Lab-Tek Products, Division of Miles Laboratories, Inc., Naperville, Ill.

WIN-3000 (ion-exchange resin): Winthrop-Stearns, Inc., 1450 Broadway, New York, N.Y.

Appendix B

MISCELLANEOUS PROCEDURE CHART

How to remove cover slips from old slides or broken slides

1. Hold the slide at end with long forceps and dip briefly into liquid nitrogen. The cover slip will loosen immediately. Allow the slide to warm up and place in several changes of xylene to ensure removal of old mounting medium.
2. *Alternate method.* Soak off cover slip by immersion of the slide in xylene, which may take hours to days. *Do not pull* cover slip off, since it might damage the tissue.

How to repair broken slides

1. Place the slide pieces on a new slide with the use of mounting medium. *Do not clean off excess* until the new slide is dried hard.
2. Dry the slide flat for several hours on a hot plate or at the flat end of a Lipshaw slide dryer.
3. After slide is thoroughly dry, remove excess mounting medium with a razor blade.

How to restore faded hematoxylin slides

1. Remove cover slips with liquid nitrogen method.
2. Remove old mounting medium with several changes of xylene.
3. Take slides through 1-minute changes of two absolute alcohols, two 95% alcohols and two 80% alcohol down to water.
4. Wash in running tap water for 5 minutes.
5. Decolorize in acid alcohol to remove old stain.
6. Wash in running tap water for 5 minutes and proceed with new stain.

Alternative method (McCormick 1959)

1. After tissues are in running water, place slides in 0.5% aqueous solution of potassium permanganate for 5 minutes.
2. Rinse in tap water.
3. Bleach in 0.5% solution of oxalic acid for 2 to 3 minutes.
4. Wash in running tap water for 5 minutes. If the stain is not removed, repeat steps 1 to 4.
5. Use dilute stains or shorter times for staining when restaining with hematoxylin or aniline nuclear dyes.

How to restore basophilic properties to tissue (AFIP) leuco

Poorly stained nuclei can be caused by:
1. Long storage in acid formalin or other fixative.
2. Overexposure to decalcifying solution.
3. Dried tissue.
4. Burned tissue.

The following three methods are used with varying results. If one does not work, try no. 2 and then no. 3 in sequence.

Method 1

1. Deparaffinize and hydrate slides.
2. Place slides in 5% aqueous sodium bicarbonate solution from 4 hours to overnight.
3. Wash in tap water for 5 minutes.
4. Stain as desired.

Method 2

In step 2, use a 5% aqueous solution of ammonium sulfide overnight.

Method 3

In step 2, use a 5% aqueous solution of periodic acid overnight.

How to remove silver stains

Silver stains are removed from hands with permanent-wave solution.

Appendix C

DOS AND DON'TS FOR STAINING

1. When bulk staining is being done in large baskets, check a slide microscopically from each basket after use of hematoxylin to be sure the nuclei are well stained.
2. Never allow the tissues to dry at any point in the staining process.
3. If ammonia water is used to blue the hema- toxylin, do not agitate the slides, since it will loosen the tissue.
4. If tissues have been in fixative for a longer time than normal, they require additional staining time in hematoxylin.
5. For autopsy tissues, increase the staining times in hematoxylin and eosin by one third.

Appendix D

ECONOMIC WAY TO DIGEST SEVERAL TISSUES WITH SMALL AMOUNT OF ENZYME

1. Deparaffinize slide down to water.
2. Equilibrate in proper buffer.
3. Draw a circle around specimen with a wax pencil.
4. Slides are placed in a 13 × 9 inch cake pan that comes with a clear plastic lid. Rubber sponge pad, the kind that is used for rugs, is cut the size of the pan and dampened with distilled water. The slides are placed on the damp sponge. The damp sponge keeps the slides from drying out.
5. A drop of enzyme dissolved in proper buffer is dropped on each tissue; make sure tissue is completely covered.
6. Put a drop of buffer on control slides. Place slides side by side, cover with plastic lid, and digest at proper temperature.

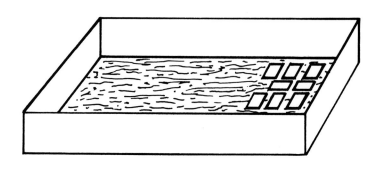

Index

A

Absolute alcohol–chloroform mixture, 260
Absorbent, 355
Absorption, 355
    antiserum, in immunofluorescence methods, 315
Absorption theory for staining, 126
Accession, record of, 399
Acetaldehyde as fixative modifier, 42
Acetate buffer, 94
    Walpole's, 151
Acetic acid, 47, 222, 223, 228, 229
    for decalcification, 91
    for fixation, 45
    in fixative mixture, 42
    glacial, 47, 48
    preparation of molar and normal solutions of, from concentrated acid solutions, 388
Acetocarmine, 119, 138
Acetolacmoid, 138
Acetone
    citrate-buffered, for fixing smears in enzyme histochemistry, 295
    for dehydration, 60, 61, 131
    as fixative modifier, 42
Aceto-orcein, 138
Achromatic objectives, 19
Acid alcohol solution, 239
Acid aniline dye mixtures with picric acid
    for collagen and muscle, 189
    fixatives for, 53
Acid chlorides, 371, 373
Acid decalcification method, 90
Acid decalcifying agents, 91
    formulas for, 92
Acid dyes, 122
Acid-fast inclusion bodies, Ziehl-Neelsen method for, fixatives for, 55
Acid-fast stain, Kinyoun's, for tubercle bacillus, 156
Acid-fast technics
    for bacteria, 235-239
    stains for, 50
Acid formaldehyde hematein, 46
Acid fuchsin stain, 103, 190, 215
    Bujard's, for mast cell granules, 282
Acid hematein, 220
    fixatives for, 58
Acid hematein method for phospholipids, Baker's, 208-209
    fixatives for, 54
    Mowry's alcian blue method for, fixatives for, 52
    stains for, 52

Acid mucosubstances, 160-161
    alcian blue technics to demonstrate, 172-174
    demonstration of, 163
        methods for, 168-169
    distribution of, Prussian blue reaction to indicate, 171
    fixatives for, 164
    hyaluronidase digestions to identify, 174-175
    iron diamine methods to demonstrate, 175
    metachromasia in, at controlled pH, 170
    mucins and, metachromatic methods for demonstration of, 169-170
    Müller-Mowry colloidal iron technic for, 171-172
Acid phosphatase, 298-300
Acid polychrome methylene blue, Terry's
    for fixed frozen sections, 150
    for fresh unfixed frozen sections, 150
Acid silver nitrate argentaffin reaction for melanin, 222
Acid solutions
    concentrated, preparation of molar and normal acid solutions from, 387-392
    decalcification methods using, 90-92
    molar and normal, preparation of, from concentrated acid solutions, 387-392
Acidic and neutral lipids, Nile blue sulfate technic for, 207-208
Acidic salts, 353
Acidified permanganate solution, 104
Acids, 42, 352; see also specific acid
    and bases, 353
Acidulated water, 240
Acridine orange fluorescent method for deoxyribonucleic acid and ribonucleic acid, 152-153
Acridine orange solution, 153
Actinomyces, 233
Actinomyces bovis, staining technics for, 244
Activators and enzymes, 293
Acyl group, 373
Addison's disease, melanin in, 220
Addition, 359
Adenohypophysis, 267-268
    aldehyde thionin–Luxol fast blue–periodic acid Schiff method for, 270-271
Adenosine triphosphatase, 302-304
Adjective stain, 124
Adrenal glands, 274-276
    stains for, 50-51
    fixatives for, 50
Adrenal insufficiency, melanin in, 220

447